Traumatic Disorders
of the Knee

John M. Siliski

Editor

Traumatic Disorders
of the Knee

Line Illustrations by Laurel Cook Lhowe

With 380 Figures in 680 Parts

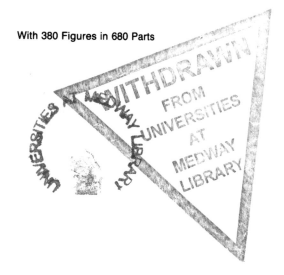

Springer-Verlag
New York Berlin Heidelberg London Paris
Tokyo Hong Kong Barcelona Budapest

John M. Siliski, M.D.
Wang Ambulatory Care Center
Massachusetts General Hospital
Harvard Medical School
Boston, MA 02114, USA

Cover illustration: Detail from Fig. 9.6, p. 131, of a comminuted tibial plateau fracture.

Library of Congress Cataloging-in-Publication Data

Traumatic disorders of the knee / [edited by] John M. Siliski.
    p. cm.
  Includes bibliographical references and index.
  ISBN 0-387-94171-1.—ISBN 3-540-94171-1
  1. Knee—Wounds and injuries. 2. Knee—Surgery. I. Siliski,
John M.
  [DNLM: 1. Knee Injuries—surgery. WE 870 T777 1994]
  RD561.T73   1994
  617.5'82—dc20
  DNLM/DLC
  for Library of Congress   93-46007

Printed on acid-free paper.

Production coordinated by Chernow Editorial Services, Inc. and managed by Theresa Kornak; manufacturing supervised by Jacqui Ashri.
Typeset by Asco Trade Typesetting Ltd., Hong Kong.
Printed and bound by Edwards Brothers, Ann Arbor, MI.
Printed in the United States of America.

9 8 7 6 5 4 3 2 1

ISBN 0-387-94171-1 Springer-Verlag New York Berlin Heidelberg
ISBN 3-540-94171-1 Springer-Verlag Berlin Heidelberg New York

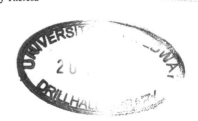

Preface

Management of knee trauma has changed rapidly over the past decade, with the acquisition of additional knowledge and new surgical techniques. At present, the optimal management of knee injuries requires the synthesis of multiple approaches drawn from orthopaedics and related surgical fields. The goal of this work is to comprehensively discuss the current state of the art in management of all types of knee trauma, including soft tissue and osteoarticular injuries. In order to take care of the patient with knee trauma, the orthopaedic surgeon must be able to assess and manage injuries of menisci, ligaments, articular surfaces, and bone, as all of these structures must work harmoniously for the knee to function properly.

This book has been organized into five major sections. The first section on fundamental principles covers anatomy, articular cartilage injury and repair, osteochondral fractures, soft tissue management, extensile exposure, external fixation, and the use of allografts in the knee. These chapters set the stage for the second section, which covers major fractures of the distal femur and tibial plateau, and the third section, where injuries of the extensor mechanism are discussed. In section four, injuries of the menisci and ligaments are covered comprehensively, including discussion of multiple ligament disruptions and knee dislocations. The final section covers late reconstructive problems and complications of knee trauma, including knee stiffness, malunions and nonunions, arthrodesis, total knee replacements for posttraumatic arthritis, fractures about total knee replacement, and extensor mechanism disruption in total knee replacements.

Throughout the book, an effort has been made to present in a comprehensive manner new techniques. Surgical approaches are included from arthroscopic techniques to extensile exposure. The use of allografts is discussed including application for collateral and cruciate ligaments, osteoarticular surfaces, menisci, and the extensor mechanism. Fracture treatment includes discussion of percutaneous techniques, indirect reduction, and ring fixators. Multiple new topics in the management of complications and late reconstructions after trauma are presented. This work is therefore meant to be a comprehensive review of the management of knee trauma, without being limited to a single approach to treatment or being diluted by discussion of nontraumatic disorders. It is my hope that it will fill a need in the orthopaedic library for the orthopaedic surgeon who manages knee trauma.

John M. Siliski, M.D.
February 1994

Acknowledgments

This book is the product of the contributions of many individuals who have given in both tangible and intangible ways. This volume is dedicated to the families of the contributors, who worked on their chapters primarily during their free family time. Especially, I wish to thank my family, including my wife Toni, and my sons Michael, Daniel, and Andrew, for the countless hours that they gave up with me so that this work could be completed.

Those who have written chapters in this book have done a superlative job combining their own personal experience and historical perspective. All of the authors are very busy surgeons and researchers, and I am very grateful that they were willing, for the love of the field, to make time in their schedules for this book.

In my office, Debbie Krudop and Toni Monteiro provided outstanding secretarial support, meeting deadlines and keeping organized the flow of paper and photographs. Laurel Cook Lhowe worked countless hours creating hundreds of line drawings that appear throughout the book. Michelle Rose and David Burnham processed the photographs that further illustrate the book. The outstanding work of all these people is greatly appreciated in the creation of this text.

I want to thank the staff at Springer-Verlag and Chernow Editorial Services, who were a pleasure to work with. I especially thank Bill Day, Zareh MacPherson Artinian, and the production staff.

John M. Siliski, M.D.

Contents

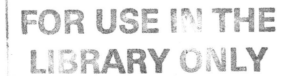

Contributors

STEVEN P. ARNOCZKY, DVM
College of Veterinary Medicine, Michigan State University, East Lansing, MI 48824-1314, USA

KENNETH S. AUSTIN, MD
Wang Ambulatory Care Center, Massachusetts General Hospital, Boston, MA 02114, USA

BERNARD R. BACH, JR., MD
Department of Orthopaedic Surgery, Rush-Presbyterian-St. Luke's Medical Center, Rush Medical College, Chicago, IL 60612, USA

FIELD T. BLEVINS, MD
University of New Mexico School of Medicine, Albuquerque, NM 87131, USA

ARTHUR L. BOLAND, MD
Harvard Medical School, Massachusetts General Hospital, Boston, MA 02114, USA

MARTIN BOUBLIK, MD
Steadman-Hawkins Denver Clinic, Englewood, CO 80111, USA

CHARLES H. BROWN, JR., MD
Kenmore Center, Harvard Community Health Plan, Harvard Medical School, Boston, MA 02181, USA

DAVID D. BULLEK, MD
Insall Scott Kelly Institute for Orthopaedics and Sports Medicine at Beth Israel Medical Center, North Division, New York, NY 10128, USA

CHARLES CARR, MD
Section of Orthopaedics, Department of Surgery, Dartmouth-Hitchcock Medical Center, Lebanon, NH 03756, USA

NICHOLAS J. CARR, MD
Vancouver General Hospital, Vancouver, British Columbia

DANIEL E. COOPER, MD
W. B. Carrell Memorial Clinic, Dallas, TX 75204, USA

JULIE DODDS, MD
Department of Surgery, College of Medicine, Michigan State University,
E. Lansing, MI 48824-1314, USA

PETER VAN EENENAAM, MD
Department of Orthopaedic Surgery, Harvard Medical School, Massachusetts General Hospital, Boston, MA 02114, USA

ROGER H. EMERSON, JR., MD
Presbyterian Hospital, Dallas, TX 75231, USA

TIMOTHY E. FOSTER, MD
Department of Orthopaedic Surgery, Boston University Medical Center,
Boston, MA 02118, USA

MARK G. FRANCO, MD
Department of Orthopaedic Surgery, Rush-Presbyterian-St. Luke's Medical
Center, Rush Medical College, Chicago, IL 60612, USA

GREGORY GALLICO, MD
Harvard Medical School, Massachusetts General Hospital, Boston, MA 02114

CHRISTOPHER D. HARNER, MD
Center for Sports Medicine and Rehabilitation, University of Pittsburgh
School of Medicine, Pittsburgh, PA 15213, USA

WILLIAM L. HEALY, MD
Department of Orthopaedic Surgery, Lahey Clinic Medical Center, Burling-
ton, MA 01805, USA

JAMES J. IRRGANG, MD
Center for Sports Medicine and Rehabilitation, University of Pittsburgh
School of Medicine, Pittsburgh, PA 15213, USA

MICHAEL A. KELLY, MD
Insall Scott Kelly Institute for Orthopaedics and Sports Medicine at Beth
Israel Medical Center, North Division, New York, NY 10128, USA

KENNETH J. KOVAL, MD
Orthopaedic Institute, Hospital for Joint Disease, New York, NY 10003,
USA

JUSTIN LAMONT, MD
Department of Orthopaedic Surgery, New York University Medical Center,
New York, NY 10016, USA

DAVID W. LHOWE, MD
Department of Orthopaedic Surgery, Harvard Medical School, Massachusetts General Hospital, Boston, MA 02114, USA

HENRY J. MANKIN, MD
Department of Orthopaedic Surgery, Harvard Medical School, Massas-
chusetts General Hospital, Boston, MA 02114, USA

JEFFREY MAST, MD
Hutzel Hospital, Detroit, MI 48201, USA

MARK S. MCMAHON, MD
Lenox Hill Hospital, New York, NY 10021, USA

LYLE J. MICHELI, MD
Children's Hospital Medical Center, Harvard Medical School, Boston, MA
02114, USA

MARK D. MILLER, MD
Center for Sports Medicine and Rehabilitation, University of Pittsburgh
School of Medicine, Pittsburgh, PA 15213, USA

FRANK X. PEDLOW, JR., MD
Harvard Medical School, Massachusetts General Hospital; Boston, MA
02114, USA

KEVIN D. PLANCHER, MD
Steadman-Hawkins Clinic, Vail, CO 81657, USA

ROY SANDERS, MD
Department of Orthopaedics, Tampa General Hospital, and Florida Orthopaedic Institute, Tampa, FL 33617-2011, USA

MICHAEL SCHMITZ, MD
Department of Orthopaedic Surgery, Lahey Clinic Medical Center, Burling-
ton, MA 01805, USA

JOHN M. SILISKI, MD
Wang Ambulatory Care Center, Harvard Medical School, Massachusetts
General Hospital, Boston, MA 02114, USA

DEMPSEY S. SPRINGFIELD, MD
Harvard Medical School, Massachusetts General Hospital, Boston, MA
02114, USA

J. RICHARD STEADMAN, MD
Steadman-Hawkins, Clinic, Vail, CO 81657, USA

MARK E. STEINER, MD
Harvard Community Health Plan, Boston, MA 02215, and Sports Medicine-
Brookline, Brookline, MA 02167, USA

GEORGE THABIT III, MD
Sports Orthopaedic and Rehabilitation Medicine Associates, Menlo Park,
CA 94025, USA

WILLIAM W. TOMFORD, MD
Department of Orthopaedic Surgery, Harvard Medical School, Massas-
chusetts General Hospital, Boston, MA 02114, USA

STEPHEN B. TRIPPEL, MD
Department of Orthopaedic Surgery, Harvard Medical School, Massas-
chusetts General Hospital, Boston, MA 02114, USA

BERTRAM ZARINS, MD
Harvard Medical School, Massachusetts General Hospital, Boston, MA
02114, USA

Part 1
Fundamental Principles

1A

Anatomy: Bony Architecture, Biomechanics, and Menisci

Martin Boublik, Field T. Blevins, and J. Richard Steadman

Bony Architecture and Biomechanics

Accurate diagnosis and successful treatment of traumatic knee disorders relies on a thorough understanding of knee anatomy and biomechanics. This is obviously true for surgical cases, but is also essential for rehabilitation of nonoperative lesions. This chapter attempts to present a comprehensive and systematic overview of knee anatomy relevant to orthopedic surgeons who treat traumatic disorders of the knee.

The description of the bony architecture is adapted from several standard anatomic and surgical texts.[1-18]

The distal femur, proximal tibia, and patella form the knee joint articulation (Fig. 1A-1). This articulation is divided into three compartments: medial tibiofemoral, lateral tibiofemoral, and anterior patellofemoral. Although the knee has traditionally and simplistically been described as a hinge joint, its motions are much more complex and consist of three translational (anteroposterior, medial-lateral, compression-distraction) and three rotational (flexion-extension, varus-valgus, internal rotation-external rotation) movements. The relative incongruence of the osseous structures is compensated by the soft tissues, especially the menisci in the medial and lateral compartments.

The rounded femoral condyles are asymmetric prominences of the distal femur, which project slightly anterior and markedly posterior to the femoral shaft. The articular surfaces viewed from the side are eccentrically curved, with a longer radius of curvature anteriorly than posteriorly. The medial condyle is more tightly curved posteriorly than the lateral condyle. Anteriorly, the confluence of the femoral condyles forms the trochlea for articulating with the patella (Fig. 1A-2). The articular surface for the patella is larger and projects 5 mm

more anteriorly on the lateral than the medial condyle. This configuration may protect against lateral patellar subluxation. The femoral condyles are separated posteriorly by the nonarticulating intercondylar area, which contains attachments for the anterior cruciate ligament, posterior cruciate ligament, and meniscofemoral ligaments.

The knee joint is parallel to the ground, and the medial femoral condyle projects approximately 0.5 cm more distal than the lateral condyle to compensate for the difference between the anatomic and biomechanical axes of the femur (Fig. 1A-3). The long (anatomic) axis of the shaft of the femur subtends an angle of approximately 6° with a line connecting the centers of the femoral head, knee joint, and ankle joint (mechanical axis) and approximately 9° with the vertical.[10,25] This angle is higher in women than in men.[25]

Viewed on end, the femoral condyles form a near trapezoid which is higher laterally than medially and wider posteriorly than anteriorly (see Fig. 1A-2). The medial wall slants at approximately 25° and the lateral wall slants at about 10°. The articular surface of the medial condyle is longer, and that of the lateral condyle is wider (see Figs. 1A-1 and 1A-2). The medial condyle has an overall greater surface area. The long axis of the lateral condyle lies along the sagittal plane; that of the medial condyle diverges about 22° from anterior to posterior.

The epicondyles are medial and lateral prominences proximal to the condyles. The medial epicondyle is more prominent than the lateral. The deep medial ligament arises just distal to the medial epicondyle. The adductor magnus inserts into the adductor tubercle just proximal to the medial epicondyle. The lateral epicondyle gives rise to the lateral collateral ligament and re-

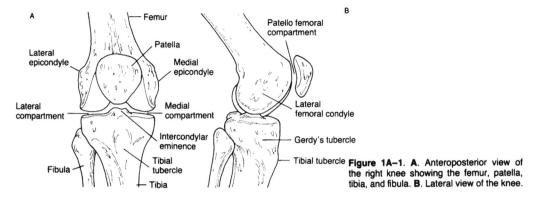

Figure 1A-1. **A.** Anteroposterior view of the right knee showing the femur, patella, tibia, and fibula. **B.** Lateral view of the knee.

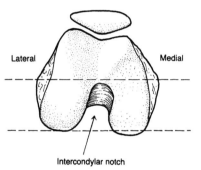

Figure 1A-2. End-on view of the right distal femur. The lateral wall of the trochlear groove is higher than the medial side, and may assist in preventing lateral subluxation of the patella. The intercondylar notch provides a space for the cruciate ligaments, and separates the medial and lateral femoral condyles. If the medial and lateral epicondyles are used as the axis of the femur when viewed from the end on, the medial femoral condyle extends farther posteriorly than the lateral condyle.

Figure 1A-3. Anteroposterior view of the right lower extremity. The anatomic axis of the tibia (---) is essentially the same as the mechanical axis, and runs from the center of the tibial plateau to the center of the ankle. The anatomic axis of the femur (· · ·) does not pass to the center of the intercondylar notch or knee joint. If extended to the distal femur, it passes through the medial side of the intercondylar notch just anterior to the insertion of the posterior cruciate ligament. The mechanical axis of the femur (---) passes from the center of the femoral head to the center of the knee joint. The angle between the anatomic and mechanical axes of the femur is approximately 6°. There is an additional 3° angle between the mechanical axis of the femur and the sagittal plane (——) drawn as a vertical line perpendicular to the knee and the ground. The resulting angle between the anatomic axis and sagittal plane is therefore 9°. The mechanical and anatomic axes of the tibia form a 3° angle with the sagittal plane. The mechanical axis from the center of the hip to the center of the ankle is nearly a straight line passing through the center of the knee.

ceives some fibers from the iliotibial tract. Distal to the lateral epicondyle, the lateral condyle is grooved by the origin of the popliteus muscle.

The proximal end of the tibia is expanded to form the medial and lateral tibial plateaus which articulate with the femoral condyles (see Fig. 1A-1). The lateral plateau is higher than the medial plateau and is convex. The medial plateau is slightly concave. Both plateaus slope posteriorly approximately 10°. The nonarticulating in-

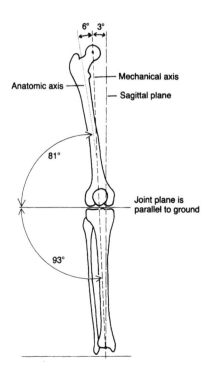

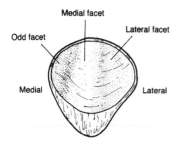

Figure 1A–4. Articular surface of the patella demonstrating the facets. The inferior pole is not covered by articular cartilage, but serves for attachment of the patellar tendon.

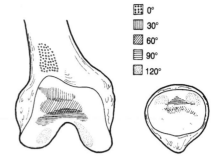

Figure 1A–5. Contact points on the patella and femur at varying degrees of knee flexion. Contact points on the femur move from proximal to distal as flexion increases, and move from distal to proximal on the patella during flexion. At higher degrees of flexion, contact splits into two areas on the femoral condyles and patellar facets.

tercondylar eminence is a prominent area that separates the tibial plateaus and contains medial and lateral spinous processes. Anteriorly and posteriorly, the plateaus are separated by the depressed triangular anterior and posterior intercondylar fossae, respectively. The intercondylar areas are the attachment sites for the menisci and the anterior cruciate ligament. The iliotibial tract inserts on the lateral (Gerdy's) tubercle of the tibia, approximately 3 cm lateral to the tibial tubercle.

The patella is the largest sesamoid bone in the body and is embedded in the tendon of the quadriceps muscle. Triangular in shape, it has a wide proximal pole and a narrow distal pole. The thick articular surface is divided into a larger lateral and smaller medial facet by a vertical ridge (Fig. 1A–4). The medial and lateral facets are each divided vertically into three facets by some authors, with a seventh odd facet on the extreme medial aspect of the patella. The patellofemoral contact area varies with the degree of flexion, with maximum contact at approximately 45° (Fig. 1A–5). As the knee is flexed from full extension to 90° of flexion, a continuous band of contact sweeps across the patella from inferior to superior. The odd facet does not contact the medial femoral condyle until about 135° of flexion. Past 90° of flexion, the quadriceps tendon also contacts the trochlea.[26]

Kapandji's description of the biomechanics of the

tibiofemoral articulation indicates that with flexion from full extension, the femoral condyles roll without sliding on the tibial plateaus during the first 10 to 15° of flexion on the medial side and the first 20° on the lateral side. Sliding then begins to occur, and in terminal flexion, the condyles slide without rolling (Fig. 1A–6).[8]

Muller has described the ratio of rolling to sliding as approximately 1:2 in early flexion and 1:4 by the end of flexion.[10] A four-bar linkage system has been proposed to explain the rolling and sliding mechanism of the knee. The bars consist of the two cruciate ligaments and the two bone segments that connect the insertion sites of the ligaments in the femur and tibia. The bars are of essentially fixed length, and motion is restricted to a pattern that accurately outlines the anatomic shape of the femoral and tibial surfaces and reproduces the known pattern of combined rolling and sliding (Fig. 1A–7).

The tibiofemoral contact area moves posteriorly throughout flexion. In terminal extension, the tibia externally rotates on the femur because of the asymmetric anatomic configuration described earlier. This "screw home mechanism" is reversed with early flexion.

Figure 1A–6. Rolling and sliding of the tibial femoral joint. A. Pure rolling would require dislocation of the knee to achieve greater than 90° of flexion. B. Pure sliding would result in impingement of the femur and tibia, limiting flexion. C. A combination of rolling and sliding results in maximal flexion while maintaining contact between the femur and tibia. The contact point on the tibia moves posteriorly with greater degrees of flexion.

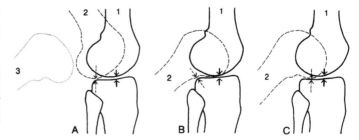

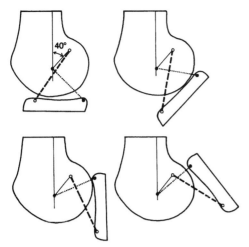

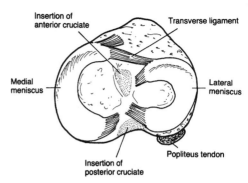

Figure 1A-8. Superior view of the tibia showing the menisci.

Figure 1A-7. Four-bar linkage system as a model that describes the shape of the articular surfaces of the femur and tibia and the rolling/sliding mechanism of motion. The anterior (---) and posterior (· · ·) cruciate ligaments form two of the bars with fixed points of insertion on the bones. The other two bars are the connections within the bones between the ligament insertion sites. Motion of the linkage system is determined by the insertion sites and lengths of the bars. The linkage system and articular surfaces are designed to work in concert, producing normal knee motion.

The Menisci

The menisci (semilunar cartilages) are two crescent-shaped fibrocartilaginous disks interposed between the femoral condyles and the tibial plateaus (Fig. 1A-8). Embryologically, the menisci appear at aproximately 45 days and are clearly defined by the eighth week of development.[22,27]

Triangular in cross section, the menisci have a thick, convex attached peripheral edge that tapers to a thin, concave unattached central edge (Fig. 1A-9). The menisci deepen the proximal tibial articular surface and have concave superior surfaces to accept the femoral condyles and flat inferior surfaces that rest on the proximal tibia.[7,28]

The medial meniscus is approximately 3.5 cm long, is semicircular, and is longer in an anteroposterior direction than the lateral meniscus (see Fig. 1A-8). The lateral meniscus is nearly circular and covers proportionately more of the tibial articular surface than does the medial meniscus. The medial meniscus is wider posteriorly than anteriorly, whereas the lateral meniscus is more consistent throughout.[7,28,29]

The anterior extent (anterior horn) of the medial meniscus is attached to the anterior intercondylar fossa of the tibia anterior to the anterior cruciate ligament. It

partially extends anteriorly off the tibial plateau. The anterior horn of the lateral meniscus is attached to the tibia anterior to the intercondylar eminence and posterior to the anterior cruciate ligament. The attachment of the lateral meniscal anterior horn often blends with the attachment of the anterior cruciate ligament.[7,28,29]

A variable fibrous band (transverse ligament) connects the two anterior horns. When present as a complete band, the transverse ligament generally connects the midportion of the medial meniscus anterior horn with the most anterior fibers of the lateral meniscus anterior horn (Ho, C. Personal communication, San Francisco Neuroskeletal Imaging Center, Daly City, CA). The posterior horn of the medial meniscus is more firmly attached than the anterior horn. It is attached to the posterior intercondylar fossa of the tibia posterior to

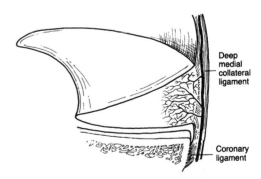

Figure 1A-9. Cross section of the medial meniscus. In cross section, it is roughly triangular, with a flat inferior surface to match the tibia and a contoured superior surface to match the femoral condyle. The mid- and inner portions of the meniscus have no vascular supply. The meniscus is attached to the deep medial collateral ligament, which is a portion of the medial capsule. Inferiorly, the meniscus is firmly attached to the tibia through the coronary ligament.

the posterior horn of the lateral meniscus and anterior to the posterior cruciate ligament. The posterior horn of the lateral meniscus is attached to the tibia posterior to the intercondylar eminence and often blends with the posterior aspect of the attachment of the anterior cruciate ligament. The anterior and posterior meniscofemoral ligaments, which pass around the posterior cruciate ligament and connect the posterior horn of the lateral meniscus and the lateral aspect of the medial femoral condyle, are described in the cruciate ligament section.[7,29] A fibrous band (Barkow's ligament) connecting the posterior horn of the lateral meniscus and the anterior horn of the medial meniscus has also been described.[29,30]

The periphery of each meniscus is attached to the femur and tibia by the joint capsule. The tibial portion of this attachment is known as the coronary ligament.[7,28] The peripheral attachment of the medial meniscus is continuous. The deep medial collateral ligament is a condensation of the joint capsule which firmly attaches the midportion of the medial meniscus to the femur and tibia. The semimembranosus muscle indirectly inserts posteromedially on the medial meniscus via the capsule and may retract the posterior horn.[28,29,31]

The peripheral attachment of the lateral meniscus is interrupted by the popliteus tendon posterolaterally. This popliteal hiatus measures approximately 1.3 cm in length and is bordered by superior and inferior meniscal fascicles.[32] Some popliteal fibers insert into the periphery of the meniscus and may retract the posterior horn.[29,31,33] Unlike the medial meniscus, the lateral meniscus does not attach to the (lateral) collateral ligament.[28]

The menisci are composed of hydrated fibrocartilaginous tissues and are approximately 75% water by weight. The solid organic component is approximately 90% collagen (predominantly type I) and 2 to 3% proteoglycan. The collagen fibers are organized primarily in circumferential bundles with small interconnecting radial fibers. The arrangement appears well suited for resisting large hoop stresses.[20]

The vascular supply to the medial and lateral menisci arises primarily from branches of the superior and inferior medial and lateral geniculate arteries, with additional contributions from the middle geniculate artery.[2,21,34] These vessels form a perimeniscal capillary plexus in the synovial and capsular tissue which supplies the peripheral 10 to 30% of the medial meniscus and 10 to 25% of the lateral meniscus.[34] The remaining inner portions of the menisci are avascular. The anterior and posterior horns are more vascular than the middle portion of the meniscus, and the posterolateral segment of the lateral meniscus adjacent to the popliteal hiatus is devoid of penetrating peripheral vessels.[34–36] The innervation of the menisci has not been as well

characterized as the vascular supply. It arises from the richly innervated perimeniscal capsular tissues and penetrates the peripheral one third of the meniscus. The nerve fibers appear to parallel only partially the vascular supply. The anterior and posterior horns are more highly innervated than the middle segment of the meniscus. Several distinct types of mechanoreceptors have been identified within the medial meniscus.[28,36–38]

The menisci move anteriorly in extension and posteriorly in flexion. This motion is produced largely by the rolling/sliding of the femoral condyles, with contributions to posterior retraction by the semimembranosus medially and the popliteus laterally.[5,23,31] Three-dimensional reconstruction of magnetic resonance images of cadaveric human menisci has shown that the posterior excursion of the lateral meniscus in flexion is greater than that of the medial meniscus and that the anterior horn segments are more mobile than the posterior horn segments bilaterally.[24,29]

Although the menisci were long felt to be vestigial structures, Fairbank in 1948 recognized degenerative changes after meniscectomy and proposed a weight-bearing function.[40] Currently, the menisci are believed to perform multiple biomechanical functions, including load transmission at the tibiofemoral articulation, shock absorption, stability (as a secondary restraint to anterior translation after anterior cruciate ligament failure), and possibly joint lubrication.[20]

References

1. Anderson JE, ed. *Grant's Atlas of Anatomy.* 7th ed. Baltimore: Williams & Wilkins; 1978.
2. Arnoczky SP, Škyhar MJ, Wickiewicz TL. Basic science of the knee. In: McGinty JB, ed. *Operative Arthroscopy.* New York: Raven Press; 1991:155–181.
3. Basmajian JV, ed. *Grant's Method of Anatomy.* 10th ed. Baltimore: Williams & Wilkins; 1980.
4. Hollinshead WH. Buttock, hip joint and thigh. In: Hollinshead WH, ed. *Anatomy for Surgeons.* Vol. 3: *The Back and Limbs.* Philadelphia: Harper & Row; 1982:619–732.
5. Hollinshead WH. Knee, leg, ankle and foot. In Hollinshead WH, ed. *Anatomy for Surgeons.* Vol. 3: *The Back and Limbs.* Philadelphia: Harper & Row; 1982:733–859.
6. Hoppenfeld S, deBoer P. *Surgical Exposures in Orthopaedics: The Anatomic Approach.* New York: JB Lippincott; 1984:389–441.
7. Insall JN. Anatomy of the knee. In: Insall JN, ed. *Surgery of the Knee.* New York: Churchill Livingstone; 1984:1–20.
8. Kapandji IA. *The Physiology of the Joints.* Vol. 2: *Lower Limb.* Edinburgh: Churchill Livingstone; 1970.
9. Main WK, Scott WN. Knee anatomy. In: Scott WN, ed. *Ligament and Extensor Mechanism Injuries of the Knee: Diagnosis and Treatment.* St. Louis: Mosby Year Book; 1991:13–32.
10. Müller W. *The Knee: Form, Function, and Ligament Reconstruction.* New York: Springer-Verlag; 1983:2–16.

11. Müller ME, Allgower M, Schneider R, et al. *Manual of Internal Fixation*. 2nd ed. New York: Springer-Verlag; 1979.
12. Reckljng FW, Munns, SW. Knee. In: Reckling FW, Reckling JB, Mohn MP, eds. *Orthopaedic Anatomy and Surgical Approaches*. St. Louis: Mosby Year Book; 1990:357–389.
13. Schatzker J. Supracondylar fractures of the femur. In: Schatzker J, Tile M, eds. *The Rationale of Operative Fracture Care*. New York: Springer Verlag; 1987:255–273.
14. Schatzker J. Fractures of the tibial plateau. In: Schatzker J, Tile M, eds. *The Rationale of Operative Fracture Care*. New York: Springer-Verlag; 1987:279–295.
15. Sisk TD. Knee injuries. In: Crenshaw AH, ed. *Campbell's Operative Orthopaedics*. 8th ed. St. Louis: Mosby Years Book; 1992:1487–1732.
16. Stockwell RA. Joints. In: Romanes GJ, ed. *Cunningham's Textbook of Anatomy*. 12th ed. New York: Oxford University Press; 1981:211–264.
17. Warren RF, Arnoczky SP, Wickiewicz TL. Anatomy of the knee. In: Nicholas JA, Hershman EB, eds. *The Lower Extremity and Spine in Sports Medicine*. St. Louis: CV Mosby; 1986:657–694.
18. Wolf-Heidegger G. *Atlas of Systemic Human Anatomy*. New York: Hafner; 1962.
19. Moreland Jr, Bassett LW, Hanker GJ. Radiographic analysis of the axial alignment of the lower extremity. *J Bone Joint Surg Am*. 1987;69:745–749.
20. Mow VC, Ratcliffe A, Chern KY, et al. Structure and function relationships of the menisci of the knee. In: Mow VC, Arnoczlcy SP, Jackson DW, eds. *Knee Meniscus: Basic and Clinical Foundations*. New York: Raven Press; 1992:37–57.
21. Scapinelli R. Studies on the vasculature of the human knee joint. *Acta Anat Basel*. 1968;70:305–331.
22. Scott WN, Insall JN. Injuries of the knee. In: Rockwood CA, Green DP, Bucholz, RW, eds. *Rockwood and Green's Fractures in Adults*. 3rd ed. Philadelphia: JB Lippincott; 1991:1799–1914.
23. Smith FB, Blair, HC. Tibial collateral ligament strain due to occult derangements of the medial meniscus: Confirmed by examination in thirty cases. *J Bone Joint Surg Am*. 1954:36–88.
24. Thompson WO, Thaete FL, Fu FH, et al. Tibial meniscal dynamics using three-dimensional reconstruction of magnetic resonance images. *Am J Sports Med*. 1991;19:210–216.
25. Yoshioka Y, Siu D, Cooke TDV. The anatomy and functional axes of the femur. *J Bone Joint Surg Am*. 1987;69:873–880.
26. Goodfellow J, Hungerford DS, Zindell M. Patellofemoral joint mechanics and pathology: Functional anatomy of the patellofemoral joint. *J Bone Joint Surg Br*. 1976;58:287–290.
27. Hosea TM, Tria AJ, Bechler JR. Embryology of the knee. In: Scott WN, ed. *Ligament and Extensor Mechanism Injuries of the Knee*. St. Louis: Mosby Year Book; 1991:1–12.
28. Arnoczky SP. Gross and vascular anatomy of the meniscus and its role in meniscal healing, regeneration and remodeling. In: Mow VC, Arnoczky SP, Jackson DW, eds. *Knee Meniscus: Basic and Clinical Foundations*. New York: Raven Press; 1992:1–14.
29. Johnson RJ. Anatomy and biomechanics of the knee. In: Chapman MW, ed. *Operative Orthopaedics*. Philadelphia: JB Lippincott; 1988:1617–1632.
30. Helfet AJ. *The Management of Internal Derangement of the Knee*. Philadelphia: JB Lippincott; 1963.
31. Kaplan EB. Some aspects of functional anatomy of the human knee joint. *Clin Orthop*. 1962;23:18–29.
32. Cohn AK, Mains DB. Popliteal hiatus of the lateral meniscus: Anatomy and measurement at dissection of ten specimens. *Am J Sports Med*. 1979;7:221–226.
33. Last RJ. Some anatomical details of the knee joint. *J Bone Joint Surg Br*. 1948;30:683–688.
34. Arnoczky SP, Warren RF. Microvasculature of the human meniscus. *Am J Sports Med*. 1982;10:90–95.
35. Danzig L, Resnick D, Gonsalves M, et al. Blood supply to the normal and abnormal menisci of the human knee. *Clin Orthop*. 1983;172:271–276.
36. Day B, Mackenzie WG, Shim SS, et al. The vascular and nerve supply of the human meniscus. *Arthroscopy*. 1985;1:58–62.
37. Kennedy JC, Alexander IJ, Hayes KC. Nerve supply of the human knee and its functional importance. *Am J Sports Med*. 1982;10:329–335.
38. Zimny ML, Albright DL, Dabeziew E. Mechanoreceptors in the human medial meniscus. *Acta Anat*. 1988; 133:35–40.
39. Fu FH, Thompson WO. Motion of the meniscus during knee flexion. In: Mow VC, Arnoczky SP, Jackson DW, eds. *Knee Meniscus: Basic and Clinical Foundations*. New York: Raven Press; 1992:75–89.
40. Fairbank TJ. Knee joint changes after meniscectomy. *J Bone Joint Surg Br*. 1948;30:664–670.

1B

Anatomy: Ligaments, Tendons, and Extensor Mechanism

Field T. Blevins, Martin Boublik, and J. Richard Steadman

Medial Structures

Structures on the medial aspect of the knee have been divided into three layers by Warren and Marshal[1] (Fig. 1B-1). Layer I, the superficial layer, is composed of the deep or crural fascia. Layer II is composed of the superficial medial ligament and ligaments of the posteromedial corner of the knee. Layer III comprises the deep medial ligament and the capsule.

Layer I is the first fascial plane encountered when a skin incision is made medially (Fig. 1B-2). The layer is defined by the fascia surrounding the sartorius muscle and tendon, and extends from the patella anteriorly to the midportion of the popliteal fossa posteriorly. Anteriorly, 1 to 2 cm in front of the anterior margin of the medial collateral ligament, it blends with layer II (see Fig. 1B-1). The two layers continue together and contribute to the patellar retinaculum. Slightly more posteriorly, the sartorius inserts into this layer. Thus, the sartorius does not have a distinct tendon of insertion as do the gracilis and semitendinosus which are deep to it.

Posterior to the parallel fibers of the superficial medial ligament, layer I is distinct and separated from the underlying gracilis, semitendinosus, and semimembranosus by a layer of adipose tissue. Farther posteriorly, layer I blends with fascia over the medial gastrocnemius. Inferiorly, layer I blends with the periosteum at the attachment of the sartorius and the deep fascia of the leg. Superiorly, it is continuous with fascia overlying the quadriceps muscles.

Layer II, consisting of the parallel fibers of the superficial medial ligament, is separated inferiorly from layer I by the semitendinosus and gracilis as they cross to their insertions on the tibia (Figs. 1B-1 and 1B-3). The anterior parallel fibers of the superficial medial ligament are roughly 11 cm long by 1.5 cm wide, arise from the medial epicondyle, and insert 4 to 5 cm distal to the joint line. They are joined by obliquely oriented posterior fibers to form a triangle with the apex located posteriorly on the joint line.

The femoral origin of the anterior parallel fibers of the superficial medial ligament is situated around the varying axis of flexion of the knee. This results in some portion of these fibers remaining under constant tension throughout range of motion. The anterior fibers are under tension in flexion, whereas the more posterior fibers are tighter in extension. Posteriorly, the oblique fibers blend in the posteromedial capsule and are indistinguishable from layer III. These fibers are taut in extension and loose in flexion. The fibers of the superficial medial ligament continue their insertion into the medial aspect of the tibia for approximately 10 cm distal to the joint line.

The term *posterior oblique ligament* refers to the combination of oblique fibers of the superficial medial ligament and fibers of the posteromedial capsule. Although Warren and Marshal suggest using two separate terms for these fibers and not combining them under the term *posterior oblique ligament*,[1] this term is commonly used. The patellofemoral ligament is an extension of layer II, extending from the medial femoral epicondyle anteriorly to the patella, deep to the vastus medialis obliquus (see Fig. 1B-3).

Layer III is made up of the true medial capsule of the knee (Figs. 1B-1 and 1B-4). Its attachment to the femur and tibia follows the margins of the articular surfaces. Anteriorly, the layer envelops the fat pad and is thin, not aiding in stability. Warren et al point out that the thin baggy true anterior capsule should be differentiated from the "surgical capsule," which includes the overlying retinacular tendons contained in layers I and II.[2]

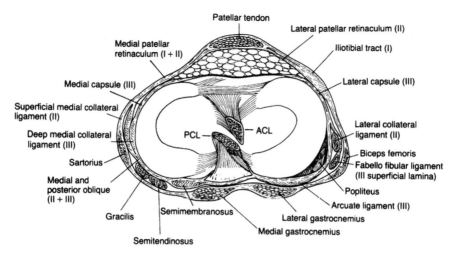

Figure 1B–1. Cross section of the knee showing the three layers comprising the medial and lateral structures. ACL, anterior cruciate ligament; PCL, posterior cruciate ligament.

Deep to the superficial medial ligament, vertical parallel fibers of layer III thicken, forming the deep medial ligament. The deep medial ligament may be divided into a meniscofemoral portion and a meniscotibial portion. The deep medial ligament originates 0.5 cm distal to the medial epicondyle and inserts on the medial meniscus. It then continues from the medial meniscus and attaches to the tibia above the attachment of the anterior slip of the semimembranosus tendon.

The fibers of the deep medial ligament are separated from the fibers of the superficial medial ligament by a bursa. Posteriorly, 1 to 2 cm behind the anterior edge of the superficial medial ligament fibers, layer III blends with layer II to form the posterior oblique ligament.

Function of the Medial Ligamentous Structures

Selective cutting studies have demonstrated that the parallel fibers of the superficial medial collateral ligament function as the primary static restraint to valgus stress.[2-5] The posterior oblique ligament, posterior capsule, and cruciate ligaments act as secondary restraints

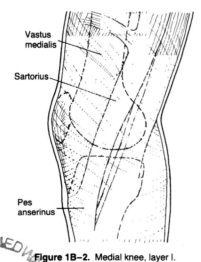

Figure 1B–2. Medial knee, layer I.

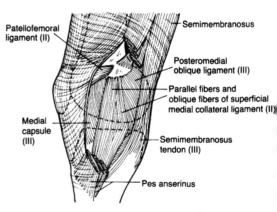

Figure 1B–3. Medial knee, layer II.

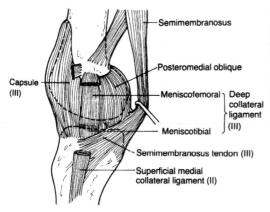

Figure 1B-4. Medial knee, layer III.

particularly near full extension.[2,4,6] The oblique portion of the superficial medial collateral ligament and the deep medial collateral ligament do not appear to play a significant role in resisting valgus stress.

The medial collateral ligament also functions in controlling rotation of the tibia on the femur. Warren et al noted that sectioning the superficial parallel fibers of the medial collateral ligament significantly increased external rotation. The increase in external rotation was greater as the knee flexed from 0 to 90°.[2] Sectioning the oblique fibers of the superficial medial collateral ligament and the deep medial collateral ligament had little effect on tibial rotation. Markolf et al and Seering et al have found the medial collateral ligament to have a greater role in resisting internal than external rotation.[5,7]

The superficial fibers of the medial collateral ligament also function as a secondary restraint to anterior tibial

translation in an anterior cruciate ligament (ACL) deficient knee. Sullivan et al found that sectioning the parallel fibers of the superficial medial collateral ligament significantly increased anterior tibial translation if the ACL had been sectioned first.[8] Sectioning the posteromedial capsule, the oblique fibers of the superficial medial collateral ligament, or the deep medial ligament had no effect on anterior tibial translation.

Muscles of the Medial Side

There are five insertions of the semimembranosus: (1) direct, (2) anteromedial tendon, (3) oblique popliteal ligament, (4) posterior capsule, (5) posterior horn of the medial meniscus (Fig. 1B-5). Warren and Marshal found that most of the semimembranosus tendon inserts on the infragleneoid tubercle of the tibia at the posteromedial corner just below the joint line.[1] The anterior, or medial, tendon is an extension of the direct insertion and continues medially along the tibial condyle, inserting beneath the superficial fibers of the medial ligament, just distal to the tibial margin of layer III.

The other three insertions of the semimembranosus are described by Warren and Marshal as extensions of the semimembranosus tendon sheath into the posteromedial and posterior parts of the capsule. The oblique popliteal ligament extends obliquely and laterally from the posteromedial tibia toward the head of the lateral gastrocnemius. At this point, it joins and combines with posterior fibers of layer II. Distal slips of the semimembranosus run inferiorly and insert on the tibia posterior to the inferior oblique portion of the superficial medial collateral ligament and blend here with its fibers.

Recognized functions of the semimembranosus include flexion of the knee, internal rotation of the tibia, and tension of the posterior capsule with knee flexion. It has been suggested that attachments of the semimembranosus to the posterior capsule and posterior horn of

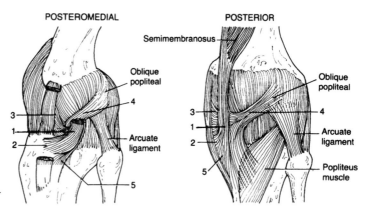

Figure 1B-5. Insertions of the semimembranosus tendon.

the medial meniscus act to tighten the posterior capsule and pull the medial meniscus posteriorly with knee flexion.

The sartorius, semitendinosus, and gracilis tendons insert along the proximal medial tibia as a conjoined tendon 2 cm distal and 2 cm medial to the apex of the tibial tubercle. They are primary flexors and internal rotators of the knee joint and dynamically act to decrease loads on the medial ligament and anterior cruciate ligament.

Lateral and Posterolateral Structures

The lateral side of the knee has been divided into three distinct layers by Seebacher et al.[9] (Figs. 1B–1, 1B–6, 1B–7, and 1B–8). The most superficial layer, layer I, is made up of the iliotibial tract with its anterior expansion and the superficial portion of the biceps with its posterior expansions (see Fig. 1B–6). The iliotibial tract inserts at two sites. Proximally, it inserts into the lateral epicondyle of the femur, and distally it inserts into the lateral tibial tubercle (Gerdy's tubercle). The iliotibial tract remains parallel to the biceps in flexion and extension, but crosses the popliteus tendon and lateral collateral ligament in flexion. It moves anterior in extension and posterior in flexion, but remains tight throughout range of motion of the knee.

Layer II is composed of the quadriceps retinaculum anteriorly and the two patellofemoral ligaments posteriorly (see Fig. 1B–7). The proximal patellofemoral ligament extends from the retinaculum to the terminal fibers of the lateral intermuscular septum. The distal patellofemoral ligament courses from the retinaculum posteriorly to the flabella, if present. When the flabella

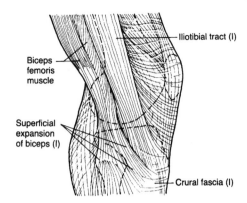

Figure 1B–6. Lateral knee, layer I.

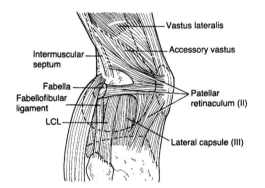

Figure 1B–7. Lateral knee, layer II.

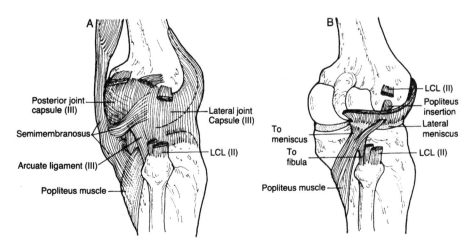

Figure 1B–8. Lateral knee, layer III. **A.** Joint capsule and arcuate ligament. **B.** Insertions of popliteus tendon.

is not present, the distal patellofemoral ligament has been found to insert into the lateral head of the gastrocnemius muscle and the iliotibial tract.[9]

Layer III, the lateral portion of the joint capsule, is attached to the tibia and femur along the lateral margins of the joint (see Fig. 1B–8). The capsule has a meniscotibial portion and a meniscofemoral portion (coronary ligaments). The popliteus tendon passes through an area devoid of meniscocapsular attachment in the posterolateral aspect of the knee. Just posterior to the iliotibial tract, layer III divides into two lamellae. The superficial branch surrounds the lateral collateral ligament and ends posteriorly in the fabellofibular ligament (short collateral ligament). The deeper lamina courses deep, forming the coronary ligament and ending at the arcuate ligament. The inferolateral geniculate vessels pass between these two lamellae.

The lateral collateral ligament, unlike the deep medial collateral ligament, is not attached to its neighboring meniscus. It extends from the lateral epicondyle of the femur to the midportion of the fibular head. It is a tight bandlike structure, easily palpated in the figure-of-four position. It is located posterior to the medial collateral ligament in the coronal plane and runs slightly posteriorly from femur to fibula. It lightens in extension and loosens in flexion, although contraction of the middle layer of the biceps insertion, which surrounds it, may maintain some tension in flexion.[10]

The main insertion of the popliteus tendon is the lateral condyle of the femur. It courses distally deep to the lateral collateral ligament before dividing just distal to the joint line. One limb continues to the posterior tibia and lateral meniscus; the other inserts onto the posterior fibula (see Fig. 1B–8)[11–13] (Maynard M, Deng X-H, Warren RF. Unpublished data).

The fabellofibular ligament (short ligament) inserts onto the flabella when present and runs parallel to the lateral collateral ligament. It attaches to the fibular head posterior to the biceps tendon and reinforces the posterolateral capsule.

The arcuate ligament also inserts into the posterior aspect of the fibular head and arches over the popliteus tendon to insert on the lateral head of the gastrocnemius on the posterior tibia where they are joined by the oblique popliteal ligament (see Fig. 1B–8). The arcuate ligament acts to reinforce the posterolateral capsule. Seebacher et al describe three variations in the posterolateral capsular structures.[9] They found arcuate ligament fibers present alone 13% of the time, fabellofibular ligament fibers present alone 20% of the time, and fibers from both ligaments present 67% of the time. They noted that when there is a large flabella, the fabellofibular ligament is large, and no arcuate ligament is present. In contrast, when the flabella is absent, there are no fabellofibular ligament fibers and there is a stout arcuate ligament.

Function of the Posterolateral Ligamentous structures

The lateral collateral ligament and popliteus–arcuate ligament complex both function as principal structures in preventing varus rotation and external rotation of the tibia.[4,5,14–17] The posterior cruciate ligament functions as a secondary restraint, limiting varus and external rotation in knees in which the lateral collateral ligament and popliteus–arcuate ligament complex have been sectioned.[14–16]

Muscles of the Lateral Aspect of the Knee

The muscle belly of the popliteus is attached to a triangular area of the posterior proximal tibia. The tendon of the popliteus attaches to the lateral femoral condyle, slightly anterior and inferior to the origin of the lateral collateral ligament (see Fig. 1B–8). It courses inferior and medially across the posterolateral aspect of the joint, deep to the lateral collateral ligament, where it fans out into the fleshy muscle belly. Secondary fascicles extend from the tendon to the fibula and the lateral meniscus[11–13] (Maynard M, Deng X-H, Warren RF. Unpublished data) (see Fig. 1B–8). Dynamically, the popliteus assists in knee flexion and internal rotation of the tibia on the femur.[12,13] It also unlocks the screw home mechanism during the first 10° to 20° of flexion.[11] The popliteus also functions to draw the posterior horn of the lateral meniscus posteriorly as the knee is flexed.[11] As noted it stabilizes the posterolateral corner of the knee, assisting the lateral collateral ligament and popliteus–arcuate complex in preventing posterolateral and varus instability.[14–17]

The biceps femoris insertions are similar to those of the semimembranosus. The muscular fibers of the long head of the biceps become tendinous 7 to 10 cm above the joint. The short head remains more muscular farther distally, and joins the long head, forming a short, thick common tendon of insertion.[10] Marshal et al found that as the common tendon passes distally it splits into three layers: superficial, middle, and deep.[10]

The superficial layer of the biceps femoris passes lateral to the lateral collateral ligament and forms an anteromedial and posterior expansion, inserting onto the anterior crural fascia, lateral collateral ligament, and head of fibula, as well as the fascia over the gastrocnemius and soleus muscles, respectively. The middle layer is thin and surrounds the distal one fourth of the collateral ligament. The deep layer of the common biceps tendon travels deep to the fibular collateral ligament and splits into the tibial attachment at Gerdy's tubercle and a fibular attachment into the head and styloid process of the fibula. A direct insertion into the posterior aspect of the tibia has also been noted. Five to seven centimeters above the joint line, a fibrous connection between the biceps and iliotibial band is described.[10]

The functions of the biceps include flexion and lateral rotation through the action of the superficial layer; tensing of the lateral collateral ligament in flexion by the middle layer; tensing of the iliotibial band in flexion by its attachment; and posterior pull of the capsule in flexion by the deep layer attachments, preventing impingement of the capsule in the joint.

Anterior Knee Structures

The anterior aspect of the knee is composed primarily of the patella and extensor mechanism, including the quadriceps insertions and patellar tendon (Fig. 1B–9). The rectus femoris tendon inserts most superficially into a 3- to 5-cm-wide proximal portion of the patella, but also sends fibers past the patella to become continuous with the patellar tendon. The middle layer is composed of tendons from the vastus lateralis and vastus medialis. The deep layer, made up of fibers from the vastus intermedius, inserts into the posterior edge of the proximal pole of the patella. Distal fibers of the vastus medialis obliquus are oblique, oriented 55° to 70° from the sagittal plane, and thus exert a medial vector on the patella. Distal fibers of the vastus lateralis are also oblique, 20° to 45°, but terminate 3 cm above the superior pole of the patella into the tendon.[18] Aponeurotic fibers of the vastus medialis and vastus lateralis contribute to the medial and lateral patellar retinaculum along the extensions of the fascia lata. On the lateral side, thickening of the fascia lata becomes the iliotibial tract and the iliopatellar band.[19] The iliopatellar band inserts onto the lateral aspect of the patella, whereas the iliotibial tract continues to Gerdy's tubercle. Deeper thickenings of the joint capsule pass from the medial and lateral epicondyles to respective sides of the patella. These patellofemoral ligaments are reported to be present in varying degrees by Reider et al and to be present most consistently laterally.[18]

The extensor mechanism attaches to the tibial tubercle via the patellar tendon. The patellar tendon averages 33 mm in width. It originates from the distal aspect of the patella, closer to the anterior than the deep surface, and inserts into the tibial tubercle by blending with periosteal fibers.

In addition to extending the knee, the extensor mechanism exerts a translational force on the tibia, depending on the position of the knee. In 0° to 70° of flexion, the extensor mechanism exerts an anterior force on the tibia and thus acts synergistically with the posterior cruciate ligament to prevent posterior tibial subluxation. In greater than 70° of flexion, the contracting quadriceps mechanism reverses its role and acts synergistically with the anterior cruciate ligament to prevent anterior subluxation.[20] Other functions of the quadriceps mechanism include stabilizing patellar tracking, tensing the anterior medial and lateral capsule, and re-

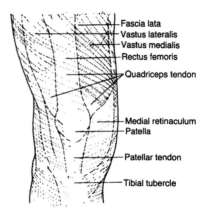

Figure 1B–9. Extensor mechanism of the knee.

ducing stress on the medial collateral ligament when valgus forces are applied.[21] The quadriceps mechanism may also act to pull the anterior horns of the medial and lateral menisci forward during extension through its capsular attachment.[22]

Synovial Plicae

The cavity of the knee joint is lined by the synovial membrane, which partly subdivides it into a number of communicating compartments. This is a result of development. Early in intrauterine life, the knee is separated into three compartments: medial, lateral, and suprapatellar. During fetal life, the thin membranes separating the compartments involute, forming a single cavity. In 20% of people, remnants of these septa remain to various degrees and have been given the name *plicae*[23] (Fig. 1B–10).

Hardaker et al have classified plicae by anatomic position, focusing on three main types: suprapatellar, medial patellar, and infrapatellar.[23] The infrapatellar plica, also known as the ligamentum mucosum, is the most common. Its attachments are the superior, anterior portion of the intracondylar notch and the infrapatellar fat pad. Although generally not considered a source of symptoms,[23] resection of a fibrotic infrapatellar plica has been associated with relief of anterior knee pain in athletes (Steadman JR. Personal communication).

The next most commonly observed plica is in the suprapatellar pouch. The suprapatellar plica either partially or, more rarely, completely divides the suprapatellar compartment from the rest of the knee. It is seen most commonly on the medial side of the pouch, originating just superior to the superior pole of the patella. It may extend inferiorly and become contiguous with the medial patellar plica. The suprapatellar plica

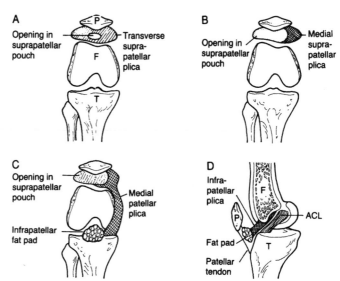

Figure 1B–10. Synovial plicae of the knee. **A, B.** Suprapatellar. **C.** Medial patellar. **D.** Infrapatellar.

may be a cause of patellar malalignment and maltracking when fibrotic.

The medial patellar plica originates from the medial suprapatellar plica and inserts on the synovial membrane covering the fat pad. It therefore lies along the medial wall of the joint. A thickened medial patellar plica may snap over the femoral condyle. Erosion of the underlying articular cartilage has been reported in advanced cases.[23] Normally, plicae appear thin, pink, and pliable and do not cause symptoms; however, they may become inflamed, thickened, and fibrotic as the consequence of trauma or overuse, resulting in clinical symptoms.[23]

The Cruciate Ligaments

The cruciate ligaments consist of regularly oriented dense connective tissue surrounded by a vascular synovial envelope. They are composed of collagen fibrils which combine to form larger fibers, larger subfasicular units, and finally fascicles. The ligaments are surrounded by a paratenon, the fascicles by an epitenon, and the fibers by an endotenon. Although the cruciate ligaments are intraarticular, because of their surrounding synovial membrane, they are extrasynovial.

The blood supply to the cruciates stems primarily from the middle genicular artery with contributions from the superior and inferior medial and lateral geniculates. Ligamentous branches of the middle genicular artery and terminal branches of the inferior genicular arteries supply the synovial plexus overlying the ligaments. According to Arnoczky, the synovial vessels contribute to a network of periligamentous vessels which surround the ligament. The periligamentous vessels give rise to smaller connecting branches which penetrate the ligament transversely, communicating with a plexus of endoligamentous vessels which run longitudinally parallel to the collagen fibers in the ligament.[24,25]

The nerve supply to the cruciate ligaments originates from the posterior articular branch of the posterior tibial nerve.[26] Most of the nerve fibers are associated with endoligamentous vessels, but some lie alone within the ligament and appear to function in proprioception. Golgi light tension receptors have been found near the origins of the cruciate ligaments. Animal studies have demonstrated that mechanoreceptors with myelinated axons are present in the ACL and provide information on its tension.[27] Decreased proprioceptive function has been observed clinically in patients with all deficient knees.[28]

Anterior Cruciate Ligament

The anterior cruciate ligament has a femoral attachment in the form of a segment of a circle on the medial surface of the lateral femoral condyle in the intercondylar notch (Fig. 1B–11A). From here, the anterior cruciate ligament passes anteriorly, medially, and distally to its insertion on the tibia (Figs. 1B–11B and 1B–12). Its tibial attachment is anterior and lateral to the anterior tibial spine, beneath the transverse meniscal ligament. It is somewhat wider and stronger than the femoral attachment.[25,29]

The anterior cruciate ligament is composed of two bands, an anteromedial band and a posterolateral band, named on the basis of their tibial attachment sites. Each

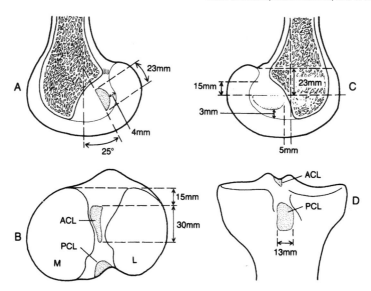

Figure 1B–11. Insertions of the cruciate ligaments. **A.** Femoral insertion of the anterior cruciate ligament. **B.** Tibial insertion of the anterior cruciate ligament. **C.** Femoral insertion of the posterior cruciate ligament. **D.** Tibial insertion of the posterior cruciate ligament.

band, in turn, is composed of numerous fascicles. When the knee is extended, the posterolateral band is tight and the anteromedial band is mildly lax. As the knee is flexed, the femoral attachment of the anterior cruciate ligament becomes more horizontal, loosening the posterolateral band and tightening the anteromedial band[25,29] (Fig. 1B–13). This corresponds with clinical findings. Injury to the anteromedial portion of the anterior cruciate ligament demonstrates more anterior laxity at 90° (drawer test).[25,29] Arnoczky, however,

points out that the division into anteromedial and posterolateral bands is an oversimplification. He states the anterior cruciate ligament is actually a continuum of fibers, a different portion of which is tight throughout the range of motion.[25]

No fibers of the anterior cruciate ligament are truly isometric. The least amount of variation in length appears to occur in the anteromedial portion (1.5 mm) during range of motion.[30]

The anterior cruciate ligament on average is 38 mm

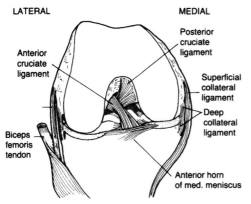

Figure 1B–12. Cruciate ligaments within the femoral notch.

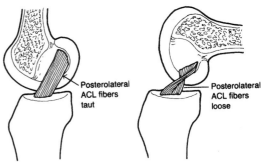

Figure 1B–13. Tension within the anterior cruciate ligament during motion. The posterolateral portion is under maximal tension in extension, and the anteromedial portion is under maximal tension in flexion.

long, 11 mm wide, and 5 mm thick. Its ultimate tensile strength in young individuals is usually quoted as 1700 to 2000 N.[31,32] The primary function of the anterior cruciate ligament is to prevent anterior displacement of the tibia and hyperextension of the knee. Secondary functions include resistance of varus/valgus stresses and internal rotation of the tibia on the femur.[4]

Posterior Cruciate Ligament

The posterior cruciate ligament attaches to the lateral surface of the medial femoral condyle in the intercondylar notch in the form of a broad (3-cm) segment of a circle[29] (see Fig. 1B–11C). The attachment is horizontally oriented and follows the curvature of the condyle, with the most distal fibers originating 3 mm proximal to the articular surface.[29] The fibers descend inferiorly, posteriorly, and laterally to insert in a groove in the posterior aspect of the tibia between the two condyles (see Fig. 1B–11D and 1B–12) The insertion site is centered approximately 1 cm below the articular surface with an average width of 13 mm.

The average length of the posterior cruciate ligament is 38 mm,[29] and its average width is 13 mm, fanning out more superiorly. It is composed of a large anteromedial portion and a small more oblique posterolateral portion.[29] These bundles, however, are not completely separable. In extension, the smaller posterolateral bundle is tight, whereas the anteromedial portion is lax. In flexion, the posterolateral bundle becomes lax and the anteromedial bundle taut[29] (Fig. 1B–14). As with the anterior cruciate ligament, this is an oversimplification as, in reality, a gradual change in tension occurs from anterior to posterior as the knee is extended.[33] None of the fibers are entirely isometric, but it appears that there is less variation in length with knee motion in the posterior fibers.[33]

The meniscofemoral ligaments, when present, reinforce the posterior cruciate ligament, but appear to play a minor role in humans.[34] (see Fig. 1B–1). The ligament of Humphry, or anterior meniscofemoral ligament, is less than one-third the diameter of the posterior cruciate ligament.[35] It runs superiorly from the posterior horn of the lateral meniscus to insert on the femur at the distal edge of the posterior cruciate ligament. The ligament of Wrisberg, or posterior meniscofemoral ligament, may be as large as one-half the diameter of the posterior cruciate ligament.[35] It arises from the posterior horn of the lateral meniscus and crosses obliquely posterior to the posterior cruciate ligament to insert on the medial femoral condyle. It has been reported to attach to the posterior capsule, or tibia, instead of the lateral meniscus.[35]

Girgis et al reported that in 30% of knees, both meniscofemoral ligaments are absent.[29] In the remaining 70%, both ligaments were never observed together. Clancy et al report that when either the ligament of Wrisberg or the ligament of Humphry is large, it can mask clinical laxity in a posterior cruciate ligament-deficient knee.[36] Other authors feel that the meniscofemoral ligaments play a minor role as secondary restraints to the posterior cruciate ligament.[34]

The posterior cruciate ligament provides over 90% of the resistance to posterior displacement of the tibia on the femur, and is believed to be the primary restraint to posterior translation from 0° to 90° of flexion.[14] The posterior cruciate ligament is a secondary restraint to varus/valgus rotation and external rotation.[14]

The strength of the posterior cruciate ligament is approximately 2000 N.[33] In cadaver knees, isolated sectioning of the posterior cruciate ligament produced increased posterior translation in all degrees of flexion.[14] The greatest translation was found between 75° and 90° of flexion.[14] Although isolated sectioning of the posterior cruciate ligament in the intact knee had no effect on varus/valgus rotation or external rotation, the posterior cruciate ligament was found to provide substantial restraint to varus rotation and external rotation of the tibia after sectioning of the posterolateral structures (arcuate complex, popliteus, and fibular collateral ligament).[14,15]

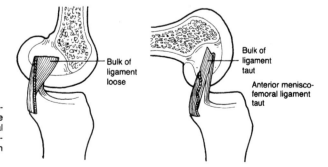

Figure 1B–14. Tension within the posterior cruciate ligament during motion. The posterolateral portion is under maximal tension in extension, and the anteromedial portion is under maximal tension in flexion.

Bulk of ligament loose

Bulk of ligament taut

Anterior meniscofemoral ligament taut

References

1. Warren LF, Marshal JL. The supporting structures and layers on the medial side of the knee. *J Bone Joint Surg Am.* 1979;61:56.
2. Warren LF, Marshal JL, Girgis F. The prime static stabilizer of the medial side of the knee. *J Bone Joint Surg Am.* 1974;56:665–674.
3. Robichon J, Romero C. The functional anatomy of the knee joint, with special reference to the medial collateral and anterior cruciate ligaments. *Can J Surg.* 1968;11:36.
4. Grood ES, Noyes FR, Butler DL, Suntay WJ. Ligamentous and capsular restraints preventing straight medial and lateral laxity in intact human cadaver knees. *J Bone Joint Surg Am.* 1981;63:1275.
5. Seering WP, Piziali RL, Nagel DA, Schurman DS. The function of the primary ligaments of the knee in varus–valgus and axial rotation. *J Biomech.* 1980;13:785–794.
6. Hughston JC, Eilers AF. The role of the posterior ligament in repairs of acute medial (collateral) ligament tears of the knee. *J Bone Joint Surg Am.* 1973;55:923–940.
7. Markolf K, Mensch J, Armsutz H. Stiffness and laxity of the knee—The contributions of the supporting structures. *J Bone Joint Surg Am.* 1976;58:583–594.
8. Sullivan D, Levy R, Sheskier S, Torzilli PA, Warren RF. Medial restraints to anterior–posterior motion of the knee. *J Bone Joint Surg Am.* 1984;66:930.
9. Seebacher JR, Ingles AE, Marshall JL, Warren RF. The structure of the posterolateral aspect of the knee. *J Bone Joint Surg Am.* 1982;64:536.
10. Marshal JL, Fakhry GG, Zelko RR. The biceps femoris tendon and its functional significance. *J Bone Joint Surg Am.* 1972;54:1444.
11. Last R. The popliteus muscle and the lateral meniscus. *J Bone Joint Surg Br.* 1950;32:93–99.
12. Basmajian JV, Lovejoy JF. Functions of the popliteus muscle in man. *J Bone Joint Surg Am.* 1971;533:557.
13. Garth WP, Pomphrey MM, Merrill KD. Isolated avulsion of the popliteus tendon: Operative repair. *J Bone Joint Surg Am.* 1992;74:130.
14. Gollehon DL, Torzilli PA, Warren RF. The role of the posterolateral and cruciate ligaments in stability of the human knee. *J Bone Joint Surg Am.* 1987;69:232.
15. Veltri DM, Deng X-H, Maynard MJ, Torzilli PA, Warren RF. The role of the popliteofibular ligament in stability of the human knee: A biomechanical study, Unpublished manuscript.
16. Markolf KL, Wascher DC, Finerman GAM. Direct in vitro measurement of forces in the cruciate ligaments. Part II. The effect of section of the posterolateral structures. *J Bone Joint Surg Am.* 1993;75:387.
17. Grood ES, Stowers SF, Noyes FR. Limits of movement in the human knee. Effect of sectioning the posterior cruciate ligament and posterolateral structure. *Joint Surg Am.* 1988;70:88–97.
18. Reider B, Marshal JL, Koslin B, et al. The anterior aspect of the knee. *J Bone Joint Surg Am.* 1981;63:351.
19. Terry GC, Hughston JC, Norwood LA. The anatomy of the iliopatellar band and iliotibial tract. *Am J Sports Med.* 1986;14:39.
20. Daniel DM, Stone M, Sachs S, et al. The quadriceps active test. Presented at the 53rd Annual Meeting of the Americal Academy of Orthopaedic Surgery; New Orleans: February 1986.
21. Pope MH, Johnson RJ, Brown DW, et al. The role of musculature in injuries to the medial collateral ligament. *J Bone Joint Surg Am.* 1979;61:398.
22. Kaplan EB. Factors responsible for stability of the knee joint. *Bull Hosp Joint Dis.* 1957;18:51.
23. Hardaker WT, Jr, Whipple TL, Bassett FH. Diagnosis and treatment of plica syndrome of the knee. *J Bone Joint Surg Am.* 62:221, 1980.
24. Arnoczky S. Blood supply to the anterior cruciate ligament and supporting structures. *Orthop Clin North Am.* 1985;17:15.
25. Arnoczky S. Anatomy of the anterior cruciate ligament. *Clin Orthop Relat Res.* 1983;172:19–25.
26. Kennedy JC, Alexander IJ, Hayes KC. Nerve supply of the human knee and its functional importance. *Am J Sports Med.* 1982;10:329.
27. Krauspe R, Schmidt M, Schaible HG. Sensory innervation of the anterior cruciate ligament. *J Bone Joint Surg Am.* 1992;74:390.
28. Barrack R, Skinner H, Buckley S. Proprioception in the anterior cruciate ligament deficient knee. *Am J Sports Med.* 1989;17:1–6.
29. Girgis FG, Marshal JL, Almonajem ARS. The cruciate ligaments of the knee joint: An anatomical, functional, and experimental analysis. *Clin Orthop Relat Res.* 1975;106:216.
30. Johnson RJ. Anatomy and biomechanics of the knee. In: Chapman M, ed. *Operative Orthopaedics.* Philadelphia: JB Lippincott; 1988:1617.
31. Noyes FR, Grood ES. The strength of the Anterior cruciate ligament in humans and rhesus monkeys. *J Bone Joint Surg Am.* 1976;58:1074.
32. Woo SL-Y, Adams D. The tensile properties of human anterior cruciate ligament and ACL graft tissues. In: Daniel D, ed. *Knee Ligaments: Structure, Function, Injury, and Repair.* New York: Raven Press; 1990.
33. Cooper DE, Warren RF, Warner JJP. The posterior cruciate ligament and posterolateral structures of the knee: Anatomy, function, and patterns of injury. In: Tullos HS, ed. *Instructional Course Lectures.* American Academy of Orthopaedic Surgeons; 1991;40(Ch 32):249.
34. Heller L, Langman J. The meniscofemoral ligaments of the human knee. *J Bone Joint Surg. Br.* 1964;46:307–313.
35. Clancy WG, Shelbourne KD, Zoellner GB, et al. Treatment of knee joint instability secondary to rupture of the posterior cruciate ligament. *J Bone Joint Surg Am.* 1983;65:310.
36. Kennedy JC, Hawkins RJ, Willis RB, et al. Tension studies of human knee ligaments: Yield point, ultimate failure, and disruption of the cruciate and tibial collateral ligaments. *J Bone Joint Surg Am.* 1976;48:350–355.

2

Articular Cartilage Injury and Repair

Stephen B. Trippel and Henry J. Mankin

Introduction

The clinical attributes and contributions of articular cartilage are readily apparent in daily orthopaedic practice. This thin layer of rubbery tissue lining the surface of joints enables the smooth, pain-free gliding that we take for granted in all skeletal motion. Its disruption can relegate an aging patient from dynamic self-sufficiency to disabled dependency or demote an athlete from star to spectator. As with any tissue subject to injury or deterioration, healing is critical to recovery of function. Yet, as is evident from clinical practice, function is not readily restored to damaged or diseased joints. For this reason, articular cartilage has been a particularly intriguing problem and one that has evoked attention for centuries. Hippocrates viewed injuries of this tissue as incurable, and over the intervening years numerous anatomists, physicians, and biologists have offered evidence and opinions in support of or against the generally held concept that wounds in articular cartilage cannot heal.[1-12]

To answer the question of whether cartilage heals or not (as will be seen in this chapter, the answer is both yes and no, depending on the circumstances) and to decipher new ways of helping the healing process, one must briefly review the information available regarding the structure, biochemistry, and metabolism of articular cartilage with special emphasis on those aspects that have a bearing on the process of healing. The first section of this chapter is devoted to such a review. The second portion of the chapter defines the current understanding of the responses of articular cartilage to trauma. The final section is devoted to projecting approaches to the problem of cartilage healing based on current understanding and ongoing research.

Normal Articular Cartilage

Anatomy

Articular cartilage is the principal "working" component of diarthrodial joints and is uniquely suited to this role. Cartilage gliding on cartilage has a coefficient of friction lower than that of a well-sharpened ice skate gliding on ice.[13] It is endowed by its high collagen content with an enormous capacity to resist shear forces applied to it during motion under load, and by its proteoglycan content to withstand the compression imposed by weight bearing and muscle contraction.[14-16] Despite the functional demands placed on it, articular cartilage generally measures less than 5 mm in thickness in mammalian joints, with considerable variation depending on the species, the joint, and the site within the joint.[17,18] Contrary to expectations raised by its low coefficient of friction and gross appearance, the surface of articular cartilage is not smooth.[19] Scanning electron microscopic studies have demonstrated gentle undulations and irregular depressions some of which appear to correspond in location and shape to cells lying beneath the surface.[20,21]

Articular cartilage is both avascular and alymphatic. In adult animals, articular chondrocytes derive their nutrition by a double diffusion system.[22-24] Nutrients must first diffuse from the vascular space into the synovial fluid and then through the dense matrix of the cartilage to the cell.[25] There are no nerves in articular cartilage, rendering the bearing surfaces of the joint dependent on capsular, synovial, subchondral bone, and muscular nerve endings for appreciation of pain and proprioception.[23] By virtue of its lack of sensory innervation, it cannot directly appreciate and report abnormal states such as blunt trauma, lacerative injury,

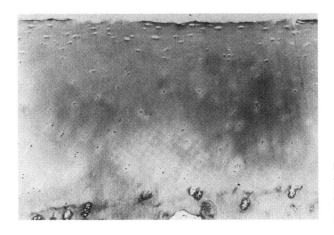

Figure 2–1. Low-power photomicrograph of adult articular cartilage. Note the preponderance of the intercellular matrix and the sparse cellularity. Contrary to initial impression, the cells are not homogeneous or randomly distributed. Hematoxylin and eosin; 100×.

mechanical overloading, and structural incongruity. By virtue of its avascular and alymphatic state, articular cartilage is for the most part dependent on the chemical composition of the synovial fluid and/or variations in joint pressure to receive signals that regulate metabolism. The avascular state is of particular importance to the issue of cartilage healing in that, as we shall see, this deprives the tissue of the inflammatory response (mediated through the vascular system) available to most tissues to facilitate repair.

Articular cartilage is remarkably hypocellular, less than 1% of its volume being composed of cells in the adult[26] (Fig. 2–1). During skeletal growth, a process that includes expansion of the articular surface, articular cartilage is relatively hypercellular; however, with growth, cell proliferation does not keep pace with matrix production and cells become progressively more widely dispersed. The distribution of chondrocytes is not random.[24] Four zones can be distinguished: (1) a tangential or gliding zone in which the cells are somewhat flattened with their long axes parallel to the articular surface; (2) a transitional zone in which cells are round or ovoid and appear randomly distributed; (3) a radial zone in which the cells appear to line up vertically in short, irregular columns; and (4) a calcified zone in which the matrix is heavily infiltrated with hydroxyapatite and is firmly attached to the subchondral bone[27,28] (Fig. 2–2). The calcified zone is separated from the radial zone superficial to it by a wavy, irregular bluish line (on hematoxylin and eosin staining) called the *tidemark* (Fig. 2–3). The tidemark appears with skeletal maturity and marks the interface between avascular cartilage, nourished from synovial fluid, and the subchondral bone with its underlying marrow and rich vascular supply.[25]

Just as the cells of articular cartilage are not random-

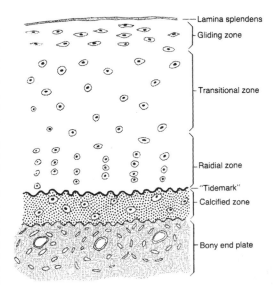

Figure 2–2. Diagrammatic representation of the zones of mature articular cartilage.

ly arranged, neither are its matrix elements. The fibrillar component of cartilage matrix was observed at least as early as the turn of the century to vary in depth with the tissue. Benninghoff, in 1902, described these fibrillar structures as "arcades," formed by fibers arising from subchondral bone, arching toward the surface and then descending back to subchondral bone.[29] Details of this collagen structure (as, for example, whether a single collagen fiber forms a complete arch) have been de-

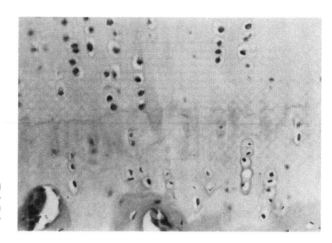

Figure 2–3. Photomicrograph of the basal layers of articular cartilage showing the "tidemark," a bluish line of hematoxylin and eosin stain, which separates the radial from the calcified zone. 250×.

bated for years and will likely be the subject of controversy for some time to come.[20,29,37] Nevertheless, it appears well established that the general orientation of collagen in the superficial layers of articular cartilage is parallel to the articular surface and that their orientation becomes more oblique in the transitional zone and then more vertical or radial in the deep zone. It is probably safe to assume that this arrangement contributes to the ability of normal articular cartilage to accommodate the shear and compressive forces under which it must function.

Matrix is also oriented with respect to the cells it encompasses. Scanning and transmission electron microscopy have demonstrated that the microenvironment of the articular chondrocyte includes a porous, feltlike "capsule" surrounding middle and deep, but not superficial, cells.[28]

Biochemistry

The biochemical composition of articular cartilage is unlike that of any other tissue. This is particularly evident in its two major structural components: collagen and proteoglycan. Although articular cartilage is 70 to 80% water,[39–42] collagen is its most prevalent organic constituent, accounting for over 50% of the dry weight.[37,43] The principal collagen of cartilage, classified as type II collagen, differs in several respects from that of skin or bone (type I collagen). Type II collagen consists of three identical α 1(II) chains in a helical arrangement. This contrasts to type I collagen in which two α 1(I) chains and one α 2(I) chain form the triple helix.[43,46] The chains of type II collagen are encoded by a different gene from those of other collagen types and differ from type I collagen in possessing an increased quantity of hydroxylysine and degree of glycosylation.[44,45]

Articular cartilage also contains small, nonfibrillar collagens. One of these, designated type IX, is a chimeric molecule that is partly collagen and partly proteoglycan.[47] Although it constitutes only 1 or 2% of articular cartilage collagen, it appears to play an important role in the molecular attachment of type II collagen to cartilage proteoglycans or other type II fibrils within the articular cartilage matrix[48,49] or in the control of type II fibril growth.[43] Another "minor" collagen is type XI, formerly termed 1α, 2α, 3α. Our understanding of this collagen is still rudimentary. It constitutes approximately 3% of total articular cartilage collagen[50] and appears to coexist in the same fibrils as type II collagen (Fig. 2–4). It has been speculated that type XI collagen is involved in controlling the diameter of type II collagen fibrils.[47]

The second most prevalent solid in cartilage is the proteoglycan known as aggrecan, a macromolecule consisting of a protein core and polysaccharide chains. These enormous (200 million daltons or more) molecules exist as aggregates[39,51,52] of four distinct molecular subtypes (Fig. 2–5). The central core of the proteoglycan aggregate is a long, thin filament of hyaluronic acid which accounts for less than 1% of the total polysaccharide within the tissue, but is critically important in maintaining its physical properties.[53] The second and third components of the proteoglycan aggregate are a linear protein ("core" protein or aggrecan[54]) approximately 180 to 210 nm long and polysaccharide chains (glycosaminoglycans).[39,52,55] The glycosaminoglycan chains are attached end-to-side to the protein core in a "bottlebrush" configuration to form proteoglycan "subunits."[39] The glycosaminoglycans are themselves of three different species: chondroitin 6-sulfate, chon-

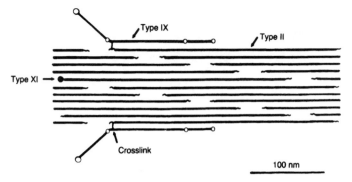

Figure 2–4. Proposed macromolecular organization of a thin collagen fibril in hyaline cartilage. Note that type II, type IX, and type XI collagens are all included within the same fibril. The location of the hydroxypyridium crosslink between the amino terminus of type II collagen and the NC3 domain of type IX collagen is shown. The location of type XI collagen in the fibril is not known, and it may be either within the fibril, as shown, or on the surface of the fibril. (Reprinted with permission from Mayne[47].)

Proteoglycan Aggregate

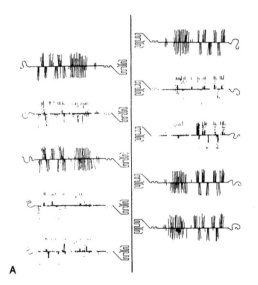

A

droitin 4-sulfate, and keratan sulfate.[39,52,55] The distribution of these species on the proteoglycan core protein varies with cartilage, age, and disease.[56] The fourth key constituent of the proteoglycan aggregate is another peptide, link protein. This protein secures or "links" the proteoglycan subunits to the hyaluronic acid, thereby stabilizing the three-dimensional structure of the aggregate.[51] In addition to aggrecan, another group of proteoglycans containing dermatan sulfate have been recently described. These molecules, decorin and biglycan, are considerably smaller in size, do not aggregate, and may play a role in healing cartilage (or at best failure to heal).[57,58]

Articular cartilage contains numerous other biologic materials in small quantities. Approximately 5 to 6% of the tissue is in the form of inorganic constituents, mostly calcium salts.[51] Lipids[59] account for approximately 1% of the dry weight. A variety of glycoproteins contribute to the matrix.[51,60,61] In addition, fibronectin, a peptide involved in cell-to-substrate attachment, has recently been identified in articular cartilage and found to be distributed principally in the superficial zone.[62,63] Approximately 20 different phosphorylated glycoproteins are made by articular chondrocytes[64]; however,

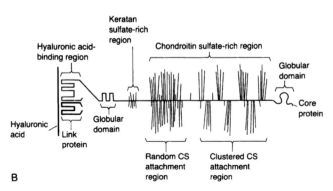

B

Figure 2-5. Proteoglycan aggregate (**A**) and its constituents (**B**). Each proteoglycan subunit consists of a core protein with globular domains, one of which serves as a binding site for hyaluronic acid. Attached to the core protein are glycosaminoglycans and chondroitin sulfate, which, in three dimensions, are thought to assume a high-volume "bottlebrush" configuration. Link protein associates with hyaluronic acid and core protein to stabilize the core protein-to-hyaluronic acid attachment. (Adapted from Muir[51] and Heinegard and Oldberg.[61] Reprinted with permission from Mankin HJ, Trippel SB, "Articular Cartilage Healing" in *Mechanisms of Surgical Diseases of Small Animals* 2nd edition, Bojrab J (ed.), Lea and Febiger, 1993).

the character and function of these remain to be defined.

Metabolism

Studies on the metabolism of articular matrix contradict the inert appearance of the tissue by demonstrating surprising rates of synthesis and degradation of the component macromolecules. Specifically, it has been clearly established by biochemical and molecular biologic techniques that articular chondrocytes are responsible for the synthesis of both the proteoglycan[51] and collagen[44,65–68] of cartilage. This responsibility is not evenly divided, and metabolic activity, at least with respect to RNA synthesis, varies among different articular chondrocyte populations.[69] Proteoglycan macromolecules turn over relatively rapidly, being degraded and replaced with freshly synthesized material.[47,70–73] Collagen is considerably more stable than the proteoglycan.[28,74] The rapid turnover of at least a small portion of the proteoglycan (far in excess of the amount likely to occur as a result of attritional loss)[71] suggests the presence of an internal remodeling system, and evidence has accumulated that this is based on the release of autodegradative enzymes which have as their principal substrate the proteoglycan.[75–78] In addition, a collagenase that degrades the collagen of cartilage has been found in tissues from osteoarthritic and, in lesser concentrations, normal human articular cartilage.[79] Both metalloproteinases and serine proteinases have been implicated in this degradative activity.[79–82] Prominent among these are collagenase[79,83]; the collagenase-activating enzyme stromelysin[83–85]; and plasmin, possibly contributed by the serum.[86–88] Regulation of these enzymes involves several mediators, including the prostaglandins,[89] interleukin-I (IL-I),[83,84,90,91] transforming growth factor beta (TGF-β),[92] and tumor necrosis factor (TNF).[93]

A central issue regarding the healing of cartilage is the potential of chondrocytes to reproduce themselves (cell replication). Light microscopic studies of immature articular cartilage disclose the presence of cells in various phases of mitosis.[94,95] This mitotic activity is found to occur in two distinct zones[94,95] (Fig. 2–6). The first is subjacent to the articular surface and presumably accounts for the growth of the cellular component of the articular portion of the cartilage mass. The second lies deep in the cartilage and comprises a narrow band of cells which morphologically resemble those of the proliferative zone of a microepiphyseal growth plate.[95] As the animal ages and approaches maturity, the pattern changes: the mitotic index decreases and a single remaining zone persists just above the zone of vascular invasion in the deep layers of the cartilage.[96] At skeletal maturity (coincident with epiphyseal plate closure in most species) mitotic activity appears to cease.[96] Care-

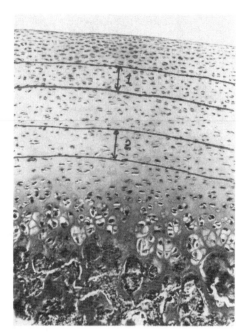

Figure 2–6. Low-power photomicrograph of the distal femur of an immature rabbit shows the two zones in which metabolic activity may be found. 100×.

ful search of the histologic sections of normal articular cartilages from adult animals of multiple species has failed to demonstrate mitotic figures and no grains were seen over the nucleus on all the radiographic studies using [³H]thymidine, an indicator of DNA synthesis.[96] On the basis of these observations it is evident that once maturity is reached, chondrocytes cease to divide. In relation to this finding it would seem essential to define whether this cessation of mitotic activity is irreversible or whether chondrocytes may, under appropriate conditions, regain the privilege of DNA synthesis and cell replication.

Using other terms the question is, Does the mature chondrocyte "break the switch" for DNA synthesis or merely "turn it off" and hence retain the capacity to turn it on again under appropriate conditions? Ample evidence now exists that the latter circumstance is the case and that chondrocytes can under appropriate conditions display brisk replicative activity. This finding is very important in considering the potential of articular cartilage for healing.

With this background, it is possible to review the experimental data regarding articular cartilage injury and repair. There are, of course, several forms of injury to the articular surface, but only the prototype, mechanical injury, is considered in the discussion that follows.

Response of Articular Cartilage to Mechanical Trauma

Pathophysiology of Trauma

The general response to injury in vascular mammalian tissues is a phasic one, so similar for most organs and structures as to be almost stereotypic. The response may be divided into three more or less distinct phases: necrosis, inflammation, and repair. The phase of necrosis begins immediately and is characterized by tissue death which varies considerably in extent depending on the type and degree of trauma, the tissue dependence on its blood supply, and the richness of the vascular bed. The second phase, inflammation, follows shortly after the first and is similar to that seen in infectious challenge in that it is almost entirely mediated by the vascular system. Vascular dilation, increased blood flow, transudation, and hematoma formation characterize this phase in which the wound fills with organized fibrin clot containing inflammatory cells. The phase of repair supervenes when the fibrin clot is invaded by blood vessels and fibroblasts begin to produce at first granulation tissue and subsequently a fibrous repair tissue that welds the wound together in the form of a scar. In certain of the body's tissues, the final phase is associated with replacement of the damaged tissue by the same tissue (eg, bone healing with bone) rather than with a fibrous scar; and in these circumstances the reparative material must also undergo a remodeling phase to restore the normal anatomy.

In considering the application of this scheme to injuries to hyaline articular cartilage, it is apparent that when subjected to trauma it undergoes necrosis, the first phase, just as would any other body tissue. Cells at the site of injury die and matrix disruption occurs consistent with the extent and type of trauma. Because no blood vessels are present, however, the second phase, which is almost entirely mediated by the vascular system, is absent. No blood escapes from ruptured vessels and no clot can be produced. There is no hyperemia, no transudation to provide plasma with its many growth factors, and no exudation to provide progenitor cells for the subsequent formation of repair tissue. All repair of superficial lacerations must be accomplished by nomadic cells in the synovial fluid or by the cartilage itself.

In consideration of deep defects, in which the injury extends not only through the articular cartilage, but through the subchondral bone as well, the marrow becomes involved in the repair process. In this circumstance the process of repair becomes dominated by the vascular system of the underlying bone, and the second

and third phases, vascular reaction and repair, are available to contribute to healing.

Types of Injury

Response of Articular Cartilage to Blunt Impact. Articular cartilage is expected, in the course of normal human activity, to accommodate a moderate, and at times high, degree of impact loading. Relatively few studies have attempted to determine at what point impact forces become harmful to the articular surface. Repo and Finlay analyzed human articular tissues subjected to impact by a "drop tower" technique using isotopic tracer studies, histology, and scanning electron microscopy (SEM).[97] All cartilage specimens loaded to 10% strain survived without apparent injury to the chondrocytes. All specimens loaded to strains of 40% or more showed some evidence of chondrocyte death. Matrix damage was first observed at strains on the order of 20 to 30%. Specimens subjected to 40 and 50% were consistently fissured, and SEM of the specimens demonstrated that the mechanism of failure involved a teasing apart of the collagen fibrin network at the point of rupture while the rest of the collagen network between fissures appeared to be quite normal.[97] There may exist species differences in tolerance for impact loading. In contrast to the preceding human data, the results of Radin et al indicate that strains of only 20% induced severe damage to metatarsophalangeal and metacarpophalangeal joints of rabbits,[98] and studies by Thompson et al showed progressive development of osteoarthritis in dogs after a single impact on the patella of 2170 newtons (N) over 2 milliseconds.[99]

Repetitive impact loading (as opposed to a single traumatic episode) may also be a source of cartilage damage that appears to be different from that sustained in a single massive impact. Lukoschek et al imposed a load of one times body weight in a rabbit knee model and found only mild cartilage changes.[100] Using electron microscopy, Broom has shown that in repetitive loading, the cartilage matrix fibers are "crimped" into a zigzag waveform[31] that contrasts with the massive fissuring seen with a single disruptive blow.

It is apparent that there exists a threshold for single or multiple impacts that articular cartilage can withstand without undergoing significant injury.[31,98,100,101] If the threshold is exceeded, however, cartilage damage ensues. Although such damage may progress to an osteoarthritis-like lesion, a recent study by Radin and co-workers suggests that these lesions may on occasion, be reversible, particularly if the injury is mild.[102]

Response of Articular Cartilage to Superficial Injury. As early as 1743 Hunter stated, "from Hippocrates to the present age it is universally allowed that ulcerated cartilage is a troublesome thing and that, once destroyed, it is not repaired."[6] Since then, scores of studies have been undertaken to define the response of articular cartilage to lacerative injury[1-3,5,7,8,11,12,17,102-108] (Rosenberg L, unpublished data). With few exceptions (eg, Redfern in 1851, who made the observation that "I no longer entertain the slightest doubt that wounds in articular cartilage are capable of perfect union by the formation of fibrous tissue out of the texture of the cut surfaces,"[109] virtually all observers have demonstrated a disappointing inability of articular cartilage to produce sufficient tissue to coapt the margins of a lacerative injury or to repair an ulcerative defect in the cartilage. As noted previously, in injuries confined to the substance of the cartilage of adult animals (not violating the junction of the calcified zone in the underlying bony end plate), the response lacks an inflammatory component because the avascular tissue has no capillary network. The ensuing reaction is independent of extent or depth of the lesion and is characterized by minimal attempts on the part of the cartilage to add cellular and matrix elements. The repair process is almost never effective in healing the defect[104,106,110] (Rosenberg L, unpublished data) (Fig. 2–7).

Several in vivo animal studies have defined the biochemical and cellular characteristics of this response. Immediately after superficial lacerative injury, a relatively intense burst of mitotic activity is noted in the cartilage adjacent to the margins of the defect.[111] This activity is associated with smaller increments in the rates of synthesis of matrix components as measured by incorporation of [^{35}S]sulfate (an indicator of glycosaminoglycan synthesis) and [^{3}H]glycine (an indicator of protein synthesis).[104,110]

The incorporation of isotopically labeled substrate accelerates through the first and second postinjury days, suggesting increments in the rates of matrix synthesis. Even more importantly, cell replication (as measured by [^{3}H]thymidine incorporation) also occurs. This process, unfortunately, is short-lived. By 1 week after trauma, the values have diminished to levels equivalent to those of cartilage samples from sham-operated or normal joints (Fig. 2–8). Such a brief response is clearly not sufficient to be of clinical value. Nevertheless, it indicates that articular cartilage does retain the capacity to mount a reparative response to injury. In terms of cartilage repair these data suggest that what is needed is a means of prolonging or enhancing this innate reparative capacity.

Examination of the degradative side of the metabolic process to trauma has been demonstrated by Thompson et al.[112] The first week after creation of a superficial lacerative lesion, there is an increase in the concentration of cathepsins. β-glucuronidase, hexuronidase and aryl sulfatase. Continued study of the tissue, however,

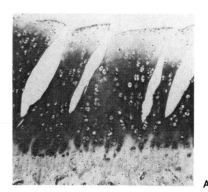

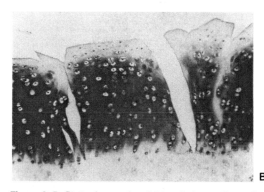

Figure 2–7. Photomicrographs of the articular cartilage of the distal femur of rabbits in which multiple slices were made. The lacerative injuries did not violate the tidemark or calcified zone. A. Appearance of the cartilage shortly after injury. B. The cartilage 1 year later. The failure of healing is readily apparent. Safranin O–fast green–iron hematoxylin; 100x. (Photographs depict the results of an unpublished experiment performed by Lawrence C. Rosenberg, MD. Reprinted with permission of the author and publisher from Mankin.[23])

showed a decline to control values for all enzymes except aryl sulfatase, which became elevated again about 16 weeks postinjury for unknown reasons.

Fuller and Ghadially created tangential partial-thickness defects in the articular cartilage of rabbits, and studied them histologically and by electron microscopy.[106] The results conformed with those of the majority in showing no repair reaction, even in young animals. The ultrastructural studies showed cell death at the margin of the wound and evidence of a heightened metabolic activity in the surviving chondrocytes, presumably directed toward the synthesis of substances necessary for maintaining the integrity of the cartilage. Nucleolar hypertrophy, increased quantities of rough

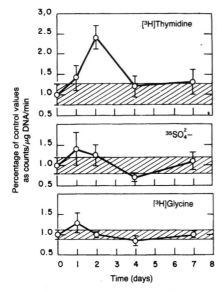

Figure 2-8. Graphic display of rates of incorporation of the labeled substrates: [³H]thymidine (an indicator of DNA synthesis), $^{35}SO_4^{2-}$ (an indicator of glycosaminoglycan synthesis); and [³H]glycine (an indicator of protein synthesis) into lacerated cartilage from rabbits at intervals after the defects had been created. As can be noted, there is a short burst of increased radioactivity at 1 to 2 days, which for thymidine is considerable. The response is short-lived, however, and all values return to normal by 4 days. (Reprinted with permission of author and editor from Mankin and Boyle.[111])

It is apparent from all these data that lacerative injuries that remain superficial (do not penetrate below the tidemark) evoke only a short-lived metabolic and enzymatic response which fails to provide sufficient numbers of new cells or matrix to repair even the simple defect created by a scalpel blade. Of further interest is the evidence that has been presented that these lesions persist as defects for at least a year and do not necessarily lead to an osteoarthritis type of degenerative process. This concept has some clinical relevance in that superficial lesions caused by trauma or surgical procedures may be considered to be of little consequence. Thus, although the long-term effects of such injuries are not known, there is reason to speculate, on the basis of the studies just described, that they are generally limited in expression and do not lead to clinical degenerative joint disease.

Response of Articular Cartilage to Full-Thickness, Penetrating Injury.

Injuries that violate the subchondral bone differ markedly from either blunt or superficial lacerative trauma in bringing to the repair process the multiple cell types and blood plasma constituents available in bone marrow. It has been demonstrated by several investigators that a deep defect almost immediately fills with blood.[10,103] The hematoma becomes organized into a fibrin clot in which are trapped red blood cells, white cells, bone marrow elements, and platelets. Progenitor cell populations multiply and lay down a bed of vascular fibroblastic tissue[23,104,111] (Fig. 2-9). The

endoplasmic reticulum, and occasionally an increased number of Golgi complexes were noted after injury, but by 6 months the defect remained, and save for some remodeling of the surface, all healing processes had ceased.[106]

Longer-term follow-up of superficial lacerative injuries has demonstrated no further attempt at healing over time, but of some interest, little evidence for progression to osteoarthritis. In 1963, Meachim described a "scarification" model in the rabbit knee, in which multiple superficial cuts were made into the articular cartilage.[113] Instead of progressing, as expected, to degenerative joint disease, these lesions remained stable and only occasionally found evidence for early osteoarthritic change[112,113] (Rosenberg L. Unpublished data). Rosenberg performed such a study and used routine histology and safranin-O staining (as a histochemical indicator of proteoglycan concentration) to observe the cartilage over time. At the end of 1 year he found the lacerative defects in the cartilage essentially unaltered. Not only was there little attempt at repair, but there was no indication of conversion of the lesions to those of chondromalacia or osteoarthritis.

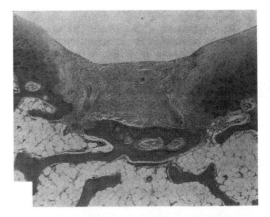

Figure 2-9. Low-power photomicrograph of the distal femoral cartilage in mature dog a short time after a "deep coring lesion" has been created. The defect has filled with fibrous tissue and shows early evidence of chondrification. Hematoxylin and eosin; 100×. (This photograph represents a study performed by Crawford Campbell, MD, who graciously consented to publication of this figure.)

fibrous tissue undergoes progressive hyalinization, becoming chondrified to produce a fibrocartilaginous mass. At the base of the lesion, in the region in contact with the injured bone, active new bone formation occurs and extends toward the joint. For reasons not yet well understood, bone formation generally stops at the margin of the old cartilage–bone junction, leaving the remaining defect to fill in with the aforementioned fibrocartilage[3,104,114] (Rosenberg L. Unpublished data). (Fig. 2–10).

At the margin of such defects, the hyaline cartilage that survived the injury undergoes a response essentially identical to that seen in the superficial lacerative injuries.[111] There is a brief burst of synthetic activity in this cartilage, but it is only sufficient to replace some of the cells and matrix destroyed by the initial wound. Although it has been suggested that the gliding zone of the old hyaline cartilage on either side of this defect slides tangentially to resurface the now filled-in deep injury,[3] there is little evidence supporting this process or its contribution to healing.

The ultimate fate of the newly formed fibrocartilaginous tissue is, of course, of considerable interest. Mitchell and Shepherd demonstrated in a rabbit articular defect model that, in the early course of repair, the primary fibrous reparative tissue was converted to a chondroid tissue which showed evidence of mitotic activity and histochemical staining consistent with the presence of a high concentration of proteoglycan.[115] Cheung et al, in a similar model, have shown that this reparative tissue appropriately contains type II collagen, consistent with the formation of true hyaline cartilage[116]; however, in Mitchell and Shepherd's studies, by 12 months postinjury the cartilaginous nature of the material was less obvious and it appeared more fibrous. The surface layer cells were more typical of fibrocartilage than of hyaline cartilage, and the tangential collagen orientation (the "skin") failed to appear. The surface became fibrillated and the subjacent matrix remained densely collagenous. Nevertheless, the site of the deep defect remained filled with a cartilage-like material and, as nearly as could be determined, function remained unimpaired. This experience paralleled those of others who have indicated that the site of an old "deep" laceration or defect may be clearly visible years after injury as a slightly discolored, roughened pit or linear groove on the otherwise smooth and quite normal surface of the adjacent hyaline articular cartilage.[1,2,8,80]

Nelson et al performed a biomechanical analysis of full-thickness osteochondral defects in adult dogs, a model in which the repair process follows a pattern remarkably similar to that described before in the rabbit. These authors found that the repair tissue was of poor mechanical quality and did not contribute appreciably to weight bearing. On the other hand, the cartilage

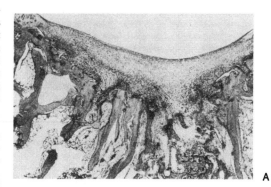

A

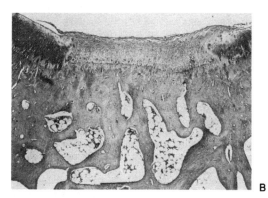

B

Figure 2–10. Low-power photomicrographs of the distal femora of two rabbits, in both of which a deep coring defect was created. A. The early response and exuberant fibroblast proliferation extend from the vascular bone in the base of the cartilage and firmly weld the cartilaginous surfaces together. Hematoxylin and eosin; 100×. B. The subsequent course is illustrated: the defect has filled in with a hyaline-like cartilage that stains poorly with Safranin-O, but nonetheless closely resembles the original cartilaginous surface. The tissue is somewhat irregular in its surface layers and shows evidence of early degeneration. Safranin-O–fast green–iron hematoxylin; 100x. (Photographs represent studies performed by Dr. Lawrence C. Rosenberg who graciously consented to the publication of these figures.)

adjacent to the defect did not experience unduly high stresses, and neither gross nor light microscopic evidence of degeneration had appeared by 11 months postinjury.[117]

Convery and associates reported an experiment in which large osteochondral defects created in the distal femora of horses were followed over time.[114] The repair of these defects generally followed the same process just described, but was in part dependent on the size of the lesions. Defects smaller than 3 mm in diameter showed complete repair after 3 months and were difficult to locate after 9 months. None of the defects 9 mm or larger showed complete repair. The repair tissue for all lesions was a variable mixture of fibrous tissue, fibrocartilage, hypercellular hyaline-like cartilage, and an occasional island in which the clots served as a framework for fibroblast proliferation, vascular invasion, and subsequent remodeling to mature scar.[114]

Implications for Repair

It is apparent from the pathophysiology of articular cartilage healing that there are two problems that hold some relevance to clinical joint disease. The first is the failure of intraarticular cartilage injuries to heal. If these could somehow be stimulated to heal, it is possible that some joint injuries could be effectively treated and, of considerable potential significance, that chondromalacia and early osteoarthritis could be ameliorated. The nonprogressive lesion created by a slice in the cartilaginous surface is of little consequence, but the progressive focal destruction, loss of proteoglycan, and fibrillation associated with early osteoarthritis are clearly of much clinical concern.

The second problem is the deep injury to cartilage. Here the difficulty lies not with repair, which is ordinarily exuberant and rapid, but with the nature of the material that ultimately fills the defect. Although this material tends to become cartilaginous, it remains more or less fibrous and does not attain the character of true hyaline articular cartilage.

In the first circumstance, efforts to achieve improved repair must address the replicative and synthetic capabilities of the articular chondrocytes themselves. In the second circumstance, multiple cell types are available and the problem is one of effectively inducing these cells to form the correct composite of cartilage proteoglycans, collagen, and other matrix constituents that make up normal articular cartilage.

If the available cells are not capable of accomplishing adequate repair, then the alternative approach of introducing new cell populations with the correct matrix structure already in place or with the capability of forming such a matrix may be required.

Approaches to the Problem of Cartilage Healing

Debridement

Before the advent of reliable joint replacement arthroplasty for degenerative joint disease, debridement was an accepted form of treatment. The technique described by Magnuson was designed to remove all irritative material from within the joint, including any abnormal synovium, osteophytes, and softened fibrillated cartilage, as well as degenerated menisci.[118] The technique

was modified by Pridie to include drilling of bone.[119] This type of operation approximated the surgical technique designed to produce repair tissue in the experimental models cited above. Although the clinical results of the procedure employed by Pridie were reported by Insall to be pleasing to the patient in 77% of 62 knees, he also found that function was improved to a lesser degree and noted that at least four of these patients required subsequent fusion.[120] The procedure fell out of favor with improvements in joint replacement arthroplasty.

Joint debridement for degenerative changes again became popular with the refinement of the arthroscope, an advance that has permitted easy access to the articular cartilage. Experience with the technique of "shaving" the roughened cartilage surfaces has led some clinicians to the opinion that, contrary to prior experimental evidence, such surgery leads to "healing" of defects,[121] whereas skeptics consider it possible that other aspects of the procedure may improve the symptoms of the patient but, in fact, have little or no effect on the cartilage surface.[122] It is important in this regard to distinguish articular cartilage shaving (debridement) from abrasion "arthroplasty" (burring or drilling into vascularized subchondral bone). The former is analogous to the earlier described superficial cartilage injury and would not be expected to be followed by cartilage healing. The latter is a form of deep injury and could, in some circumstances (see later), lead to some degree of reparative activity. As noted earlier, however, such repair is suboptimal and further investigation will be required to develop methods of improving the repair process.

Continuous Passive Motion

Prolonged immobilization of a joint has long been recognized to be deleterious to articular cartilage.[123–125] To test the hypothesis that motion may be beneficial, Salter and co-workers created coring defects through the underlying bone in the distal femora of rabbits and treated the animals in one of three ways: by plaster immobilization, by cage ambulation (obviously limiting), or by continuous passive motion (achieved by placing the rabbits in an assembly in which the firmly held extremities were passively flexed and extended at a slow rate).[126] After 4 weeks the animals were sacrificed and the cartilage defects studied. In the animals subjected to continuous passive motion (CPM), the tissue appeared by histologic and histochemical staining to more closely approximate hyaline cartilage than fibrocartilage. These data suggest that CPM materially enhances the healing of cartilage defects. A subsequent study by Palmosky and co-workers has shown that motion of the limb without weight bearing alters the chemical structure of normal rabbit articular cartilage by depleting proteoglycan, increasing water, and diminishing synthetic activity.[127] These data would seem inconsistent with Salter's theory but it is possible that the injured and uninjured surfaces behave differently in their response to passive motion.

Shimizu et al analyzed the dose–response characteristics of CPM in a rabbit knee full-thickness defect model. They found that 8 or 24 hours of CPM per day was effective in achieving cartilage repair but that only 2 hours per day was not much better than immobilization. In all instances CPM was initiated immediately after injury, and it is of some interest that delaying CPM for a week diminished its effectiveness.[128]

Electrical Stimulation

A study by Baker and co-workers introduced the possibility that an electrical field could enhance the repair of deep defects in articular cartilage.[129] Coring defects were created in the distal femora of rabbits and an electrode was placed in the bone beneath the defect through a channel created in the shaft of the bone (thus not transversing the normal cartilage on the defect). In those animals in which electrical fields were established (as compared with controls in which no electrodes were placed or controls in which the electrodes were placed but not activated), accelerated healing of the defect was noted and histologic study showed hyaline cartilage filling the gap.

Using cartilage cells in culture, Rodan et al have shown that these cells respond to oscillating electric fields by increasing their rate of DNA synthesis,[130] and Norton has documented a variety of metabolic responses, including an increase in hyaluronate and DNA, a decrease in glycosaminoglycan, and an increase in lysozyme activity.[131] Using growth plate chondrocytes as a model for cartilage responsiveness to electrical stimulation, Brighton et al have shown that exposure to electrical fields for as short a period as 3.6 minutes per 24 hours is sufficient to induce cartilage cell proliferation.[132] Despite these advances, it continues to be unclear what characteristics of the electrical signal are responsible for the stimulation or by what mechanism the signal induces its metabolic effects.

Grafting of Cartilage Defects

Tissue Grafts. Partly in response to the difficulties inherent in eliciting satisfactory cartilage repair from the cells and tissue within the injured joint, considerable attention has been turned to the use of exogenous sources of cells for repair. Long recognized to have chondrogenic potential, perichondrium has recently emerged as a popular source of tissue for filling cartilage defects.[133] Using the full-thickness rabbit knee defect model, multiple investigators have reported that

application of rib perichondrium to these defects is followed by filling with hyaline-like cartilage.[134-137]

Perichondrial grafts have now been used for several years to treat human arthritis, principally in the joints of the hand,[138,139] but results have been variable.[138,139] Seradge and colleagues reported a minimum 3-year follow-up of 36 perichondrial resurfacing arthroplasties in metacarpophalangeal and proximal interphalangeal joints. In metacarpophalangeal arthroplasties, 100% of patients in their twenties and 75% of patients in their thirties had good results; however, no good results were recorded for patients over 40 years of age.[139] Application of this technique to large joints is even more limited, but a case report from Hvid and Andersen indicates that it can be successful in the treatment of chondromalacia patella.[140]

Periosteum, like perichondrium, has chondrogenic potential, and has been similarly employed for repair of deep cartilage defects.[141-147] Rubak created full-thickness defects in the articular cartilage of rabbit patellar grooves, covered some with a periosteal graft, and left others open. Defects into which periosteum had been transplanted filled with hyaline-like cartilage by 4 weeks and retained this morphology for up to 1 year.[144] When Rubak et al interposed a filter between the periosteal graft and the cartilage defect, the repair cells were seen to arise from the graft rather than from the bone.[145] In support of these results, Zarnett et al showed, by prelabeling the graft with [³H]thymidine, that the repair tissue is derived from the cells of the periosteal graft.[147]

The durability of the periosteally regenerated tissue has been further investigated by O'Driscoll and associates.[141] After grafting, rabbits were treated by either immobilization in a cast, intermittent active motion in a cage, or 2 weeks of CPM. At 1-year follow-up, degenerative changes had occurred in 57% of immobilized knees, 73% of rabbits treated by intermittent active motion, and 22% of those treated with CPM. The beneficial effect of passive motion was statistically significant. In contrast, Woo et al, using perichondrial autografts in a similar model, analyzed the biomechanical characteristics of the repair tissue and found that although CPM applied intermittently for 2 weeks enhanced the magnitude of the shear moduli of the neocartilage, the difference between CPM and controls disappeared at longer periods.[137]

Cell Grafts. In a closely related approach to articular cartilage defect repair, isolated cells, often derived from articular cartilage, have been employed as a source of repair tissue.[148-152] The application, and perhaps effectiveness, of this technique is limited by the problem of localizing and retaining isolated cells within the cartilage defect. Grande et al, using a rabbit knee model, addressed this problem by injecting isolated articular chondrocytes into defects over which a periosteal flap had been sutured. Healing in the presence of cells and periosteum was 82%, but with periosteum alone was only 18%. Defects not covered by periosteum or treated with cells had a 16.5% healing rate.[151] These results appear to contrast with reports that periosteum alone induces defect repair, but such differences in results may reflect variations in experimental technique or design.

Glycosaminoglycans

Considerable enthusiasm has recently arisen, particularly in equine veterinary medicine, for treating joint disease with various forms of connective tissue glycosaminoglycan. Pursuing early evidence that hyaluronic acid ameliorates the symptoms of arthritis in horses,[153,154] Rose administered sodium hyaluronate to 16 horses, all of whom were clinically lame. Selection of the involved joint for injection was determined by pain on motion of the joint, distension and thickening of the joint capsule, and relief of pain and lameness after intraarticular local anesthesia. Animals with chip fractures or advanced degenerative joint disease (joint space narrowing and osteophyte production) were excluded. All animals improved following sodium hyaluronate injection and 11 continued to be sound 3 months posttreatment.[155] The mechanism of action of sodium hyaluronate remains to be fully elucidated; however, its clinical benefit appears to result more from an anti-inflammatory effect on the synovium than from a true reparative effect on the articular cartilage (Morris E. Unpublished data).

Related glycosaminoglycans have also been investigated in animal models of osteoarthritis. Glycosaminoglycan polysulfuric acid ester (GAGPS) was administered by Altman et al to dogs with surgically induced instability of the knee, an animal model for osteoarthritis. GAGPS was administered intraarticularly two times per week for 4 weeks and the joints compared with similar animals treated only with saline. The authors found that GAGPS decreased the levels of active and latent collagenase in the cartilage and increased uronic acid and hydroxyproline levels.[156] Using the same model, Howell and colleagues also reported an increase in the number of chondrocytes in the articular cartilage of treated animals.[157] In a study of horses suffering from joint disease, Tew found that the glycosaminoglycan polysulfate ester L1016 reduced the quantity of cartilage debris in the synovial fluid. The 18 horses that completed the course of nine injections over 6 weeks showed a decrease in total amount of debris from a mean of 72 mm³ prior to treatment to 21 mm³ after treatment.[158] The rate of this improvement in synovial fluid and in clinical improvement varied considerably between animals, occurring after as little as 2 weeks of treatment in some animals, but requiring as much as 6

weeks in others.[158] Although these studies do not formally document articular cartilage healing in response to glycosaminoglycans or their derivatives, they are compelling in their argument that this approach to osteoarthritis holds promise and warrants further investigation.

A first step toward such investigation has recently been taken by Raatikainen et al.[159] These investigators performed a placebo-controlled randomized study of the glycosaminoglycan polysulfate Arteperon (Luitpold, Munich) in the treatment of chondromalacia patellae. Thirty-one patients with patellofemoral pain and arthroscopically confirmed patellar cartilage lesions without other joint pathology were randomized to either 12 injections of glycosaminoglycan polysulfate given intramuscularly twice a week for 6 weeks or physiologic saline injections given according to the same schedule. Twenty-six patients were available for rearthroscopy at 1-year follow-up. According to both clinical and arthroscopic parameters, the treatment group improved to a greater degree than the placebo group. Visualized articular cartilage damage at 1 year in the treatment group was worse in eight patients, unchanged in five, and improved in eight. In the placebo group, damage was worse in three, unchanged in seven, and improved in three patients. The mechanism underlying this observed effect remains unknown. Although this investigation is of limited size and duration, its results are optimistic in suggesting that enhancement of articular cartilage repair is clinically feasible.

Cartilage repair may also be governed by matrix molecules that are endogenous in articular cartilage. It has recently been suggested that two forms of dermatan sulfate proteoglycans, DSPG I or biglycan and DSPG II or decorin, may be involved in the inhibition of tissue repair.[58] These proteoglycans bind to the surface of collagen fibrils, inhibiting collagen fiber formation[160,161]; they bind to the linkage molecule fibronectin, thereby interfering with cell adhesion[162]; and they bind to the cell regulatory peptide TGF-β, inhibiting its mitogenic effect.[163] The presence of DSPGs in articular cartilage may help explain why lesions in this tissue fail to heal.[58] Thus, it appears that certain matrix constituents may have to be removed to achieve effective cartilage repair.

Growth Factors

Perhaps the most recently explored approach to articular cartilage healing is the use of low-molecular-weight peptides known as growth factors. Efforts to understand how cell multiplication and differentiation are regulated led cell biologists to the discovery that growth factors often serve as the messengers that instruct cells to engage in a particular behavior (eg, division). These messenger molecules bind to specific receptors on the surface membrane of their target cells. This messenger–

receptor interaction initiates a complex series of intracellular events leading to the cell response. Growth factors may stimulate not only cell proliferation but differentiated activities including, in the case of chondrocytes, matrix synthesis. Although many of the known growth factors were named for their ability to stimulate a particular cell type (eg, fibroblast growth factor [FGF]), their discovery in a specific tissue (eg, platelet-derived growth factor [PDGF]), or their initially investigated activity (eg, insulin-like growth factor [IGF]), most of them are now known to influence a broad distribution of target cells and to induce a variety of cellular effects. Cartilage is a known target tissue for many of these peptides, including FGF,[164–167] TGF-β,[158] IGF-I,[165,170–175] PDGF,[166,167] and epidermal growth factor (EGF),[165–167] among others.[165,167] With the exception of TGF-β, whose effects appear to be highly situation specific, virtually all of the effects of these growth factors on cartilage have been anabolic. For this reason it has been speculated that these factors may be capable of stimulating articular cartilage repair.

Using rabbit articular chondrocytes in monolayer culture, Prinz et al tested the ability of PDGF, EGF, and FGF to influence both DNA synthesis and matrix synthesis.[166,167] PDGF, FGF, and EGF each stimulated [³H]thymidine incorporation into DNA and [³⁵S]sulfate uptake into matrix glycosaminoglycans, whereas insulin stimulated matrix but not DNA synthesis. Osborn et al tested the responsiveness of adult articular cartilage in organ culture, a system in which chondrocytes are retained in situ within their matrix.[165] These authors demonstrated that insulin, EGF, FGF, and low concentrations of IGF-I stimulated matrix synthesis as reflected in [³⁵S]sulfate incorporation. In contrast, of these four factors, only FGF, used individually, enhanced [³H]thymidine incorporation into DNA. Interestingly, when used in concert, certain of these factors generated additive or synergistic stimulation. IGF-I enhanced the [³⁵S]sulfate stimulation of EGF and FGF in an additive fashion. Insulin and EGF, though having no effect on [³H]thymidine incorporation when used individually, markedly stimulated DNA synthesis when used in concert. A similar synergistic effect on [³H]thymidine was also generated by insulin and FGF (Fig 2–11).

It is evident from these data and the results of multiple other studies[164,169,172,173] that growth factors augment the cellular activities required for repair in articular chondrocytes, at least in vitro.

The capacity of growth factors to induce articular cartilage repair in vivo has to date been investigated principally with the basic form of FGF (bFGF). Using FGF purified from bovine brain (a standard source of native bFGF), Wellmitz et al were able to enhance repair of intrachondral (not penetrating subchondral bone) cartilage defects in rabbit knees.[176] By measuring the cartilage cell types constituting the repair tissue, these

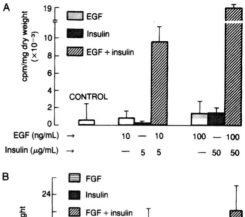

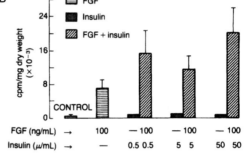

Figure 2–11. A. Effect on [³H]thymidine incorporation of EGF and insulin acting individually and in combination on adult bovine articular cartilage in organ culture. The vertical bars indicate isotope incorporation per milligram weight of lyophilized cartilage. The numbers beneath the bars indicate the dose of each growth factor. Neither EGF nor insulin used alone is significantly stimulatory. In combination, their effect is synergistic, with stimulation at both high doses ($P < 0.0055$) and low doses ($P < 0.001$). **B.** Effect on [³H]thymidine incorporation of FGF and insulin acting individually and in combination. The stimulatory effect of FGF is enhanced by the addition of insulin, although insulin alone produces no effect at any dose tested. The effect of insulin (50 μg/ml) and FGF is greater than the effect of FGF alone ($p < 0.005$). (Reprinted with permission from Osborn et al.[165])

authors also demonstrated that the effect of FGF, compared with saline treatment (control), was to increase the number of chondrocyte clones or "clusters," but not the number of cells per clone or the number of individual hypertrophic or degenerative chondrocytes. Cuevas et al recently reported on the use of bacterially produced (recombinant) bFGF in an intrachondral rabbit knee defect model of articular cartilage damage.[177] At 20 days following surgery, healing of the defects was observed in the FGF-treated animals, but not in saline-treated controls.

All of these experimental studies are, from a clinical perspective, quite preliminary and an ability to effectively intervene in cases of articular cartilage failure is not yet within our grasp. The data clearly demonstrate, however, that articular cartilage is capable of responding positively to both exogenous and endogenous stimuli. Through pursuit of research problems suggested by these leads, it is possible that in the future our understanding of cartilage physiology and pathophysiology will be sufficient to improve our treatment of cartilage injury and disease.

Acknowledgments. The authors thank Mrs. Brenda White for expert assistance in preparing the manuscript. Research for this chapter was supported in part by USPHS Grant AR-31068.

References

1. Bennett GA, Bauer W. Further studies concerning the repair of articular cartilage in dog joints. *J Bone Joint Surg.* 1935;17:141.
2. Bennett GA, Bauer W, Maddock SJ. A study of the repair of articular cartIlage and the reaction of normal joints of adult dogs to surgically created defects of articular cartilage, "joint mice" and patellar replacement. *Am J Pathol.* 1932;8:499.
3. Calandruccio RA, Gilmer WS Jr. Proliferation, regeneration and repair of articular cartilage of immature animals. *J Bone Joint Surg Am.* 1962;44:431.
4. Geis T. Histologische und experimentelle studien uber gelenkkrankheiten IV. Uber hellung von knorpelwuden. *Dtsch Z Chir.* 1882;18:2.
5. Haebler C. Experimentelle untersuchungen uber die regeneration des gelenkknorpels. *Beitr Klin Tuberk.* 1925;134:602.
6. Hunter W. On the structure and diseases of articulating cartilage. *Philos Trans R Soc Lond.* 1743;42:514–521.
7. Ito LK. The nutrition of articular cartilage and its method of repair. *Br J Surg.* 1924;12:31.
8. Key JA. Experimental arthritis: The changes in joints produced by creating defects in the artIcular cartilage. *J Bone Joint Surg.* 1931;13:725.
9. Kuettner KE, Eisenstein R, Sorgente N. Lysozyme in calcifying tissues. *Clin Orthop.* 1975;112:316.
10. Meachim G, Roberts C. Repair of the joint surface from subarticular tissue in the rabbit knee. *J Anat.* 1971; 109:317.
11. Paget J. Healing of cartilage. *Lect Surg Pathol (Lond).* 1853;1:263.
12. Shands AR Jr. The regeneration of hyaline cartilage in joints: An experimental study. *Arch Surg.* 1931;22:137.
13. Simon SR. Biomechanics of joints. In: Kelly WN, Harris ED, Ruddy S, Sledge CB, eds. *Textbook of Rheumatology.* Philadelphia: WB Saunders; 1981:194.
14. Harris ED Jr, Parker MG, Radin EL, Krane SM. Effects of proteolytic enzymes on structural and mechanIcal properties of cartilage. *Arthritis Rheum.* 1972;15:497.
15. Kempson GE. Mechanial properties of articular cartilage. In: Freeman MAR, ed. *Adult Articular Cartilage.* New York: Grune & Stratton; 1977:196.
16. Kempson GE, Muir H, Pollard C, Tuke M. The tensile properties of the cartilage of human femoral condyles related to the content of collagen and glycosaminoglycans. *Biochim Biophys Acta.* 1973;297:456.
17. Meachim G. Effect of age on thickness of adult articular cartilage at the shoulder joint. *Ann Rheum Dis.* 1971;30:43.
18. Simon W. Scale effects in animal joints. I. Articular cartilage thickness and compressive stress. *Arthritis Rheum.* 1970;12:244.
19. Redler I, Zimny ML. A scanning electron microscopic study of human, normal and osteoarthritic articular cartilage. *Clin Orthop.* 1974;102:262.
20. Clark IC. Articular cartilage: A review and scanning electron microscopic study. I. The interterritorial fibrillar architecture. *J Bone Joint Surg Br.* 1971;53:732.
21. Clark IC. Articular cartilage: A review and scanning electrong microscopic study. II. The territorial fibrillar architecture. *J Anat.* 1974;118:261.
22. Barnett CH, Davies DV, MacConnaill MA. *Synovial Joints: Their Structure and Mechanics.* Springfield, IL: Charles C Thomas; 1961.
23. Mankin HJ. The reaction of articular cartilage to injury and osteoarthritis. *N Engl J Med.* 1974;291:1285.
24. Stockwell RA, Meachim G. The chondrocytes. In: Freeman MAR, ed. *Adult Articular Cartilage.* New York: Grune & Stratton; 1973.
25. McKibben B, Holdsworth FS. The nutrition of immature joint cartilage in the lamb. *J Bone Joint Surg Br.* 1966;48:793.
26. Hamerman D, Schubert M. Diarthrodial joints, an essay. *Am J Med.* 1962;33:555.
27. Green WT Jr, Martin GN, Evans ED, Sokoloff L. Microradiographic study of the calcIfied layer of articular cartilage. *Arch Pathol.* 1970;90:151.
28. Repo RU, Mitchell N. Collagen synthesis in mature articular cartilage of the rabbit. *J Bone Joint Surg Br.* 1971;53:541.
29. Benninghoff A. Form und bau der gelenkknorpel in ihren beziehungen zur funktion, zweiter teil: Der aufbau des gelenknorpels in seinen beziehungen zur funktion. *Z Zellforsch Mikrosk Anat.* 1925;2:183.
30. Broom ND. Further insights into the structural principles governing the function of articular cartilage. *J Anat.* 1984;139:275.
31. Broom ND. Structural consequences of traumatizing articular cartilage. *Ann Rheum Dis.* 1986;45:225.
32. Bullough P, Goodfellow J. The significance of th fine structure of articular cartilage. *J Bone Joint Surg Br.* 1968;50:852.
33. Meachim G, Denham D, Emery IH, Wilkinson PM. Collagen alignments and articular splits at the surface of human articular cartilage. *J Anat.* 1974;118:101.
34. Mow VC, Lai WM, Eisenfeld J, Redler I. Some surface characteristics of articular cartilage. II. On the stability of articular surface and a possible biomechanical factor in etiology of chondro-degradation. *J Biomech.* 1974; 7:457.
35. Speer DP, Dahners L. The collagenous architecture of articular cartilage. Correlation of scanning electron microscopy and polarized light microscopy observations. *Clin Orthop.* 1979;139:267.
36. Weiss C. Ultrastructural characteristics of osteoarthritis. *Fed Am Soc Exp Biol.* 1973;32:1459.
37. Weiss C, Rosenberg L, Helfet AL. An ultrastructural study of normal young adult human articular cartilage. *J Bone Joint Surg Am.* 1968;50:663.
38. Poole CA, Flint MH, Beaumont BW. Chondrons in cartilage. Ultrastructural analysis of the pericellular microenvironment in adult human articular cartilage. *J Orthop Res.* 1987;5:509.

39. Muir H, Hardingham TE. Structure of proteoglycans. In: Whelan WJ, ed. *MIP International Review of Science: Biochemistry Series One*. Vol. 5: *Biochemistry of Carbohydrates*. Baltimore: University Park Press; 1975.
40. Lindahl O. Ueber den wassergehalt des knorpels. *Acta Orthop Scand*. 1958;17:134.
41. Mankin HJ, Thrasher AZ. Water content and binding in normal osteoarthritic human cartilage. *J Bone Joint Surg Am*. 1975;57:76.
42. Miles JS, Eichelberger J. Biochemical studies of human cartilage during the aging process. *J Am Geriatr Soc*. 1964;12:1.
42. Lane JM, Weiss C. Current comment: Review of articular cartilage collagen research. *Arthritis Rheum*. 1975; 18:553.
44. Miller EJ. A review of biochemical studies in the genetically distinct collagens of the skeletal system. *Clin Orthop*. 1973;92:260.
45. Miller EJ, Matukas VJ. Chick cartilage collagen: A new type of alpha I chain not present in bone or skin of the species. *Proc Natl Acad Sci USA*. 1969;64:1264.
46. Miller EJ, Vanderkorst JK, Sokoloff L. Collagen of human and costal cartilage. *Arthritis Rheum*. 1969;12:21.
47. Mayne R. Cartilage collagens. What is their function and are they involved in articular disease? *Arthritis Rheum*. 1989;32:241.
48. Eyre DR, et el. Collagen type IX: Evidence for covalent linkage to type II collagen in cartilage. *FEBS Lett*. 1987;220:337.
49. Konomi H, Seyer JM, Ninomiya Y, Olsen BR. Peptide-specific antibodies identify the α2 chain as the proteoglycan subunit of type IX collagen. *J Biol Chem*. 1986;261:6792.
50. Wu JJ, Eyre BR. Cartilage type XI collagen is cross-linked by hydroxypyridinium residues. *Biochem Blophys Res Commun*. 1984;123:1033–1039.
51. Muir IHM. Biochemistry. In: Freeman MAR, ed. *Adult Articular Cartilage*. 2nd ed. Kent: Pitman; 1973.
52. Rosenberg L. Structure of cartilage proteoglycan. In: Burleigh PMC, Poole AR, eds. *Dynamics of Connective Tissue Macromolecules*. New York: American Elsevler; 1975.
53. Hardingham TE, Muir H. Hyaluronic acid in cartilage. *Biochem Soc Trans*. 1973;1:282.
54. Doege KJ, Sasaki M, Kimura T, Yamada Y. Complete coding sequence and deduced primary structure of the human cartilage large aggregating proteoglycan aggrecan. *J Biol Chem*. 1991;266:894–902.
55. Rosenberg L, Hellman W, Kleinschmidt AK. Electron microscopic studies of proteoglycan aggregates from bovine articular cartilage. *J Biol Chem*. 1975;250:1877.
56. Mankin HJ, Lippiello L. The glycosaminoglycans of normal and arthritic cartilage. *J Clin Invest*. 1971;50:1712.
57. Bianco P, Fisher LW, Young MF, Termine JD, Robey PG. Expression and localization of two small proteoglycans, byglycan and decorin, in developing human skeletal and non-skeletal tissues. *J Histochem Cytochem*. 1990;38:1549–1563.
58. Rosenberg LC. Structure and function of dermatan sulfate proteoglycans in articular cartilage. In: Kuettner K, et al, eds. *Articular Cartilage and Osteoarthritis*. New York: Raven Press; 1992:45–63.
59. Bonner WM, Jonsson H, Malanos C, Bryant M. Changes in the lipids of human articular cartilage with age. *Arthritis Rheum*. 1975;18:461.
60. Fife RS, Palmoski MJ, Brandt KD. Metabolism of a car-

tilage matrix glycoprotein in normal and osteoarthritic canine articular cartilage. *Arthritis Rheum*. 1986;29:1256.
61. Heinegard D, Oldberg A. Structure and biology of cartilage and bone matrix non-collagenous macromolecules. *FASEB J*. 1989;3:2042.
62. Jones KL, Brown M, Ali SY, Brown RA. An immunohistochemical study of fibronectin in human osteoarthritic and disease free articular cartilage. *Ann Rheum Dis*. 1987;46:809.
63. Wurster NB, Lust G. Synthesis of fibronectin in normal and osteoarthritic articular cartilage. *Biochim Biophys Acta*. 1984;800:52.
64. Anderson RS, Schwartz ER. Phosphorylation of proteoglycans from human articular cartilage. *Arthritis Rheum*. 1984;27:58.
65. Benya PD, Padill SR, Nimni ME. Independent regulation of collagen types by chondrocytes during the loss of differentiated function in culture. *Cell*. 1978;15:1313.
66. Benya PD, Shaffer JD. Dedifferentiated chondrocytes reexpress the differentiated collagen phenotype when cultured in agarose gels. *Cell*. 1982;30:215.
67. Goldring MB, et al. Interleukin-I suppresses expression of cartilage-specific types II and IX collagens and increases types I and III collagens in human chondrocytes. *J Clin Invest*. 1988;82:2026.
68. Goldring MB, Sandell LJ, Stephenson ML, Krane SM. Immune interferon suppresses levels of procollagen in RNA and type II collagen synthesis in cultured human articular and costal chondrocytes. *J Biol Chem*. 1986;261:9049.
69. Trippel SB, Ehrlich MG, Lippiello L, Mankin HJ. Characterization of chondrocytes from bovine articular cartilage. I. Metabolic and morphological experimental studies. *J Bone Joint Surg Am*. 1980;62:816.
70. Mankin HJ, The metabolism of articular cartilage in health and disease. In: Burleigh PMC, Poole AR, eds. *Dynamics of Connective Tissue Macromolecules*. New York: American Elsevler: 1975.
71. Mankin HJ, Lippiello L. The turnover of adult rabbit articular cartilage. *J Bone Joint Surg Am*. 1969;51:1591.
72. Roden L, Schwartz NB. Biosynthesis of connective tissue proteoglycans. In: Whelan WJ, ed. *MIP International Review of Science, Biochemistry, Series One*. Vol 5: *Biochemistry of Carbohydrates*. Baltimore: University Park Press; 1975.
73. Sandy JD, Plaas AMK. Age-related changes in the kinetics of release of proteoglycans from normal rabbit cartilage explants. *J Orthop Res*. 1986;4:263.
74. Lippiello L, Hall D, Mankin HJ. Collagen synthesis in normal and osteoarthritic human cartilage. *J Clin Invest*. 1977;59:593.
75. Ali SY. The degradation of cartilage matrix by an intracellular protease. *Biochem J*. 1964;93:611.
76. Ehrlich MG, Armstrong AL, Treadwell BV, Mankin HJ. Degradatlve enzyme systems in cartilage. *Clin Orthop*. 1986;213:62.
77. Sapolsky AI, Altman RD, Woessner JF Jr, Howell DS. The action of cathepsin D in human articular cartilage. *J Clin Invest*. 1973;52:624.
78. Sapolsky AI, Howell DS, Woessner JF Jr. Neutral proteinases and cathepsin D in human articular cartilage. *J Clin Invest*. 1974;53:1044.
79. Ehrlich MG, et al. Collagenase and collagenase inhibitors in osteoarthritic and normal human cartilage. *J Clin Invest*. 1977;59:226.
80. Campbell IK, et al. Recombinant human interleukin-I

stimulates human articular cartilage to undergo resorption and human chondrocytes to produce both tissue- and urokinase-type plasminogen activator. *Biochim Biophys Acta.* 1988;967:183.
81. Martel-Pelletier J, et al. Neutral proteases capable of proteoglycan digestion activity in osteoarthritic and normal human articular cartilage. *Arthritis Rheum.* 1984;27:305.
82. Meats JE, et al. Enhanced production of prostaglandins and plasminogen activator during activation of human articular chondrocytes by products of mononuclear cells. *Rheumatol Int.* 1984;4:143.
83. Stephenson ML, et al. Stimulation of procollagenase synthesis parallels increases in cellular procollagenase mRNA in human articular chondrocytes exposed to recombinant interleukin-I beta on phorbol ester. *Biochem Biophys Res Commun.* 1987;144:583.
84. Dodge GR, Poole AR. Immunohistochemical detection and immunochemical analysis of type II collagen degradation in human normal rheumatological and osteoarthritic articular cartilages and in explants of bovine articular cartilage culture with interleukin-I. *J Clin Invest.* 1989;83:627.
85. Gunja-Smith Z, Nagase H, Woessner JF Jr. Purification of the neutral proteoglycan degrading metalloproteinase from human articular cartilage tissue and its identification as stromelysin matrix metalloproteinase-3. *Biochem J.* 1989;258:115.
86. Cruwys SC, Davies DE, Pettipher ER. Cooperation between interleukin-I and the fibrinolytic system in the degradation of collagen by articular chondrocytes. *Br J Pharmacol.* 1990;100:631–635.
87. Werb Z, Mainardi CL, Vater CA, Harris ED Jr. Endogenous activation of latent collagenase by rheumatoid synovial cells. Evidence for a role of plasminogen activator. *N Engl J Med.* 1977;296:1017–1023.
88. Treadwell BV, Pavia M, Towle CA, Cooley VJ, Mankin HJ. Cartilage synthesizes the serine protease inhibitor PAI-I: Support for the involvement of serine proteases in cartilage remodeling. *J Orthop Res* 1991;9:309–316.
89. Bunning RAD, Russell RGG. The effect of tumor necrosis factor alpha and gamma interferon on the resorption of human articular cartilage and on the production of prostaglandin R and of caseinase activity by human articular chondrocytes. *Arthritis Rheum.* 1989;32:780.
90. Treadwell BV, et al. Stimulation of the synthesis of collagenase activator protein in cartilage by a factor present in synovial conditioned medium. *Arch Biochem Biophys.* 1986;251:724.
91. Frisch SM, Ruley HE. Transcription from the stromelysin promotor is induced by interleukin-I and repressed by dexamethasone. *J Biol Chem.* 1987;262:16302.
92. Chandrasekhar S, Harvey AK. Transforming growth factor-β is a potent inhibitor of IL-I induced protease activity and cartilage proteoglycan degradation. *Biochem Biophys Res Commun.* 1988;157:1352–1359.
93. Saklatvala J. Tumour necrosis factor alpha stimulates resorption and inhibits synthesis of proteoglycan in cartilage. *Nature* 1986;322:547.
94. Mankin HJ. Localization of tritiated thymidine in articular cartilage of rabbits. I. Growth in immature cartilage. *J Bone Joint Surg Am.* 1962;44:682.
95. Mankin HJ. The calcified zone (base layer) of articular cartilage of rabbits. *Anat Rec.* 1963;145:73.
96. Mankin HJ. Localization of tritiated thymidine in articular cartilage of rabbits. III. Mature articular cartilage. *J Bone Joint Surg Am.* 1963;45:526.

97. Repo RV, Finlay JB. Survival of articular cartilage after controlled impact. *J Bone Joint Surg Am.* 1977;59:1068.
98. Radin EL, Paul IL, Lowy M. A comparison of the dynamic force transmitting properties of subchondral bone and articular cartilage. *J Bone Joint Surg Am.* 1970; 52:444.
99. Thompson RC Jr, Oegema TR, Lewis JL, Wallace L. Osteoarthritic changes after acute transarticular load. *J Bone Joint Surg Am.* 1991;73:990–1001.
100. Lukoschek M, et al. Comparisons of joint degeneration models. Surgical instability and repetitive impulse loading. *Acta Orthop Scand.* 1986;57:349.
101. Afoke NYP, Byers PD, Hutton WC. Contact pressures in the human hip joint. *J Bone Joint Surg Br.* 1987;69:536.
102. Radin EL, et al. Effect of repetitive impulsive loading on the knee joint of rabbits. *Clin Orthop.* 1978;131:288.
103. Campbell CJ. The healing of cartilage defects. *Clin Orthop.* 1969;64:45.
104. DePalma AF, McKeever CD, Subin DK. Process of repair of articular cartilage demonstrated by histology and autoradiography and tritiated thymidine. *Clin Orthop.* 1966;48:229.
105. Fisher T. Some researches into the physiological principles underlying the treatment of injuries and diseases of the articulations. *Lancet.* 1923;2:541.
106. Fuller JA, Ghadially FN. Ultrastructural observations on surgically produced partial-thickness defects in articular cartilage. *Clin Orthop.* 1972;86:193.
107. Landells JW. The reactions of injured human articular cartilage. *J Bone Joint Surg Br.* 1957;39:548.
108. Puhl W, Dustmann HO, Quasdorf U. Tierexperimentelle untersuchungen zur regeneration des gelenkknorpels. *Arch Orthop Unfallchir.* 1973;74:352.
109. Redfern P. On the healing of wounds in articular cartilages, and on the removal of these structures after amputations at the joints, with remarks on the relation which exists between the diseases of cartilage and ulceration and inflammation in other textures. *Month J Med Soc.* 1852;13:201.
110. Mankin HJ, Boyle HC. The acute effects Gf lacerative injury on DNA and protein synthesis in articular cartilage. In: Bassett CAL, ed. *Cartilage Degradation and Repair.* Washington, DC: National Academy of Sciences, National Research Council; 1967.
111. Mankin HJ. Localization of tritiated thymidine in articular cartilage of rabbits. II. Repair in immature cartilage. *J Bone Joint Surg.* 1962;44:688.
112. Thompson RC Jr. An experimental study of surface injury to articular cartilage and enzyme responses within the joint. *Clin Orthop.* 1975;107:239.
113. Meachim G. The effect of scarification on articular cartilage in the rabbit. *J Bone Joint Surg.* 1963;45:150.
114. Convery FR, Akeson WK, Krown GH. The repair of large osteochondral defects in experimental study of horses. *Clin Orthop.* 1972;82:253.
115. Mitchell N, Shepard N. The resurfacing of adult rabbit articular cartilage by multiple perforations through the subchondral bone. *J Bone Joint Surg Am.* 1976;58:230.
116. Cheung HS, Lynch KL, Johnson RP, Brewer JP. *In vitro* synthesis of tissue specific type II collagen by healing cartilage. I. Short-term repair of cartilage by mature rabbits. *Arthritis Rheum.* 1980;23:211.
117. Nelson BH, Anderson DD, Brand RA, Brown TD. Effect of osteochondral defects on articular cartilage. Contact pressures studied in dog knees. *Acta Orthop Scand.* 1988;59:574.

118. Magnusen PB. Joint debridement. Surgical treatment of degenerative arthritis. *Surg Gynecol Obstet.* 1941;73:1.
119. Pridie KH. A method of resurfacing osteoarthritic knee joints. *J Bone Joint Surg Br.* 1959;41:618.
120. Insall JN. Intra-articular surgery for degenerative arthritis of the knee. A report of the work of late K. H. Pridie. *J Bone Joint Surg Br.* 1967;49:211.
121. Johnson LL. Arthroscopic abrasion arthroplasty historical and pathologic perspective: Present status. *Arthroscopy.* 1986;2:54.
122. Dandy DJ. Abrasion chondroplasty. *Arthroscopy.* 1986;2:51.
123. Evans EB, Eggers GWN, Butler JK, Blumel J. Experimental immobilization and remobilization of rat knee joints. *J Bone Joint Surg Am.* 1960;42:737.
124. Langenskiold A, Michelsson J-E, Videman T. Osteoarthritis of the knee in the rabbit produced by immobilization. *Acta Orthop Scand.* 1979;50:1.
125. Palmoskey MJ, Perrlone E, Brandt KD. Development and reversal of a proteoglycan aggregation defect in normal canine knee cartilage after immobilization. *Arthritis Rheum.* 1979;22:508.
126. Salter RB, et al. The effect of continuous passive motion on the healings of articular cartilage defects. *J Bone Joint Surg Am.* 1975;57:570.
127. Palmosky MJ, Coyler RA, Brandt KD. Joint motion in the absence of normal loading does not maintain normal articular cartilage. *Arthritis Rheum.* 1980;23:325.
128. Shimizu T, Videman T, Shimazaki K, Mooney V. Experimental study on the repair of full-thickness articular cartilage defects: Effects of varying periods of continuous passive motion, cage activity, and immobilization. *J Orthop Res.* 1987;5:187.
129. Baker B, Becker RO, Spadaro J. A study of electrochemical enhancement of articular cartilage repair. *Clin Orthop.* 1974;102:251.
130. Rodan GA, Bourret LA, Norton LA. DNA synthesis in cartilage cells is stimulated by oscillating electric fields. *Science.* 1978;199:690.
131. Norton LA. Effect of a pulsed electromagnetic field on a mixed chondroblastic tissue culture. *Clin Orthop.* 1982;167:280.
132. Brighton CT, et al. Proliferative and synthetic response of bovine growth plate chondrocytes to various capacitively coupled eletrical fields. *J Orthop Res.* 1989;7:759.
133. Tizzoni G. Sulla istologia normale e patholgisa delle cartilagini ialine. *Arch Sci Med.* 1978;2:27.
134. Engkvist O, Johansson SH, Ohlsen K, Skoog T. Reconstruction of articular cartilage using autologous perichondrial grafts. *Scand J Plast Reconstr Surg.* 1975; 9:203.
135. Engkvist O, Wilander E. Formation of cartilage from rib perichondrium grafted to an articular defect in the femur condyle of the rabbit. *Scand J Plast Reconstr Surg.* 1979;13:371.
136. Skoog T, Ohlsen L, Sohn SA. Perichondrial potential for cartilaginous regeneration. *Scand J Plast Reconstr Surg.* 1972;6:123.
137. Woo SL-Y, et al. Perichondrial autograft for articular cartilage. Shear modulus of neocartilage studied in rabbits. *Acta Orthop Scand.* 1987;58:510.
138. Engkvist O, Johansson SH. Perichondrial arthroplasty. A clinical study in twenty-six patients. *Scand J Plast Reconstr Surg.* 1980;14:71.
139. Seradge H, et al. Perichondral resurfacing arthroplasty in the hand. *J Hand Surg [Am].* 1984;9:880.
140. Hvid I, Andersen LI. Perichondrial autograft in traumatic chondromalacia patellae. *Acta Orthop Scand.* 1981;52:91.
141. Niedermann B, et al. Glued periosteal grafts in the knee. *Acta Orthop Scand.* 1985;56:457.
142. O'Driscoll SW, Keeley FW, Salter RB. Durability of regenerated articular cartilage produced by free autogenous periosteal grafts in major full-thickness defects in continuous passive motion. A follow-up report at one year. *J Bone Joint Surg Am.* 1988;70:595.
143. O'Driscoll SW, Salter RB. The induction of neochondrogenesis in free intra-articular periosteal autografts under the influence of continuous passive motion. An experimental investigation in the rabbit. *J Bone Joint Surg Am.* 1984;66:1248.
144. Rubak JM. Reconstruction of articular cartilage defects with free periosteal grafts. An experimental study. *Acta Orthsp Scand.* 1982;53:175.
145. Rubak JM, Poussa M, Ritsila V. Chondrogenesis in repair of articular cartilage defects by free periosteal grafts in rabbits. *Acta Orthop Scand.* 1982;53:181.
146. Rubak JM, Poussa M, Ritsila V. Effects of joint motion on the repair of articular cartilage with free periosteal grafts. *Acta Orthop Scand.* 1982;53:187.
147. Zarnett R, Delaney JP, O'Driscoll SW, Salter RB. Cellular origin and evolution of neochondrogenesis in major full-thickness defects of a joint surface treated by free autogenous periosteal grafts and subjected to continuous passive motion in rabbits. *Clin Orthop.* 1987;222:267.
148. Bentley G, Green R. Homotransplantation of isolated epiphyseal and articular chondrocytes into joint surfaces of rabbits. *Nature* 1971;230:385.
149. Bentley G, Smith AV, Mukerjhee R. Isolated epiphyseal chondrocytes allografts into joint surfaces. An experimental study in rabbits. *Ann Rheum Dis.* 1978;37:449.
150. Chesterman PJ, Smith AV. Homotransplantation of articular cartilage and isolated chondrocytes. An experimental model in rabbits. *J Bone Joint Surg Br.* 1968;50:184.
151. Grande DA, Singh IJ, Pugh J. Healing of experimentally produced lesions in articular cartilage following chondrocyte transplantation. *Anat Rec.* 1987;218:142.
152. Green WT Jr. Articular cartilage repair: Behavior of rabbit chondrocytes during tissue culture and subsequent grafting. *Clin Orthop.* 1977;124:237.
153. Asheim A, Lindblad G. Intra-articular treatment of arthritis in race horses with sodium hyaluronate. *Acta Vet Scand.* 1976;17:379.
154. Rydell NW, Butler J, Balays EA. Hyaluronic acid in synovial fluid. VI. Effect of intra-articular injection of hyaluronic acid on the clinical symptoms of arthritis in track horses. *Acta Vet Scand.* 1970;11:139.
155. Rose RJ. The intra-articular use of sodium hyaluronate for the treatment of osteoarthritis in the horse. *N Z Vet J.* 1979;27:5.
156. Altman RD, Dean DD, Muniz OE, Howell DS. Prophylactic treatment of canine osteoarthritis with glycosaminoglycan polysulfuric acid ester. *Arthritis Rheum.* 1989;32:759.
157. Howell DS, Muniz OE, Carreno MR. Effect of glycosaminoglycan polysulfate ester on proteoglycan-degrading enzyme activity in an animal model of osteoarthritis. *Adv Inflam Res.* 1986;11:197.
158. Tew WP. Demonstration by synovial fluid analysis of the efficacy in horses of an investigational drug (L-1016). *J Equine Vet Sci.* 1982;2:42.

159. Raatikainen T, Vaananen K, Tamelander G. Effect of glycosaminoglycan polysulfate on chondromalacia patellae. A placebo-controlled one year study. *Acta Orthop Scand*. 1990;61:443–448.
160. Scott JE. Proteoglycan–fibrillar collagen interactions. *Biochem J*. 1988;252:313–323.
161. Vogel KG, Trotter JA. The effect of proteoglycans on the morphology of collagen fibrils formed in vitro. *Collagen Relat Res*. 1987;7:105–114.
162. Lewandowska K, Choi HU, Rosenberg LC, Zardi L, Culp LA. Fibronectin-mediated adhesion of fibroblasts: Inhibition by dermatan sulfate proteoglycan and evidence for a cryptic glycosaminoglycan-binding domain. *J Cell Biol*. 1987;1105:1443–1454.
163. Yamaguchi Y, Mann DM, Ruoslahti E. Negative regulation of transforming growth factor-β by the proteoglycan decorin. *Nature*. 1990;346:281–284.
164. Jones KL, Addison J. Pituitary fibroblast growth factor as a stimulator of growth in cultured rabbit articular chondrocytes. *Endocrinology*. 1975;97:359
165. Osborn KO, Trippel SB, Mankin HJ. Growth factor stimulation of adult articular cartilage. *J Orthop Res*. 1989;7:35.
166. Prins APA, Lipman JM, McDevitt CA, Sokoloff L. Effect of purified growth factors on rabbit articular chondrocytes in monolayer culture. II. Sulfated proteoglycan synthesis. *Arthritis Rheum*. 1982;25:1228.
167. Prins APA, Lipman JM, Sokoloff L. Effect of purified growth factors on rabbit articular chondrocytes in monolayer cultures. I. DNA synthesis. *Arthritis Rheum*. 1982;25:1217.
168. Sachs BL, Goldberg VM, Moskowitz RW, Malemud CJ. Response of articular chondrocytes to pituitary fibroblast growth factor (FGF). *J Cell Physiol* 1982;112:51.
169. Morales TI, Roberts AB. Transforming growth factor beta regulates the metabolism of proteoglycans in bovine cartilage organ cultures. *J Biol Chem*. 1988;263:12828.
170. Hill DJ, et al. Increased thymidine Incorporation into fetal rat cartilage *in vitro* in the presence of human somatomedin, epidermal growth factor and other growth factors. *J Endocrinol*. 1983;96:489.
171. Luyten FP, et al. Insulin-like growth factors maintain steady-state metabolism of proteoglycans in bovine articular cartilage explants. *Arch Biochem Biophys*. 1988;267:416.
172. McQuillan DJ, et al. Stimulation of proteoglycan biosynthesis by serum an insulin-like growth factor I in cultured bovlne articular cartilage. *Biochem J*. 1986;240:423.
173. Trippel SB, et al. Effect of somatomedin C/insulin-like growth factor and growth hormone on cultured growth plate and articular chondrocytes. *Pediatr Res*. 1989;25:76.
174. Trippel SB, VanWyk JJ, Foster MB, Svoboda ME. Characterization of a specific somatomedin-C receptor on isolated bovine growth plate chondrocytes. *Endocrinology*. 1983;112:2128.
175. Watanabe N, et al. Characterization of a specific insulin-like growth factor/somatomedin-C (IGF/SM-C) receptor on high density primary monolayer cultures of bovine articular chondrocytes: Regulation of receptor concentration by somatomedin, insulin and growth hormone. *J Endocrinol*. 1985;107:275.
176. Welellmitz G, et al. A bovine brain fraction with fibroblast growth factor activity inducing articular cartilage regeneration *in vivo*. *Acta Biol Med Germ*. 1980;39:967.
177. Cuevas P, Burgos J, Baird A. Basic fibroblast growth factor (FGF) promotes cartilage repair *in vivo*. *Biochem Biophys Res Commun*. 1988;156:611.

3

Osteochondral and Chondral Fractures of the Knee

David D. Bullek and Michael A. Kelly

Introduction

Acute knee injuries resulting in locking hemarthrosis or knee instability are not necessarily the result of meniscal or ligamentous injury. Fractures of the articular surface of the knee have been reported to occur in approximately 10% of acute traumatic hemarthrosis.[1-8] Meniscal and ligamentous injuries have readily lent themselves to repair or resection. Articular cartilage lesions are quite the opposite, with satisfactory surgical outcomes less reliably achieved. Early diagnosis and treatment are necessary to avoid early arthritis in the involved compartment and loose-body formation.

Osteochondral and chondral injuries are due primarily to rotational or direct blow trauma.[3] Osteochondral fractures are usually diagnosed by careful physical and radiologic examination because of the underlying bony component. Pure chondral lesions are much more difficult to diagnose. The physical examination of a patient with a chondral lesion can be quite unimpressive. Hemarthrosis may not occur when subchondral bone is not violated. Early symptoms of both chondral and osteochondral fractures can often be obscure in that the immediate disability is slight but there may be progression to a significant chronic disability.[9]

Although chondral and osteochondral lesions may present in similar fashion, chondral lesions are quite different and must be considered separately. Pure chondral injuries usually occur in the skeletally mature patient, whereas osteochondral fractures are more common in the adolescent.[10] It is postulated that this occurs because of force transmission differences in mature cartilage. Articular cartilage changes with age; the basilar layer calcifies as we exit adolescence. This basilar layer, the "tidemark," separates calcified from noncalcified cartilage. It creates a stress riser and is the line of fracture cleavage with shear stress in the adult. The adult therefore sustains a chondral fracture.[11-14] Adolescents have very little calcified cartilage. Shearing forces are transmitted along the subchondral bone in these young patients, resulting in an osteochondral fracture.

Osteochondral fractures are due primarily to patellar subluxation or dislocation.[1,14] The mechanism of the injury is shearing of the inferomedial patella against the lateral femoral condyle on reduction of a patellar dislocation (Fig. 3-1). Reduction force is usually due to a strong quadriceps contraction. This results in a fracture of the patella or lateral femoral condyle in approximately 5% of cases.[15]

Matthewson and Dandy also noted lateral femoral condyle osteochondral injuries secondary to shear forces of the lateral femoral condyle and the lateral tibial plateau as the knee pivots in extension[16] (Fig. 3-2). Osteochondral fractures elsewhere are rare except for direct blow injuries.

The incidence of pure chondral lesions is unknown. Johnson-Nurse and Dandy found chondral lesions in older patients on the weight-bearing surface of the medial femoral condyle[10] (Fig. 3-3). They concluded these injuries to be secondary to shearing while pivoting on an extended knee. Terry found a high incidence of posterior medial femoral condyle chondral fractures that mimic meniscal tears and could be easily missed on arthroscopic examination if the knee was not flexed adequately.[17] He noted the posterior location to correspond to an injury with the knee flexed. Bauer and Jackson, in their review of 167 patients with chondral fractures, found that these fractures occur predominantly on weight-bearing surfaces in the medial compartment of the knee.[3]

Several classification systems for chondral lesion have been set forth. Bauer and Jackson classified chondral

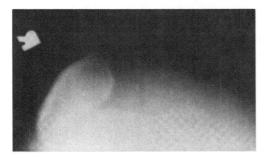

Figure 3–1. Patellar dislocation may cause an osteochondral fracture of the patella or lateral femoral condyle. Merchant view.

lesions by appearance[3] (Fig. 3–4). They identified six groups and remarked on their location and mechanism of injury. A type I (linear crack-type) lesion is a crack of variable depth in the articular surface usually found in a weight-bearing area and thought to be caused by a shearing force. A type II (stellate fracture-type) lesion is a system of diverging cracks with a central flaking of cartilage. These lesions were noted primarily in weight-bearing areas and thought to result predominantly from direct trauma. Type II lesions were the most common lesions seen. The type III (flap-type) lesion is a flap of articular cartilage with an attached base. These were predominant in weight-bearing areas and seen in pivot injuries in competitive athletes. Type IV (crater-type) lesions consist of a full-thickness defect of cartilage. These lesions are usually found in weight-bearing areas and are associated with loose bodies. Type V (fibrillation-type) lesions are characterized by fine fibrillations of the cartilage surface, are usually partial-thickness, and are found most frequently on the lateral femoral condyle in weight-bearing areas. This type is thought to represent early degenerative arthritis. Type VI (degrading-type) are frayed, soft cartilage found in weight-bearing areas. Posteromedial changes are often associated with posterior horn tears or the medial meniscus and represent localized arthrosis.

Although Bauer and Jackson's classification is a superb descriptive categorization, location and size are not taken into account. Dzioba put forth a classification in 1988 that categorized lesions by age, size, depth, and location[18] (Table 3–1). This classification includes both osteochondral and chondral lesions. Dzioba found that younger patients with small, partial-thickness lesions had the best prognosis. Noyes and Stable[19] put forth a classification system that categorized chondral lesions by surface description, extent of involvement, size, location, and degree of knee flexion in weight bearing. This is the most complete classification to date (Table 3–2).

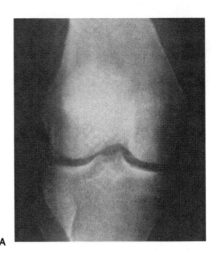

A

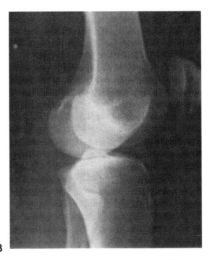

B

Figure 3–2. Anteroposterior (**A**) and lateral (**B**) x-rays of a small osteochondral fracture of the lateral femoral condyle in a young ballet dancer.

Information on chondral lesions, including diagnosis, treatment, and prognosis, is in a process of change. The clinical usefulness of an elaborate classification is sometimes cumbersome but the information gained by use of specific classification in future prospective investigations will better clarify the natural history of these lesions. These gains will assist the clinicians in more successful management of these patients in the future.

Chondral and osteochondral fractures are important but often overlooked clinical entities. The purpose of

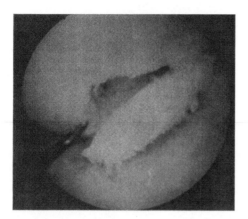

Figure 3–3. Flap-type chondral lesion of the medial femoral condyle. (Reprinted with permission from Scott WN, ed. *Arthroscopy of the Knee.* Philadelphia: WB Saunders; 1990.)

Table 3–1. Classification of Acute Articular Cartilage Lesions

Age of lesion
  Acute: treated within 3 weeks
  Acute or chronic: previously treated
  Chronic: prolonged history
Size of lesion
  Small: < 1 cm
  Medium: 1–3 cm
  Large: > 3 cm
Depth of lesion
  1. Superficial (an arthroscopic scrape)
  2. Partial thickness: separation of the tidemark
  3. Full thickness: to subchondral plate
  4. Osteochondral
Local of lesion
  1. Weight-bearing femoral condyle
  2. Submeniscal, tibial
  3. Intercondylar, non-weight bearing

Data taken from Dzioba.[15]

this chapter is to review the clinical presentation, objective evaluation, and operative management of chondral and osteochondral fractures in the knee. Successful evaluation and treatment of traumatic injury to articular cartilage require a basic understanding of articular cartilage anatomy, function, and response to injury.

Basic Science

Hunter, in 1743, noted that "cartilage once destroyed is not repaired."[20] The ability of articular cartilage to re-

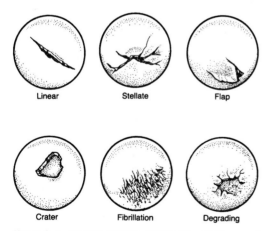

Figure 3–4. Articular cartilage classification of Bauer and Jackson. (Adapted with permission from Scott WN, ed. *Ligament and Extensor Mechanism Injuries of the Knee.* St. Louis: Mosby Year Book; 1991.)

spond to injury has been continuously investigated since that time. The majority of these studies demonstrate that cartilage is repaired under certain conditions, but typically, the repair tissue lacks the composition, the material properties, and the durability of normal articular cartilage. Similarly, the quantity and quality of this repair tissue following a specific cartilage injury cannot be reliably predicted.

Articular cartilage does not respond to injury with an inflammatory response because of its avascular nature. The effect of injury on matrix composition and structure is critical to the normal function of articular cartilage. Mechanical injures related to the cartilage layer elicit a different response and result than injuries extending to the subchondral bone that trigger an inflammatory and vascular response. The location, volume, and surface area of such an injury may also influence the repair process.[21] Most recent evidence indicates that chondrocytes respond to injuries related to the cartilage by proliferating and increasing their synthetic activity[22]; however, typically they fail to restore a normal matrix even if the lesion or defect is small. This repair response may also decrease with age as the cell numerical density and the capacity of the cells to respond to injury decrease.[22]

Injuries to the knee may extend through articular cartilage into the underlying subchondral bone. When a full-thickness articular cartilage defect is created, marrow cells capable of an inflammatory response have access to the defect. Some full-thickness defects may undergo repair during the first 2 months following injury even without treatment.[22] Although this repair tissue may give the appearance of normal articular cartilage, the composition of this tissue is not identical. Often the integrity of these reparative tissue is not maintained with the gradual development of tissue fibrillation and degenerative changes. Examination of

Table 3–2. New Classification Articular Cartilage Lesions

Surface description	Extent of involvement	Diameter (mm)	Location	Degree of knee flexion
1. Cartilage surface intact	A. Definite softening with some resilience remaining	<10 ≤15 ≤20	Patella A. Proximal 1/3 Middle 1/3 Distal 1/3	Degree of flexion where the lesion is in weight-bearing contact (eg, 20–45°)
	B. Extensive softening with loss of resilience (deformation)	≤25 >25	B. Odd facet Middle facet Lateral facet	
2. Cartilage surface damaged: cracks, fissures, fibrillation, or fragmentation	A. <Half thickness B. ≥Half thickness		Trochlea Medial femoral condyle A. anterior 1/3 B. middle 1/3 C. posterior 1/3	
3. Bone exposed	A. Bone surface intact B. Bone surface cavitation		Lateral femoral condyle A. anterior 1/3 B. middle 1/3 C. posterior 1/3 Medial tibial condyle A. anterior 1/3 B. middle 1/3 C. posterior 1/3 Lateral tibial condyle A. anterior 1/3 B. middle 1/3 C. posterior 1/3	

Data taken from Noyes and Stabler.[50]

the repair matrix demonstrates that the cells do not differentiate into normal chondrocyte.[22] The extracellular matrix of normal articular cartilage contains type II collagen and a high concentration of cartilage-type proteoglycans and does not contain type I collagen.[22] In contrast, the repair tissue formed in full-thickness defects contains large amounts of type I collagen and a lower concentration of proteoglycans, despite the close resemblance of this tissue to articular cartilage histologically.

The differences between the repair of injuries restricted to articular cartilage and those extending into subchondral bone raise the possibility that bone matrix may contain growth and differentiation factors governing cartilage and bone formation that may have a critical role in cartilage repair.[22] An injury penetrating subchondral bone may release these factors, whereas those injuries restricted to articular cartilage will not. The significance of such a response may vary with lesion size.[23]

The mechanical properties of cartilage repair tissue require additional investigation. Work by Whipple and co-workers evaluating the biphasic material properties of repair cartilage suggests that repair cartilage was more permeable and less stiff than normal articular cartilage.[24] A number of methods of promoting cartilage repair or chondrogenesis have been and are currently under investigation. These techniques include laser stimulation of chondrocytes, matrix proteoglycans, or stimulating factors and the use of periosteal and perichondrial grafts.[22,25–28] Currently recognized techniques to promote cartilage repair consist of perforation or abrasion of the exposed subchondral bone, initial protection of the tissue from excessive load with no or limited weight bearing, and often continuous passive knee joint motion (CPM). The perforation or abrasion of the subchondral bone elicits the repair process, including formation of fibrin clot and vascular invasion of the repair tissue.[29,30] Mitchell and Shepard demonstrated in rabbits that areas of articular cartilage can be repaired by multiple perforations into subchondral bone.[31] The repair tissue grows from the holes and spreads over the surface. The tissue appears to become more fibrous over time with a tendency to fibrillation and breakdown. DePalma and associates noted that early range of motion and weight bearing provided a beneficial result on repair of full-thickness cartilage defects.[32] Investigations of the effects of continuous passive motion on articular cartilage were reported by Salter and co-workers.[33] They noted no benefit of CPM on lesions restricted to the cartilage surface; however, in defects 1 mm in diameter that penetrated the subchondral bone, CPM improved repair and produced a hyaline-like tissue.[33] The effect of CPM on defects of larger dimensions such as those seen in human osteochondral injuries is difficult to predict.

History and Physical

Typically, the patient with an osteochondral fracture presents after an acute injury to the knee from a twisting valgus or varus injury or direct blow. The patient may report a history of patellar subluxation or dislocation. Rorabeck and Bobechko reported that osteochondral fractures complicate 5% of all acute dislocations of the patella.[15] Occasionally, the patient may report an audible "crack" at the time of injury along with sudden onset of pain and immediate swelling. Acutely, the symptoms mimic those of a meniscal tear: joint line pain and tenderness, popping or crepitus with motion, and locking. In those patients with patellar dislocation, medial retinacular pain and positive apprehension sign are common. Pain usually precludes weight bearing. The effusion, unlike those with meniscal tears, occurs immediately; fluid on aspiration is bloody and may be laden with fat globules. The finding of fat globules is an important clue to the clinician to the presence of an osteochondral fracture. Physical examination may also show associated ligamentous or meniscal injury. Noyes and Bassett demonstrated a significant association between anterior cruciate ligament (ACL) tears, meniscal tears, and osteochondral fractures.[7] Patients presenting after acute symptoms resolve reveal quadriceps atrophy, recurrent effusions, popping, clicking, and occasional locking. This symptom complex is common to all patients with loose bodies regardless of their etiology.

Pure chondral injuries have a different presentation. Usually they do not have an acute hemarthrosis because the fracture does not extend to vascular subchondral bone. Acute hemarthrosis can accompany chondral fractures associated with ligament tears. Late presentation of chondral injury presents in similarly to loose body in the knee as discussed earlier. Multiple authors have emphasized the difficulty in initial diagnosis of these articular cartilage injuries. Morscher attributed a low diagnostic accuracy to a history of apparently insignificant trauma, failure of the clinician to appreciate the seriousness of a hemarthrosis in an adolescent, and failure to obtain adequate radiographic examination.[34] He noted misdiagnosis to be more frequent in the group with pure chondral lesions from direct trauma than in the patient groups with osteochondral lesions resulting from patellar subluxation or dislocation.

Radiography

Diagnosis of osteochondral and chondral fractures of the knee requires the clinician to maintain a high index of suspicion. Standard radiographs are usually inadequate to fully evaluate a patient suspected of an articular cartilage injury. Osteochondral fractures in the adolescent may only show a small fleck of bone that may seem innocuous but can grossly underestimate the true size of the chondral fragment (see Fig. 3–2). Chondral injury in the adult will not be evident on plain radiographs. DeHaven found the incidence of osteochondral fracture when the osseous component is not visible on radiographs to be 6% of all hemarthroses evaluated.[35]

At our institution routine radiographic evaluation of acute knee injury includes standing anteroposterior (AP), lateral, and patellar axial views. The patellar axial view we prefer is a modified Merchant view. In our experience, this patellar view is useful in localizing osteochondral fractures. Most of the osteochondral fractures seen at our institution originate either from the lateral femoral condyle or from the medial facet of the patella. Tunnel views are helpful in the diagnosis of lesions in the intercondylar notch. We found the tunnel view to be more useful in those patients with suspected osteochondritis dissecans. Oblique views may occasionally be indicated in suspected cases.

Arthrography, both single and double contrast, has been used in the past to evaluate both osteochondral and chondral lesions. Single-contrast arthrography uses water-soluble iodinated contrast media to help view intraarticular structures. Double-contrast arthrography uses carbon dioxide gas combined with contrast media for better resolution.[36] Large fragments are localized, but accuracy in detecting small fragments is limited by both methods. Both single-contrast and double-contrast arthrography are limited because of their invasive nature. Single-contrast arthrography is also limited by impaired visualization of the fragment by the contrast material used. Double-contrast arthrography using gas has been reported to produce high false-positive interpretations as a result of gas bubbles.[37] Although arthrography is useful in the evaluation of osteochondral fractures, the advent of magnetic resonance imaging (MRI) has greatly enhanced its present role in diagnostic imaging.

Computerized Axial Tomography (CATSCAN) and MRI have been used extensively in the detection of intraarticular pathology of the knee. CATSCAN can detect bony lesions as small as 3 mm, especially with intraarticular injection of contrast material, but pure chondral lesions are difficult to detect. MRI has supplanted other modalities in the evaluation of osteochondral and chondral fractures.[38] MRI of hemarthroses and osteochondral fractures show fat, with a high signal on T1, rising to the highest point of the effusion, and an articular cartilage defect.[39] Mink and Deutsch have shown that these fractures are easily missed on routine MRI.[40] Multiple techniques for delineation of articular cartilage by MRI are currently being investigated. Fast scan gradient echo techniques show cartilage with a high signal intensity. Gradient echo imaging distinguishes articular cartilage most easily from subchondral bone and adjacent fluid. Heron and Calvert noted "perfect" correlation between arthroscopic examination and gradient image MRI techniques for grades II and III articular cartilage changes.[41] The injection of intraarticular fluid or Gd-DTPA allows detection of lesions as small as 2 to 3

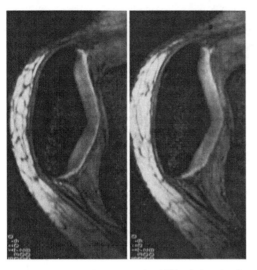

Figure 3-5. Hyaline fat suppression MRI technique to show articular cartilage. (Courtesy of Dr. Alejandro Gonzalez Sosa and Dr. Donald Resnick.)

mm. Intraarticular fluid serves to enhance contrast difference between cartilage and joint cavity.[42] A technique referred to as fat suppression MRI has been reported to have excellent resolution of cartilage lesions. Chandnani and co-workers reported that spin-echo fat suppression imaging was superior to both conventional spin-echo and magnetic resonance arthrography in the evaluation of articular cartilage.[43] Hadler and co-workers concurred with these conclusions and remarked on this technique's simplicity and accuracy.[44] Most recently, Tl-weighted hybrid fat suppression sequence MRI has been reported to be superior to all other types of fat suppression imaging.[45] Ho and co-workers found that hybrid fat suppression imaging clearly demonstrated gross anatomic findings of hyaline cartilage thinning, surface irregularity, and focal defects in a study of goat knees.[46] An example of this technique on a human patella is shown in Figure 3-5. Fat suppression magnetic resonance shows articular cartilage as a high-intensity signal. The accuracy of MRI in the detection of hyaline cartilage defects is increasing rapidly. Clinically useful techniques in the immediate future will surely expand our diagnostic accuracy. Despite advances in radiographic technique, arthroscopy remains the "gold standard" for the detection of osteochondral and chondral fractures. Clinical suspicion, especially in the acute knee injury with hemarthrosis, should encourage an aggressive approach to detect and treat injuries to the articular cartilage.

Treatment

Arthroscopy is the mainstay of diagnosis and treatment in both osteochondral and chondral fractures. Complete arthroscopic examination is necessary when an articular surface injury is suspected. Multiple portals and the use of a 70° arthroscope are helpful in the evaluation of the suprapatellar, posteromedial, and posterolateral compartments. The treatment of osteochondral and chondral fractures differs significantly and is discussed separately.

Osteochondral Fractures

Once the diagnosis of an osteochondral fracture has been established, surgical treatment is required. A loose fragment will cause mechanical symptoms and may lead to further injury to the articular cartilage. Treatment depends on the time since injury and the location and size of fracture. Initially, a decision must be made on whether to replace the fragment into its bed. A small or fragmented piece should be excised. Scott advised removal of smaller fragments in non-weight-bearing areas and repair of fractures greater than 25% of a joint surface (Fig. 3-6).

The acute fracture is best suited for repair. With the passage of time the bed fills with fibrous or fibrocartilaginous tissue and the fragment rounds as a result of mechanical abrasion. Multiple authors found 2 weeks to be the time limit for replacement of an osteochondral fracture.[9,11,16,47] At our institution we evaluate the fit of the fragment after removal of soft tissue and make our decision based on arthroscopic examination. We concur that after several weeks it is more difficult to replace the fragment.

The location of the fragment and the skill of the arthroscopist determine whether the fragment can be replaced by an open or arthroscopic technique. Osteochondral fractures originating from the undersurface of the patella or posterior condyles are quite difficult to replace arthroscopically and usually require an open technique.

Multiple methods of fixation have been advised for fixation of osteochondral fragments: smooth wires, screws, bone pegs, Herbert compression screws, biodegradable pins, and fibrin adhesive substance. The success of any internal fixation device depends on secure fixation of the fragment to the underlying bone. There are advantages and disadvantages to each method. Obviously, screws provide better fixation than smooth pins. Pins also tend to migrate but can be used in smaller fragments. Any metallic device must be removed prior to the beginning of weight bearing. Absorbable devices do not require removal but the strength of fixation is unknown.

The reported results on all of the aforementioned

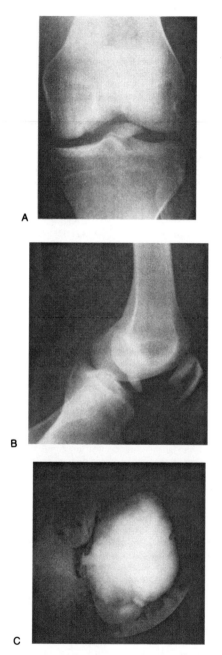

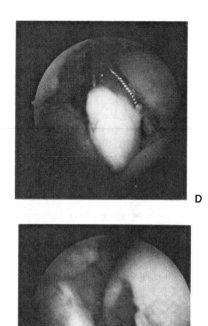

Figure 3–6. Osteochondral loose body from medial femoral condyle, shown on anteroposterior (**A**) and lateral (**B**) radiographs. Arthroscopic view (**C**) is shown with removal by grasper (**D**). Defect remains after removal of loose body (**E**).

fixation devices are good but usually documented on small patient populations. Cortical bone pegs have been used successfully by several authors, but on a small number of patients.[48,49] Our experience is limited with this technique and we refer the reader to the referenced work for guidance.

Arthroscopic cannulated screw fixation was reported by Johnson in 1984.[50] Although fixation is quite good, the screw must be removed prior to initiation of weight bearing. There have been several reports of success with the use of the Herbert compression screw in the fixation of large osteochondral fragments and osteochondritis dissecans. The Herbert screw, originally designed for fixation of scaphoid fractures and nonunions, can be inserted arthroscopically and recessed beneath the articular cartilage surface.[50–52] This may obviate the need for removal of this fixation device.

Bioabsorbable pins have recently been introduced for treatment of osteochondral lesions. There are no long-term studies to support their use at present.

An alternative to conventional fixation is the use of fibrin glue. The fibrin adhesive system is composed of a two-component fibrin sealant which is applied to dried bone and held for 5 minutes with a bone clamp. The joint is then immobilized without weight bearing for 6 weeks. This procedure requires an open technique and is in its early stage of development. Its true clinical application is unknown at this early juncture.[53,54]

Advances in the fixation of osteochondral lesions are directed toward biologically compatible secure fixation. At present, we strive for rigid fixation that allows immediate postoperative motion. We prefer absorbable fixation but find that secure fixation is not always possible.

Chondral Fractures

The treatment options in chondral fractures are much different from those presented for osteochondral fractures. Articular cartilage lesions without associated bone have little option to repair. Historically, treatment of chondral lesions has consisted primarily of debridement of loose cartilage, drilling or abrading of bone, CPM, and no weight bearing for several months, waiting for ingrowth of fibrocartilage. Work on the transplantation of cartilage and grafting of costal perichondrium has been reported. The natural history of chondral fractures and the effects of present treatments are unknown.

Chondral lesions are treated arthroscopically in a standard fashion. After complete inspection of the joint for loose fragments of cartilage, the lesion is debrided of all loose borders to a stable rim of hyaline cartilage. The side walls of the lesion should be perpendicular to the subchondral surface. We believe the early relief of symptoms after arthroscopy is due to adequate removal of loose bodies and debridement of cartilage flaps that cause mechanical symptoms and synovitis. Magnuson first discussed the effect of debridement of "mechanical irritants" in the short-term improvement of patients with osteoarthritis.[55] Pridie[29,30,55,56] modified Magnuson's technique by drilling through the subchondral plate to allow ingrowth of fibrocartilage. Surgical defects in cartilage will not be replaced by fibrocartilage unless a defect in the subchondral plate is created.[57,58] As discussed in the section on articular cartilage, fibrocartilage is a poor substitute for normal hyaline cartilage. Whether to drill the subchondral bone or abrade the surface is a question yet unanswered. After arthroscopy the patient is usually maintained non-weight bearing for at least 2 months to allow for ingrowth.

There are multiple reports on the results of this treatment regimen. Dzioba reported 69% good results at 2-year follow-up, and he reported several prognostic indicators.[18] Those patients with the best prognosis had these lesional characteristics: small to medium size (small equals less than 1 cm, medium equals 1–3 cm), acute duration, partial thickness, non-weight-bearing location, and osteochondral nature. Patients less than

45 years old had the best chance of satisfactory results. In fact, he found 95% of patients with these types of lesions to have good results. He noted that the tidemark served a "protective" effect and these patients had good results after treatment. Poor prognostic lesional characteristics included large size (more than 3 cm), full-thickness lesions with loss of tidemark, chronic duration, and submeniscal and/or weight-bearing location. Older, obese patients had poorer results. Long-term studies of the results of treatment of these lesions are necessary to further define the natural history and long-term success of our present treatment modalities.

Investigations of alternative techniques in the treatment of weight-bearing cartilage defects in younger patients with cartilage transplantation, and perichondral and periosteal grafts have been reported with variable results. Meyers and co-authors reported their results of transplanted fresh osteochondral allograft to resurface patella, tibial plateau, and femoral condyles.[59] The results were favorable in the treatment of posttraumatic defects of the patella, tibial plateau, and femoral condyle at greater than 3 years follow-up. They set forth eight criteria that must be met for osteochondral allografts to be successful:

1. The osteochondral allograft must be fresh and include no more than 0.5 to 1.0 cm of subchondral bone.
2. The graft must be orthotopic and taken from bone of exact size to ensure good fit and articular congruity.
3. Chips of autologous bone may be used to lift the graft to provide maximal contact between host bone and allograft.
4. A firm press fit must obtained, except in the patella, where screws can be used for fixation.
5. The joint must be stable.
6. The synovial membrane must be closed to prevent ingrowth of granulation tissue and enhance nutrition of cartilage by containment of synovial fluid.
7. Weight bearing must be restricted until bone is completely incorporated.
8. Joint motion must be initiated early.

The authors admit the fate of the graft is unknown and that this technique may be useful in the young patient with a unicompartmental traumatic defect who is not a candidate for total knee arthroplasty.[59]

Gross and co-authors had less convincing results.[60] Of 78 small-fragment transplantations with fresh osteochondral allograft, 26 patients required further surgery. Patients with osteochondritis dissecans had the best results; those with bipolar grafts had the worst results. They advised that this procedure be limited to young patients with limited injury.[60] The fate of the cartilage in these osteochondral allografts is unknown. Some authors have found failed allograft cartilage to be replaced by fibrocartilage.[4] Kandel and co-authors found some viable cartilage in a pathologic study of 42 failed allografts.[61] Further investigations as to the pathophysiology of transplantation of osteochondral allografts are necessary to determine the long-term outcome and clinical usefulness of this modality.

O'Driscoll and co-workers reported an alternative method of resurfacing the articular cartilage defects with autogenous periosteal grafts. In a study in rabbits they found that periosteal grafts placed over full-thickness articular cartilage defects and treated with CPM resulted in tissue that resembled articular cartilage at 4 weeks.[27] The cambium layer of the periosteal graft must face outward away from the subchondral bone for success. There are no reports on the use of periosteal grafts in humans in the orthopedic literature.

Perichondral grafts have also been suggested for use in full-thickness chondral defects. Homminga and co-workers in The Netherlands reported their results using an autologous strip of costal perichondrium fixed to subchondral bone with fibrin glue.[62] At 1-year follow-up the Hospital for Special Surgery (HSS) knee score was increased from 73 to 90. In 28 of 30 lesions the defects were filled in with tissue resembling articular cartilage. Their early results were quite encouraging, but long-term studies and histopathology are necessary to fully evaluate their usefulness in clinical practice.

Summary

Early detection and treatment of chondral and osteochondral lesions are essential for optimal outcome using conventional treatment methods. Investigative techniques of osteochondral allografts, and periosteal and perichondral grafts may hold some promise to salvage the young patients with these injuries. As our knowledge of the articular cartilage physiology increases, new gains will surely reveal new techniques to resurface damaged articular surfaces.

References

1. Ahstrom JT. Osteochondral fracture in the knee joint associated with hypermobility and dislocation of the patella. *J Bone Joint Surg Am.* 1965;47:1491–1502.
2. Armstrong CG, Mow VC. Variations in the intrinsic mechanical properties of human articular cartilage with age, degeneration and water content. *J Bone Joint Surg Am.* 1982;64:88–94.
3. Bauer M, Jackson RW. Chondral lesions of the femoral condyles: A system of arthroscopic classification. *Arthroscopy.* 1988;4(2):97–102.
4. Brown KLB, Cruess RL. Bone and cartilage transplantation in orthopedic surgery. *J Bone Joint Surg Am.* 1982;64:270–277.
5. Butler JC, Andrews JR. The role of arthroscopic surgery in the evaluation of acute traumatic hemarthrosis of the knee. *Clin Orthop.* 1988;228:150–152.
6. Gillquist J, Hagberg G, Oretorp N. Arthroscopy in

7. acute injuries of the knee joint. *Acta Orthop Scand.* 1977;48:190–196.
8. Noyes RF, Bassett RW, Grood, ES, Butler DL. Arthroscopy in acute hemarthrosis of the knee. *J Bone Joint Surg Am.* 1980;62:687–695.
9. Sandberg R, Balkfors B. Traumatic hemarthrosis in stable knees. *Acta Orthop Scand.* 1986;57:516–517.
10. O'Donoghue DH. Chondral and osteochondral fractures. *J Trauma.* 1966;6:469–481.
11. Johnson-Nurse C, Dandy DJ. Fracture separation of articular cartilage in the adult knee. *J Bone Joint Surg Br.* 1985;67:42–43.
12. Kennedy JC, Grainger RW. Osteochondral fractures of the femoral condyles. *J Bone Joint Surg Br.* 1966;48:436–440.
13. Landells JW. The reactions of injured human articular cartilage. *J Bone Joint Surg Br.* 1957;39:548–561.
14. Milgram JE. Tangential osteochondral facture of the patella. *J Bone Joint Surg.* 1943;25:271–280.
15. Rosenberg NJ. Osteochondral fracture of the lateral femoral condyle. *J Bone Joint Surg Am.* 1964;46:1013–1026.
16. Rorabeck CH, Bobechko WP. Acute dislocation of the patella with osteochondral fracture. *J Bone Joint Surg Br.* 1976;58:237–240.
17. Matthewson MH, Dandy DJ. Osteochondral fracture of the lateral femoral condyle: A result of indirect violence to the knee. *J Bone Joint Surg Br.*1978;60:199–202.
18. Terry GC, Flandry F, Van Manen JW, Norwood LA. Isolated chondral fractures of the knee. *Clin Orthop.* 1988;234:170–177.
19. Dzioba RB. The classification and treatment of acute articular cartilage lesions. *Arthroscopy.* 1988;4(2):72–80.
20. Noyes FR, and Stabler CL. A system for grading articular cartilage lesions at arthroscopy. *Am J Sports med.* 1989;17(4):505–513.
21. Hunter W. On the structure and diseases of articulating cartilage. *Philos Trans R Soc London Biol.* 1743;9:267.
22. Convery FR, Akeson WH, Keown GH. The repair of large osteochondral defects: An experimental study in horses. *Clin Orthop.* 1972;82:253–262.
23. Buckwalter JA, Rosenberg LC, Hunziker EB. Articular cartilage: Composition, structure, response to injury, and methods of facilitating repair. In: Ewing JW, ed. *Articular Cartilage and Knee Joint Function: Basic Science and Arthroscopy.* New York: Raven Press; 1990.
24. Buckwalter JA, Hunziker E, Rosenberg LC, Coutts R, Adams M, Eyre O. Articular cartilage: Composition and structure. In: Woo SL, Buchwalter JA, eds. *Injury and Repair of the Musculoskeletal Soft Tissues.* Park Ridge: American Academy of Orthopaedic Surgeons; 1988:405–425.
25. Whipple RR, Gibbs MC, Lai WM, et al. Biphasic properties of repaired cartilage at the articular surface. *Trans Orthop Res Soc.* 1985;10:340.
26. Dunn AR, Sampsen, R. Regrowth of articular cartilage by direct hormonal induction with growth hormone following full-thickness surgical debridement. Presented at the 53rd Annual Meeting of the American Academy of Orthopaedic Surgeons, New Orleans, February 25, 1986.
27. Kwan MK, Woo SL-Y, Amiel D, et al. Neocartilage generated from rib perichondrium: A long-term multidisciplinary evaluation. *Trans Orthop Res Soc.* 1987;12:277.
28. O'Driscoll SW, Keeley FW, Salter RB. The chondrogenic potential of free autogenous periosteal grafts for biological resurfacing of major full-thickness defects in joint surfaces under the influence of continuous passive motion. *J*

Bone and Joint Surg Am. 1986;68:1017–1035.
29. Insall JN. Intra-articular surgery for degenerative arthritis of the knee. A report of the work of the late K. H. Pridie. *J Bone Joint Surg Br.* 1967;49:211–228.
30. Pridie KH. A method of resurfacing osteoarthritic knee joints. *J Bone Joint Surg Br.* 1959;41:618.
31. Mitchell N, Shepard N. The resurfacing of adult rabbit articular cartilage by multiple perforations through the subchondral bone. *J Bone Joint Surg Am.* 1976;58:230–233.
32. DePalma AF, McKeever CD, Sudin DK. Process of repair of articular cartilage demonstrated by histology and autoradiography with tritiated thymidine. *Clin Orthop.* 1966;48:229–242.
33. Salter RB, Simmonds DF, Malcolm BW, et al. The biological effect of continuous passive motion on the healing of full-thickness defects in articular cartilage: An experimental investigation in the rabbit. *J Bone Joint Surg Am.* 1980;62:1232–1251.
34. Morscher E. Cartilage–bone lesions of the knee joint following injury. *Reconstr Surg Traumatol.* 1971;12:2–26.
35. DeHaven KE. Diagnosis of acute knee injuries with hemarthrosis. *Am J Sports Med.* 1980;8:9–14.
36. Stoler DJ. Arthrography of the knee. In: Aichroth PM, Cannon WD Jr, Patel DV, eds. *Knee Surgery.* London: Martin Dunitz Limited; 1992.
37. Staple TW. Extrameniscal lesions demonstrated by double contrast arthrography of the knee. *Radiology.* 1971;102:311–319.
38. Gylys-Morin VM, Hajek PC, Sartoris DJ, Resnick D. Articular cartilage defects. Detectability in cadaver knees with MR. *Am J Radiol.* 1989;48:1153–1157.
39. Mink JH, Reicher MA, Crues JV. *MRI of the knee.* New York: Raven Press; 1987:128–129.
40. Mink JH, Deutsch AL. Occult cartilage and bone injuries of the knee: Detection, classification, and assessment with MR imaging. *Radiology.* 1989;170:823–829.
41. Heron CW, Calvert PT. Three dimensional gradient echo MR imaging of the knee. *Radiology.* 1992;183:839–844.
42. Wojtys E, Wilson M, Buckwalter K, Braunstein E, Martel W. Magnetic resonance imaging of the knee hyaline cartilage and intraarticular pathology. *Am J Sports Med.* 1987;15:455–463.
43. Chandnani VJ, Ho C, Chu P, Trudell D, Resnick D. Knee hyaline cartilage evaluated with MR imaging: A cadaveric study involving multiple imaging sequences and intraarticular injection of gadolinium and saline solution. *Radiology.* 1991;178:557–561.
44. Hadler J, Trudell D, Pathria MN, Resnick D. Width of the articular cartilage of the hip: Quantification by using fat-suppression spin-echo MR imaging in cadavers. *Am J Radiol.* 1992;159:351–355.
45. Szumowski J, Eisen JK, Vinitski S, Haake PW, Plewes DB. Hybrid methods of chemical-shift imaging. *Magn. Reson. Med.* 1989;9:379–388.
46. Ho C, Cervilla V, Kjellin I, et al. Magnetic resonance imaging in assessing cartilage changes in experimental osteoarthrosis of the knee. *Invest radio.* 1992;27:84–90.
47. Locht RC, Gross AE, Langer F. Late osteochondral allograft resurfacing for tibial plateau fractures. *J Bone Joint Surg Am.* 1984;66:328–335.
48. Johnson EW Jr, McLoed TL. Osteochondral fragments of the distal end of the femur fixed with bone pegs. *J Bone Joint Surg Am.* 1977;59:677–679.
49. Lindholm S, Pylkkanen P. Internal fixation of the fragment of osteochondritis dissecans in the knee by means of bone pins. A preliminary report on several cases. *Acta Chir Scand.* 1974;140:626–629.
50. Johnson L. Arthroscopic repair of osteochondritis. In: *Arthroscopy Video Digest.* Okemos, MI: Instrument Makar; August 1984.
51. MacNamer PB, Bunker TD, Scott TD. The Herbert Screw for osteochondral fractures: Brief report. *J Bone Joint Surg Br.* 1988;70:145–146.
52. Thomson NL. Osteochondritis dissecans and osteochondral fragments managed by Herbert compression screw fixation. *Clin Orthop.* 1987;224:71–78.
53. Meyer MH, Herron M. A fibrin adhesive seal for the repair of osteochondral fracture fragments. *Clin Orthop.* 1984;182:258–263.
54. Visur T, Timo K. Fixation of large osteochondral fractures of the patella with fibrin adhesive system. *Am J Sports Med.* 1989;17(6):842–845.
55. Magnuson PB. Joint debridement. Surgical treatment of degenerative arthritis. *Surg Gynecol Obstet.* 1941;73:1.
56. Insall JN. The Pridie debridement operation for osteoarthritis of the knee. *Clin Orthop.* 1974;101:62–67.
57. Calandruccio RA, Gilmer WS Jr. Proliferation, regeneration, and repair of articular cartilage of immature animals. *J Bone Joint Surg Am.* 1962;44:431–455.
58. Carlson H. Reactions of rabbit patellary cartilage following operative defects. A morphological and Autoradiographic study. *Acta Orthop Scand Suppl.* 1957;28.
58. Schultz RJ, Krishnamurthy, S, Thelmo W, et al. Effects of varying intrinsic of laser energy on articular cartilage: A preliminary study. *Lasers Surg Med.* 1985;5:577–588.
59. Meyers MH, Akeson W, Convery FR. Resurfacing of the knee with fresh osteochondral allograft. *J Bone Joint Surg Am.* 1989;71:704–713.
60. Gross AE, McKee NH, Pritzker KPH, Langer F. Reconstruction of skeletal deficits at the knee. *Clin Orthop.* 1983;174:96–106.
61. Kandel RA, Gross AE, Grand A, McDermott AGP, Langer F, Pritzker KPH. Histopathology of failed osteoarticular shell allografts. *Clin Orthop.* 1985;197:103–110.
62. Homminga GN, Bulstra SK, Bouwmeester PSM, Van Der Linden AJ. Perichondral grafting for cartilage lesions of the knee. *J Bone Joint Surg Br.* 1990;72:1003–1007.

Bibliography

Mow, VC, Fithian DC, Kelly MA. Fundamentals of articular cartilage and meniscus biomechanics. In: Ewing JW, ed *Articular Cartilage and Knee Joint Function: Basic Science and Arthroscopy.* New York: Raven Press; 1990.
Mow VC, Holmes MH, Lai WM. Fluid transport and mechanical properties of articular cartilage: A review. *J Biomech.* 1984;27:377–394.
Mow VC, Proctor CS, Kelly MA. Biomechanics of articular cartilage. In: Nordin M, Frankel V, eds. *Basic Biomechanics of Locomotor System.* Philadephia: Lea & Febiger; 1989.
Mow VC, Lai WM, Redler I. Some surface characteristics of articular cartilage. I. A scanning electron microscopy study and a theoretical model for the dynamic interaction of synovial fluid and articular cartilage. *J Biomech.* 1976;7:449.

4

Soft Tissue Injuries and Management About the Knee

Nicholas J. Carr and Gregory Gallico

Oh, Adam was a gardener, and God who made him sees
That half a proper gardener's work is done upon his knees.
Rudyard Kipling (1865–1936)
The Glory of the Garden

As it is with gardeners so it is with us all. From the scrapes of childhood to the mechanized encounters of adulthood, our knees bear much of the trauma. Soft tissue injury about the knee may occur in isolation, but frequently is part of more extensive trauma involving articular and periarticular musculoskeletal structures. The prognosis for functional knee recovery following trauma is determined not only by the success with which musculoskeletal anatomy is restored, but also by the timely provision of soft tissue coverage. Indeed, other than initial bony stabilization, formal musculoskeletal reconstruction must be held in abeyance pending soft tissue closure.

The goals of management of soft tissue injury about the knee are the expedient provision of closure that is viable, durable, aesthetically acceptable, and, where possible, sensate. This should be done while minimizing functional and cosmetic sacrifice of donor sites. Occasionally, reconstructive goals will vary according to specific clinical needs and these special situations are discussed.

Soft Tissue Anatomy About the Knee

Unlike the situation in the thigh where the femur is cloaked circumferentially by a myofascial envelope, the knee joint is a subcutaneous structure surrounded by the iliotibial tract and tendons of the quadriceps, hamstring, and gastrocnemius muscle groups. The popliteal fossa is invested by a superficial fascia deep to which, in a layer of loose fat, run the tibial nerve, popliteal vein,

and popliteal artery in order from superficial to deep and lateral to medial.

The knee is supplied by a rich vascular plexus with horizontal arcades originating from the popliteal artery interrupted by anastomoses with longitudinal vessels issuing from the thigh and leg.[1] Level with the proximal edge of the femoral condyles, the popliteal artery gives off superior genicular arteries which lie deeply supplying the joint capsule, but also giving off cutaneous perforators. The middle genicular artery supplies the cruciate ligaments and synovium alone. The superior medial genicular artery runs deep to the semimembranosus and semitendinosus muscles anastomosing with the articular branch of the descending genicular artery and supplying the lower fibers of vastus medialis as well as the skin superior and medial to the patella. The superior lateral genicular artery runs deep to the tendon of biceps femoris, giving branches to vastus lateralis and the skin of the superior and lateral borders of the patella (Figs. 4–1 to 4–4).

The inferior genicular arteries arise from the popliteal artery approximately level with the joint line. The inferior medial vessel runs deep to the medial head of the gastrocnemius and the tibial collateral ligament, branching superficial and deep to the ligamentum patellae to join the cutaneous patellar plexus. In similar fashion, the inferior lateral genicular artery runs deep to the lateral gastrocnemius and fibular collateral ligament, supplying skin inferolateral to the patella and contributing to the patellar plexus.

Three named vessels ascend from the leg to contribute to the cutaneous patellar plexus.[2] The anterior recurrent artery arises from the anterior tibial artery and pierces tibialis anterior coursing up the lateral knee; the circumflex fibular and posterior tibial recurrent arteries

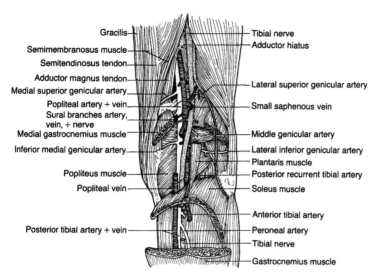

Gracilis
Semimembranosus muscle
Semitendinosus tendon
Adductor magnus tendon
Medial superior genicular artery
Popliteal artery + vein
Sural branches artery, vein, + nerve
Medial gastrocnemius muscle
Inferior medial genicular artery
Popliteus muscle
Popliteal vein
Posterior tibial artery + vein

Tibial nerve
Adductor hiatus
Lateral superior genicular artery
Small saphenous vein
Middle genicular artery
Lateral inferior genicular artery
Plantaris muscle
Posterior recurrent tibial artery
Soleus muscle
Anterior tibial artery
Peroneal artery
Tibial nerve
Gastrocnemius muscle

Figure 4–1. Vascular anatomy of the posterior knee.

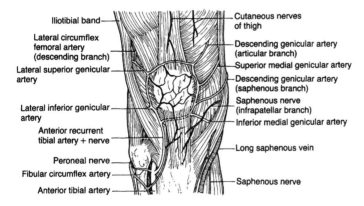

Iliotibial band
Lateral circumflex femoral artery (descending branch)
Lateral superior genicular artery
Lateral inferior genicular artery
Anterior recurrent tibial artery + nerve
Peroneal nerve
Fibular circumflex artery
Anterior tibial artery

Cutaneous nerves of thigh
Descending genicular artery (articular branch)
Superior medial genicular artery
Descending genicular artery (saphenous branch)
Saphenous nerve (infrapatellar branch)
Inferior medial genicular artery
Long saphenous vein
Saphenous nerve

Figure 4–2. Vascular anatomy of the anterior knee.

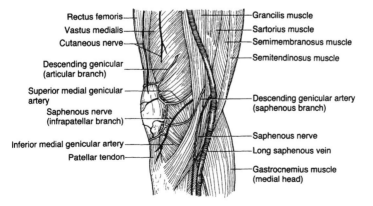

Rectus femoris
Vastus medialis
Cutaneous nerve
Descending genicular (articular branch)
Superior medial genicular artery
Saphenous nerve (infrapatellar branch)
Inferior medial genicular artery
Patellar tendon

Grancilis muscle
Sartorius muscle
Semimembranosus muscle
Semitendinosus muscle
Descending genicular artery (saphenous branch)
Saphenous nerve
Long saphenous vein
Gastrocnemius muscle (medial head)

Figure 4–3. Vascular anatomy of the medial knee.

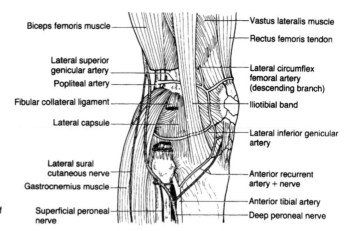

Biceps femoris muscle

Lateral superior
genicular artery

Popliteal artery

Fibular collateral ligament

Lateral capsule

Lateral sural
cutaneous nerve

Gastrocnemius muscle

Superficial peroneal
nerve

Vastus lateralis muscle

Rectus femoris tendon

Lateral circumflex
femoral artery
(descending branch)

Iliotibial band

Lateral inferior genicular
artery

Anterior recurrent
artery + nerve

Anterior tibial artery

Deep peroneal nerve

Figure 4–4. Vascular anatomy of
the lateral knee.

are septocutaneous perforators branching proximally from their parent arteries.

Originating from the superficial femoral artery cephalad to the adductor hiatus, the descending genicular artery passes deep to sartorius, giving off a deep musculoarticular branch and a superficial saphenous branch. The latter, in company with the saphenous nerve and long saphenous vein, continues into the upper medial leg, giving off a significant infrapatellar branch which joins the patellar plexus. The lateral knee receives contributions from the descending branch of the lateral circumflex femoral artery and the terminal perforating branch of the profunda femoris artery which anastomose with the superior lateral geniculate artery. Posteriorly, the medial superficial sural artery arises from the popliteal artery or, on occasion, from the sural muscular arteries and supplies the superior calf fascia. An unnamed popliteal branch ascends from the popliteal fossa to supply the posterior thigh fascia and is the basis for a fasciocutaneous flap to be described later.

The venous anatomy about the knee consists of the popliteal vein and its continuation, the superficial femoral vein, which connect via transfascial perforating veins with the short saphenous vein posteriorly and the long saphenous vein medially. Paired vena comitantes accompany named arteries and drain into the deep venous system.

Cutaneous innervation about the knee is provided by branches of the lateral femoral cutaneous nerve (L-2,3), femoral nerve (L-2,3,4), obturator nerve (L-2,3,4), and posterior femoral cutaneous nerve (S-1,2,3). The anterior knee receives sensory innervation from the patellar plexus, which is formed by the anterior branch of the lateral femoral cutaneous nerve and the intermediate, medial, and infrapatellar branches of the femoral nerve.

The medial side of the knee receives cutaneous innervation from the subsartorial plexus made up of branches from the medial femoral cutaneous nerve, saphenous nerve, and anterior cutaneous branch of the obturator nerve. The posterior femoral cutaneous nerve supplies the skin over the popliteal fossa.

The knee is represented by the L-3 dermatome medially, L-4 anteriorly, L-5 laterally, and S-1 and S-2 posteriorly.

Classification of Soft Tissue Injuries About the Knee

The nature of lower extremity soft tissue injury is highly correlated with the mechanism of causation.[3] Low-energy wounds produce lacerations and abrasions with a well-circumscribed zone of injury. High-energy trauma produces diffuse soft tissue avulsion and crush with a poorly defined zone of injury. From the point of view of reconstruction, these wounds may be classified on the basis of the absence or presence of full-thickness skin loss. In the former situation, direct suture or skin graft is adequate whereas in the latter case, some form of flap reconstruction is required. In high-energy wounds, the determination of whether skin loss has occurred must await stabilization of the zone of injury and subsequent assessment of soft tissue viability.

High-energy trauma often produces underlying musculoskeletal trauma in concert with overlying soft tissue damage. Wounds may communicate with intact cortical surfaces, fractures, or the knee joint. In addition, there may be associated vascular or neurologic injuries. Specific types of soft tissue trauma that are considered in this chapter are skin avulsions, gunshot wounds, open joint injuries, prosthetic exposure, and amputation stump coverage (Table 4–1).

Table 4–1. Classification of Soft Tissue Injury About the Knee

I. Low-energy wounds
  A. Laceration
  B. Abrasion
    1. Partial thickness
    2. Full thickness
II. High-energy wounds
  A. Skin avulsion
  B. Compound wounds
    1. Exposed patella
    2. Compound fracture
    3. Open joint
    4. Gunshot wounds
III. Special situations
  A. Vascular injury
  B. Nerve injury
  C. Exposed prosthesis
  D. Amputation stump coverage

Principles of Management of Soft Tissue Trauma

The management of the trauma victim must proceed in an orderly fashion beginning with a primary survey and attention to the lifesaving ABCs of airway, ventilation, circulation, and control of hemorrhage. Following initial stabilization, a careful secondary survey for major injury reveals the specifics of extremity trauma including soft tissue, neurovascular, and musculoskeletal injuries.[4] The mechanism and energy of the injury and details of significant medical history must be determined.

Emergency room management of extremity trauma consists of x-ray, wound culture, sterile dressing, fracture reduction and splintage, and tetanus and antibiotic prophylaxis. Fasciotomy must be considered in the setting of high-energy closed or open leg trauma, penetrating trauma, or vascular injury and, where necessary, performed expeditiously. Vascular injury must also be diagnosed emergently as the consequences of missed diagnoses are limb threatening. Angiography is indicated on clinical grounds in the presence of pallor, reduced distal capillary refill, coolness, or decreased or absent pulses in contrast to the uninjured limb. Injuries such as knee dislocation and periarticular fractures, bumper crush, and gunshot wounds with a high probability of subclinical vascular trauma should also be studied angiographically. The risks and benefits of a formal biplane angiogram must be weighed against the more limited, but expeditious information available from an intraoperative study.[5] In the severely injured limb, judgment must be made as to limb viability and the potential for functional salvage. Scoring systems have been developed to assist the clinician with the difficult decision of primary amputation.[6] When possible, however, amputation is best deferred until discussed with the patient following the initial surgery.

Once stable, the patient should be taken to the operating room for fixation of skeletal injuries, evaluation of the zone of injury, and formal debridement. Wounds should be irrigated with large volumes of saline (10 L+) by jet pulse lavage. Skin is excised until bleeding dermis is obtained and muscle viability is judged on the basis of color, bleeding, and contractility. All bone fragments without periosteal attachment are excised.[7] Following debridement and irrigation, repeat wound cultures should be taken. Broad-spectrum parenteral antibiotics are administered for 3 days[8] and subsequent to this are given on a culture-specific basis as required. Low-energy, minimally contaminated wounds may be closed primarily by suture or immediate skin graft, but the majority of wounds should be packed with saline gauze in anticipation of delayed primary closure. Saline dressings may be changed on the ward, saline may be infused into dressings at a low rate, or an occlusive cover may be applied over the dressing. The specific manner of dressing is not important as long as wound desiccation is prevented. Antibiotic-impregnated methyl methacrylate beads under an occlusive dressing with a closed suction drain provide a useful method of maintaining wound sterility without desiccation.[9,10] At intervals of about 48 hours, the patient should be returned to the operating room for repeat examination of wounds with debridement as necessary. This process of sequential examination and debridement permits the recognition of all devitalized tissue and definition of the zone of injury in three dimensions.[11] Neurovascular structures exposed by serial debridement must be preserved and demand urgent coverage with healthy soft tissue. Wound closure must not be pursued until the wound is controlled both bacteriologically and with respect to a stable zone of injury.[12]

Significant debate exists in the literature over appropriate timing for soft tissue coverage of lower extremity wounds. Most of this research is specifically directed at free flap coverage of osteocutaneous tibial defects. Despite the fact that this work does not directly reference the knee, certain lessons still apply. A consistent correlation has been demonstrated between earlier soft tissue closure and lower rates of flap failure and secondary osteomyelitis.[1–16] This concept has been taken to its extreme with immediate free flap closure of complex posttraumatic wounds, and a number of series support the validity of this approach.[17] Logistics dictate that some patients will present in a delayed fashion and in this situation meticulous serial debridement in the manner outlined earlier can be expected to permit acceptable flap and wound complication rates, even in the face of subacute or chronic wounds with their attendant bacterial colonization. The actual time postinjury that soft tissue coverage is appropriate varies according to the degree of devitalization and contamination. A realistic goal is to provide coverage following two or three debridements spaced at 48 hours, and on this basis wound closure should be generally attainable in the first week postinjury.

Selecting a Method of Soft Tissue Reconstruction

The concept of the reconstructive ladder is based on selection of the simplest method of wound closure available and therefore sequentially considers direct closure, grafts, flaps, and free flaps. Posttraumatic soft tissue surgery must not only provide wound closure but also must take into account future reconstructive demands. A wound may be graftable, but if this prohibits requisite arthroplasty or bone grafting, flap coverage may be indicated primarily. A corollary to this approach is that if a more complex method of reconstruction will provide a better functional outcome, it should be selected despite the availability of simpler methods. This latter situation most commonly arises when comparing local with free flap options for reconstruction. The following section reviews the soft tissue reconstructive techniques available about the knee.

Direct Wound Closure

Wounds with minimal or no skin loss should be managed by direct reapproximation of their margins. The timing of the closure is a matter of judgment and should be based on consideration of wound contamination and tissue viability. Where a single irrigation and debridement is judged to control both of these factors, primary closure at the time of presentation may be appropriate. With the exception of low-energy trauma, however, the conditions for primary closure are rarely met.

Closure should be delayed if any uncertainty regarding contamination or tissue viability exists at the time of the initial debridement. The main prerequisite of a dressing is that it prevent wound desiccation, and despite many choices the most effective is frequent saline dressings. Repeat debridement should be performed at intervals of about 48 hours, and once viability is ensured delayed primary closure should be performed. The principles of direct suturing of wounds are minimal undermining, layered closure without tension, and splinting to avoid traction on the wound edges.

Skin Grafts

Wounds will be encountered where, in addition to the normal retraction of wound edges, there is a net skin loss. This type of wound results from skin avulsions, abrasions, and scything or burst-type lacerations with loss or debridement of the resulting traumatic flaps. Analysis of these wounds must consider the surface area of skin loss, the wound substrate, and future reconstructive needs.

In rare circumstances, if the area of skin loss is sufficiently small (on the order of 1 cm or less edge to edge), it may be appropriate to allow healing by secondary intention. Similarly, in abrasive wounds, if on inspection residual dermis remains, the wound may be dressed expectantly while awaiting reepithelialization from the epidermal appendages. In the remainder of these skin loss situations, a judgment must be made as to whether the wound is skin graftable. This entails an assessment of the wound bed with grafting possible on tissue with intact capillary circulation including fascia, paratenon, perichondrium, and periosteum. Skin grafts applied to deep musculoskeletal structures do not provide an "operative window" for surgical exposure, and flap coverage is preferred if further reconstruction is likely.

The mechanism of injury usually determines the appropriate timing for skin grafting. Clean avulsion injuries as well as surgically created wounds should be grafted immediately. Wounds with crushed and devitalized tissue should undergo staged debridements until healthy tissue with capillary bleeding is encountered. Alternatively, wounds with heavy contamination or avascular areas may be treated with wet dressings until granulation tissue develops. Although granulation tissue is colonized with bacteria, this usually is not an impediment to skin graft survival unless *Pseudomonas* or group A *Streptococcus* is present or the bacterial load exceeds 10^5 per gram of tissue.[18]

The depth at which a skin graft is harvested may vary from split to full thickness depending on whether part or all of the donor dermis is taken. Thinner grafts offer the advantage of greater reliability and rapidity of graft take but, compared with full-thickness grafts, are less durable and more prone to dryness, contracture, and pigmentation. The appropriate graft for lower extremity trauma is almost always a split-thickness graft.

With little practice, excellent skin grafts can be harvested using electric or air power dermatomes. Preferred harvest sites are the upper thighs or buttocks, with care to avoid areas of potential flap harvest or prosthesis contact. Medium-thickness grafts in the range 0.01 to 0.015 in. represent a reasonable compromise of the qualities discussed earlier and create a donor site that will heal in 10 to 14 days. Donor sites may be covered by a variety of gauzes, but heal more rapidly and comfortably under an occlusive dressing.

A number of choices exist with respect to manner of skin graft application. The graft may be sheet or meshed and may be applied immediately on harvest or delayed. The significance of these strategies relates to the adequacy of hemostasis in the wound bed. From an aesthetic standpoint, the best graft appearance is achieved with sheet graft, which is often applied after a delay following the final wound debridement to avoid subgraft hematoma. The advantages of meshed skin graft are an expanded area of coverage, egress of blood and wound exudate, and more ready contouring to difficult three-dimensional wounds.[19] A graft nearly comparable in appearance to sheet graft may be obtained by the immediate application of nonexpanded meshed skin graft. This strategy allows debridement of the wound and application of skin graft under the same anesthetic with expectation of excellent appearance and graft take.

The skin graft should be compressively dressed for 5 to 7 days postapplication. Generally a circumferential dressing suffices, but if the graft traverses a concavity, a tie-over dressing is necessary. The limbs should be elevated and splinted following graft application, but leg dependency with elastic bandage support may be initiated as early as 1 week postoperatively if no mitigating factors exist.

Flaps

A flap can be defined as a segment of vascularized tissue transported to a site distant from its origin. Flaps are classified on the basis of their movement, vascularity, or tissue composition. The earliest use of flaps was as skin and subcutaneous flaps based on their random dermal circulation. These random flaps were classified according to the manner in which they were transported and, on this basis, they consisted of either pivot or advancement flaps.

A more encompassing view of flaps is obtained if they are classified by their vascular supply. By this taxonomy there are random and axial flaps. Unlike the limitations of random flaps, axial flaps based on a known blood vessel function independently of length–width constraints. Axial flaps may be cutaneous flaps based on a direct cutaneous artery, fasciocutaneous flaps, or muscle flaps. An example of the former is the groin flap based on the superficial circumflex iliac artery; however, with the exception of some occasionally used free flaps, this group of flaps has little application about the knee. The following section discusses random flaps, fasciocutaneous flaps, and muscle flaps in soft tissue reconstruction of the knee. In addition free flaps and cross-leg flaps are axial flaps transported from distant as opposed to regional sites and are also included in this section.

The indications for flap coverage have been briefly discussed already. The most common indication is coverage of a wound with vascularity inadequate to support a skin graft. Other indications include provision of an "operative window" for future surgical exposure or the need for specific tissues in reconstruction such as osteocutaneous and functional muscle–tendon composites.

Random Flaps. Random flaps consist of skin and subcutaneous tissue that receive their blood supply through the subpapillary and deep dermal plexi and subcutaneous vessels of the flap pedicle (Fig. 4–5). These flaps are not reliable beyond a length:width ratio of 1:1. Many designs are possible, but can be broadly grouped as advancement or pivot based on their movement. Within the advancement group are included pure advancement and V–Y flaps; the pivot group includes rotation, transposition, rhomboid, and bilobed flaps. The majority of these flaps require skin graft closure of the flap donor site as there is minimal skin laxity surrounding the knee. Apart from the occasional small wound, particularly about the prepatellar area, random skin flaps have little application in soft tissue recon-

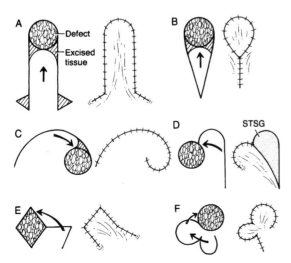

Figure 4–5. Random flaps. **A.** Pure advancement. **B.** V–Y advancement. **C.** Rotation. **D.** Transposition. **E.** Rhomboid. **F.** Bilobed. (STSG, split-thickness skin graft.)

struction about the knee. A variant that may occasionally prove useful is the deepithelialized turnover flap in which a deepithelialized flap paralleling the wound is hinged at the wound margin, the deep side of the flap and donor site being skin grafted in continuity.[20]

The use of soft tissue expansion to resurface chronically unstable wounds or to correct contour defects is another variant of the random skin flap with some relevance about the knee.[21–24] One or more silicone expanders are placed in a subcutaneous plane beneath unscarred skin. The expanders are gradually inflated over a period of about 3 months, after which a flap fashioned from the expanded skin and subcutaneous tissue is used to resurface the unstable wound. The presence of an open wound at the level of the knee is a contraindication to soft tissue expansion, as it is almost uniformly associated with infection of the expander or wound dehiscence.[25]

Fasciocutaneous Flaps. The fasciocutaneous arterial system consists of perforators that pass through intermuscular septae to fan out on the superficial surface of the deep fascia, giving branches to the subcutaneous tissue and skin.[26] The concept of fasciocutaneous flaps was introduced by Ponten in 1981 and, by including the fascia in his "super flaps," he was able to produce proximally based leg flaps with an average length:width ratio of 2.5:1 without need for delay.[27] Further work has shown the fascial plexus in the leg to be supplied by perforators from the anterior and posterior tibial and peroneal arteries passing along their adjacent intermuscular septae.[28,29] These perforators branch radially on the superficial surface of the fascia, anastomosing with adjacent perforators and producing longitudinally oriented anastomotic arcades aligned with each of the intermuscular septae.[30] This basic pattern of cutaneous supply is augmented by the saphenous and sural arteries coursing within the subcutaneous layer and musculocutaneous perforators from the gastrocnemius muscles.[26] A similar system of fasciocutaneous perforators exist in the thigh based on the superficial and profunda femoris arteries.

Fasciocutaneous flaps for soft tissue reconstruction about the knee have received considerable recent attention. In general terms, they can be based proximally with skin taken from the leg or based distally with skin taken from the thigh. Cormack and Lamberty have classified these flaps according to their pattern of vascularization, which may be via single or multiple fasciocutaneous perforators entering at the flap base or multiple septocutaneous perforators entering the length of the flap from an underlying deep artery.[31]

Conditions favoring the choice of a fasciocutaneous flap are appropriate wound geometry, mitigating medical conditions prohibitive of a more complex procedure,

local muscle injury or vascular damage, and the need for a salvage flap. Fasciocutaneous flaps are particularly useful for coverage of small to moderate-sized wounds containing exposed bone, tendon, nerve, or vessels.[32] Deadspace within deep recessed wounds is better obliterated by a muscle flap. In secondary reconstruction, fasciocutaneous flaps provide thin supple cover for the release of contractures or unstable scars. In the setting of osteomyelitis, muscle flaps are generally preferred, although some evidence suggests fasciocutaneous flaps may be efficacious.[33,34] Similarly, in the presence of exposed hardware, fasciocutaneous flaps have a high complication rate,[35] although some disagree with this premise.[36]

The advantages of fasciocutaneous flaps in comparison to random cutaneous flaps are reliability, with length:width ratios up to 3:1 based proximally or distally without need for delay. Dissection is rapid, simple, and relatively bloodless, taking place in what Haertsch has termed the "surgical plane" of the leg.[37] In comparison to muscle or musculocutaneous flaps, the contrast in ease and speed of dissection is even more marked. Additionally, fasciocutaneous flaps are less bulky and do not sacrifice muscle function.[38] The significant disadvantages of fasciocutaneous flaps are poor malleability in obliterating wound contours, questionable efficacy in dealing with exposed hardware or infected bone, and requisite donor site skin graft resulting in greater disfigurement than with muscle flaps.

The simplest fasciocutaneous flaps about the knee are local skin flaps raised subfascially and incorporating random fascial vessels in their pedicle (Fig. 4–6). These flaps are most useful for small defects over the anterior knee and are generally designed as transposition or advancement-type flaps, with skin grafting usually necessary at the donor site.[39–41]

A variety of larger fasciocutaneous flaps based on constant direct cutaneous vessels and septocutaneous

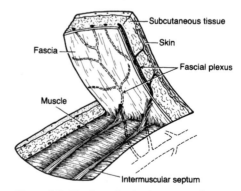

Figure 4–6. Simple random fasciocutaneous flap.

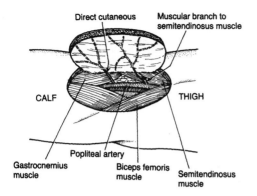

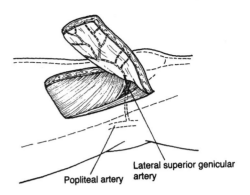

Figure 4–7. Popliteoposterior thigh flap.

Figure 4–8. Lateral genicular artery flap.

perforators in the thigh and leg have recently been described. Two flaps consisting of thigh skin pedicled on a single distally based vessel at the knee have been described. The posterior thigh skin from gluteal crease to the popliteal fossa may be pedicled as a fasciocutaneous flap based on an ascending perforator from the popliteal artery which originates between the semimembranosus and biceps femoris muscles 11 cm cephalad to the plane of the knee joint. This flap has been variably named the popliteoposterior thigh[42] or suprapopliteal flap (Fig. 4–7).[43] The second thigh fasciocutaneous flap of use about the knee is based on a constant cutaneous perforator of the superior lateral genicular artery which exits a triangular space defined by the lateral femoral condyle, vastus lateralis, and the short head of biceps femoris (Fig. 4–8). Based on this vessel, the lateral thigh skin from the femoral condyle midway to the greater trochanter can be pedicled to reach all except medial knee defects. The nutrient vessel to this flap courses

midway in the subcutaneous layer. Therefore the flap is not by necessity fasciocutaneous; however, inclusion of fascia lata can facilitate quadriceps mechanism repair. This flap has been named the lower posterolateral thigh flap[44] or lateral genicular artery flap.[45]

A variety of proximally based fasciocutaneous flaps from the leg useful in knee coverage have been described (Fig. 4–9). These consist of three types corresponding to Cormack and Lamberty's classification.[31] Type A flaps contain multiple fasciocutaneous vessels in their pedicle and are designed to capture maximally the longitudinally arranged arcades of the septocutaneous perforating vessels. Ponten's "super flaps" are of this type and, with lengths of up to 22 cm, can reach some knee defects albeit with creation of significant "dog ear" deformity at the flap rotation point.[27]

Type B flaps are based on a single fasciocutaneous perforator and are represented by flaps based on the saphenous, sural, and anterior tibial septocutaneous

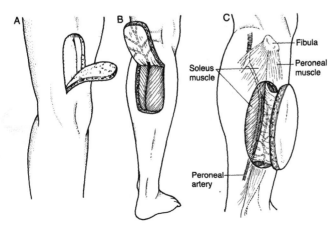

Figure 4–9. Proximally based fasciocutaneous flaps from the leg. **A.** Type A flap based on multiple fasciocutaneous vessels. **B.** Type B flap based on a single fasciocutaneous perforator. The example shown is a posterior calf (sural) flap. **C.** Type C flap based on a series of septocutaneous perforators from an underlying artery. Example shown is a peroneal island flap.

arteries. The saphenous artery is the continuation in the leg of the descending genicular artery, which arises from the superficial femoral artery above the adductor hiatus and passes deep to sartorious to supply skin overlying the medial knee. The saphenous flap can be pedicled over a limited arc about the anterior knee, but is of limited application other than as a free flap.[46]

The posterior calf flap[47,48] or sural fasciocutaneous flap[49,50] is a type B flap based on the superficial sural artery which arises from the popliteal, medial, or lateral sural arteries and supplies a fasciocutaneous territory of the posterior calf extending to the midaxial lines and junction of the middle and distal thirds of the leg. This flap readily reaches the anterior knee, but requires sacrifice of the sural nerve.

The anterior tibial flap[51,52] and anterolateral leg island flap[53] are type B fasciocutaneous flaps based on a constant septocutaneous perforator of the anterior tibial artery passing through the anterior crural septum 7 to 11 cm caudad to the fibular head. Based on this constant vessel, the skin overlying the anterior crural septum in the lower half of the leg can be pedicled to reach defects of the anterior knee.

Type C flaps of Cormack and Lamberty consist of a fasciocutaneous flap connected by a series of septocutaneous perforators to an underlying artery in an arrangement akin to a ladder on edge. The peroneal island flap is of this design and, by division of the peroneal artery distally, can create a pedicle of sufficient length to carry a small skin island to any aspect of the knee.[54]

In summary, a considerable variety of fasciocutaneous flaps applicable to soft tissue reconstruction about the knee exist. Their development is recent and they have not yet assumed the frequency of use they are likely to have in the future.

Muscle and Musculocutaneous Flaps. Selection of soft tissue coverage for knee wounds should generally be predicated on the simplest method capable of providing durable cover with minimum functional compromise. In most situations a cutaneous or fasciocutaneous flap best serves this purpose; however, in some cases a muscle flap may be indicated.

Muscle flaps have been demonstrated experimentally and clinically to be more resistant to soft tissue infection than random pattern skin flaps and are therefore the preferred form of coverage in contaminated or infected wounds.[55,56] In high-energy wounds with comminuted segmental fractures where the need for bone grafting is anticipated, the vascularity conferred by a muscle flap augments the bone healing potential of the wound.[57] Muscle flaps offer a degree of flexibility in obliterating the deadspace of complex three-dimensional wounds that is not found with cutaneous flaps. Rarely, a muscle flap may be indicated to provide functional restoration

of a muscle–tendon unit, most frequently the quadriceps mechanism. In this role the muscle may serve as a carrier for restoration of a tendon segment or may reestablish functional muscle.

Muscle flaps may be transferred as musculocutaneous composites carrying an overlying skin segment nourished by the musculocutaneous perforating vessels. Alternatively, the muscle may be transferred in isolation and skin grafted. In circumstances where muscle flap coverage is indicated but no local muscle is satisfactory, free flap transfer becomes the procedure of choice and this is discussed in the next section.

Muscles available for pedicled coverage of knee defects may be carried on proximally based pedicles from the leg or distally based pedicles from the thigh. The gastrocnemius muscle constitutes the former group and is the only local muscle of significant utility in knee coverage. The thigh muscles are occasionally helpful in coverage of small defects, but have very limited application and a poor track record with respect to reliability.

The medial and lateral heads of the gastrocnemius muscle arise from their respective femoral condyles, fuse in the midline, and insert with the soleus into Achilles tendon. Medial and lateral sural arteries with paired vena comitantes enter the deep surface of each head within the popliteal fossa. The two heads receive separate innervation by branches of the tibial nerve which enter the muscle with the vascular pedicles. Both heads of the gastrocnemius are type I muscles after the classification of Mathes and Nahai.[58] This means that they each receive a single dominant vascular pedicle and the muscle completely survives elevated on that pedicle. From a practical point of view, this means that the full length of either head can be elevated and its arc of rotation is determined by the sural pedicle in the popliteal fossa.

Selection of the appropriate head of the gastrocnemius muscle permits coverage of moderate-sized wounds on any aspect of the knee.[59] The lateral gastrocnemius is shorter, narrower, and flatter than the medial head. Its arc of rotation is therefore somewhat less, but it has the advantage of providing a less bulky reconstruction with less donor deformity in appropriately situated wounds.[60] The posterior calf skin is vascularized by direct cutaneous, septocutaneous, and musculocutaneous arteries. The latter arise overlying the proximal gastrocnemius heads and run longitudinally, supplying skin to within 5 and 10 cm cephalad to the medial and lateral malleoli, respectively.[59] As this skin territory extends well beyond the caudal limit of the muscle, a musculocutaneous flap prolonged with a fasciocutaneous extension provides a flap of greater length and breadth.[61] In rare circumstances, either the medial or lateral gastrocnemius musculocutaneous flaps may prove useful, but in general their use is avoided because of their bulk and significant donor site deformity. Use

56 — Nicholas J. Carr and Gregory Gallico

of the muscle flap without overlying skin permits primary donor site closure and only a slight contour deformity results. A useful variation of the gastrocnemius musculocutaneous flap is a muscle flap containing a small skin island which provides full-thickness subcutaneous cover for small knee wounds while still allowing primary donor site closure.[62] The two heads of the gastrocnemius together with the soleus form the triceps surae responsible for plantar flexion. It is preferable to harvest only one of these three heads, but where necessary both heads of the gastrocnemius may be elevated without noticeable functional disturbance.[63,64]

Traumatic defects of the knee may have associated vascular injuries particularly in circumferential injuries such as preoperative bumper crush.[65] Angiography is advisable when vascular injury or preexisting disease is suspected.[66,67] The gastrocnemius muscle is harvested under tourniquet with the patient in the semi- or full lateral position. A longitudinal incision is made somewhat posterior to the midaxis of the leg. After incision of the deep muscular fascia, the correct plane of dissection between gastrocnemius and soleus is established by identifying the plantaris tendon. The muscle is then split beginning distally by taking a small cuff of the tendinous insertion to facilitate suturing. The midline raphe between the two heads is not discrete, but can be established by using the superficially located short saphenous vein and sural nerve as markers. Once fully mobilized, the muscle can be passed through a subcutaneous tunnel to its destination, or, alternatively, the harvest incision can be connected with the knee wound. The wound edges are undermined and the gastrocnemius flap sutured deep to the wound margin (Fig. 4–10). A medium-thickness skin graft is then meshed, but not expanded, and immediately applied to the raw muscle surface using a tie-over dressing. The patient is confined to bed with the leg splinted for about 1 week prior to initiating leg dependency. The common peroneal nerve must be protected during harvest of the lateral gastrocnemius, but otherwise the technique is similar with either head.

With large or complex wounds, certain maneuvers may be necessary. To increase the arc of rotation the neurovascular pedicle may be isolated and the femoral condylar origin of the muscle divided, thereby creating a true island flap. If the muscle falls slightly short in reach or transverse width, the fascia may be scored or excised, permitting some expansion of the flap. The muscle may be split at its leading edge, creating independent flaps useful in obliterating small osseous defects. If the knee has been fused, the flap may pass directly through bone to fill an osseous defect.[63] Contour at the proximal rotation point may be improved by thinning the muscle.[68]

Muscle flaps harvested from the thigh have not gained popularity in reconstruction of the knee. In

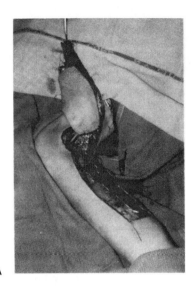

A

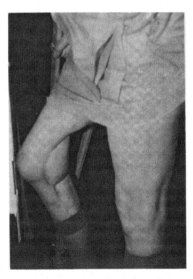

B

Figure 4–10. Medial gastrocnemius flap. **A.** Flap being raised from the posteromedial calf and being swung proximally to cover a defect behind the posteromedial knee. **B.** Final result showing flap over posteromedial knee, with skin graft covering the donor defect.

general, they provide little tissue, reach only the anterior–superior knee, and are unreliable. The most useful of these flaps is the vastus medialis, which can be advanced on its segmental pedicles to cover patellar defects.[69] A variant of this flap has been described whereby a composite of vascularized quadriceps femoris tendon, functional muscle, and overlying skin is used to reconstruct segmental loss of the quadriceps mechanism.[70] Vastus lateralis can be turned down as a distally based flap carried on the superior lateral genicular artery, but this flap requires sacrifice of part of the quadriceps mechanism, routinely undergoes partial necrosis, and should therefore be a clear second choice to the lateral gastrocnemius flap for lateral knee defects.[71] Distally based sartorious[72] and delayed gracilis[73] flaps have been used for coverage of small superior patellar defects.

Free Flaps. Not infrequently the situation arises where a compound wound exists about the knee and local fasciocutaneous or muscle flaps are either inadequate or unavailable because of associated trauma. In this circumstance, composite blocks of remote tissue can be transferred to the site needed and then revascularized using microsurgical anastomosis to local vascular supply. This technique confers the ability to customize soft tissue cover with provision of well-vascularized tissue supplying specific needs. Free flaps can be classified according to the constituents of the tissue composite transferred. The most common of these flaps contains skin and subcutaneous tissue, muscle, and bone in a variety of combinations according to need. Other tissues such as tendon and nerve may also be transferred as components of the vascularized flap if specifically required in reconstruction.

Age is not a specific contraindication to free flap surgery, there being significant experience reported in the literature in both children[74] and the elderly.[75,76] Likewise, preexisting occlusive vascular disease does not preclude microsurgical reconstruction, although simultaneous or staged arterial bypass reconstruction may be a necessary adjunct.[77,78] The general health of the patient must be sufficient to withstand an operation that typically requires at least 5 hours of general anesthesia.

Reported success rates for free tissue transfer to the lower extremity are on the order of 90% in recent series.[79,80] A direct relationship between free flap success and degree of lower extremity trauma and contamination has been demonstrated.[81-83] Survival and complication rates for free flaps are comparable to those for pedicled muscle flaps,[84] whereas morbidity, length of hospitalization, and cost show clear advantage over cross-leg flaps.[85] Postoperative microsurgical complications necessitate reoperation in 8 to 34% of reported series, with successful flap salvage in 75 to 100%.[86]

The issues of wound preparation and flap timing were discussed in a previous section. In summary, flap coverage should not proceed until a stable wound with bacteriologic control and a defined zone of injury has been obtained. Lower extremity angiography is generally indicated,[87] and in the case of free flaps with pedicle variability donor site angiography is prudent as well.

The attendant details are multiple and necessary to ensure the success of transfer. Preoperatively the patient must be well hydrated and premedicated with acetosalicylic acid as prophylaxis against thrombosis.[88] Intraoperative positioning of the patient is critical to avoid nerve traction and pressure sore complications. Despite multiple surgical fields, the patient can usually be positioned so that minimal or no intraoperative repositioning is required. Microsurgical anastomoses must be performed outside the zone of injury, this being established both by angiography and by examination of the tissues at surgery.[81,89] To this end, donor flaps of appropriate pedicle length must be selected and, where necessary, elongated by use of vein interposition grafts. For free flap coverage about the knee, depending on the wound and flap specifics, the superficial femoral,[90] popliteal,[91] or sural[92] arteries may be used. The vascular anastomoses may be end-to-end or end-to-side; however, particularly with respect to the artery, the latter is preferred for reasons of preservation of distal flow, reduction of vessel spasm, and demonstrated lower rates of thrombosis where size-discrepant vessels are involved.[93-95] The passage of the flap pedicle must be through a nonconstricting subcutaneous tunnel, although if necessary, skin graft may be applied directly to the pedicle.[96] Free flap margins should be meticulously sutured to the wound defect prior to recirculation of the flap as immediate flap edema otherwise makes contouring difficult. Muscle flaps should be advanced beneath undermined wound margins and the use of closed suction drainage is routine.

It is critical that all members of the medical team know the pedicle location and whether flow is affected by limb positioning. Postoperative care involves avoidance of limb dependency for about 2 weeks, euthermia, volume maintenance, a hemoglobin ideally in the range 100 g/dL to balance rheologic and oxygen-carrying considerations, and avoidance of nicotine products. Heparin is often used in single-bolus fashion intraoperatively, but is usually not continued postoperatively in uncomplicated elective microsurgery. Low-molecular-weight dextran has rheologic, antithrombotic, and vascular expansion benefits and is often infused in the first postoperative week.[97,98]

A large variety of modalities exist for monitoring free flaps postoperatively.[99] The critical period in terms of risk of pedicle thrombosis is the first week prior to endothelialization of the anastomotic sites. Monitoring devices may assess flap viability at the level of the pedicle or the terminal circulation within the flap, but the key to all methods is the ability to provide reliable, early detection of pedicle thrombosis allowing timely salvage. The most common flap monitoring systems in clinical use are clinical evaluation, Doppler evaluation of arterial and venous pedicle flow,[100] surface temperature monitoring,[101,102] and laser Doppler flowmetry[103-105] of the distal flap circulation.

Free flap selection must be based on wound requirements with consideration of size, specific contour needs, and other composite elements requiring reconstruction. The thinnest, vascularized covering can be provided by fascial flaps such as the temporoparietal fascial flap covered with skin graft; however, these do not confer the advantages of durability and pliability associated with skin or muscle flaps and are therefore not generally indicated. Pure skin and subcutaneous flaps exemplified by the scapular[106,107] and parascapular[108,109] flaps or fasciocutaneous flaps such as the radial forearm[110] provide superb patches to fill small, flat subcutaneous defects.[7] The most versatile coverage of large, nongraftable soft tissue defects about the knee, however, is obtained with free muscle flaps. When first used these were most often musculocutaneous units, but for reasons similar to those given with the respect to the gastrocnemius flap, the most common application today is a pure muscle flap with immediate skin graft coverage.[111-113] The skin-grafted muscle provides durable and pliable cover and, with the expected atrophy of 1% per day for 60 days, provides excellent contour restoration.[114,115] Significant experience with delayed bone grafting has shown free flaps to be reliable "operative windows" providing surgical access to underlying structures. Where this need is anticipated, an antibiotic-impregnated methyl methacrylate spacer should be placed at the initial flap surgery. Transferred tissue is also capable of providing a stable soft tissue envelope through which bone lengthening by the Ilizarov distraction method can be performed.[116]

The advantages of muscle free flaps are their potential size, ability to contour and fill wound deadspace, augmentation of fracture healing, and demonstrated efficacy in contaminated wounds and osteomyelitis.[117-123] The appropriately selected muscle–tendon unit also has the potential to replace missing tendon segments and, where required, to restore function by means of a reinnervated functional muscle transfer.[120] Restoration of sensibility in free flaps has been achieved by suture of recipient site nerves to cutaneous sensory nerves within skin flaps or to motor nerves in the case of muscle flaps.[121] The former method is clearly the most effective, but neither has proven necessary to prevent late flap ulceration. Without nerve suture, sufficient protective sensibility is achieved by a combination of peripheral neurotization of the flap and deep-pressure sensation.

The most commonly used free muscle flap about the knee is the latissimus dorsi because of its large size and relative thinness which allows contouring (Fig. 4–11).[90,122,123] It possesses a long vascular pedicle of wide internal diameter and its internal vascular anatomy allows partial harvest with functional preservation of the remaining muscle or segmental splitting of the transferred muscle.[124,125] For smaller defects, the rectus abdominis[126] and gracilis[127] muscles often suffice.

Cross-Leg Flaps. Prior to the advent of pedicled muscle and free flaps, cross-leg flaps represented the only method to close large, nongraftable lower extremity defects. With the flap armamentarium now available, cross-leg flaps have few indications. Situations in which this technique may still find application are inadequate recipient site vasculature, previous failed free tissue transfer, or patient refusal to undergo free tissue transfer.

Earlier reviews of experience with cross-leg flaps reported exceptionally high complication rates, with flap necrosis in 40% of cases, infection in 28% and nerve compression due to plaster fixation in 10%.[128] Recent series using the principles of fasciocutaneous blood supply[129] and immobilization with external fixators[130] have reported lower complication rates, with successful tissue transfer in 90% of cases.[131]

A variant of the cross-leg flap is the cross-leg free flap whereby a free flap is anastomosed to recipient vessels on the contralateral leg and pedicled at the same stage into the ipsilateral leg wound. The pedicle is divided between 4 and 6 weeks. Indications for this procedure are the presence of a wound of sufficient size and depth to require free tissue transfer with no available local recipient vasculature because of trauma or vascular occlusive disease.[132]

Management of Specific Soft Tissue Problems

Skin Avulsion

Skin avulsion injuries are produced by the application of tangential forces to the skin surface which produce shearing between the relatively mobile subcutaneous tissue and fixed muscular fascia. This severs the fasciocutaneous and musculocutaneous perforators to the skin, effectively producing random pattern flaps of varying dimension.[133] In addition, there is usually a crush component to the injury that further compromises the skin circulation. Major skin avulsions are most frequently seen in the lower extremity and are usually the product of pedestrian "run over" injuries, often involving the double rear tires of heavy vehicles.

Two forms of skin avulsion injury have been described.[134] In the common avulsion injury the open wound involves most of the undermined area, whereas in the atypical presentation the open wound is small and extensively undermined areas are concealed. Both types of presentation are associated with damage to under-

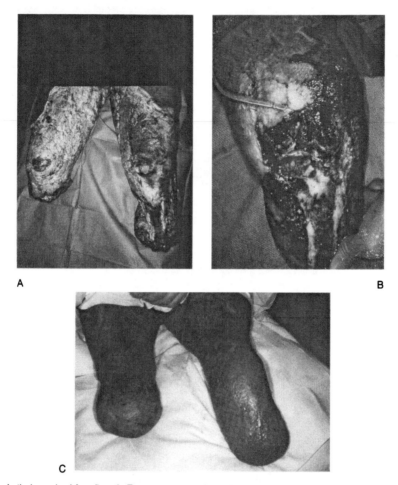

Figure 4–11. Latissimus dorsi free flap. **A**, Traumatic amputations of both lower extremities with associated burns and skin loss. **B**. Closeup of left below-knee amputation, with exposed anterior half of remaining tibia. A free flap was used to cover the tibia to preserve a below-the-knee amputation. **C**. Final appearance after free muscle flap and skin grafting.

lying muscle, with fractures present in greater than 80%. Multiple fractures in the involved limb are present in more than half of cases and these tend to cluster around the knee.[135,136] Coexistent life-threatening trauma is present in two thirds of cases.

Initial management involves consideration of the need for angiography and fasciotomy followed by bony stabilization. The extent of the degloved skin must then be determined by operative exploration. In atypical avulsion injuries, incisions for exposure should be made cognizant of the patterns of cutaneous blood supply. With this pattern of injury it is important to recognize the considerable potential for buried necrotic tissue on the deep aspect of the subcutaneous plane. Devitalized muscle and ecchymotic skin should be excised. Skin with briskly bleeding dermis should be preserved. Difficulty is encountered in determining skin viability in areas intermediate between these extremes. Intravenous fluorescein injection (15 mg/kg) with excision of poorly or nonfluorescing skin adds some measure of quantitation. Similarly, quantitative dermofluorometry using smaller repetitive doses of fluorescein and a fluorometer for analysis has been suggested as a more precise method to gauge viability, but experience is limited.[134] Generally, skin showing poor dermal bleeding or spotty fluorescence should be primarily debrided.

Closure of degloved skin is a serious mistake and results in progressive flap necrosis and high risk of sepsis. Following debridement, many of these wounds are suitable for immediate closure. Full-thickness skin graft harvested from the degloved skin produces greater than 90% graft take and any remaining areas can be covered by meshed split-thickness skin graft harvested from noninjured skin. In some cases the underlying zone of injury is diffuse and serial debridement with delayed primary closure is appropriate. Skin grafts harvested from avulsed skin can be refrigerated for up to 2 weeks in this scenario.

Vascular Injury

Diagnosis of vascular injury is based on hard signs such as arterial bleeding, absent or diminished pulses, expanding or pulsatile hematoma, bruit, pallor, paresthesia, and coolness of the extremity. These signs are individually associated with a 75% likelihood of major vascular injury and greater than 90% likelihood if multiple signs are present.[137] Soft diagnostic signs are proximity of penetrating injury to a major neurovascular bundle, anatomically related neurologic deficit, unexplained shock, and hematoma adjacent to a major vessel. In patients with documented vascular injury, 10 to 15% have intact pedal pulses and 10 to 27% show no signs of vascular injury on initial examination.[138]

Angiography is performed if the preceding signs are present or in injuries with a high probability of vascular trauma, such as knee dislocation and gunshot wound. A formal biplane study is indicated unless other injuries, shock, limb ischemia, or compartment syndrome necessitates immediate exploration. In this case, a single-shot intraoperative study can be performed. In the case of a stable patient with a questionable vascular injury, angiography should be performed followed by exploration if positive and serial physical examination if negative.

Penetrating trauma is the most common cause of popliteal artery trauma followed by blunt injury secondary to fractures and dislocation.[139] Approximately one third of knee dislocations have associated vascular trauma,[140] and the most common anterior form of dislocation has the highest associated risk. Even in low-velocity dislocation such as occurs in athletics there is sufficient risk of popliteal artery trauma to justify angiography despite the presence of normal pedal pulses.[141] Penetrating trauma tends to produce partial or complete transection arterial injury with or without associated venous injury. Blunt trauma, in addition to transection injuries, frequently causes arterial contusion with intimal tear, and it is this injury that is made difficult to diagnose by the frequent preservation of distal flow. Less common vascular lesions are acute arterial venous fistulas and missile emboli.

Collateral circulation does not adequately sustain leg perfusion in the presence of popliteal artery disruption. Military experience has shown that failure to reestablish popliteal flow within 8 hours of injury is associated with an 86% amputation rate, whereas repair within 8 hours results in 80% salvage.[142] The essentials of operative management of popliteal vascular trauma are four-compartment leg fasciotomy, skeletal reduction and stabilization, temporary vascular shunts where life-threatening injuries supersede, liberal use of saphenous vein interposition grafts, popliteal vein repair, and completion angiography.

Nerve Injury

Knee trauma may be associated with a variety of lesions of the sciatic, tibial or peroneal nerves. A variety of mechanisms account for nerve lesions at the knee level, including penetrating trauma, gunshot wounds, fracture shards or displaced fractures, knee dislocation, varus or hyperextension injuries, and iatrogenic accidents. With knee trauma it is important to establish whether the nerve deficit was immediate or delayed, the latter suggesting an ischemic rather than disruptive etiology. Partial nerve deficits in the setting of penetrating trauma should be explored; however, following blunt trauma partial deficits suggest a nerve injury in continuity, and delayed exploration is justified. Peroneal neuropathy is the most common lower extremity palsy; when partial, the deep division is most frequently affected, giving rise to "foot drop." With tibial neuropathy above the branches to the gastrocnemius muscles, ankle plantar flexion is extremely weak, but in injury distal to the popliteal fossa, the main deficit is plantar anesthesia.

Seddon classified traumatic nerve injuries as neuropraxia with localized ischemic demyelination, axonotmesis with intact endoneural tubes but interrupted axons, and neurotmesis with nerve severance.[143] Neuropractic lesions tend to recover spontaneously and fairly completely by 4 months. They are characterized by lack of Wallerian degeneration in the nerve segment distal to the zone of injury, and for this reason nerve conduction studies show maintenance of distal conduction. By distinction, all higher grades of nerve injury experience Wallerian degeneration with loss of distal conduction at about 72 hours. Axonal regrowth occurs from the node of Ranvier proximal to the site of injury at a rate of 1 mm per day, with patient age the chief limiting factor. Axonotmetic lesions maintain fascicular alignment, and therefore do not require early operative intervention and tend to recover better than neurotmetic lesions where there is discontinuity. This schema is somewhat of an oversimplification, but provides a useful reference in decision making.

Penetrating knee trauma tends to produce neurotmesis. The incidence of peroneal nerve palsy following knee dislocation is 16 to 18% and about one quarter of these have associated arterial injury.[144] Knee dislocation is associated with neuropraxia, axonotmesis, or neurotmesis of an avulsive nature with a wide zone of injury within the nerve. Similarly, gunshot wounds can create all three types of nerve injury.

A neurologic deficit in the setting of penetrating trauma should undergo early exploration and repair. The results of acute nerve repair are better than generally believed. If studies prior to 1975 are excluded, functional success rates for common peroneal and tibial nerve repairs are greater than 80%.[11] Primary nerve repair should be performed before the onset of Wallerian degeneration at 72 hours postinjury to allow intraoperative fascicular testing for fascicular alignment. Only in contaminated or high-energy wounds should repair be delayed.

Judgments with respect to neurologic deficit associated with knee dislocation are more difficult because of the traction mechanism and varied nerve pathology. If operative intervention is mandated for other reasons, most frequently vascular repair, the major nerves must be explored to examine their continuity. Lesions with the nerve in continuity should be followed expectantly for an advancing Tinel's sign or functional return for 6 months prior to exploration and possible nerve grafting.[145] Discontinuity lesions should be sutured to adjacent soft tissue to prevent retraction and definitively repaired, usually by interposition nerve graft, at about 3 weeks postinjury when the zone of injury has demarcated.[146] In the case of postdislocation nerve deficits that have not been explored, nerve conduction studies after 72 hours will distinguish neuropraxia from higher-grade lesions. The problem is then to distinguish whether the nerve is in continuity. Results of nerve grafting have been so poor that many surgeons feel exploration is unwarranted. Studies of functional return in appropriately timed nerve grafts at the popliteal level are few and show variable results with occasional functional motor recovery, but poor sensory return.[147] According to Wood, graft lengths of 8 cm or less have a reasonable expectation for recovery when done within 6 months of injury.[145] Our position, based on the high probability of peroneal nerve avulsion, is to recommend early exploration in all cases and then follow the regimen outlined earlier depending on nerve continuity.

Gunshot Wounds

The wounding power of a missile relates to its transmitted energy, which is determined by the equation kinetic energy $= \frac{1}{2}mv^2$. As predicted by this relationship, bullet velocity is the most important determinant of energy imparted to the tissues. Civilian firearms are generally low-velocity weapons, with muzzle velocity in the range 200 to 300 m/s. Military rifles are high-velocity weapons, with velocities of 800 to 1000 m/s and correspondingly greater wounding potential. Damage is also determined by the size, shape, and stability of the missile and the density of the structures it contacts.[133]

Missiles damage tissue by laceration, crushing, and cavitation. The permanent bullet tract roughly approximates missile size, but with high-velocity missiles the temporary cavity can reach 30 times missile size, leaving a large zone of tissue contamination and devitalization. The amount of tissue damage from the temporary cavitation is directly proportional to tissue density and inversely proportional to tissue elasticity.[148] Muscle and bone, which are relatively dense, sustain significant damage, whereas the elasticity of skin may produce a small entrance wound disguising profound underlying injury.

Shotgun injuries have been classified by the depth of pellet penetration, which is determined by the weapon distance.[149] Type I injuries inflicted at more than 7 m rarely penetrate the deep fascia. Type II injuries inflicted between 3 and 7 m produce deep wounds, with bone and joint injury in 50% and vascular injury in 35%. Type III injuries produced at less than about 3 m produce maximum tissue destruction and tend to carry shell wadding and clothing into the wound.[150]

Low-velocity wounds are treated similarly to other penetrating trauma. Angiography and wound exploration are performed on the basis of functional deficit, and injured structures are repaired primarily. If there is no functional deficit the wound is debrided, irrigated by jet pulse lavage, and allowed to heal by delayed primary closure or secondary intention.[133]

High-velocity missile injuries and close-range shotgun wounds require assessment of limb viability. Massive injuries are best treated with early definitive amputation.[151,152] Limb salvage requires debridement of devitalized tissue on a serial basis until the zone of injury is defined. Constricting fascial envelopes which impair the vascularity of edematous muscle must be incised. In shotgun wounds the zone of injury can be predicted by the radiographic distribution of pellets. Fractures are stabilized by external fixation. Debridement includes the inspection of potentially involved neurovascular structures. Major vessels require repair which often involves extraanatomic bypass outside the zone of injury. Nerves are examined under magnification and are resected only if clearly damaged. Transected nerve ends are sutured to adjacent soft tissue to prevent retraction. Remaining neurovascular structures are covered by any available healthy local tissue. Following serial debridement delayed primary wound closure is performed, which often requires flap coverage. Definitive nerve repair should be performed as soon as stable wound coverage is obtained.

Open Joint Injuries

Of all open joint wounds, the knee is the major joint most frequently involved.[153,154] In a civilian population, the majority of these are caused by vehicular trauma or gunshot wounds. An open joint injury may occur by direct penetrating trauma or by extension into the knee through compound periarticular fractures. Knee dislocations are open in 20 to 30% of cases.[142] The criteria for diagnosis of an open joint include a visible wound, palpable opening into the joint, air or foreign body in the joint on x-ray, and saline extravasation through the wound during arthrocentesis. A classification of open joint injuries has been proposed based on the extent of injury to both extracapsular soft tissue and intraarticular structures.[153]

Initial treatment requires wound culture and broad-spectrum antibiotics. Meticulous debridement of the wound including formal arthrotomy, irrigation of the knee joint, and possibly arthroscopy is required. Free cartilage pieces and foreign bodies are removed from the joint. In clean, debrided wounds the synovium and joint capsule are closed. If the adequacy of debridement is uncertain or the time since injury exceeds 12 hours, joint closure is delayed. The overlying wound, but not the joint cavity, is packed with saline dressings. In all cases, a delayed primary closure of the subcutaneous tissue and skin is performed.

Closed systems of irrigation and suction drainage have not been found to yield superior results and are associated with a significant risk of iatrogenic joint contamination.[154] Intraarticular antibiotic instillation is likewise unnecessary as parenteral antibiotics achieve bactericidal levels in joint fluid. Use of a closed suction drain for 24 to 48 hours to allow egress of residual contaminated joint fluid is considered prudent.[153] Antibiotics are continued for 72 hours and then discontinued or changed to culture-specific therapy for 2 weeks in the event of established joint infection. The degree of associated soft tissue injury determines the required period of knee immobilization, but where soft tissue allows, and particularly in the presence of cartilaginous injury or intraarticular fracture, early passive motion may reduce arthrofibrosis and improve results. In the situation of delayed presentation of an open knee joint, function may be salvageable using treatment as outlined up to 10 weeks postinjury.[155]

Definitive soft tissue closure of the open knee joint follows the guidelines already established with respect to the reconstructive ladder. Closure should proceed only if there is no evidence of joint infection. Open joint wounds require flap coverage, which, depending on the defect and extent of trauma, may consist of local fasciocutaneous[36,39] or muscle flaps. The medial[156] and lateral[60,157] gastrocnemius, vastus medialis[69,70] and lat-eralis,[71] and sartorius[72] muscles have all been used for this purpose. For large wounds free tissue transfer may be required.[90,158]

Exposed Prosthesis

Hardware may become exposed in the posttraumatic knee as a result of skin necrosis or flap loss. The exposed prosthesis may be a plate or a joint prosthesis. Osteomyelitis is the most serious consequence of plate exposure and can lead to infected nonunion. In knee arthroplasty, infection can necessitate prosthesis removal and lead to loss of bone substance and interference with subsequent procedures.

An exposed plate in the periarticular area should be dealt with by culture-specific antibiotics, debridement, and flap coverage. This should be done without delay, although there is not a clear association between length of exposure and likelihood of success. There is, however, a strong correlation between a positive wound culture and a negative outcome which likely relates to the inadequecy of debridement when hardware is retained.[159] Adequate debridement frequently requires removal of the hardware with subsequent stabilization by other methods, such as an external fixator. The issue of how best to deal with an exposed joint prosthesis has been examined by a number of authors. Failure to respect preexisting lacerations and surgical incisions appears to be a common causative factor. The problem may present as impending exposure with superficial skin necrosis or frank exposure with a joint sinus, deep dehiscence, or visible prosthesis.[160] It is important to have a clear understanding of whether wound breakdown is the primary event or merely a sequela of prosthetic infection.[147] In the latter case, successful salvage is not as likely.[161] Management of impending or frank exposure consists of knee immobilization and culture-specific antibiotics. As is the case with exposed plates, there is no apparent correlation between duration of exposure and successful salvage,[162] although early intervention is recommended.[163] It is generally agreed that attempts at secondary suture or skin graft are unlikely to be successful.[161,164] In the absence of frank infection and where skin loss is minimal, local fasciocutaneous flaps are adequate.[36,160,165] For more extensive wounds or frankly infected prostheses, antibiotic joint irrigation and gastrocnemius muscle flap coverage are recommended.[160,162,163,166]

Amputation Stump Coverage

Compared with a more proximal amputation, the below-knee amputation has decreased work of ambulation, more natural gait, and less complex prosthetic fitting. It is possible to fit a prosthesis to a short below-knee stump with as little as 6 cm of tibial shaft. For these reasons, limb salvage surgery should direct considerable effort to the preservation of a below-knee level for amputation.

At the time of the initial trauma, the concept of "spare parts" surgery may permit below-knee stump preservation. The plantar skin from the amputated leg has been used for stump coverage as either a pedicled[167] or a free tissue[168] transfer. Local muscle coverage of the stump may be obtained by a musculocutaneous V–Y advancement of the gastrocnemius remnant.[63] Both heads of the muscle are detached and anterior advancement of 3 cm with primary closure of overlying skin is possible.[120] The vastus lateralis turndown flap is also occasionally useful in stump coverage.[72,120]

Free flap transfer to preserve a below-knee level has been demonstrated worthwhile.[168,169] Free skin flaps have a lower incidence of late ulceration than does skin-grafted muscle, but use of a sensory flap does not appear necessary as all patients develop deep-pressure sensibility. The development of flap redundancy secondary to muscle atrophy correlates with late ulceration, and for this reason the initial flap inset must be well tailored. Tissue expansion of adjacent skin and subcutaneous tissue may be helpful in late below-knee stump resurfacing.[24]

References

1. Cormack GC, Lamberty BGH. *The Arterial Anatomy of Skin Flaps.* Edinburgh: Churchill Livingstone; 1986:224–225.
2. Clemente CD, ed. *Gray's Anatomy.* Philadelphia, Lea & Febiger; 1985:1229–1232.
3. Yaremchuk MJ, Brumback RJ, Manson PN, et al. Acute and definitive management of traumatic osteocutaneous defects of the lower extremity. *Plast Reconstr Surg.* 1987;80:1–12.
4. *Advanced Trauma Life Support Manual.* Chicago: Committee on Trauma, American College of Surgeons; 1983.
5. McAndrew MP, Lantz BA. Initial care of massively traumatized lower extremities. *Clin Orthop.* 1989;243:20–29.
6. Helfet DL, Howey T, Sanders R, et al. Limb salvage versus amputation: Preliminary results of the mangled extremity severity score. *Clin Orthop.* 1990;256:80–86.
7. Arnez ZM. Immediate reconstruction of the lower extremity—An update. *Clin Plast Surg.* 1991;19:449–457.
8. Patzakis MJ, Wilkins J, Moore TM. Use of antibiotics in open tibial fractures. *Clin Orthop.* 1983;178:31–35.
9. Calhoun JH, Mader JT. Antibiotic beads in the management of surgical infections. *Am J Surg.* 1989;157:443–449.
10. Henry SL, Ostermann PAW, Seligson D. The prophylactic use of antibiotic impregnated beads in open fractures. *J Trauma.* 1990;30:1231–1238.
11. Walton RL, Rothkopf D. Judgement and approach for management of severe lower extremity injuries. *Clin Plast Surg.* 1991;18:525–543.

12. Brumback RJ. Wound debridement. In: Yaremchuk MJ, Burgess AR, Brumback RJ, eds. *Lower Extremity Salvage and Reconstruction.* New York: Elsevier Science; 1989:71–80.
13. Byrd HS, Cierny G, Tebbetts JD. The management of open tibial fractures with associated soft-tissue loss: External pin fixation with early flap coverage. *Plast Reconstr Surg.* 1981;68:73–79.
14. Godina M. Early microsurgical reconstruction of complex trauma of the extremities. *Plast Reconstr Surg.* 1986;78:285–292.
15. Francel TJ, Vander Kolk CA, Hoopes JE, et al. Microvascular soft-tissue transplantation for reconstruction of acute open tibial fractures: Timing of coverage and long-term functional results. *Plast Reconstr Surg.* 1992;89:478–487.
16. Fischer MD, Gustilo RB, Varecka Tf, et al. The timing of flap coverage, bone-grafting, and intramedullary nailing in patients who have a fracture of the tibial shaft with extensive soft-tissue injury. *J Bone Joint Surg Am.* 1991;73:1316–1322.
17. Chen SHT, Wei F-C, Chen H-C, et al. Emergency free-flap transfer for reconstruction of acute complex extremity wounds. *Plast Reconstr Surg.* 1992;89:882–888.
18. Robson MC, Krizek TJ. Predicting skin graft survival. *J Trauma.* 1973;13:213–217.
19. Salisbury RB. Use of the mesh skin graft in treatment of massive casualty wounds. *Plast Reconstr Surg.* 1967;40:161–162.
20. Ramakrishnan EM, Jayaraman V, Ramachandran K, et al. De-epithelialized turnover flaps in burns. *Plast Reconstr Surg.* 1988;82:262–266.
21. Rees RS, Nanney LB, Fleming P. et al. Tissue expansion: Its role in traumatic below-knee amputations. *Plast Reconstr Surg.* 1986;77:133–137.
22. Filho PTB, Neves RI, Gemperli R, et al. Soft-tissue expansion in lower extremity reconstruction. *Clin Plast Surg.* 1991;18:593–599.
23. Weinzweig N, Dowden RV, Stulberg BN. The use of tissue expansion to allow reconstruction of the knee: A case report. *J Bone Joint Surg Am.* 1987;69:1238–1240.
24. May JW, Sheppard J. Reconstruction of the stump after below-the-knee amputation. Soft-tissue expansion and local muscle rotation flaps: A case report. *J Bone Joint Surg Am.* 1987;69:1240–1245.
25. Manders EK, Oaks TE, Au VK, et al; Soft-tissue expansion in the lower extremity. *Plast Reconstr Surg.* 1988;81:208–217.
26. Cormack GC, Lamberty BGH. *The arterial anatomy of skin flaps.* Edinburgh: Churchill Livingstone; 1986:93.
27. Ponten B. The fasciocutaneous flap: Its use in soft-tissue defects of the lower leg. *Br J Plast Surg.* 1981;34:215–220.
28. Haertsch PA. The blood supply to the skin of the leg: A post-mortem investigation. *Br J Plast Surg.* 1981;34:470–477.
29. Barclay TL Cardoso E, Sharpe DT, et al. Repair of lower leg injuries with fasciocutaneous flaps. *Br J Plast Surg.* 1982;35:127–132.
30. Carriquiry A, Costa MA, Vasconez LO. An anatomic study of the septocutaneous vessels of the leg. *Plast Reconstr Surg.* 1985;76:354–361.
31. Cormack GC, Lamberty BGH. A classification of fasciocutaneous flaps according to their pattern of vascularization. *Br J Plast Surg.* 1984;37:80–87.
32. Fix RJ, Vasconez LO. Fasciocutaneous flaps in recon-

struction of the lower extremity. *Clin Plast Surg*. 1991; 18:571–582.

33. Mathes SJ, Alpert BS, Chang N. Use of the muscle flap in chronic osteomyelitis: Experimental and clinical correlation. *Plast Reconstr Surg*. 1982;69:815–828.

34. Bailey MH, Mossie RD, Yungbluth M, et al. The interaction of transferred tissue and osteomyelitis in the rabbit. *Surg Forum*. 1987;38:629–633.

35. Dickson WA, Dickson MG, Roberts AHN. The complications of fasciocutaneous flaps. *Ann Plast Surg*. 1987;19:234–237.

36. Lewis VL, Mossie RD, Stulberg DS. The fasciocutaneous flap: A conservation approach to the exposed knee joint. *Plast Reconstr Surg*. 1990;85:252–257.

37. Haertsch P. The surgical plane in the leg. *Br J Plast Surg*. 1981;34:464–469.

38. Tolhurst DE, Haeseker B, Zeeman RJ. The development of the fasciocutaneous flap and its clinical applications. *Plast Reconstr Surg*. 1983;71:597–605.

39. Moscona AR, Govrin-Yehudain J, Hirshowitz B. The island fasciocutaneous flap: A new type of flap for defects of the knee. *Br J Plast Surg*. 1985;38:512–514.

40. Maryuama Y. Bilobed fasciocutaneous flap. *Br J Plast Surg*. 1985;38:512–517.

41. Hallock GG. Local knee random fasciocutaneous flaps. *Ann Plast Surg*. 1989;23:289–296.

42. Maruyama Y, Iwahira Y. Popliteo-posterior thigh fasciocutaneous island flap for closure around the knee. *Br J Plast Surg*. 1989;42:140–143.

43. Satoh K, Gyoutoku H, Usami Y. Suprapopliteal flap. *Ann Plast Surg*. 1990;24:459–466.

44. Laitung JKG. The lower posterolateral thigh flap. *Br J Plast Surg*. 1989;42:133–139.

45. Hayashi A, Maryuama Y. The lateral genicular artery flap. *Ann Plast Surg*. 1990;24:310–317.

46. Acland RD, Schusterman M, Godina M, et al. The saphenous neurovascular free flap. *Plast Reconstr Surg*. 1981;67:763–774.

47. Walton RL, Bunkis J. The posterior calf fasciocutaneous free flap. *Plast Reconstr Surg*. 1984;74:76–85.

48. Walton RL, Matory WE, Petry JJ. The posterior calf fascial free flap. *Plast Reconstr Surg*. 1985;76:914–924.

49. Satoh K, Fukuya F, Matsui A, et al. Lower leg reconstruction using a sural fasciocutaneous flap. *Ann Plast Surg*. 1989;23:97–103.

50. Li Z, Liu K, Lin Y, et al. Lateral sural cutaneous artery island flap in the treatment of soft tissue defects at the knee. *Br J Plast Surg*. 1990;43:546–550.

51. Rocha JFR, Gilbert A. The anterior tibial flap. In: Strauch B, Vasconez LO, Hall-Findlay EJ, eds. *Grabb's Encyclopedia of Flaps*. Boston: Little, Brown; 1990: 1761–1764.

52. Morrison WA, Shen TY. Anterior tibial artery flap: Anatomy and case report. *Br J Plast Surg*. 1987;40:230–235.

53. Torii S, Namiki Y, Hayashi Y. Anterolateral leg island flap. *Br J Plast Surg*. 1987;40:236–240.

54. Yoshimura M, Shimada T, Imura S, et al. Peroneal island flap for skin defects in the lower extremity. *J Bone Joint Surg Am*. 1985;67:935–941.

55. Ger R. Muscle transposition for treatment and prevention of chronic post-traumatic osteomyelitis of the tibia. *J Bone Joint Surg Am*. 1977;59:784–791.

56. Chang N, Mathes SJ. Comparison of the effect of bacterial inoculation in musculocutaneous and random-pattern flaps. *Plast Reconstr Surg*. 1982;70:1–9.

57. Richards RR, McKee MD, Paitich CB, et al. A comparison of the effects of skin coverage and muscle flap coverage on the early strength of union at the site of osteotomy after devascularization of a segment of canine tibia. *J Bone Joint Surg Am*. 1991;73:1323–1330.

58. Mathes SJ, Nahai F. Classification of the vascular anatomy of muscles: Experimental and clinical correlation. *Plast Reconstr Surg*. 1981;67:177–187.

59. McCraw JB, Fishman JH, Sharzer LA. The versatile gastrocnemius myocutaneous flap. *Plast Reconstr Surg*. 1978;62:15–23.

60. Elsahy NI. Cover of the exposed knee joint by the lateral head of the gastrocnemius. *Br J Plast Surg*. 1978; 31:136–137.

61. Feldman JJ, Cohen BE, May JW. The medial gastrocnemius myocutaneous flap. *Plast Reconstr Surg*. 1978; 61:533–539.

62. Kroll SS, Marcadis A. Aesthetic considerations of the gastrocnemius myocutaneous flap. *Plast Reconstr Surg*. 1987;79:67–71.

63. Arnold PG, Mixter RC. Making the most of the gastrocnemius muscles. *Plast Reconstr Surg*. 1983;72:38–438.

64. McCraw JB, Arnold PG. Gastrocnemius muscle and musculocutaneous flaps. In: *McCraw and Arnold's Atlas of Muscle and Musculocutaneous Flaps*. Norfolk: Hampton Press; 1986:491–543.

65. Yaremchuk MJ, Manson PN. Local and free flap donor sites for lower-extremity reconstruction. In: Yaremchuk MJ, Burgess AR, Brumback RJ, eds. *Lower Extremity Salvage and Reconstruction*. New York: Elsevier Science; 1989;117–157.

66. Alpert BS, Nahai F, Vasconez LO. Lower extremity complications. In: Mathes SJ, Nahai F, eds. *Clinical Applications for Muscle and Musculocutaneous Flaps*. St. Louis: CV Mosby; 1982;581–584.

67. Guzman-Stein G, Fix RJ, Vasconez LO. Muscle flap coverage for the lower extremity. *Clin Plast Surg*. 1991;18:545–552.

68. Kroll SS. Radical thinning of the pedicle of a gastrocnemius musculocutaneous flap. *Ann Plast Surg*. 1989; 23:363–368.

69. Arnold PG, Prunes-Carrillo F. Vastus medialis muscle flap for functional closure of the exposed knee joint. *Plast Reconstr Surg*. 1981;68:69–72.

70. Tobin GR. Vastus medialis myocutaneous and myocutaneous tendinous composite flaps. *Plast Reconstr Surg*. 1985;75:677–684.

71. Swartz WM, Ramasastry SS, McGill JR, et al. Distally based vastus lateralis muscle flap for coverage of wounds about the knee. *Plast Reconstr Surg*. 1987;80:252–263.

72. Petty CT, Hogue RJ. Closure of an exposed knee joint by use of a sartorius muscle flap. *Plast Reconstr Surg*. 1978;62:458–461.

73. Mathes SJ, Vasconez LO. Lower extremity: Reconstruction. In: Mathes SJ, Nahai F, eds. *Clinical Applications for Muscle and Musculocutaneous Flaps*. St. Louis: CV Mosby; 1982:532–580.

74. Banic A, Wulff K Latissimus dorsi free flaps for total repair of extensive lower leg injuries in children. *Plast Reconstr Surg*. 1987;79:769–775.

75. Dabb RW, Davis RM. Latissimus dorsi free flaps in the elderly: An alternative to below-knee amputation. *Plast Reconstr Surg*. 1984;73:633–640.

76. Chick LR, Walton RL, reus W, et al. Free flaps in the elderly. *Plast Reconstr Surg*. 1992;90:87–94.

77. Colen LB. Limb salvage in the patient with severe

peripheral vascular disease: The role of microsurgical free-tissue transfer. *Plast Reconstr Surg.* 1987;79:389–395.
78. Chowdary RP, Celani VJ, Goodreau JJ, et al. Free-tissue transfers for limb salvage utilizing in situ saphenous vein bypass conduit as the inflow. *Plast Reconstr Surg.* 1991;87:529–534.
79. Khouri RK, Shaw WW. Reconstruction of the lower extremity with microvascular free flaps: A 10-year experience with 304 consecutive cases. *J Trauma.* 1989; 29:1086–1094.
80. Melissunos EG, Parks DH. Post-trauma reconstruction with free tissue transfer—Analysis of 442 consecutive cases. *J Trauma.* 1989;29:1095–1103.
81. Weiland AJ, Moore JR, Daniel RK. The efficacy of free-tissue transfer in the treatment of osteomyelitis. *J Bone Joint Surg Am.* 1984;66:181–193.
82. Swartz WM, Mears DC. The role of free-tissue transfers in lower-extremity reconstruction. *Plast Reconstr Surg.* 1985;76:364–373.
83. Byrd HS, Spicer TE, Cierney G. Management of open tibial fractures. *Plast Reconstr Surg.* 1985;76:719–728.
84. Zook EG, Russell RC, Asaadi M. A comparative study of free and pedicle flaps for lower extremity wounds. *Ann Plast Surg.* 1986;17:21–33.
85. Serafin D, Georgiade NG, Smith DH. Comparison of free flaps with pedicle flaps for coverage of defects of the leg or foot. *Plast Reconstr Surg.* 1977;59:493–499.
86. Lineaweaver WC, Buncke HJ. Complications. In: Buncke HJ, ed. *Microsurgery: Transplantation–Replantation: An Atlas–Text.* Philadelphia: Lea and Febiger; 1991:722–728.
87. Grotting JC. Prevention of complications and corrections of postoperative problems in microsurgery of the lower extremity. *Clin Plast Surg.* 1991;18:485–489.
88. Lineaweaver WC, Valauri FA. Pharmacology. In: Buncke HJ, ed. *Microsurgery: Transplantation–Replantation: An Altas–Text.* Philadelphia: Lea and Febiger; 1991:696–714.
89. Serafin D, Sabatier RE, Morris RL, et al. Reconstruction of the lower extremity with vascularized composite tissue: Improved tissue survival and specific indications. *Plast Reconstr Surg.* 1980;66:230–241.
90. Fisher J, Cooney WP. Designing the latissimus dorsi free flap for knee coverage. *Ann Plast Surg.* 1983;11:554–562.
91. Godina M, Arnez ZM, Lister GD. Preferential use of the posterior approach to blood vessels of the lower leg in microvascular surgery. *Plast Reconstr Surg.* 1991; 88:287–291.
92. Johnson PE, Harris GD, Nagle DJ, et al. The sural artery and vein as recipient vessels in free flap reconstruction about the knee. *J Reconstr Microsurg.* 1987; 3:233–241.
93. Parsa FD, Spira M. Evaluation of anastomotic techniques in the experimental transfer of free skin flaps. *Plast Reconstr Surg.* 1979;63:696–699.
94. Godina M. Preferential use of end-to-side arterial anastomoses in free flap transfers. *Plast Reconstr Surg.* 1979;64:673–682.
95. Rao VK, Morrison WA, Angus JA. Comparison of vascular hemodynamics in experimental models of microvascular anastomoses. *Plast Reconstr Surg.* 1983; 71:241–247.
96. McDonald HD, Buncke HJ, Goodstein WA. Split thick-

ness skin grafts in microvascular surgery. *Plast Reconstr Surg.* 1981;68:731–736.
97. Davidson SF, Brantley SK, Das SK. Comparison of single-dose antithrombotic agents in the prevention of microvascular thrombosis. *J Hand Surg.* 1991;16A:585–589.
98. Ketchum LD. Pharmacological alterations in the clotting mechanism: Use in microvascular surgery. *J Hand Surg.* 1978;3:403–415.
99. Buncke HJ, Lineaweaver WC, Valauri FA, et al. Monitoring. In: Buncke HJ. ed. *Microsurgery: Transplantation–Replantation: An Atlas–Text.* Philadelphia: Lea and Febiger; 1991:715–721.
100. Harrison DH, Girling M, Mott G. Methods of assessing the viability of free flap transfer during the postoperative period. *Clin Plast Surg.* 1983:10:21–36.
101. Kaufman T, Granick MS, Hurwitz DJ, et al. Is experimental muscle flap temperature a reliable indicator of its viability? *Ann Plast Surg.* 1987;19:34–41.
102. Khouri RK, Shaw WW. Monitoring of free flaps with surface-temperature records: Is it reliable? *Plast Reconstr Surg.* 1992;89:495–499.
103. Walkinshaw M, Holloway A, Bulkley A, et al. Clinical evaluation of laser doppler blood flow measurements in free flaps. *Ann Plast Surg.* 1987;18:212–217.
104. Jenkins S, Sepka R, Barwick WJ. Routine use of laser doppler flowmetry for monitoring autologous tissue transplants. *Ann Plast Surg.* 21:423–426.
105. Clinton MS, Sepka RS, Bristol D, et al. Establishment of normal ranges of laser doppler blood flow in autologous tissue transplants. *Plast Reconstr Surg.* 1991; 87:299–309.
106. Gilbert A, Teot L. The free scapular flap. *Plast Reconstr Surg.* 1982;69:601–604.
107. Urbaniak JR, Koman LA, Goldner RD, et al. The vascularized cutaneous scapular flap. *Plast Reconstr Surg.* 1982;69:772–778.
108. Nassif TM, Vidal L, Bovet JL, et al. The parascapular flap: A new cutaneous microsurgical free flap. *Plast Reconstr Surg.* 1982;69:591–600.
109. Koshima I, Soeda S. Repair of a wide defect of the lower leg with the combined scapular and parascapular flap. *Br J Plast Surg.* 1985;38:518–521.
110. Swanson E, Boyd JB, Manktelow RT. The radial forearm flap: Reconstructive applications and donor-site defects in 35 consecutive patients. *Plast Reconstr Surg.* 1990;85:258–266.
111. May JW, Lukash FN, Gallico GG. Latissimus dorsi free muscle flap in lower-extremity reconstruction. *Plast Reconstr Surg.* 1981;68:603–607.
112. Nahai F, Mathes SJ. Musculocutaneous flap or muscle flap and skin graft? *Ann Plast Surg.* 1984;12:199–203.
113. Lineaweaver W, Clapson B, Alpert B, et al. Immediate skin grafting on microvascular free tissue transfers. *Ann Plast Surg.* 1988;21:124–126.
114. Hagerty R, Bostwick J, Nahai F. Denervated muscle flaps: Mass and thickness changes following denervation. *Ann Plast Surg.* 1984;12:171–176.
115. May JW, Savage RC. Free muscle flaps with split thickness skin grafts for contoured closure of difficult wounds. In: Strauch B, Vasconez LO, Hall-Findlay EJ, eds. *Grabb's Encyclopedia of Flaps.* Boston: Little, Brown; 1990:1779–1782.
116. Jupiter JB, Kour AK, Palumbo MD, et al. Limb reconstruction by free-tissue transfer combined with the Ilizarov method. *Plast Reconstr Surg.* 1991;88:943–951.

117. Peat BG, Liggins DF. Microvascular soft tissue reconstruction for acute tibial fracture—Late complications and the role of bone grafting. *Ann Plast Surg.* 1990;24;517–520.
118. Anthony JP, Mathes SJ, Alpert BS. The muscle flap in the treatment of chronic lower extremity osteomyelitis: Results in patients over 5 years after treatment. *Plast Reconstr Surg.* 1991;88:311–318.
119. May JW, Jupiter JB, Gallico GG, et al. Treatment of chronic traumatic bone wounds—Microvascular free tissue transfer: A 13 year experience in 96 patients. *Ann Surg.* 1991;214:241–252.
120. Swartz WM, Jones NF. Soft tissue coverage of the lower extremity. *Curr Prob Surg.* 1985;22(6):1–59.
121. Hermanson A, Dalsgaard D-J, Arnander C, et al. Sensibility and cutaneous reinnervation in free flaps. *Plast Reconstr Surg.* 1987;79:422–425.
122. May JW, Lukash FN, Gallico GG. Latissimus dorsi free muscle flap in lower extremity reconstruction. *Plast Reconstr Surg.* 1981;68:603–607.
123. May JW, Gallico GG, Lukash FN. Microvascular transfer of free tissue for closure of bony wounds of the distal lower extremity. *N Engl J Med.* 1982;306:253–257.
124. Tobin GR, Mobert AW, Dubou RH, et al. The split latissimus dorsi myocutaneous flap. *Ann Plast Surg.* 1981;7:272–280.
125. Elliot LF, Raffel B, Wade J. Segmental latissimus dorsi free flap: Clinical applications. Ann Plast Surg. 1989;23:231–238.
126. Bunkis J, Walton RL, Mathes SJ. The rectus abdominis free flap for lower extremity reconstruction. *Ann Plast Surg.* 1983;11:373–380.
127. Tamai S, Buncke HJ, Alpert BS. Vascularized muscle transplantation and gracilis muscle transplantation. In: Buncke HJ, ed. *Microsurgery: Transplantion–Replantation: An Atlas–Text.* Philadelphia: Lea and Febiger; 1991:368–393.
128. Dawson RL. Complications of the cross-leg flap operation. *Proc R Soc Med.* 1972;65:626–629.
129. Barclay TL, Cardoso E, Sharpe DT, et al. Repair of lower leg injuries with fasciocutaneous flaps. *Br J Plast Surg.* 1982;35:127–132.
130. Calhoun JH, Gogan WJ, Beraja V, et al. Dynamic axial fixation for immobilization of cross-leg flaps in chronic osteomyelitis. *Ann Plast Surg.* 1989:23:354–356.
131. Hodgkinson DJ, Irons GB. Newer applications of the cross-leg flap. *Ann Plast Surg.* 1980;4:381–390.
132. Brenman SA, Barber WB, Pederson WC, et al. Pedicled free flaps: Indications in complex reconstruction. *Ann Plast Surg.* 1990;24:420–426.
133. Yaremchuk MJ. Special injuries. In: Yaremchuk MJ, Burgess AR, Brumback RJ, eds. *Lower Extremity Salvage and Reconstruction.* New York: Elsevier Science; 1989;41–58.
134. Hidalgo DA. Lower extremity avulsion injuries. *Clin Plast Surg.* 1986;13:701–710.
135. Hudson DA, Knottenbelt JD, Krige JE. Closed degloving injuries: Results following conservative surgery. *Plast Reconstr Surg.* 1992;89:853–855.
136. Kudsk KA, Sheldon GF, Walton RL. Degloving injuries of the extremities and torso. *J Trauma.* 1981;21:835–839.
137. Smith PL, Lim WN, Ferris EJ, et al. Emergency arteriography in extremity trauma: Assessment of indications. *AJR.* 1981;137:803–807.
138. Khalil IM, Livingston DH. Management of lower limb vascular injuries. *Clin Plast Surg.* 1986;13:711–722.
139. Lim LT, Michuda MS, Flanigan DP, et al. Popliteal artery trauma: 31 consecutive cases without amputation. *Arch Surg.* 1980;115:1307–1313.
140. Green NE, Allen BL. Vascular injuries associated with dislocation of the knee. *J Bone Joint Surg Am.* 1977;59:236–239.
141. McCoy GF, Hannon DG, Barr RJ, et al. Vascular injury associated with low-velocity dislocations of the knee. *J Bone Joint Surg Br.* 1987;69:285–287.
142. Leffers D. Dislocations and soft tissue injuries of the knee. In: Browner BD, Jupiter JB, Levine AM, et al, eds. *Skeletal Trauma: Fractures, Dislocations, and Ligamentous Injuries.* Philadelphia: WB Saunders; 1992:1717–1744.
143. Seddon HJ. Three types of nerve injury. *Brain.* 1946;66:237–288.
144. Siegel DB, Gelberman RH. Peripheral nerve injuries associated with fractures and dislocations. In: Gelberman RH, ed. *Operative Nerve Repair and Reconstruction.* Philadelphia: JB Lippincott; 1991:619–633.
145. Wood MB. Peripheral nerve injuries to the lower extremity. In: Gelberman RH, ed. *Operative Nerve Repair and Reconstruction.* Philadelphia: JB Lippincott; 1991: 489–504.
146. Aldea PA, Shaw WW. Lower extremity nerve injuries. *Clin Plast Surg.* 1986;13:691–699.
147. Gallico GG, May JW. Discussion. *Plast Reconstr Surg.* 1989;83:97–99.
148. Amato JJ, Billy LJ, Lawson NS, et al. High velocity missile injury: An experimental study of the retentive forces of tissue. *Am J Surg.* 1974;127:454–459.
149. Sherman RT, Parrish RA. Management of shotgun injuries: A review of 152 cases. *J Trauma.* 1963;3:76–86.
150. DeMuth WE. The mechanism of shotgun wounds. *J Trauma.* 1971;11:219–229.
151. Wiss DA, Gellman H. Gunshot wounds to the musculoskeletal system. In: Browner BC, Jupiter JB, Levine AM, et al, eds. *Skeletal Trauma: Fractures, Dislocations, and Ligamentous Injuries.* Philadelphia: WB Saunders; 1992;367–400.
152. Omer GE. Nerve injuries associated with gunshot wounds of the extremities. In: Gelberman RH, ed. *Operative Nerve Repair and Reconstruction.* Philadelphia: JB Lippincott; 1991:655–670.
153. Collins DN, Temple SD. Open joint injuries: Classification and treatment. *Clin Orthop.* 1989;243:48–56.
154. Patzakis MJ, Dorr LD, Ivler D, et al. The early management of open joint injuries: A prospective study of one hundred and forty patients. *J Bone Joint Surg Am.* 1975;57:1065–1071.
155. Gallico GG, Bartlett SP, May JW. Flap coverage of exposed and infected large joints. Presented at the American Society of Plastic & Reconstructive Surgeons' Annual Meeting, Los Angeles, California, October 1986.
156. Asko-Seljavaara S, Haajanen J. The exposed knee joint: Five case reports. *J Trauma.* 1982;22:1021–1025.
157. Barfod B, Pers M. Gastrocnemius-plasty for primary closure of compound injuries of the knee. *J Bone Joint Surg Br.* 1970;52:124–127.
158. Gordon L, Buncke HJ, Alpert BS. Free latissimus dorsi muscle flap with split-thickness skin graft cover: A report of 16 cases. *Plast Reconstr Surg.* 1982;70:173–178.
159. Gault DT, Quaba A. Is flap cover of exposed metalwork worthwhile? A review of 28 cases. *Br J Plast Surg.* 1986;39:505–509.
160. Laing JH, Hancock K, Harrison DH. The exposed total

knee replacement prosthesis: A new classification and treatment algorithm. *Br J Plast Surg.* 1992;45:66–69.

161. Johnson DP, Bannister GC. The outcome of infected arthroplasty of the knee. *J Bone Joint Surg.* 1986; 68:289–291.

162. Sanders R, O'Neill T. The gastrocnemius myocutaneous flap used as a cover for the exposed knee prosthesis. *J Bone Joint Surg Br.* 1981;63:383–386.

163. Greenberg B, Lakossa D, Lotke PA, et al. Salvage of jeopardized total-knee prosthesis: The role of the gastrocnemius muscle flap. *Plast Reconstr Surg.* 1989;83:85–89.

164. Bengston S, Carlsson A, Relander M, et al. Treatment of the exposed knee prosthesis. *Acta Orthop Scand.* 1987;58:662–665.

165. Hallock GG. Salvage of total knee arthroplasty with lo-cal fasciocutaneous flaps. *J Bone Joint Surg Am.* 1990;72:1236–1239.

166. Lesavoy MA, Dubrow TJ, Wackym PA, et al. Muscle-flap coverage of exposed endoprostheses. *Plast Reconstr Surg.* 1989;83:90–96.

167. Hamm JC, Stevenson TR, Mathes SJ. Knee joint salvage utilizing a plantar musculocutaneous island pedicle flap. *Br J Plast Surg.* 1986;39:249–254.

168. Gallico GG, Ehrlichman RJ, Jupiter J, et al. Free flaps to preserve below-knee amputation stumps: Long term evaluation. *Plast Reconstr Surg.* 1987;79:871–877.

169. Shenag SM, Krouskop T, Stal S, et al. Salvage of amputation stumps by secondary reconstruction utilizing microsurgical free-tissue transfer. *Plast Reconstr Surg.* 1987;79:861–870.

5

Extensile Exposure of the Knee

Kenneth S. Austin and John M. Siliski

Recent advances in orthopaedic surgery, including arthroscopy, fluoroscopy, closed intramedullary nailing, and external fixation, have permitted the use of limited and even percutaneous surgical approaches. If a surgical goal can be met with minimal soft tissue dissection, there are many potential benefits. Decreased operating and anesthesia time, less scarring, and quicker rehabilitation are certainly advantageous; however, certain surgical problems about the knee cannot be solved with limited exposure. It is the goal of this chapter to review extensile exposure about the knee, including techniques and indications for use in trauma and posttraumatic reconstruction.

Several factors must be considered during the preoperative assessment of the knee. A history of previous surgery and preexisting scars must be incorporated into any decision process. Fracture pattern, soft tissue injuries, and timing of surgery will affect exposure. An attempt should be made to perform fracture reconstruction as early as possible. The longer the delay, the more difficult restoration of length and accuracy of reduction become. As time passes after a fracture, soft tissue stiffness and early healing of cancellous bone become increasingly problematic.[1] For joint reconstruction, such as osteotomy and total knee arthroplasty, the range of motion of the knee must also be taken into consideration. Stiffness limits exposure and requires soft tissue releases to improve final motion. It is important to choose an approach prior to entering the operating room that addresses these needs and allows for extension of the exposure as required during the progress of the surgical procedure.

There are several basic tenets to be considered when performing a surgical approach to the knee. According to Henry, straight incisions generally tend to do better than curved incisions.[2] Straight incisions have subse-

quently been shown to have fewer complications, especially with regard to total knee replacement. Many incisions, like the "triradiate" incision, can no longer be recommended because of wound healing problems.[3] One incision is usually better than two incisions. Insall stresses that one long incision is better than two short incisions as long as the amount of undermining is minimized.[1] One must be aware that when planning the original incision the possibility of repeat surgical procedures exists. Incisions should be chosen that minimize risk, maximize exposure, allow for extension, and allow for revision.

Internal fixation of simple unicondylar and supracondylar fractures of the distal femur, most tibial plateau fractures, and primary total knee replacements may be performed with relatively limited exposure; however, more complex fracture patterns, particularly those with extensive intraarticular comminution, may require more exposure than the standard approaches provide. Additionally, delayed fracture cases often require more extensive surgical exposure because of soft tissue stiffness and adherence of fracture fragments.

Another indication for extensile exposure is reconstruction after trauma, including osteotomies, the treatment of nonunions, and the release of adhesions. More complex total knee replacements, such as revisions or those performed after trauma, will frequently require more extensive exposures.

The exposures preferred for trauma and reconstruction of the knee can generally be grouped into two distinct groups: anterior and lateral approaches.

Anterior Approaches to the Knee

The anterior approach is the workhorse approach to the knee. It is the preferred incision for primary total knee

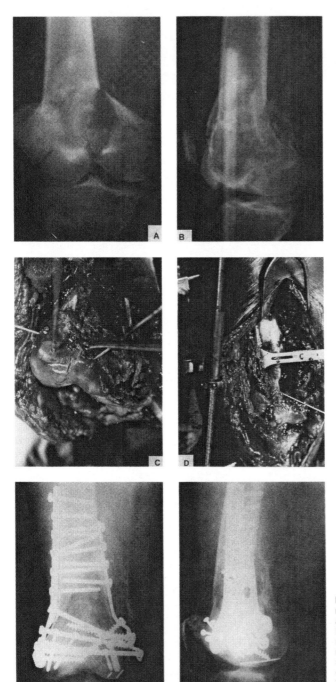

Figure 5–1. Anterior approach to a comminuted distal femoral fracture. **A.** Preoperative anteroposterior (AP) x-ray. **B.** Preoperative lateral x-ray. **C.** Intraoperative exposure with reduction and interal fixation of articular fragments of distal femur. **D.** Intraoperative exposure with femoral distractor in place, and reduction, bone grafting, and double plating of the metaphyseal fracture line in progress. **E** Postoperative AP x-ray. **F.** Postoperative lateral x-ray.

arthroplasty and most tibial plateau fractures.[4] It is also a useful approach for comminuted intraarticular fractures restricted to the distal femur (Fig. 5–1). Articular fragments can be fixed with various interfragmentary screws and the supracondylar portion can be reduced and fixed with one or two plates. The anterior approach is generally not used for femoral fractures with proximal extension beyond 20 cm from the joint line or fractures requiring a 95° blade plate or condylar screw for fixation.[5]

The skin incisions can vary according to individual surgeon preferences. A straight midline anterior incision is most common. It leaves the medial and lateral skin flaps equally dependent on the blood supply that originates from the posterior side of the knee. Medial or lateral parapatellar incisions are also acceptable. A preexisting anterior skin incision should be reused rather than a second anterior incision made. If a localized soft tissue injury exists anteriorly, the skin incision can be adjusted medially or laterally to pass through healthy tissue. Most authors agree, however, that the medial parapatellar capsular incision is the procedure of choice when approaching the knee anteriorly.[4]

Medial Parapatellar Arthrotomy

Medial parapatellar arthrotomy consists of incising the skin and subcutaneous tissue to expose the quadriceps tendon and medial joint capsule. The amount of undermining medially should be just enough to visualize a small cuff of medial retinacular tissue. The quadriceps should be incised approximately 5 cm proximal to the patella in the center of the tendon. The incision is extended distally to the superior-medial border of the patella, where it is curved distally around the medial patella. It is preferable to leave a small cuff of tissue medial to the patella and patellar tendon for later closure. It is important to be aware of the anterior insertion of the medial meniscus if it is to be preserved (Fig. 5–2).

This incision is often sufficient to allow eversion and lateral dislocation of the patella and flexion of the knee to perform either reconstruction of the knee or fracture fixation of the distal third of the femur. It is important to avoid excessive tension on the patellar tendon. Repair of an avulsed patellar tendon is quite difficult (see Chapters 12 and 25).

If difficulty arises in dislocating the patella, several options exist. The quadriceps tendon can be split further proximally. The extension should be just lateral to the medial border of the tendon. It is also possible to carefully detach the proximal third of the patellar tendon. For joint arthroplasty, a medial release at this time permits tibial external rotation and facilitates patellar eversion.

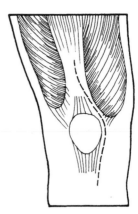

Figure 5–2. Diagram of deep incision for a medial parapatellar arthrotomy. The incision is kept 1 cm medial to the edge of the patellar tendon to leave tissue flaps for closure.

Lateral Release

If the patella cannot be everted and retracted, and the lateral retinaculum is tight, a lateral release should be performed as part of the exposure. Incising the lateral retinacular structures at this time may potentially eliminate the need for more extensile exposure (Fig. 5–3). The importance of the superior lateral geniculate artery to the vascularity of the patella is controversial[6,7]; however, the artery should be isolated and preserved during a lateral release when possible.

These techniques are sufficient in the majority of cases to allow eversion of the patella, flexion of the knee, and exposure of the joint.

V and V-Y Exposures

If there is still difficulty everting the patella and exposing the joint, two options exist. One involves doing a tibial tubercle osteotomy[4,5,8–10] (Chandler H. Unpublished data). This is discussed in detail in a separate section of this chapter. The other technique involves variations and modifications of the inverted V exposure or the V-Y type of quadricepsplasty.[1,5,11–14] These exposures are generally used during late knee arthroplasty or other late reconstructive surgeries.

Coonse and Adams originally described the V exposure (Fig. 5–4).[11] The initial indication was for open reduction and internal fixation of intraarticular fractures of the distal femur. Currently, this approach has limited use for acute fracture repair. Their experience, however, showed this to be a useful extensile approach with no reported complications and no significant quadriceps weakness.

Insall modified the V exposure to allow extensile exposure with a more limited tendinous incision (Fig. 5–5).[1]

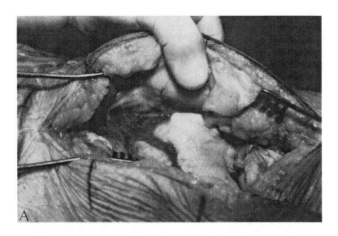

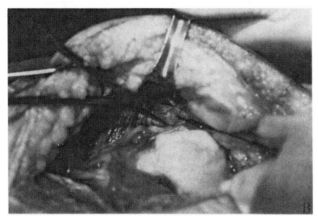

Figure 5–3. Lateral release performed from within the joint, with preservation of the superior lateral geniculate vessels. **A.** Patella could not be everted. **B.** Lateral release before arthroplasty to allow patellar eversion and exposure of the joint.

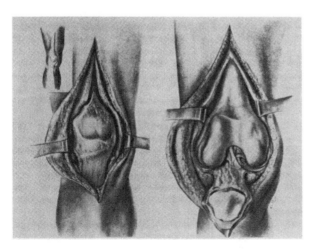

Figure 5–4. V exposure of Coonse and Adams. (Reprinted with permission from Coonse K, Adams JD. A new operative approach to the knee joint. *Surg Gynecol Obstet.* 1943;77:344.)

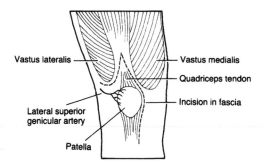

Vastus lateralis ——
Vastus medialis ——
Quadriceps tendon ——
Incision in fascia ——
Lateral superior genicular artery ——
Patella ——

Figure 5–5. V incision in the quadriceps tendon to improve exposure of the knee. Only as much of the lateral incision is made as is necessary to achieve the required exposure.

This technique allows for extension in gradations as the individual case requires. If, during the course of the exposure, only a small amount of additional release is required, a small inverted V incision can be placed in the quadriceps tendon. This can subsequently be extended to a more formal V turndown as needed, but often only a limited extension of a few centimeters into the lateral quadriceps tendon is required.

The V-Y quadricepsplasty is most useful in knees that are stiff in extension, generally with less than 60° of flexion. It allows up to 2 cm of lengthening during closure to improve flexion (Fig. 5–6). When necessary, this can be combined with a formal lateral release while preserving the superior lateral geniculate artery (Figs. 5–7 and 5–8).

In a series of seven patients with stiff knees undergoing total knee arthroplasty, Scott and Siliski noted an increase in motion of 52° when using a V-Y quadricepsplasty.[12] Postoperatively, an extensor lag was always present, but usually resolved within 6 months of surgery.

Figure 5–6. V-Y quadricepsplasty. The lateral incision is curved distally around the margin of the vastus lateralis. During closure the patella is advanced distally by up to 2 cm. **1.** The medial arthrotomy is sutured. **2.** The proximal quadriceps tendon is sutured to itself. **3.** The lateral incision is closed, unless closure interferes with patellar tracking.

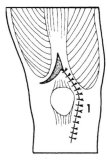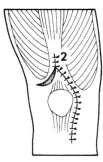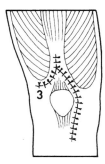

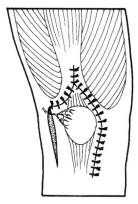

Figure 5–7. V-Y quadricepsplasty combined with a lateral release. The superior lateral geniculate vessels are preserved.

Aglietti et al used a V-Y quadricepsplasty in 11 of 26 stiff or ankylosed knees undergoing total knee arthroplasty.[13] They noted an increase of 46° in the arc of motion comparing pre- with postoperative levels. The postoperative rehabilitation in these patients was delayed 3 weeks. The authors advocated the V-Y technique because of its safety, simplicity, speed, no requirements for additional instrumentation, avoidance of any tibial bone stock problems, and avoidance of tibial stems for reconstructive procedures. They mention several disadvantages of the procedure including the potential for patellar devascularization, quadriceps dehiscence, and short-term extensor lag.

Closure of the V-Y quadricepsplasty can allow up to 2 cm of lengthening of the quadriceps tendon. During closure of the V-Y advancement, the lateral extension may be left open as for a lateral release to improve patellar tracking (see Figs. 5–6 and 5–7).

Postoperatively, these repairs can be rehabilitated

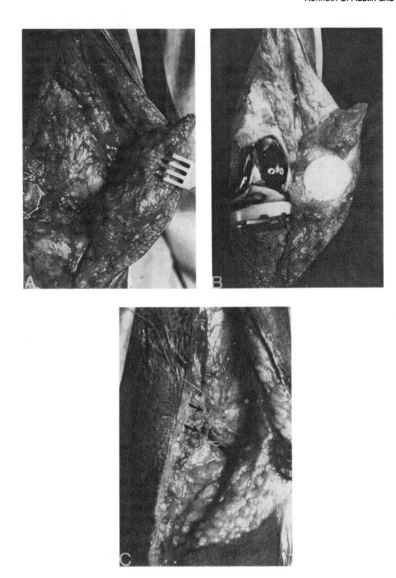

Figure 5-8. Total knee arthroplasty secondary to posttraumatic arthritis. **A**. V-Y quadricepsplasty. **B**. Components in place. **C**. Closure. Arrows note advancement of quadriceps.

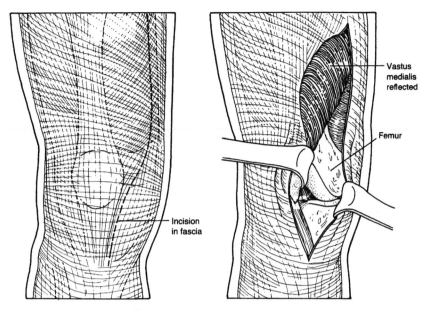

Vastus
medialis
reflected

Femur

Incision
in fascia

Figure 5–9. Medial subvastus approach.

with gentle quadriceps exercises and straight-leg raises
in a knee immobilizer. A continuous passive motion
machine may be used. An immobilizer should be worn
at night. Ambulation is permitted with partial weight
bearing with the knee locked in extension until the extensor lag is less than 15°.[12]

Medial Subvastus Approach

The subvastus or Southern approach for primary total
knee arthroplasty is also commonly used.[15] It provides
good exposure and preserves much of the extensor
mechanism and the blood supply to the patella. It can
be performed through a straight anterior skin incision,
with the deep incision passing through the superficial
facia and underneath the muscle belly of the vastus
medialis obliquus (Fig. 5–9). The vastus medialis is then
raised off the intermuscular septum, bluntly lifting the
extensor mechanism anteriorly and laterally. A curvi-
linear medial arthrotomy is then made from the superior patellar pouch around the patella to the tibial tubercle. This allows eversion of the patella. Mobilization of
the muscle belly of the vastus medialis may be required
proximally to decrease the tensile stresses on the patellar tendon and decrease the risk of avulsion. This
approach is adequate for primary knee arthroplasty or
fixation of medial femoral condyle fractures; however,
it is relatively contraindicated in revision arthroplasty,

stiff knees, or more extensive fractures as it offers
less flexibility than the standard medial parapatellar
incision.

Exposure of Tibial Plateau Fractures

The majority of tibial plateau fractures should be
approached through an anterior skin incision that
can also be used for any future reconstructive
procedure.[16,17] The capsular incision should be horizontal and inferior to the menisci, which should be retracted superiorly to allow exposure of the plateau itself
(see Chapter 9). As most plateau fractures occur laterally, a majority of tibial plateau reconstructions will require lateral arthrotomy with minimal dissection of the
patellar tendon.

Occasionally, a comminuted bicondylar plateau fracture will require more exposure. In these cases medial
and lateral horizontal capsular incisions may be used.
This usually provides sufficient exposure to allow for internal fixation; however, the wide dissection combined
with the use of medial and lateral plates may increase
the risk of skin slough. This problem has led to the increased use of external fixation devices or small plating
medially to minimize dissection of the medial soft tissues. For those cases when this still does not provide
sufficient exposure, Schatzker has recommended a Z incision of the patellar tendon (Fig. 5–10).[16] The resuture

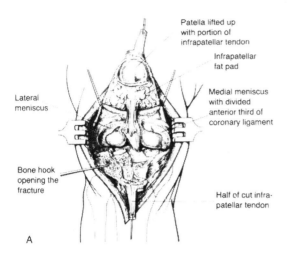

Patella lifted up
with portion of
infrapatellar tendon

Infrapatellar
fat pad

Lateral
meniscus

Medial meniscus
with divided
anterior third of
coronary ligament

Bone hook
opening the
fracture

Half of cut infra-
patellar tendon

A

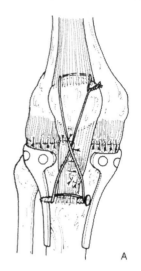

A

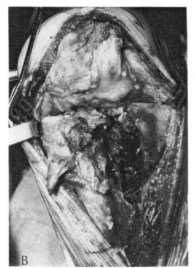

B

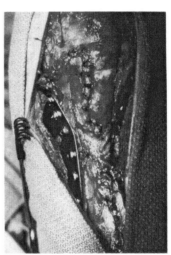

B

Figure 5–10. A. Diagram of the Z exposure through the patellar tendon. The medial and lateral capsule is divided below the menisci, and the patella, capsule, and menisci are retracted proximally. (Reprinted with permission from Schatzker J. Supracondylar fracture of the femur. In: Schatzker J, Tile M, eds. *The rationale of operative fracture care.* New York: Springer-Verlag; 1987.) **B.** Example of intraoperative Z approach to a comminuted bicondylar tibial plateau fracture.

Figure 5–11. A. Diagram of closure of the Z incision, with a tension band wire to protect the suture line of the patellar tendon and reattachment of the capsule and menisci. (Adapted with permission from Schatzker J. Supracondylar fracture of the femur. In: Schatzker J, Tile M, eds. *The rationale of operative fracture care.* New York: Springer-Verlag; 1987.) **B.** Intraoperative photograph of closure with interrupted sutures in patellar tendon and tension band in place.

of the tendon is protected by a tension band (Fig. 5–11). This approach allows excellent exposure of the proximal tibia, but the repair must be protected to permit healing of the tendon.

Lateral Approach to the Knee

The lateral approach to the distal femur is an excellent choice for exposure of distal femoral fractures.[3,16,18–20] It can be extended distally and curved somewhat anterior in the direction of the tibial tubercle to provide exposure for intraarticular fractures. This approach is adequate for an overwhelming majority of fractures of the distal femur and permits easy insertion of a 95° fixation device. If further exposure is required, a tibial tubercle osteotomy can be performed.[18–20] Two main indications exist for adding a tibial tubercle osteotomy to this approach.[5] The first is comminution of the medial femoral condyle that cannot be adequately addressed from the simple lateral approach. The second is a fracture with comminution of the medial metaphysis requiring a medial buttress plate.

The lateral approach to the distal femur should be performed with the patient in the supine position. A tourniquet may be used if the incision will not extend too far proximally. If possible, the iliac crest should be prepped and draped as part of the procedure in case a

bone graft is required. The leg should be draped free to allow for knee flexion over bolsters during the procedure. The skin incision follows the line between the greater trochanter and the lateral epicondyle (Fig. 5–12). The length of the incision depends on the extent of the fracture. For extraarticular fractures, distal extension to the joint line should be sufficient. For intraarticular fractures the incision is extended distally to the lateral edge of the tibial tubercle. The deep incision is made through the iliotibial band just anterior to the intermuscular septum. If necessary, the incision is extended distally through the lateral retinaculum. The vastus lateralis is reflected anteriorly and medially (Figs. 5–13 and 5–14) Arterial perforators should be identified between the intermuscular septum and muscle for ligation. If necessary, the tibial tubercle can be osteotomized and everted medially (Fig. 5–15). The soft tissue attachments on the medial side of the tubercle should be left intact. It is possible to perform a double plating through this approach, eliminating the necessity of a second incision.

In a study by Siliski et al, 52 supracondylar-intracondylar fractures of the femur were repaired through the lateral approach, with only one case requiring a tubercle osteotomy for adequate exposure.[18] Mize et al reported use of eight tibial tubercle osteotomies in the exposure of 30 intraarticular distal femoral fractures. The lateral approach, with or without tubercle osteotomy, may also be used for distal femoral

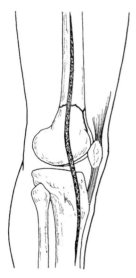

Figure 5–12. Lateral approach to the distal femur: skin incision.

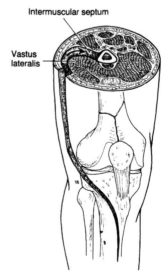

Intermuscular septum

Vastus lateralis

Figure 5–13. Lateral approach to the distal femur: reflection of vastus lateralis from the intermuscular septum.

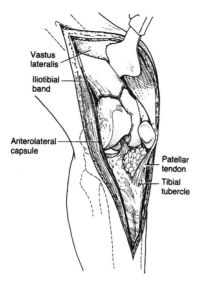

Figure 5–14. Lateral approach to the distal femur: retraction of the extensor mechanism medially.

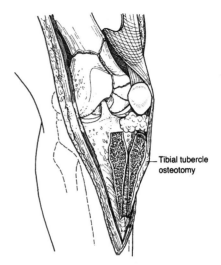

Figure 5–15. Lateral approach to the distal femur: addition of a tibial tubercle osteotomy to increase access to the medial metaphysis and condyle. The medial soft tissue attachments are left intact.

osteotomy, treatment of extra- and intraarticular femoral nonunions, and even total knee replacement for posttraumatic arthritis (Fig. 5–16).

Tibial Tubercle Osteotomy

Tibial tubercle osteotomies add additional exposure and can be used to improve patellar tracking if a transfer is performed during closure. The osteotomy may be performed with either an anterior or lateral approach as previously discussed[3,5,8,10,16,18–20] (Chandler H. Unpublished data).

Whiteside et al used tibial tubercle osteotomies in 71 total joint replacements.[8] The majority of these were revisions. He created an 8- to 10-cm-long block of bone using an oscillating saw. The patella was everted laterally, leaving lateral soft tissue attachments of the tubercle intact. They performed this through an anterior approach and reattached the osteotomy with double wiring. Postoperative early range of motion and full weight bearing were allowed. At final follow-up, this group of knees had an average of 97° of flexion, with only one case of migration of the osteotomy. Whiteside et al concluded that the osteotomy provided safe, wide exposure. Early rehabilitation with no special wound care was possible.

Whiteside and co-workers point to the biomechanical advantage of addressing difficult exposures by looking at the tensile forces in the quadriceps and patellar tendon.[8] The forces are higher in the quadriceps than in

the patellar tendon. Therefore, failures in tension should be lower when osteotomies are done distal to the patella. Further, healing of the osteotomy relies on bone-to-bone healing, leaving the extensor mechanism intact while retaining the blood supply to the patella. The V-Y quadricepsplasty relies on tendon-to-tendon healing, with suture fixation in the quadriceps where the tensile loads are higher.

Wolf et al reported 26 total knee arthroplasties in which a tibial tubercle osteotomy was performed.[10] Three of these osteotomies displaced. All three had a bone block less than 3 cm long, and all were fixed with only one screw. There was one case of patellar tendon rupture with an extensor lag and two cases of skin slough that required flaps.

H.M. Chandler (unpublished data) reviewed 36 total knee arthroplasties performed with tibial tubercle osteotomies. He used a large bone block measuring 1½ × 1 × 7 cm. He fixed the tubercle with two cancellous lag screws engaging the posterior cortex, and did not modify his usual postoperative rehabilitation. The only complication was a fracture at the proximal drill hole in one osteotomy. He reported no cases of lost fixation or extensor problems.

Osteotomy of the tibial tubercle does provide excellent extensile exposure of the knee; however, it is not without risk as described. Thus, it is important to pay attention to the skin condition over the knee and the bone stock of the tibia.

Tibial tubercle osteotomy is best performed by taking

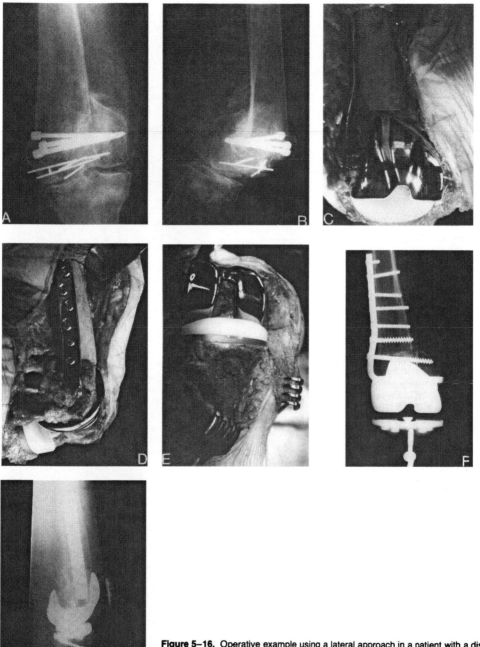

Figure 5–16. Operative example using a lateral approach in a patient with a distal femoral malunion undergoing simultaneous osteotomy and total knee replacement. A preexisting lateral incision was reused and extended with a tibial tubercle osteotomy. **A.** Preoperative AP x-ray. **B.** Preoperative lateral x-ray. **C.** Anterior view of knee. **D.** Lateral view of knee. **E.** Tibial tubercle osteotomy fragment retracted medially. **F.** Postoperative AP x-ray. **G.** Postoperative lateral x-ray.

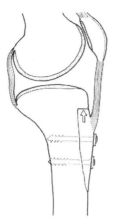

Figure 5–17. Lateral view of a tibial tubercle osteotomy demonstrating the proximal cut, leaving a shelf of intact tibia to resist proximal migration of the osteotomy.

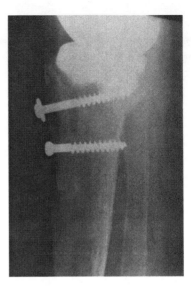

Figure 5–18. Fixation of a tibial tubercle osteotomy using two 6.5-mm cancellous screws (same case as in Fig. 5–16).

a large fragment of bone to provide solid fixation options. Minimally, the osteotomy fragment should be 2.5 cm wide and 5 cm long. The fragment should be at least 1 cm thick. The osteotomy can be performed with an oscillating saw and/or osteotome. When performed through the lateral approach, the medial soft tissues and the fat pad should be left attached to the tubercle to preserve vascularity. When the osteotomy is performed through an anterior approach, the patella is usually everted laterally, leaving the lateral soft tissue attachments intact. If the proximal cut of the osteotomy is performed at 90° to the cortex, it may be snapped back into place under the intact shelf of the tibia (Fig. 5–17). This aids in preventing proximal migration. The osteotomy fragment should be reattached to the tibia with multiple implants. An option is the use of two 6.5-mm cancellous screws, with or without washers. These may carefully engage the posterior tibial cortex to enhance fixation (Fig. 5–18). The passage of any instrument or implant through the posterior tibial cortex should be done very carefully to avoid injury to the adjacent neurovascular structures. Another fixation option is the multiple wiring technique used by Whiteside et al.[8]

Tibial Tubercle Osteotomy Versus V-Y Quadricepsplasty

The V-Y quadricepsplasty and the tibial tubercle osteotomy provide the ultimate exposure of the knee. The V-Y quadricepsplasty is preferred in knees that are extremely stiff in extension with less than 60° of preoperative flexion. It avoids problems with tibial bone

deficiency or poor skin vascularity over the tibia associated with trauma or old scars. Further, it allows advancement of the quadriceps.

Tibial tubercle osteotomies are used more commonly in those knees with greater than 60° of preoperative flexion, good tibial bone stock, and healthy skin. The osteotomy has the advantage of a relatively low complication rate with minimal disruption of the quadriceps tendon and minimal limitations of rehabilitation. Disadvantages include necrosis, loss of fixation, and inability to lengthen the quadriceps to improve flexion.

References

1. Insall JN. Surgical approach to the knee. In: *Surgery of the Knee*. New York: Churchill Livingstone; 1994;41–54.
2. Henry AK. *Extensile Exposures*. 2nd ed. Edinburgh: Churchill Livingstone; 1973.
3. Bunker T. Fractures around the knee. In: Aichroth PM, Cannon WD Jr., Patel DV, eds. *Knee Surgery—Current Practice*. New York: Raven Press; 1992.
4. Hoppenfeld S, deBoer P. *Surgical Exposures in Orthopaedics*. Philadelphia: JB Lippincott; 1984.
5. Siliski JM, Brinken B. Extensile exposure of the distal femur. Presented at the Orthopaedic Trauma Association Annual Meeting Poster Exhibit, 1992.
6. Scott RD, Turoff N, Ewald FC. Stress fractures of the patella following duopatellar total knee arthroplasty with patellar resurfacing. *Clin Orthop*. 1982;170:147–151.
7. Ritter M, Campbell ED. Postoperative patellar complication with or without lateral release during total knee arthroplasty. *Clin Orthop*. 1987;219:163.

8. Whiteside LA, Ohl MD. Tibial tubercle osteotomy for exposure of the difficult total knee arthroplasty. *Clin Orthop.* 1990;260:6.
9. Dolin NG. Osteotomy of the tibial tubercle in total knee replacement. *J Bone Joint Surg Am.* 1983;65:74.
10. Wolff AM, Hungerford DS, Krackow KA, Jacobs MA. Osteotomy of tibial tubercle during total knee replacement. *J Bone Joint Surg Am.* 1989;71:848.
11. Coonse K, Adams JD. A new approach to the knee joint. *Surg Gynecol Obstet.* 1943;77:344.
12. Scott R, Siliski JM. The use of V-Y quadricepsplasty during total knee replacement. *Orthopaedics.* 1985;8:45–48.
13. Aglietti P, Windsor RE, Buzzi R, Insall JN. Arthroplasty for the stiff or ankylosed knee. *J Arthroplasty.* 1989;4:1.
14. Scott RD. The decision to operate. In: Scott WN, ed. *Total Knee Revision Arthroplasty.* Orlando, FL: Grune and Stratton; 1987.
15. Hoffman AA, Plaster RL, Murdock LE. Subvastus (Southern) approach for primary total knee arthroplasty. *Clin Orthop.* 1991;269:70–77.
16. Schatzker J. Supracondylar fracture of the femur. In: Schatzker J, Tile M, eds. *The Rationale of Operative Fracture Care.* New York: Springer-Verlag; 1987.
17. Müller ME, Allgower M, Schneider R, Willenegger J. *Manual of Internal Fixation.* 3rd ed. Berlin: Springer-Verlag; 1991.
18. Siliski JM, Mahring M, Hofer P. Supracondylar–intercondylar fractures of the femur: treatment by internal fixation. *J Bone Joint Surg Am.* 1989;71:95.
19. Olerud S. Operative treatment of supracondylar fractures of femur. *J Bone Joint Surg Am.* 1972;54:1015–1032.
20. Mize RD, Bucholz RW, Grogan DP. Surgical treatment of displaced comminuted fractures of the distal end of the femur. *J Bone Joint Surg Am.* 1982;64:871.

6

External Fixation of the Knee

Justin Lamont

Introduction

The primary purpose of this chapter is to discuss the indications and applications of various external fixation devices for the knee. Early attempts at external fixation began in France in the mid-1800s. In 1897 Dr. Clayton Parkhill of Denver, Colorado, reported on the use of a modern type of external fixator with pins and a frame with clamps.[1] In 1902, Albin Lambotte started using an external fixator of his own design in Europe.[2] Anderson of Seattle worked on using pins and plaster and external fixation in the 1930s and 1940s.[3] Raoul Hoffman published results of his external fixation system from Switzerland in 1938.[4] The initial use of external fixation for fracture care was due in part to metallurgy problems with plates and screws. Infection and the lack of antibiotics were also factors. Unfortunately, pin infections remained a problem, despite some good clinical results. After a wave of enthusiasm, complications resulted in the decline of widespread use of external fixation devices in the United States until the 1970s.

The main reason for the resurgence of use of external fixators was the high complication rate associated with the use of internal fixation with severe soft tissue injuries, especially with the tibia. Open tibial shaft fractures became a common indication for external fixation. Half-pins and transfixation pins of varying diameters were used with both bar and ring frames. The use of transfixation pins gradually decreased and half-pins were favored because of their soft tissue-sparing application. Biomechanical and clinical union studies supported the use of half-pins.[5,6]

With the widespread introduction of Ilizarov's work with ring fixators,[7,8] transfixation pins returned. Some of the early proponents of thin-wire transfixation pins have switched back to half-pin frames.[9] External fixa-tors are now used for acute fracture care, the treatment of osteomyelitis, fusions, correction of deformities (both congenital and acquired), as well as the management of some soft tissue problems such as dislocations and burns. The ability to perform bone transport and obtain regenerate bone formation, as described by Ilizarov, stimulated renewed interest in the use of external fixation.

There has been increased interest in the combined use of thin-wire ring frame and half-pin bar frame technology. These so called "hybrid" frames are proving to be very useful for proximal and distal tibial fractures.

Evaluation

Evaluation of knee injuries must be taken in the context of the clinical setting. Multiple injuries and polytrauma patients demand attention to more basic but vital needs initially. Later, a more complete workup can proceed. One factor important in both the isolated knee injury and the polytrauma patient is the vascularity of the lower limb. Severe soft tissue disruptions with gross displacement of the knee joint place the vessels tethered in the popliteal fossa at great risk. The usual priority of injury treatment with life-threatening injuries followed by limb-threatening injuries requires a rapid workup.

The history of the injury can be very important. Associated injuries such as electrical burns are easy to underestimate or even miss if a history is lacking. The kinetic energy of the injury is easier to appreciate if items such as the size of an object, estimated speed of travel, height of fall, or degree of presenting limb deformity are included in a history. The ambulance crews are often able to provide this information, even with patients who cannot give a history. Penetrating injuries will require debridement and lavage of the knee joint.

Arthroscopic evaluation can be useful. This includes the so-called "dry scope," an arthroscope inserted into the joint capsule without irrigation fluid and the usual formal arthroscopic setup. Arthroscopy is also useful for judging articular reductions without more damaging arthrotomies.

The most fundamental aspect of an evaluation of a significant knee injury is assessment of circulation and possible compartment syndrome. Vascular disruptions must be dealt with promptly. Delays of more than 6 to 8 hours result in a dramatic increase of the amputation rate. Doppler studies are helpful with absent pulses.[10] Palpable pulses can be misleading because of the transmitted pressure waves but no flow.[11] When available, a timely vascular surgery consult is usually appropriate with severe knee injuries.

Checking the neurologic status of an awake patient should be done to help define the extent of the injury. Peroneal nerve injuries are important and must be checked. Even if a patient cannot move a limb, an examiner can feel a muscle group contract. This rough assessment indicates at the least some nerve function. Partial nerve injuries may be difficult to assess accurately during emergency treatment. It is important not to forget problems with the central nervous system as a cause for motor weakness on examination of the knee after an injury. Incomplete patterns may not be obvious in the face of severe skeletal trauma during a cursory exam.

External fixation will usually be employed for fractures or dislocations, often with associated severe soft tissue injuries. Crush injuries can be deceiving when an apparently healthy skin envelope covers ischemic or degloved tissue underneath. Severe swelling and blistering are obvious danger flags when an open reduction and internal fixation are being considered. Proper splinting, elevation, and waiting are time-honored methods of dealing with this problem. External fixation can be used as a "soft tissue-sparing" fracture fixation technique. Care must be taken to achieve and maintain proper reductions.

With grossly unstable knees after dislocations and severe soft tissue injuries, external fixators can be used to protect the knee and vital structures after vascular evaluation and before or during definitive treatment.

Angiography studies can be done in the operating room or radiology suite depending on the urgency and detail of information needed. Surgical exploration of vascular injuries must be coordinated with possible orthopedic surgical approaches that might be needed.

Plain x-rays will normally be enough to determine whether or not an external fixator will be used for a knee injury. Tomography may be useful to define the depth, location, and extent of tibial plateau depression.[12] Although he has used tomography in the past, the author does not usually find this necessary for surgical decision making. Magnetic resonance imaging can be helpful for occult fracture and soft tissue injuries, but these injuries do not usually require external fixation for treatment.

Classification

The exact classification of fractures about the knee is usually not a major factor in deciding on the use of external fixation. The soft tissue classification is more relevant; however, the relevance is usually restricted to one of two categories: "bad enough" or "not bad enough." Although more precise classifications of soft tissue injuries may aid in deciding on other treatment measures, the use of the external fixator is based on the actual soft tissue loss or the potential loss from further surgical damage during exposure.

Learning to assess soft tissue damage is an art. Experience is the best teacher. Various methods of evaluating blood flow have been used to help. These have included the administration of intravenous fluorescent dye and a Wood's UV lamp to aid in determining the viability of skin and some soft tissue. Preoperative tetracycline labeling of bone and the use of ultraviolet lamps can help show gross viability of bone. Laser doppler flow studies as described by Swiontkowski[13] can measure blood flow in small amounts if the proper equipment is used. The problem is often marginal tissue that is not necrotic, but rather traumatized and ischemic. This is further complicated by the ability of different tissue types to recover by different amounts from similar injuries. Recovery of the different tissue types is dependent on the inherent circulation. The richer the natural blood supply, the more liberal one can be when its viability is questionable. Muscle tissue can appear dusky initially and later return to normal color and function. This principle assumes a "second-look" operation to reevaluate the tissues in 1 to 2 days. Muscle viability can also be judged grossly by its contractility. In the absence of paralyzing agents, gentle mechanical stimulus will produce contraction in healthy muscle.[14]

Newer classifications of open fractures are evolving into more complex structures involving more extensive and detailed soft tissue components.[15] The idea is to better understand the so-called "personality" of the fracture. A classification should help in at least three areas. It should define the injury, suggest a treatment method, and give some expectation of outcome.

Principles of Treatment

Indications

Various indications for the use of external fixation of the knee are dislocations, open fractures, vascular injuries, closed fracture with significant soft tissue injuries, fusions, thermal injuries, and children's fractures. The risks and benefits of external fixation must be compared with those of internal fixation. Except in children, the main issue is soft tissue management. Properly done in experienced hands, internal fixation is accurate and effective,[16] but the risk of internal fixation must be considered in relation to the soft tissue status of each case.

Dislocations and vascular injuries associated with severe fractures can be very unstable. The frames used for these injuries must be multiplanar. Ring fixators lend themselves to many pins in a given length of bone at the expense of greater chance of neurovascular impalement and muscle tendon irritation. Vascular shunts can be used to rapidly revascularize an ischemic limb. Bony stabilization can then be accomplished followed by definitive vascular repair.

Fusions may be needed in the face of severe loss of bone stock. This loss can be secondary to debridement for infection or wear from loose prostheses. Leg length is also usually an issue in knee fusions because of bone loss from trauma. External fixators can be used as positioning devices that provide compression while fusion is occurring. They can also be used to lenghten limbs during or after fusions. Transport frames can make up for bone loss of diaphyseal or metaphyseal bone.

Fractures with thermal injuries and contused closed injuries make the risk of acute extensive surgical exposure unacceptable. In severe cases malunion will occur before complete soft tissue healing. Rapid closed or percutaneous reduction and stabilization with external fixation can permit early knee motion and help to decrease the effects of massive scarring.

Young children with open growth plates can be managed with skeletal pin traction. External fixation can be used as "portable traction." Open fractures in children treated with external fixation are more accessible for soft tissue procedures such as debridement and skin grafts than traction and splints or casts. External fixation can stabilize physeal injuries without surgical exposure for plating or the risk of penetrating the physis.

In general, fractures of the distal femur are more often treated with internal fixation or traction rather than external fixation, as compared with the proximal tibia. The geometry and fracture patterns of the distal femur do not lend themselves readily to safe external fixation. Distal femoral pins near the joint would be intraarticular and thus at risk for sepsis of the knee joint. It is possible to bridge the knee and place pins well above and below it, thus bypassing the zone of injury. Thigh pins tether large muscle groups. Pain restricts active motion. This plus scarring contribute to the most common problem of external fixation in the thigh, loss of knee motion.

Operating Room Case Setup

The use of radiolucent operating room tables permits the use of image intensifiers during frame application.

The ability to see all necessary parts of the limb must be verified with the image prior to prepping and draping. An offending bar or other piece of the table can obscure an important part of the field of view during the case. Plain x-rays can be used to verify joint surfaces depending on image resolution. It is easy with an image intensifier to obtain several quick oblique views to ensure that no hardware is in the joint when tolerances are tight. This is especially important with percutaneous supplemental screw fixation.

The timing and coordination in polytrauma cases should be agreed on by the trauma team prior to the start of surgery. Contaminated and clean portions of the case require reprepping and redraping. Adequate stock of sizes must be checked prior to the start of the procedure. Very large or very small sizes should be available. Redundancy is useful protection for accidentally stripping or bending a part. Separately wrapped extra instruments are handy for the ones that happen to fall off the sterile field most often. Antibiotic irrigation and method of delivery should be based on surgeon preference and local protocols.

Both immediate and planned soft tissue procedures must be kept in mind in deciding on the type and configuration of frame to be used. Some pin placements make local rotation flaps difficult at best. Debridement of necrotic or infected tissue should precede hardware placement. An exception might be with temporarily used devitalized shaft fragments to aid in estimating alignment and rotation during reduction. Xenografts and synthetic materials can be used as "biologic dressings" for wound protection between initial debridement and definitive coverage.

Bone grafting is needed for bone loss, comminution, and cavities made by elevating compressed cancellous bone. The timing of bone grafting for loss or comminution will depend on the status of the wound and risk of infection. After open contaminated wounds, grafting is best done after stable soft tissue coverage. This will usually be several weeks after flaps and skin grafting. The type of graft material, such as autograft, allograft, and other bone substitutes, should be based on a surgeon's experience and preference.[17] The availability of allograft or instruments for harvesting autograft also should be verified prior to the start of surgery.

Hardware

Hardware choices are many but general patterns exist. Pins can be broken down into half or transfixtion types. Other factors are diameter and threaded versus smooth. Thin smooth wires are used with ring frames. Washers or beads welded on the shaft of the thin wires can be used to compress or shift bone for reductions. Thin wires are tensioned to provide rigidity to the ring segment. Larger-diameter (usually greater than 4 mm) transfixation pins are not tensioned and are threaded in

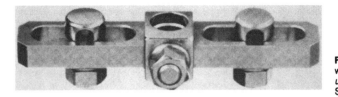

Figure 6–1. AO transverse clamp. (Reprinted with permission from Müller ME, et al. *Manual of Internal Fixation*, 3rd ed. New York: Springer Verlag, 1991)

the center area. These threads are intended for cortical purchase and will not hold as well in soft cancellous bone. Half-pins are available in self-drilling and self-tapping varieties. Sharp cutting flutes help decrease heat during insertion. Power insertion will cause thermal necrosis in hard bone.

Frames with ball joint or universal joint connectors for the bars have the advantage of easy correction of deformity and easier reductions. They are more "user friendly." Clamps with fewer degrees of freedom demand accurate reduction prior to pin insertion. Ring fixators are able to gain purchase in short segments of bone because of their ability to fan out pins horizontally over a short axial distance. There are anatomic restraints on possible safe pin placement with transfixation pins. Half-pins also have "safe corridors" for placement.[18]

Isolated fracture fragments of the proximal tibia can be adequately held by half-pins. Avoiding the patella ligament necessitates straddling it with pins that are held by some type of T-clamp (Fig. 6–1). Any fracture lines should be stabilized by supplementary screws to help counteract half-pin loosening by bending forces on pins in the bone near or through fracture lines. Ring fixators with multiple tensioned thin pins do the job of holding the segment of bone and pinning together the fracture lines at the same time. Supplementary screws can also be used, however.

Ring fixators on the shafts of long bones have the disadvantage of tethering muscle tendon units and possibly skewering nerves or blood vessels. To avoid this, a ring on the knee can be combined with a bar and half-pins on the shaft. These "hybrid" frames combine the advantage of both types of systems and are available from a variety of manufacturers. Care must be taken when using transfixation pins in the very distal femur. These pins will be intraarticular because of the anatomy of the knee joint capsule. The possibility of knee joint sepsis exists. On the tibial side, pins can be placed close to the joint line and still be extracapsular.

Knee fusions can be done with both half-pin and transfixation pin-type frames with either rings or bars. Stability is important. There should be at least two planes of pins used on bar-type frames. When ring-type frames are used, two rings per segment of bone should

be used. This helps to ensure adequate control of bony segments.

A variety of materials are available for use. Two advantages to look for are strong lightweight materials and the ability to x-ray through the material and see bone detail. Carbon fiber rods and pin clamps are available. Care must be taken not to strip carbon fiber pin clamps with wrenches during application. Ring frames on the knee used in fracture care should have an open section in the back to facilitate knee flexion. Lightweight, open-section, radiolucent ring frames have proved elusive. Carbon fiber rings are usually closed rings and the open-section rings are usually metal. The placement of pin clamps and hence ring placement can be varied depending on what the surgeon needs to see most on x-ray (Fig. 6–2).

More recent developments include the use of absorbable fracture fixation implants and motorized transport frames. Problems with adverse inflammatory reactions with drainage have occurred with some absorbable implants. Increased bulk is necesary for mechanical strength. Cannulated metal screws are safer to insert and are easier to verify extraarticular placement on x-ray. This is important when placement very close to the joint is necessary because of small fracture fragment size. Motorized transport frames will be a convenience to the patient. United States Federal Drug Administration approval has not been forthcoming on early models. Successful bone transport is certainly possible without motorized transport.

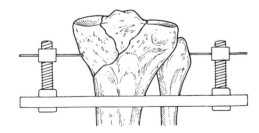

Figure 6–2. Pin clamps on top side of ring permit x-ray view of the tibial plateau.

Techniques

Good clinical outcomes with external fixation require, among other things, avoiding errant pin placement. A sound knowledge of cross-sectional anatomy is necessary. A good reference is the text by Faure and Merloz.[19] This book gives detailed drawings by section at various levels in the limbs. Copies of the diagrams can be used as templates for drawing out planned pin placements. Thus, it is possible to preassemble frame components on ring fixators. Minor adjustments will be necessary in the operating room. Half-pin placement on the tibia should be performed using the "safe corridors."[18] A frequent problem with use of external fixation on the femur is muscle tethering and the resulting knee stiffness. Soft tissue inflammation and muscle contractures are a problem with ring fixators in shaft applications. This is especially true with bone transport cases.

Another aspect of successful clinical outcome involves the appropriate selection of frame configuration. Adequate stability with a minimum of soft tissue trauma is the goal. Stability is enhanced by pins in multiple planes, thicker pins, increased pin spread in bone segment, shorter "working length" of pin, increased number of pins, stiffer frame materials, and increased cross-linking of frame components.[20,21] When using ring fixators, spreading pin clusters away from each side of the ring will increase stability (Fig. 6–3). This is, however, difficult to achieve in the proximal tibia. The knee joint cavity is on one side of the ring and the peroneal nerve by the fibula neck is on the other side of the ring near a typical pin placement site. For this reason, only a single plane of pins can be inserted, which ideally is done with three pins spaced as widely apart as the structures in the popliteal fossa will permit. The pes anserine bursa and medial gastrocnemius muscle are severely irritated when pierced by pins.

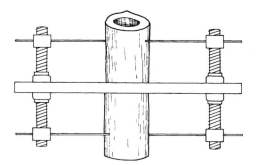

Figure 6–3. Pins on each side of ring increase stability.

Skin incisions for half-pin placement should be done in a manner to prevent tenting of the skin by the pins. The skin on the exit side of a transfixation pin can be slightly shifted prior to penetration by the pin to prevent tenting. Sleeves can be used to prevent soft tissue damage by drills or pins. Thin wires are sharp and should be inserted, tensioned, cut, and capped one at a time to prevent injury to the surgical team.

Preassembly of ring fixators will significantly decrease operative time. With tube or bar fixators, caps at the ends prevent clamps from sliding off prior to tightening. It is important to place the most distal and the most proximal pins first with bar-type fixators. Otherwise, the last pin may not be over the bone because of slight divergence of the bar with respect to the axis of the tibia.

In fracture cases, reduction of fragments is achieved before or during frame application. It is important to verify adequate reduction prior to committing oneself with extensive hardware placement. Percutaneously placed K-wires can be used for provisional fixation for tibial plateau fractures. In cases of joint and shaft fractures with large fragments, the joint surfaces should be aligned first. This is because the last pieces assembled, in this case the shaft segment, will tend to have the greatest stepoff. Although alignment is important, small incongruities of the shaft surfaces are not as critical as joint surface incongruities.

Closed reductions are best done as soon as possible. Organizing hematomas and soft tissue swelling will impede reduction maneuvers. When accurate closed reductions are not possbile, percutaneous instrumentation may make the difference between successful reduction and failure. Small elevators can lever pieces into position. The judicious use of bone hooks can help pull segments together. Steinman pins can be used to spear fragments and then steer them into position. This is sometimes referred to as a "joystick" maneuver.

One commonly used frame for proximal tibial fractures is the T-frame (Fig. 6–4). Half-pins are used to secure the bony fragments to bars and clamps. A transverse clamp is parallel to the knee joint and perpendicular to the long axis of the bone. The pins are oriented perpendicular to the long axis of the bone on the lateral view. The pins should be placed through the clamps which are already on the bars. This ensures the frame can be fitted to the pins. The most distal and the most proximal pins should be inserted first to prevent missing the bone at one end. After the proximal pin group is inserted within the transverse clamp, the fracture is reduced and then the most distal shaft pin is inserted. Prestressing of the pins by bending was described by the AO group but, now, they advocate radial preloading of pins.[22]

When there are fractures of the tibia extending near or into the knee joint, hybrid frames can be used (Fig. 6–5). A ring is used near the joint and half-pins and

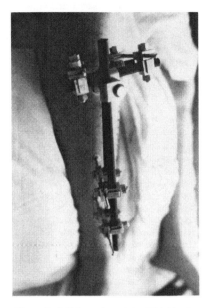

Figure 6–4. T-frame for proximal tibial fracture.

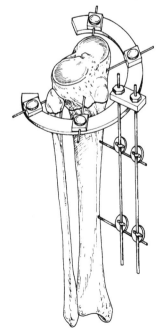

Figure 6–5. Hybrid frame for proximal tibial fracture.

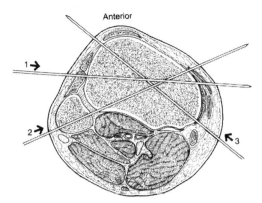

Fig 6–6. Transverse pin location shown on cross section of proximal tibia.

bars are used on the shaft. Thin wires are inserted and tensioned across a ring just below the joint. They are placed approximately at the level of the fibular head. The horizontal orientation follows a fairly consistent pattern (Fig. 6–6). Supplementary cannulated screws can be used to help lag fracture fragments together. The thin wires themselves act to hold the fractures together because they cross at angles to one another. The best pin to insert first is the transverse pin through the mid-tibia (Fig. 6–7). The image intensifier is used to verify placement. The rings are connected to a bar or tube by clamps which offer a wide range of adjustment. These clamps are used to help correct varus or valgus deformities. Correction of recurvatum or procurvatum is much more limited and these deformities must be guarded against. This is done by observing the position of the leg in the lateral view while inserting the pins. The pins should appear perpendicular to the long axis of the bone.

Frames for knee fusion usually involve pins in the anteroposterior and lateral planes. Transfixation pins in the lateral plane and half-pins in the anteroposterior plane constitute a common configuration (Fig. 6–8). Connecting the anterior bar and the side bars with cross-linking bars increases the stability. Missing the bone posteriorly with the mediolateral pins or overpenetrating with the anteroposterior pins can have catastrophic vascular consequences. When the fusion is done for a failed knee prosthesis, bone stock is often a problem. Factors to be considered are contact surface area, compressive force, stability, and vascularity of remaining bone. Large amounts of graft will take a long time to heal, incorporate, or dissolve. Based on the principle of polar moment of inertia, the bone graft is best placed around the cortical periphery rather than at the center of the joint. Ring frames offer little advantage for a

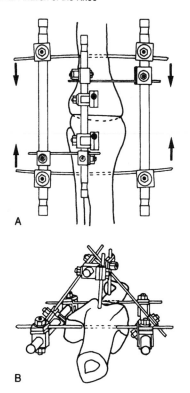

Figure 6–7. Example of knee fusion frame showing two planes of pins. (Reprinted with permission from *Manual on the AO-ASIF Tubular External Fixator.*)

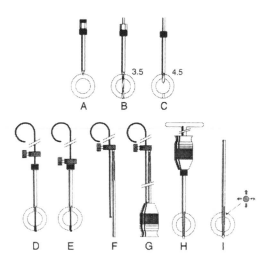

Figure 6–8. Depth gauge and sleeve system for external fixator pins. (Reprinted with permission from Müller ME, et al. *Manual of Internal Fixation*, 3rd ed. New York: Springer Verlag, 1991)

routine fusion. If there is a significant leg length shortening, a ring frame can be used for lengthening. Because of possible loss of proper limb alignment during transport, the frame should be capable of the widest range of adjustment possible. Ball joints lend themselves to easy correction. Muscle tethering of the quadriceps is not a concern with knee fusion. The bulk of a ring fixator between a patient's legs can interfere with ambulation.

Postoperative Management

The initial postoperative care usually focuses on the soft tissue injury and pin site wound care. Wounds may require various dressing changes such as wet to dry with normal saline, Dakin's solution, Silvadene, or continuing moist normal saline with exposed bone and tendon. Skin grafts may involve the use of heat lamps on donor sites and pressure antishear dressings on the graft bed. Free tissue transfers will need temperature probe monitoring and should be readily accessible to check

color and capillary refilling. Pin wounds are dressed according to surgeon preference. Bolster-type dressings that limit excessive skin motion on pins seem to help decrease inflammation. Although the incidence of reported pin tract infection varies widely, chronic osteomyelitis is uncomon.[23] As the 1-cm or so wounds around the pins are healing, it is important to prevent a buildup of dried blood and crust which will block the egress of serous drainage. Although dilute hydrogen peroxide solution is popular and effective at loosening crust, it is irritating to exposed tissue. Plain normal saline is safer when used with sterile applicators several times a day, depending on the amount of drainage. Any use of antibiotic ointments must not prevent free drainage of serous fluid. The skin will eventually wrap around the shaft of the pin as healing progresses.[24] If kept clean, pins can be kept in subcutaneous bone positions for many months. The thicker the muscle envelope the pins are going through, the higher the incidence of pin inflammation. Local injection of antibiotic solution has been used in addition to systemic administered medication. Removal, exchange, and surgical debridement should be done in the face of persistent purulent drainage. Obvious bony changes such as ring sequestra require overdrilling and curettage.

With the exception of all-ring fixator frames, most external fixators of the knee are not intended for full weight bearing. This includes hybrid frames. Testing of the hybrid frames and the resulting data need to be compared with existing data. The issue is based on the stability of the frame and the instability caused by the

injury. Massive soft tissue disruption, severe comminution, and segmental loss all put heavy demands on the
frame's strength and rigidity. Touch-down weight bearing makes ambulation easier than non-weight bearing
because of balancing and is permissible as the stresses
on the bone–external fixator construct are tolerable.
Prolonged loading of the pin sites will cause loosening
unless healing of the injury progresses. Some physicians
leave external fixators on to union with fractures, gradually destabilizing the frame as healing progresses.
The other option is to remove the frame and place the
patient in a cast or brace.

The timing of frame removal is easier to evaluate
with fractures than nonunions because of x-ray changes.
Fractures with soft tissue injuries are usually treated
empirically based on the surgeon's experience, with 6 to
8 weeks being a common number. If the frame is removed before complete fracture healing, a determination based on x-ray and physical examination of stability is made as to whether a cast or removable brace is
needed. A hinged brace permits knee motion but unless
the brace is polycentric and perfectly positioned, the
brace can accentute stress on the injured knee. There
must be enough fracture healing with some clinical stability to justify a hinged fracture brace in cases of early
frame removal.

Complications and Pitfalls

Pin Insertion

The two issues with pin problems are where you put it
and how you put it in. Knowledge of the cross-sectional
anatomy is needed to prevent "getting lost" during insertion. It is important to remember that the anatomic
references deal with uninjured limbs. Trauma may con-
vert a foreleg to a "one-vessel" limb. Surgical trauma
to what may ordinarily be one of three vessels can
necessitate prompt vascular repair or reconstruction.
Violated vessels can require repair, patching, or grafting. The surgical "team" should have these capabilities
on call before proceeding with pin insertion with
accompanying vascular trauma. Angiograms can also
show anomalies, although these would usually be done
before reconstructive procedures only if vascular injury
is not suspected. Errant drill bits and fixation pins will
wrap up nearby soft tissues. Placing sleeves to the near
cortex of the bone and avoiding overpenetration prevent injury with half-pins. Transfixation pins are "on
their own" in passage through the limb after the far cortex is passed. The selection of where to put the pins
should be based on how close to vital structures the pins
will pass. Fortunately, the metaphyseal areas of the distal femur and proximal tibia have wide "safe corridors."

The size and the number of pins used should be
based on the size of the patient and the type of frame
configuration. In an adult tibia and femur, 4.5- or 5.5-

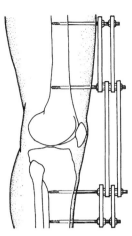

Figure 6–9. Unilateral half-pin frame over the anterior surface of the knee may be used for short-term management of
soft tissue problems about the knee.

mm half-pins are usually selected. Transfixation pins
that are not tensioned are usually 4.0 mm. Tensioned
thin wires are usually 1.8 to 2.0 mm. Two pins per bony
segment is normally sufficient in fracture cases if properly spaced. X-rays need to be checked intraoperatively to look for fracture lines propagating from pin sites
which will cause loosening in short order.

The technique of pin insertion will determine the incidence of thermal necrosis in hard cortical bone.[25,26] It
is easy to exceed the approximately 50°C needed to cause
the death of bone around the pin site. Dull drill bits and
the use of power for insertion of pins will increase the
chances of finding ring sequestra on follow-up x-rays.
Power insertion of half-pins makes it hard to estimate
depth of insertion. With sleeves, depth gauges, and
fixture of length of pin exposed in a Jacob's chuck instrument, it is possible to insert a pin to the desired
depth in a reproducible manner (Fig. 6–9). With the
thread pitches found on most half-pins and the average
cortical thicknesses of adult tibias, it is possible to count
five revolutions after the far cortex is encountered to
obtain the proper insertion depth. Self-tapping pins
must be inserted deep enough so the tap flutes are
through the far cortex for maximal purchase. X-ray
confirmation of pin depth is easy with an image intensifier.

Reduction Problems

Difficulty in obtaining reduction will depend on the instability present and soft tissue interposition. Multiple
forceful attempts at reduction are unwise. If a reduction
can be achieved but quickly slips, provisional fixation

with K-wires is helpful. If a closed reduction cannot be obtained, the soft tissue must be evaluated for open reduction. Small incisions can cause big problems when carried out in the zone of injury. Any preexisting circulatory impairment compounds the problem. Although this is germane in most geriatric trauma, a history of vascular disease must be checked for in younger patients.

The combination of very small "stab" wounds and an image intensifier can be used to steer pieces of bone into position. Normal anatomic relationships are altered with soft tissue disruption and extra care must be taken to avoid trapping nerves and vessels during the reduction process. Small blunt elevators are well suited for this use. X-rays should be obtained to check for surprises before completing definitive fixation. Displacement of unsuspected fractures and errant hardware placement are two important possible findings. Large bone reduction clamps placed percutaneously are especially helpful with split fragments of bone. The arms of the clamps must be bent to prevent crushing underlying soft tissues.

Sepsis

Pin tract infections occur in about 8.5% of cases.[27] In cases of bone transport, virtually every case will have some pin inflammation and drainage. With regular pin care and prompt intervention, chronic deep infection is rare. Superficial pin tract infections take on another dimension when present near incisions and wounds. Deep infection is best treated with early debridement and deep cultures to establish identity of the organisms causing the infection. Debridement may need to include removal of bone graft, necrotic flap tissue, or missed necrotic tissue from the injury. It is therefore important to properly debride and reexamine a wound to establish its readiness to accept bone graft and tissue coverage. A wound is initially contaminated and then becomes colonized and eventually infected. Soft tissue coverage should be done once all necrotic tiissue is debrided to prevent a colonized wound from becoming infected. Definitive coverage by 3 to 5 days is possible and desirable.[28] It is subsequent tissue death from operating in a zone of injury or missed necrotic tissue during coverage procedures that cause sepsis.

Prophylactic antibiotics are not needed beyond 3 to 5 days.[29,30] Recent studies have started to look at shorter times. Prolonged prophylactic antibiotics serve little except to select out resistant organisms. Methicillin-resistant staphylococcal infections have been increasing and the proper use of systemic antibiotics for the treatment of infections based on culture results is mandatory. Antibiotic-impregnated beads and staged bone grafts of defects have helped decrease infection of massive open wounds with bone loss.[31] The beads help to

maintain a space for the graft while the natural contraction of surrounding soft tissues occurs.

Soft Tissue Problems

Soft tissue coverage of large knee wounds can involve rotation flaps and free tissue transfers depending on location. Gastrocnemius flaps can be mobilized enough to cover the proximal tibia. The distal femoral area would require a free tissue transfer for large wounds. Skin grafting over granulating wounds or muscle flaps completes the coverage. The knee joint must be covered rapidly to prevent loss of articular cartilage. Closure of the joint capsule over a drain acutely and moist dressings with normal saline can be used until definitive coverage. Desiccation of the cartilage must be prevented. The problem of stabilization with external fixators is that they get in the way. Complex ring configurations create formidable obstacles to access for soft tissue coverage procedures. Unilateral half-pin frames are much better in this regard but not as well suited to stabilizing the knee joint. As a temporary bridging frame, a unilateral half-pin frame can be used until soft tissues have been healed and then definitive bony work can be accomplished.[32]

Prudent delays of 3 to 5 days with closed injuries before contemplated open procedures give the true extent of the soft tissue injury a chance to unfold. Severe swelling and blister formation should be treated as a burn. Bloody blisters have a worse prognosis with respect to depth of tissue loss.[33] Proximal tibia fractures that can be reduced with closed or percutaneous methods are amenable to treatment with hybrid frames. The hybrid frame can also be used as a neutralization plate with percutaneously placed interfragmentary compression screws. Long dissections and stripping of fracture fragments can be avoided in this manner. Soft tissue degloving injuries create random islands of ischemic tissue based on marginal blood supply. Incisions that would be safe in normal tissue can wreak havoc. The larger incisions required for open reduction and internal fixation of distal femur fractures have to be made through suitable tissues. Traction or external fixation bridging the area can be used as temporizing measures.

Care must be taken to not place the pins where a pin tract infection will compromise a site of definitive fixation. This also applies to limb salvage situations where pin tract infections occur above amputaion levels if the salvage fails. If placement is unavoidable, prompt removal and exchange or a switch to traction should be done for infected pins.

Loss of Fixation

Possible causes of loss of fixation include displacement of fracture lines near pins, hardware failure, sepsis, cutout of pins from bone, and aseptic loosening as a result of mechanical loading causing the pin to work loose in the bone. Patient compliance is important in preventing hardware failure. Early failure is usually due to the strength of the implants and frame; late failure is due to fatigue. Serial x-rays will show gradual loosening as a result of mechanical loosening. Infected pins are usually obvious from the drainage, pain, and erythema. Fever is not usually present if the pin is draining freely. Bone erosion by an infected pin site requires pin removal and debridement. If the frame must still be used, a new pin site must be chosen for insertion. Patients with problems of immunosuppression are at risk for multiple pin infections, which can be difficult to control with antibiotics. The author has had several patients with an HIV infection who required amputation despite aggressive treatment.

Another cause of fixation loss is failure to adequately tighten or recheck tightness of components. It is important to check all components for wrench tightness prior to taking the final films. In patients who are ambulating on the frames, instructions should be given to check tightness and report any problems promptly. Patients need to be cautioned against making any "modifications" of their frames.

Salvage

Salvage procedures for failed attempts at external fixation of the knee include revision of fixation (either external or internal), arthrodesis, traction, and arthroplasty. The age of the patient and presence of infection may be relative contraindications to some of the preceding options. Except in the early stages of care of a polytrauma patient or patient with severe pulmonary injury, traction can usually be resorted to with its attendant risks. Skin breakdown, especially in the elderly, tremendously increases the cost of medical care as well as the risk of further complications. Risk assessment and appropriate bed and mattress selection along with defined skin care protocols have been shown to decrease decubiti and their complications.

If a switch to internal fixation for definitive care is being considered, external fixation should be removed and, if necessary, traction instituted as soon as the soft tissues will permit. The length of time needed between pin removal and subsequent internal fixation is controversial. Absence of significant pin tract infections and clean, dry pin wounds are certainly recommended. A simple half-pin frame put on acutely to stabilize a knee for soft tissue care can be converted to a more stable frame for fusion if the joint is not salvageable. As more experience is gained with converting arthritic knees to total knee replacements after an external fixator has been used for high tibial osteotomies and

angular correction, the question of old pin sites and infection with prostheses can be better answered. This method of correction and fixation needs more time and several large series to validate the recommendation of its use.

External fixators are often resorted to for salvage procedures after failed knee arthroplasties requiring arthrodesis. Bone grafting is often required. Shortening results from bone loss from mechanical destruction, sepsis, or surgical debridement. The limited experience with lengthening in association with fusions has shown an increased complication rate. The use of a shoe lift is safer for most limb length inequalities.

Results

The literature on external fixation of the knee deals primarily with fusions and frames bridging the knee in severe injuries. Use of the Wagner device for distal femur fractures has been reported.[34] These did not involve the knee joint, however. Use on the femur is usually for limb salvage situations. Very little has been published on the use of hybrid frames.[35] At the time of this writing, early reports of series with hybrid frames have been presented at meetings[36]; these include the author's, which will be described.

The literature reports a success rate of approximately 50 to 80% for knee arthrodesis after failed knee arthroplasty depending on the type of prosthesis.[37] The more bone loss involved, the higher the failure rate. Results with frames crossing the knee are not well documented with respect to specific aspects of the external fixator. The outcome in these cases usually depends on revascularization, soft tissue coverage, and extent of articular damage. All of these are complex issues, and separating out the particulars on the use of external fixation is difficult at best. It clearly has been successful when everything else has worked.

The author's experience reflects the literature with respect to limited use of external fixation on the femur. I prefer to use internal fixation combined with aggressive debridement and early soft tissue coverage. I have favored internal fixation for knee fusion except in the face of infection. The carbon fiber components with two planes of pins spread between 60° and 90° have been successful and well tolerated by patients for knee arthrodesis. Debridement and staged bone grafts after clean and dry wounds are usually used. Computed tomography (CT) scans are helpful to pinpoint the location of small sequestra within the medullary cavity of a proposed knee arthrodesis.

The use of the hybrid frame for periarticular fractures of the tibia is being reported by the author and several colleagues.[38] Illustrated are cases showing the use of the

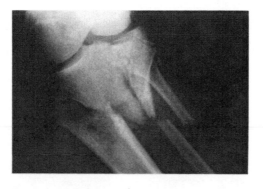

A

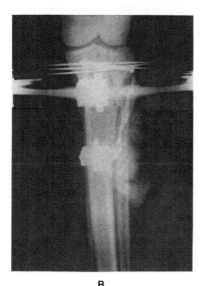

B

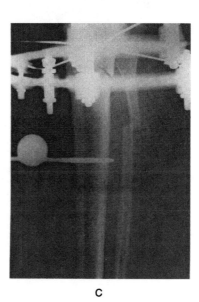

C

Figure 6–10. A. Shatzker type VI tibial plateau fracture. **B.** AP view showing percutaneous fixation with interfragmentary screw and hybrid frame. **C.** Lateral view.

hybrid frame (Figs. 10–10 to 10–12). In an early series from 1989, seventeen proximal tibia fractures were included. The final average knee motion was approximately 3° to 105°. Seven cases required supplemental internal fixation. Three were done percutaneously, three through a limited arthrotomy, and one through a formal midline approach to the knee. There were no deep infections, although we acknowledge a significant risk with pins transversing intraarticular fracture lines.

Work is continuing with hybrid frames to define their role for both open and closed injuries. The ability to achieve reduction with limited arthrotomies and at what cost are questions that need to be answered with more data. The initial experience has been encouraging. The author recommends the use of hybrid frames for periarticular fractures of the tibia when open reduction and internal fixation are precluded because of soft tissue conditions.

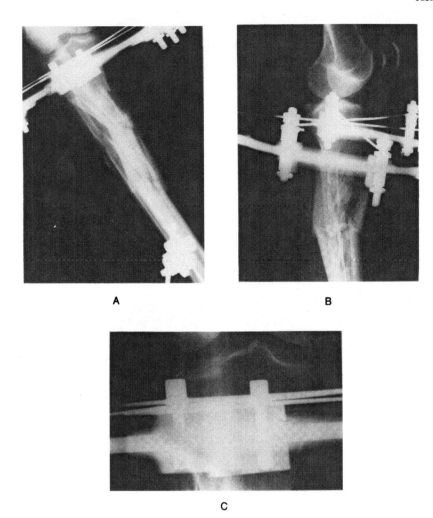

A   B

C

Figure 6–11. Comminuted proximal tibial fracture stabilized with hybrid external fixator. **A.** AP view. **B.** Lateral view. **C.** Tibial plateau visible above external fixator.

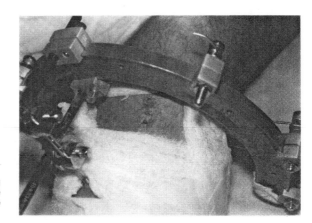

Figure 6–12. Hybrid external fixator with open ring and thin transverse wires at the upper end of the tibia, and connecting rod with half-pins over the mid- and distal tibia.

References

1. Parkhill C. A new apparatus for the fixation of bones after resection and in fractures with a tendency to displacement. *Trans Am Surg Assoc.* 1897;15:251–256.
2. Lambotte A. *Chirurgie Operatoire des Fractures.* Paris: Masson & Cie; 1913.
3. Colton CL. The history of fracture treatment. In: Browner BD, Jupiter JB, Levine AM, Trafton PG. *Skeletal Trauma Fractures, Dislocations. Ligamentous Injuries.* Philadelphia: WB Saunders; 1992:23.
4. Hoffman R. Rotules a os pour la reduction dirigee, nonsanglante, des fractures (osteotaxis). *Helv Med Acta.* 1938;6:844–850.
5. Behrens F. General theory and principles of external fixation. *Clin Orthop.* 1989;241:15–23.
6. Behrens F, Searls K. External fixation of the tibia. Basic concepts and prospective evaluation. *J Bone Joint Surg Br.* 1986;68:246.
7. Ilizarov GA. The tension–stress effect on the genesis and growth of tissues: Part I. The influence of stability of fixation and soft-tissue preservation. *Clin Orthop.* 1989; 238:249–281.
8. Ilizarov GA. The tension–stress effect on the genesis and growth of tissues: Part II. The influence of the rate and frequency of distraction. *Clin Orthop.* 1989;239:263–285.
9. Green SA. The Ilizarov method: Rancho technique. *Orthop Clin North Am.* 1991;22:677–688.
10. Cone JB. Vascular injury associated with fracture-dislocations of the lower extremity. *Clin Orthop.* 1989; 243:30–35.
11. Damron T, McBeath A. Diagnosis and management of vascular injuries associated with skeletal trauma. *Orthop Rev.* 1991;20:12–19.
12. Raffi M, LaMont JG. CT evaluation of tibial plateau fractures. *Crit Rev Diagn Imaging.* 1987;2:91.
13. Swiontkowski MF. Criteria for bone debridement in massive lower limb trauma. *Clin Orthop.* 1989;243:41–47.
14. Behrens F. Fractures with soft tissue injuries. In: Browner BD, Jupiter JB, Levine AM, Trafton PG, *Skeletal Trauma Fractures, Dislocations, Ligamentous Injuries.* Philadelphia: WB Saunders; 1992:318.
15. Suedkamp NP, Tscherne H. Hannover fracture scale: A new concept for evaluation of fractures with concomitant soft-tissue injury. Presented at the Orthopaedic Trauma Association annual meeting, Minneapolis, 1992.
16. Benirschke SK, Agnew SG, Mayo KA, Santoro VM, Henley MB. Immediate internal fixation of open complex tibial plateau fractures: Treatment by a standard protocol. *J Othrop. Trauma.* 1992;6:78–86.
17. Bucholz RW, Carlton A, Holmes R. Interporous hydroxyapatite as a bone graft substitute in tibial plateau fractures. *Clin Orthop.* 1989;240:53–62.
18. Green SA. *Complications of External Skeletal Fixation. Causes, Prevention, and Treatment.* Springfield, IL: Charles C Thomas; 1981.
19. Faure C, Merloz Ph. *Transfixation Atlas of Anatomical Sections for the External Fixation of Limbs.* New York: Springer-Verlag; 1987:66–119.
20. Chao EYSL, An K-A. Stress and rigidity analysis of external fracture fixation devices. In: Brooker A, Edwards C, eds. *External Fixation: The Current State of the Art.* Baltimore: Williams & Wilkins; 1979;691–711.
21. Tencer AF, Claudi B, Pearce S. Development of a variable stiffness external fixation system for stabilization of segmental defects of the tibia. *J Orthop Res.* 1984;1:395–404.
22. Perren SM. Improved effectiveness of external fixator pins. In: Muller ME, Allgower M, Schneider R, Willenegger H, eds. *Manual of Internal Fixation Techniques Recommended by the AO-ASIF Group.* New York: Springer-Verlag; 1991:80.
23. Roomens PM, Broos PLO, Stappaerts K, Gruwez JA. Internal stabilization after external fixation of fractures of the shaft of the tibia: Sense or nonsense? *Injury.* 1989;19:432–435.
24. Burny F. The pin as a percutaneous implant: General and related studies. *Orthopedics.* 1984;7:610–615.
25. Harkess JW, Ramsey WC, Harkess JW. Techniques of drilling holes in bone. In: Rockwood RA, Green DP, Buchloz RW, eds. *Rockwood and Green's Fractures in Adults.* Philadelphia: JB Lippincott; 1991:118–119.
26. Matthews LS, Green CA, Goldstein SA. The thermal effects of skeletal fixation—Pin insertion into bone. *J Bone Joint Surg Am.* 1984;66:1077.

27. Green SA. Complications of pin and wire external fixation. In: Greene WB, ed. *American Academy of Orthopaedic Surgeons Instructional Course Lectures, XXXIX.* Park Ridge: American Academy of Orthopaedic Surgeons; 1990: 219–228.
28. Godina M. Early microsurgical reconstruction of complex trauma of the extremities. *Clin Plast Surg.* 1986;13:619–620.
29. Dellinger EP, Miller SD, Wertz MJ. Risk of infection after open fracture of the arm or leg. *Arch Surg.* 1987;123:1320–1327.
30. Patzakis MF, Wilkins J, Moore TM. Considerations in reducing the infection rate of open tibial fractures. *Clin Orthop.* 1983;178:36–41.
31. Henry SL, Popham GJ. Management of bone defects with staged bone grafting and antibiotic impregnated beads. *Tech Orthop.* 1992;7:47–54.
32. Rogge D. External articular transfixation for joint injuries with severe soft tissue damage. In: Tscherne H, Gotzen L, eds. *Fractures With Soft Tissue Injuries.* New York: Springer-Verlag; 1984:103–117.
33. Zuckerman JD, Giordano C. The clinical significance and histology of fracture blisters. Presented at the Orthopaedic Trauma Association annual meeting, Minneapolis, 1992.
34. Seligson D, Kristiansen TK. Use of the Wagner apparatus in complicated fractures of the distal femur. *J Trauma.* 1978;18:795.
35. Reith HB, Boddekar W, Pelzer C, Kozuschek W. "Ring fixator" for treatment of lower leg fractures. A review of 30 cases treated by a new external fixation system. *Int Surg.* 1988;73:170–172.
36. Browner BD, et al. Treatment of complex tibial plateau fractures with circular external fixators. Presented at the American Academy of Orthopaedic Surgeons annual meeting, San Francisco, 1993.
37. Russell TA. Arthrodesis of lower extremity and hip. In: Crenshaw AH, ed. *Campbell's Operative Orthopaedics.* St. Louis: CV Mosby; 1987:1106–1108.
38. Carter AT, Lamont JG, Uhl RL, Murphy MD. Use of a circular half-pin hybrid fixator for peri-articular tibia fractures. In preparation.

7
Bone and Cartilage Allografts in the Knee Joint

Peter van Eenenaam and William W. Tomford

Introduction

Bone and cartilage allografts have traditionally been used in the the knee for the treatment of tumors and failed joint replacement; however, there are several other indications for allograft arthroplasty of this joint. These include traumatic injuries, osteochondritis dissecans, osteonecrosis, patellofemoral disease, and post-traumatic arthritis. For the treatment of trauma, because anatomic restoration of injured tissues is the traditional goal, the use of allografts has generally been reserved for failures of one or even two attempts at this ideal. For the treatment of other conditions, applications of bone and cartilage allografts may primarily restore knee function.

In using allografts, one must consider the appropriate type of allograft to be transplanted, the biologic characteristics of allografts, and the methods of application. This chapter reviews different types of allografts useful in knee joint injuries and conditions, the biologic function of these different types, and their various applications. Recommendations are made regarding appropriate use of allografts in the knee joint, and the advantages and disadvantages of different types of allografts, as well as their procurement, are discussed.

Allografts

Allograft types include bone, cartilage, and combinations of bone and cartilage which are known as osteoarticular or osteochondral allografts. Various methods of processing and preparation as well as different methods of storage constitute important distinguishing characteristics among these types.

Bone allografts may be obtained either freeze-dried or frozen. Freeze-dried allografts usually consist of crushed or chipped cancellous or cortical bone. These grafts are most frequently supplied as cubes about 1 cm on a side (Fig. 7–1). These chips are cut from bone obtained from areas such as the metaphyses of long bones or iliac crests. Cortical struts are usually cut from the diaphyses of long bones and measure 1 to 2 cm wide and from 3 to 10 cm long.

After they are cut to size, freeze-dried allografts are washed thoroughly to remove marrow and blood and are then placed into bottles. Crushed or chipped bone is usually packaged in quantities of 30 to 60 mL. Cortical struts are usually packaged in quantities of two or three. The bones are then lyophilized (freeze-dried) in the bottles. This process removes up to 95% of the water from the bone. Bottles are sealed with large rubber stoppers and vacuum packed to allow long-term storage without refrigeration.

Frozen bone allografts may also be used in the knee joint. These types of grafts are usually confined to femoral heads and large diaphyseal or metaphyseal segments. Although femoral heads are available as freeze-dried bones, there is no advantage to the use of a freeze-dried femoral head. It is predominantly a cancellous graft, and freeze-dried cancellous chips are much easier to use. Femoral heads are usually packaged in plastic wraps or jars and must be kept frozen until the time of use. Metaphyseal or diaphyseal segments are usually cut at the time of procurement as the proximal or distal half of a long bone. Because these segments are used solely for bone grafting without the need to preserve articular cartilage, these grafts are frequently processed by washing the medullary canal and then storing them after wrapping and sealing in plastic. Grafts frozen at −80° may be stored several years.

A third type of graft useful in the treatment of knee trauma and other conditions is a frozen osteochondral

Peter van Eenenaam and William W. Tomford

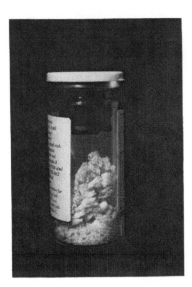

Figure 7-1. Freeze-dried cancellous allograft bone provided in sterile, dry form.

graft. This graft is stored frozen but is not processed. The articular cartilage of an osteochondral graft is cryoprotected by treating it with a cryopreservative such as glycerol or dimethyl sulfoxide prior to freezing. This method has been shown to preserve chondrocytes in articular cartilage. Osteochondral allografts stored by freezing are wrapped sterilely at the time of procurement and stored at −80°C until the time of surgery.

A similar type of cartilage graft also used in the knee is a fresh osteochondral allograft. This type of graft is removed from the donor and placed into a recipient within 48 hours of procurement. These grafts offer the advantage of transplanting large numbers of viable chondrocytes in the cartilage portion of the graft. Between procurement and transplantation, the graft is stored under refrigeration at 4°C. Recipients are required to be on call to receive this type of transplant.

Advantages and Disadvantages of Allografts

There are advantages as well as disadvantages to the use of each type of allografts that are independent of their applications. It is important for surgeons to be aware of these characteristics so that the decision to use an allograft may be based on an understanding of the risk inherent to allograft use as well as the benefit of its ability to replace anatomic structures.

The major advantage of freeze-dried allografts is that

they are least likely to transmit disease agents. Because these grafts are cut into small pieces that can be thoroughly washed free of marrow and blood elements, viruses that can be transmitted in blood such as human immunodeficiency virus (HIV) and hepatitis B virus may be removed.[1] In addition, many tissue banks that process freeze-dried bone also rinse it with bleach as an additional precaution because this chemical is highly toxic to infectious agents.

Another advantage of freeze-dried allografts is their ease of storage. As long as the vacuum remains intact, the bottle may be stored on a shelf at room temperature. In contrast, bones stored by freezing require large freezers that must be maintained at very low temperatures.

The major disadvantage of freeze-drying is that it is not useful for preserving long bones. Several weeks are usually required to freeze-dry a large, whole, diaphyseal or metaphyseal segment of a long bone. In addition, the hoop or circumferential strength of a long-bone allograft may be compromised by the drying process.[2] Furthermore, vacuum packing of large segments of long bones is difficult. Consequently, freeze-dried bone allografts are usually small chips which are most useful for packing or for supplementing autograft bone.

The major advantage of freezing is that large portions of long bones, such as distal or proximal femurs and femoral diaphyseal segments, may be easily preserved by freezing. This process results in little or no damage to tissues, and storage may extend several years as long as the tissue remains frozen. Although the choice of temperature is somewhat arbitrary, the material should be maintained at least as cold as −40°C. The lower the temperature, the longer the storage time.

The major disadvantage of using frozen long bones is that they may more easily transmit disease agents than freeze-dried bone.[3] This disadvantage is not due to the difference in storage methods. Instead, it is related to the fact that although long bones may be washed prior to freezing, it is impossible to remove all blood and marrow from a medullary canal.[4] Although the risk of disease transmission is not high if donors of long bones are properly screened, frozen bones, whether processed or unprocessed, may contain blood, and any bone that contains blood may transmit diseases.

Osteochondral allografts are advantageous because they provide a means of replacement of articular cartilage; however, these types of grafts also contain blood and marrow. Because blood products cannot be completely removed from the metaphyseal portion of an osteochondral graft, these types of allografts are among the most risky of the grafts reviewed.

Fresh osteochondral grafts also provide the possibility of replacement of articular cartilage. Some authors have suggested that fresh cartilage grafts are superior to cryopreserved grafts because they contain larger numbers of viable chondrocytes that may remain alive several months following transplantation.[5]

Fresh osteochondral allografts are associated with a slightly higher risk of disease transmission than frozen osteochondral allografts. First, they contain fresh blood and may therefore transmit viral disease agents. Second, they may also carry bacterial organisms into their recipients. Cultures of frozen allografts are usually held a minimum of 7 days; however, transplantation of an allograft within 48 hours does not allow sufficient time for evaluation of culture results.

Biology of Allograft Incorporation

The allografts discussed here are incorporated by host bone in different ways. Knowledge of the method, extent, and time of incorporation is helpful in deciding on which type of graft should be used for a specific application.

Freeze-dried allograft bone chips are usually incorporated rapidly if they are used in an area with a good blood supply. For example, when used to supplement autograft bone in a depressed tibial plateau fracture, the freeze-dried bone chips are quickly surrounded by blood vessels and pluripotential bone cells. New bone is laid down on the chips, which are gradually replaced by host bone within a few months. Conversely, freeze-dried bone chips should not be used in areas in which the blood supply is poor. If used as the sole bone graft in treatment of a nonunion of a midshaft tibial fracture, they will virtually never be incorporated by the host. In areas with a poor blood supply, autograft bone should be used in conjunction with freeze-dried allograft.

Large frozen bones such as a distal femur or proximal tibia are incorporated much more slowly than small freeze-dried chips. Large allografts rely on ingrowth of vessels from the periphery of the graft to invade the cortex, remove old bone, and supply new bone in the process of incorporation. For incorporation to occur, it is important that these grafts are surrounded by a thick muscle cuff that can supply vessels for ingrowth. This is a very long-term process, and many long bone allograft segments take years to be incorporated.

Osteochondral allografts, whether frozen or fresh, are incorporated in a combination of the processes involving freeze-dried and frozen bone. Osteochondral grafts consist of cartilage and a small portion of metaphyseal bone. The cartilage is of course not replaced by the host. It is theoretically capable of survival in the absence of a direct blood supply, obtaining nourishment from the surrounding synovial fluid; however, host vessels invade and replace the metaphyseal and subchondral necrotic bone through a process of creeping substitution and revascularization.[6,7] This bone is trabecular although not particulate as are freeze-dried chips.

During the process of incorporation, host vessels infiltrate the metaphyseal bone of the graft and surround it as if it were cortical bone in the process of replacement. The metaphyseal bone of an osteochondral allograft is not, however, as thick as the cortex of a long bone. Therefore, invasion and infiltration of the allograft bone by host vessels occurs more rapidly. The process of incorporation takes several months as compared with the several years required for incorporation of a long-bone allograft.

The biologic fate of the cartilage portion of an osteochondral allograft in the knee joint appears to be related to several factors. Stable graft fixation and a closely congruent anatomic fit with opposing and adjacent joint surfaces are important requirements for graft survival.[8-18] The presence of significant ligamentous laxity has been shown to lead to early graft failure.[13,18,19] Thickness of subchondral bone is also believed to be important in the timing of graft incorporation and avoidance of collapse. Pap and Krompecher showed that graft thickness greater than about 5 mm resulted in rapid disintegration after transplantation.[20] Others have demonstrated the importance of bone thickness in timely incorporation.[6,11,12] Gross and coworkers suggested that the ultimate fate of an osteochondral graft was most dependent on the fate of the underlying subchondral bone rather than the thickness of the cartilage portion of the graft.[21] Use of thin subchondral bone has been recommended by most of these authors to enhance and maximize bone incorporation.

Perhaps the most important factor in minimizing cartilage wear following osteochondral transplantation is correction of any malalignment of the limb.[9,10,18,21,22] If forces across the cartilage exceed normal physiologic forces, the cartilage will rapidly break down. Therefore, prior to cartilage grafting in the knee joint, the mechanical alignment of the hip–knee–ankle must be normal. If alignment is normal, both fresh and frozen cartilage allografts appear to be capable of providing satisfactory joint function for several years.

Applications of Allografts in the Knee Joint

Bone allografts applied in the area of the knee joint have been uniformly successful in the treatment of bone loss due to fractures. The metaphyseal area of the femur and the tibia is highly vascularized and is therefore an ideal area for the use of allograft bone. In condylar and plateau fractures, freeze-dried chips as well as frozen femoral heads successfully provide restoration of crushed host bone (Figs. 7–2 and 7–3).

Osteochondral allografts including both bone and cartilage have been of more historic interest and significance to surgeons because of their unique capability of replacing damaged cartilage. The first extensive use

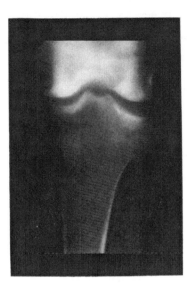

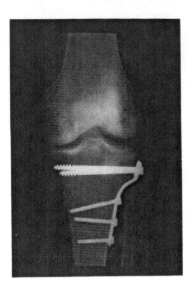

Figure 7–2. Split-depression fracture of the lateral tibial plateau as seen on tomogram of left knee.

Figure 7–3. Tibial plateau fracture elevated and packed with cancellous allograft placed under the lateral tibial plateau. Internal fixation has been performed as supporting the lateral tibial plateau and allograft.

of osteochondral allografts about the knee joint was reported by Lexer in 1925.[23] Most of Lexer's cases involved the treatment of septic joints, although several of his cases were traumatic injuries. He transplanted fresh allografts removed from knee joints procured from cadavers or amputations shortly before transplantation. Most of the transplants were shell allografts that replaced the condylar femoral surface as well as the tibial plateau. He was able to follow up about 50% of his cases, and noted good results in most of these.

Lexer made several important observations on the use of osteoarticular allografts in the knee joint. He reported that in whole-joint transplants, in which allografts were used to replace the distal femur as well as the proximal tibia, the articular cartilage remained intact for up to 2 years and then began to deteriorate. He found, however, that patients with these types of transplants did not complain of pain despite joint narrowing and degeneration noted on radiographic examinations. Lexer also found on pathologic analysis that subchondral collapse occurred at about 2 years and led to joint degeneration. For this reason, he developed an apparatus designed to reduce weight bearing across the transplanted joint and recommended that recipients use his brace for up to 2 years after transplant. It is likely that this brace substituted in part for surgical treatment of malalignment as currently recommended by surgeons

today; however, the brace also functioned as a means of reducing normal physiologic forces across the joint. In light of the fact that osteochondral allografts are incorporated several months after transplantation, this approach may provide time for the bone portion of the transplant to become sufficiently strong to withstand normal forces and thereby prevent premature collapse.

Following Lexer's reports, interest in cartilage and bone transplantation waned until Burwell reported his discovery in 1963 of diminished immunogenicity following freezer storage of these types of grafts.[24] Several authors reported their experience with the use of osteochondral allografts in the knee joint over the next two decades. Ottolenghi reported several successful cases of allograft treatment of knee injuries in 1972.[25] The grafts used were stored by freezing to −20°C. Similar to Lexer, Ottolenghi noted osteonecrosis and collapse of the subchondral bone within 2 years of transplantation. He called this phenomenon "neuropathic arthropathy" and believed it was similar to a Charcot type of joint disintegration. In 1966, and again in 1973, Parrish reported his experience with the use of frozen osteochondral allografts in tumor patients.[26,27] He noted extensive bone resorption in the subchondral portions of the grafts which led to joint degeneration, but he did not believe that immunologic responses were functional in the destruction of the grafts.

In 1976, Mankin et al published their first report on

the use of cryopreserved large osteoarticular allografts which included several cases of distal femoral and proximal tibial grafts.[28] Through numerous subsequent reports, they noted that the best results were obtained in cases in which the primary diagnosis was a benign neoplasm or traumatic injury. An average of 10% of these grafts required prosthetic replacement after 3 years because of subchondral collapse and subsequent joint destruction.[29]

Fresh osteochondral and cartilage grafts have been extensively used and studied by Mahomed et al. They recently reported on the long-term success of fresh, small osteochondral allografts used to replace intraarticular traumatic defects in the knee joint.[30] They found that grafts that replaced either the distal femur or proximal tibia had a better result than those that replaced both simultaneously, and they noted a 67% survival of grafts up to 14 years. Mahomed et al also noted that these types of grafts fared better in people younger than 60 and that normal joint alignment was crucial to joint survival. Although they used these types of grafts in cases involving other diagnoses such as degenerative joint disease and tumors, they noted their best results in traumatic injuries.

Several other authors have reported on the results of treatment of articular deficiencies in the knee joint. Using osteochondral shell allografts in 100 procedures followed for an average of 3.8 years, McDermott et al concluded that the best results were obtained with bone loss and osteonecrosis secondary to trauma.[9] They found that results of treatment of steroid-induced osteonecrosis and osteoarthritis were much poorer. Meyers and co-workers confirmed the generally poor results in osteoarthritis, reporting only a 30% success rate after 2 to 10 years of follow-up, but many of the failures were considered technical rather than physiologic.[17,18] They did note good results in the treatment of osteochondritis dissecans, osteonecrosis, and trauma to the femoral condyle, as well as posttraumatic arthritis of the tibial plateau. Their results with patellar resurfacing were also good. Osteonecrosis involving large portions of the femoral condyle have also been successfully treated with bulk osteochondral allografts.[14] Unlike Meyers' and Gross' groups, both of which used fresh allografts,[17,18,21] Flynn et al, studying frozen grafts, found that 70% of 17 knees were rated as good or excellent at an average follow-up of 4.2 years.[14] About one half of the patients had steroid-induced osteonecrosis.

The authors' personal experience with the use of osteochondral allografts in the knee is similar to that reported by other investigators. Several principles have become evident that have led to specific guidelines in the use of these grafts.[31] First, with the use of frozen osteochondral grafts, the limb must be aligned normally or perhaps even realigned to reduce forces across the graft as much as possible and, conversely, to place as much force as feasible on the more normal joint compartment. If normal alignment for a particular individual is abnormal compared with the general population, such as the excessive valgus that is encountered in some females and the excessive varus in some males, this individual's alignment must be corrected even though it is not excessive compared with the normal alignment for that particular individual.

Second, reduction of weight-bearing forces across the graft, even though alignment is normal or surgically corrected to normal, is important. Current protocol involves the use of a long-leg hinged brace measured and applied preoperatively. The purpose in using the brace is to place the anatomic alignment of the lower leg into varus or valgus compared with the upper leg. The direction depends on the location of the graft and the need to direct joint forces across the opposite side of the joint. The bone portion of the graft usually heals within 6 to 9 months, and the brace should be worn at least this length of time.

Third, the presence of mild to moderate degenerative changes in the opposite joint compartment or in the patellofemoral joint, as long as these changes are not accompanied by malalignment of the limb at the joint, is not a contraindication to the use of an osteochondral allograft. Despite these changes, as long as some articular cartilage remains, the use of an osteochondral graft is generally worthwhile. These types of grafts can provide pain relief even if other compartments demonstrate degenerative changes.

Fourth, osteochondral grafts, or at least frozen cryopreserved grafts, last about 4 to 5 years. Deterioration at that time will probably require revision to another graft or a joint replacement.

Obtaining Allografts

Numerous tissue banks that provide the types of allografts discussed in this chapter now exist throughout the United States. It is important to ensure that the tissue bank from which grafts are obtained follows current standards of tissue banking as promulgated by the American Association of Tissue Banks (AATB, McLean, Virginia) or other tissue banking associations. Now that a reasonable supply of most tissues is available, competition exists among tissue banks, and it is imperative that the surgeon be acquainted with the reputation and ideally some of the personnel of the bank. The AATB has a toll-free number (1–800–635–AATB, extension 2282) from which advice on ordering allografts may be obtained.

Acknowledgment. Work reviewed in this article was partially supported by National Institutes of Health Grant AR-21896.

References

1. Tomford WW. Disease transmission, sterilization, and the clinical use of musculoskeletal allografts. In: Tomford WW, ed. *Musculoskeletal Tissue Banking*. New York: Raven Press; 1993; 1993:213–218.

2. Bright R, Burchardt H. The biomechanical properties of preserved bone grafts. In: Friedlaender GE, Mankin HJ, Sell KW, eds. *Osteoarticular Allografts: Biology, Banking, and Clinical Applications*. Boston: Little, Brown; 1981:241–247.

3. Simonds RJ, Holmberg SD, Hurwitz RL, et al. Transmission of human immunodeficiency virus type I from a seronegative organ and tissue donor. *N Engl J Med*. 1992;326:726–732.

4. Horowitz MC, Friedlaender GE. Induction of specific T-cell responsiveness to allogenic bone. *J Bone Joint Surg Am*. 1991;73:1157–1168.

5. Oakeshott RD, Farine I, Pritzker KPH, et al. A clinical and histologic analysis of failed fresh osteochondral allografts. *Clin Orthop*. 1988;233:283–294.

6. Herndon CH, Chase SW. The fate of massive autogenous and homogenous bone grafts including articular surfaces. *Surg Gynecol Obstet*. 1954;98:273–290.

7. Campbell CJ, Ishida A, Takahashi H, et al. The transplantation of articular cartilage. *J Bone Joint Surg Am*. 1963;45:1579–1592.

8. Langer F, Gross AE, West M, et al. The immunogenicity of allograft knee joint transplants. *Clin Orthop*. 1978;132:155–162.

9. McDermott GP, Langer F, Pritzker KPH, et al. Fresh small fragment osteochondral allografts. *Clin Ortho*. 1985;197:96–102.

10. Kandel RA, Gross AE, Ganel A, et al. Histopathology of failed osteoarticular shell allografts. *Clin Orthop*. 1985;197:103–110.

11. Rodrigo JJ, Sakovich L, Travis C, et al. Osteocartilaginous allografts as compared with autografts in the treatment of knee joint osteocartilaginous defects in dogs. *Clin Orthop*. 1978;134:342–349.

12. DePalma AF, Tsaltas TT, Mauler GG. Viability of osteochondral grafts as determined by uptake of S^{35}. *J Bone Joint Surg Am*. 1963;45:1565–1578.

13. Convery FR, Meyers MH, Akeson WH. Fresh osteochondral allografting of the femoral condyle. *Clin Orthop*. 1991;273:139–145.

14. Flynn JM, Springfield DS, Mankin HJ. Osteoarticular allografts to treat distal femoral osteonecrosis. Accepted for publication, 1993.

15. Hamilton JA, Barnes R, Gibson T. Experimental homo-grafting of articular cartilage. *J Bone Joint Surg Br*. 1969;51:566.

16. Aicroth P, Burwell RG, Laurence M. Transplantation of synovial joint surfaces: An experimental study. *J Bone Joint Surg Br*. 1972;54:747.

17. Meyers MH. Resurfacing of the femoral head with fresh osteochondral allografts. *Clin Orthop*. 1985;197:111–114.

18. Meyers MH, Akeson W, Convery RF. Resurfacing of the knee with fresh osteochondral allograft. *J Bone Joint Surg Am*. 1989;71:704–713.

19. Entin MA, Alger JR, Baird RM. Experimental and clinical transplantation of autogenous whole joints. *J Bone Joint Surg Am*. 1962;44:1518–1536.

20. Pap K, Krompecher S. Arthroplasty of the knee. Experimental and clinical experience. *J Bone Joint Surg Am*. 1961;43:523–527.

21. Gross AE, McKee NH, Pritzker KPH, et al. Reconstruction of skeletal deficits at the knee. *Clin Orthop*. 1983;174:96–106.

22. Gross AE, Silverstein EA, Falk J, et al. The allotransplantation of partial joints in the treatment of osteoarthritis of the knee. *Clin Orthop*. 1975;108:7–14.

23. Lexer E. Joint transplantation and arthroplasty. *Surg Gynecol Obstet*. 1925;40:782–809.

24. Burwell RG. Studies in the tranplantation of bone. *J Bone Joint Surg Br*. 1963;45:386–401.

25. Ottolenghi CE. Massive osteo- and osteoarticular bone grafts: Technique and results of 62 cases. *Clin Orthop*. 1972;87:156–164.

26. Parrish FF. Treatment of bone tumors by total excision and replacement with massive autologous and homologous grafts. *J Bone Joint Surg Am*. 1966;48:968–990.

27. Parrish FF. Allograft replacement of all or part of the end of a long bone following excision of a tumor. *J Bone Joint Surg Am*. 1973;55:1–22.

28. Mankin HJ, Fogelson FS, Thrasher AZ, et al. Massive resection and allograft transplantation in the treatment of malignant bone tumors. *N Engl J Med*. 1976;294:1247–1255.

29. Waber BA, Tomford WW, Mankin HJ. Long-term results of osteoarticular allografts in weight-bearing joints. In: Aebi M, Regazzoni R, eds. *Bone Transplantation*. Berlin: Springer-Verlag; 1989:275–283.

30. Mahomed MN, Beaver RJ, Gross AE. The long-term success of fresh, small fragment osteochondral allografts used for intraarticular post-traumatic defects in the knee joint. *Orthopaedics*. 1992;15:1191–1199.

31. Tomford WW, Springfield DS, Mankin HJ. Fresh and frozen articular cartilage allografts. *Orthopaedics*. 1992;15:1183–1188.

Part 2
Major Fractures

8
Distal Femoral Fractures

John M. Siliski

Fractures of the distal femur constitute a heterogenous group of injuries affecting the knee. Many reports in the past have included fractures in the distal one third of the femur, thereby mixing diaphyseal, metaphyseal, and intraarticular fractures in the same series. Even knowing the distribution of fracture types in these series may not be helpful in understanding the best treatment or the prognosis for the different fracture patterns grouped under the title distal femoral fracture. In addition to a wide variety of fracture patterns, fractures of the distal femur commonly have associated injuries such as open wounds, patellar fractures, and ligament disruption. High-energy injuries tend to occur in young males, and low-energy injuries in elderly females. After consideration these factors, fractures of the distal femur must be considered a diverse group of injuries requiring thoughtful evaluation and a variety of treatments for optimal outcome. Although in the past these fractures were treated primarily by nonoperative methods, the current trend is to operate on most of these injuries. This chapter reviews the anatomy, classification, evaluation, associated injuries, treatment, and results of this group of fractures.

General Principles

Anatomy

Lower extremity alignment and knee anatomy are reviewed in Chapters 1A and 1B. The reader is referred to those chapters for topics of anatomic and mechanical alignment, general bone anatomy, extensor mechanism structure, and neurovascular anatomy.

The relevant anatomy of the distal femur as it relates to the treatment of distal femoral fractures is discussed here in three views: anterior, lateral, and end on.

On an anterior view of the distal femur, the weight-bearing surfaces of the femoral condyles are separated in the center by the femoral notch, which extends approximately 1.0 cm proximally from the articular surface (Fig. 8–1). Consequently, any internal fixation device must be inserted at a minimum of 1.5 cm proximal to the articular surface of the distal femur to avoid penetration of the joint. The anatomic axis of the femur drawn as a line down the center of the femoral shaft subtends an angle of 99° with the subchondral line of the femur; however, the lateral cortex of the distal femur subtends an angle of only 95° with the subchondral line. Consequently, fixed-angle devices that are made for insertion parallel to the subchondral line of the distal femur are usually made with an angle of 95° between the plate and the intraosseous blade or screw.

On the lateral view of the distal femur, the subchondral bone of the femoral notch is noted as a curved line overlying the femoral condyles and connecting the anterior and posterior cortices (Fig. 8–2). Any fixation device that crosses in a lateral–medial direction in the femur must be contained within the outline of these landmarks to remain intraosseous and to avoid penetration of the joint or egress into the soft tissues. Also on the lateral view, it is important to note that a line extended from the posterior cortex divides the femoral condyles into an anterior two thirds and a posterior one third. A line drawn down the center of the medullary canal of the femur marks the track of intramedullary rods and extramedullary plates used for treatment of distal femoral fractures.

When viewed from end on, the femur is a four-sided structure (Fig. 8–3); however, none of the resulting angles are right angles. If the posterior condyles are used as a line of reference, the anterior margin is noted to have a 10° slope when passing from lateral to medial.

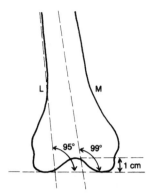

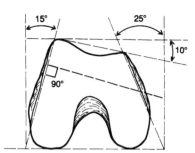

Figure 8–3. End-on view of the distal femur, showing slopes of the anterior, lateral, and medial surfaces, using the posterior condyles as reference.

Figure 8–1. Anterior view of the distal femur. A line drawn down the anatomic axis subtends an angle of 99° with the subchondral line, whereas a line extended from the lateral cortex subtends a 95° angle. The femoral notch extends into the distal femur approximately 1.0 cm. L, lateral; M, medial.

The medial margin has a 25° angle, and the lateral margin a 15° angle, from the perpendicular drawn from the posterior margin. Additional irregularities of the distal femur are created by the presence of the intercondylar notch posteriorly, the trochlear groove anteriorly, and the epicondyles medially and laterally. Fixation devices that are placed into the distal femur must remain confined to the outline of the cortices.

Epidemiology

Fractures of the distal femur constitute 4%[1] to 7%[2] of femoral fractures; however, if intertrochanteric and neck fractures are excluded, fractures of the distal femur constitute 31%[3] of femoral fractures.

There are two distinct groups that sustain distal femoral fractures.[1,3,4] The younger (younger than 40) group is composed predominantly of males who sustain high-energy injuries, mostly motor vehicle related. They commonly have associated knee injuries, such as patellar fractures and open wounds. They also commonly have multiple other injuries, both visceral and

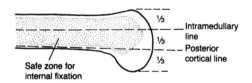

Figure 8–2. Lateral view of the distal femur. A line drawn down the intramedullary canal divides the condyles into an anterior one third and posterior two thirds. The "safe zone" for internal fixation, which crosses the femur from lateral to medial, is outlined by the cortical margins.

skeletal. The older (older than 60) group is composed mostly of females who sustain low-energy injuries, typically slips and falls. They usually sustain isolated, closed fractures, although the fracture patterns in the distal femur are not distributed differently than in the younger group.[4] This most likely is due to the osteoporotic bone in the elderly that may develop a comminuted fracture pattern even with minimal trauma.

Classification

Several classification systems have been proposed for distal femoral fractures. The classification of Neer et al has been commonly used since its publication in 1967 (Fig. 8–4).[5] This system was developed at a time when nonoperative treatment was the standard, and the fracture pattern and alignment in the metaphysis were of more importance than the articular surface. This classification, although simple, is currently not sufficiently comprehensive, instructive, or prognostic to be recommended. It is, however, important to know for understanding prior literature on the subject of distal femoral fractures.

A classification proposed by Seinsheimer divided distal femoral fractures into four types and eight subtypes.[6] This classification focuses attention on intraarticular fracture patterns. It is more comprehensive than that of Neer, but is not systematic and easy to use.

The Association for the Study of Internal Fixation (ASIF) has developed a classification that is both comprehensive and prognostic.[7] Fractures of the distal femur are divided into three basic groups: type A are extraarticular, type B are unicondylar, and type C are supracondylar–intercondylar (Fig. 8–5). Within each type, the complexity of the fracture pattern may be identified by a numeric subgrouping. If even further detail in classification is needed, each of the 9 subgroups shown in Fig. 8–5 can be divided into 3, resulting in a system of 27 fracture patterns. The reader is referred to Muller et al for a complete description of the ASIF

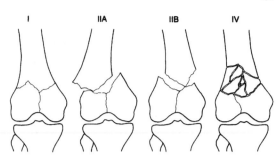

Figure 8–4. Classification of Neer for distal femoral fractures.

fracture classification, including that of distal-femoral fractures.[7] For most purposes, the nine-subgroup classification in Fig. 8–5 is sufficiently comprehensive while remaining simple and logical in design. As well, this classification integrates with the surgical techniques and

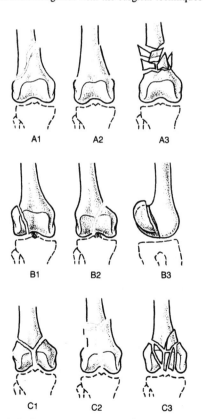

Figure 8–5. Classification of distal femoral fractures of the Association for the Study of Internal Fixation. Type A are supracondylar, type B are unicondylar, and type C are supracondylar–intercondylar. (Reprinted with permission from Müller et al.[7])

implants now commonly used in treatment. This classification is used throughout this chapter.

Associated Injuries

There are frequently knee ligament injuries associated with femoral fractures. Walling et al noted this association, and the difficulty of making a diagnosis of ligamentous knee injury until an extraarticular femoral fracture is surgically stabilized.[8] Conversely, intraarticular distal femoral fractures commonly have ipsilateral skeletal trauma. Siliski et al, in a series of 52 type C fractures, noted the following ipsilateral fractures: patella (10), tibial shaft (5), ankle and foot (4), femoral shaft (3), proximal femur (2), tibial plateau (1), and acetabulum (1).[4] The essential point is that knee injuries are commonly associated with other ipsilateral lower extremity trauma, and careful evaluation is necessary.

Neurologic and vascular injuries have been reported with distal femoral fractures, but they are much less common than with dislocation of the knee (see Chapter 17). The major angulation and displacement in distal femoral fractures are in the distal diaphysis and metaphysis. At this level the diameter of the bone is smaller, and the neurovascular structures are free to angulate with a fracture. These factors appear to protect the nerves and vessels in most, but not all, distal femoral fractures.

Ligament injuries frequently occur in association with distal femoral fractures.[4] Most commonly these are isolated anterior cruciate ligament injuries, and of these most are avulsions with bone fragments from the femoral insertion. The fracture pattern commonly passes through the femoral attachment of the anterior cruciate ligament, but less commonly affects the posterior cruciate ligament, which inserts more anteriorly in the notch to the medial condyle. Rarely, an intraarticular distal femoral fracture is part of a complex fracture dislocation of the knee with multiple ligamentous disruptions. These cases usually have a relatively simple fracture pattern, and most of the energy of injury is probably dissipated in the ligamentous disruption.

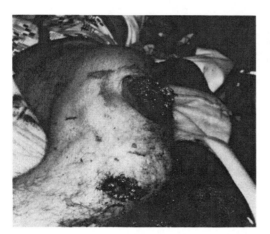

Figure 8–6. Open left distal femoral fracture with the femoral shaft protruding through the extensor mechanism. There is an abrasion over the patellar tendon which was the site of initial impact of the flexed extremity. (Courtesy of Martin Mahring.)

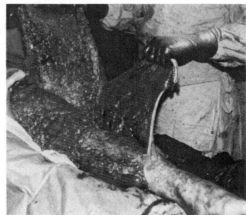

Figure 8–7. Degloving injury of left thigh and knee associated with a distal femoral fracture.

Meniscal injuries are uncommon in association with distal femoral fractures,[4] as the menisci are more closely fixed to the tibia. It is also uncommon to find a tibial plateau fracture associated with an intraarticular distal femoral fracture; however, patellar fractures are very common associated injuries. Many if not most distal femoral fractures occur as the result of a force delivered to the end of the flexed knee. The patella is the intervening structure, and it receives the same loading force as the distal femur.

Open wounds occur in approximately one third of type C fractures, predominately in association with high-energy injuries.[4] Most of these open wounds are anterior through the distal portion of the extensor mechanism (Fig. 8–6). During the process of the injury, the distal femoral fragment is displaced, and the remaining sharp end of the femur is driven through the extensor mechanism and skin. Wound contamination occurs if the protruding femur impacts against the ground, vegetation, or similar surfaces. Occasionally a distal femoral fracture occurs as the result of a crushing injury, which is more likely to produce a degloving injury or deep soft tissue loss (Fig. 8–7).

Evaluation

Physical Examination

A history of injury may be lacking if the patient is obtunded as a result of an associated medical event or multiple trauma. Soft tissue injury, swelling, deformity, and crepitation are all signs of an injury in the region of the knee. The limb should be splinted, and x-rays

obtained. The entire lower extremity should be examined for signs of associated fracture, dislocation, soft tissue wounds, compartment syndrome, and neurovascular injury. If indicated, additional workup of these associated injuries should be performed.

A thorough search should be made for open wounds communicating with the fracture. Although open wounds with distal femoral fractures are most commonly anterior, where they are easily seen, they can be over the posterior surface of the thigh and knee.

Radiographic Examination

Anteroposterior and lateral radiographs are usually sufficient to make the diagnosis of a distal femoral fracture; however, the initial set of films is often inadequate to fully assess the fracture and determine treatment. More information is often obtained by obtaining a second set of radiographs with the fracture in improved rotation and alignment, held either in skeletal traction or manually by the examiner. Oblique views may be very helpful in identifying nondisplaced intercondylar fracture lines and fractures in the oblique planes. Radiographs should be studied for the presence of associated patellar and tibial plateau fractures.

Tomography, computed tomography, and magnetic resonance imaging are not routinely used in the evaluation of these fractures, but they may occasionally be helpful in equivocal cases to assess minor amounts of displacement, number of fragments, and associated soft tissue injuries.

The pelvis and proximal femur should be evaluated in all cases of distal femoral fracture to rule out associated bone and hip joint injury.

A radiograph of the contralateral femur may be taken to use as a template for preoperative planning.

Treatment

Historical Overview

Nonoperative Treatment. The early treatment of distal femoral fractures was the same as for femoral shaft fractures. The goal of treatment was maintenance of the leg in extension with splints.[9,10] Percival Pott proposed that fractures should be immobilized in a position that relaxed the surrounding muscles which produced forces that deform the fracture.[9] Buck introduced skin traction for femoral fractures in 1861.[11] Russell combined skin traction with positioning of the hip and knee in flexion in 1921.[12]

Skeletal traction was added to the treatment of femoral fractures to counteract the strong pull of the thigh muscles. Steinmann in 1907 and Kirschner in 1909 described techniques for applying single-pin traction for femoral fractures.[13,14] Mahorner and Bradburn in 1933 reported the results of treatment of 308 femoral fractures. The best results were obtained after skeletal traction, although fractures of the distal femur had poorer results than shaft fractures.[15]

Tees in 1937 discussed the difficulty encountered in management of supracondylar femoral fractures because of limited control of the distal fragment.[16] Modlin in 1945 described double-pin traction, adding a second pin in the distal femoral fragment to counteract the pull of the gastrocnemius muscle[17] (Fig. 8–8). Hampton in 1951 and Wiggins in 1953 subsequently reported good results with this method of treatment[18,19]; Watson-Jones in 1955, however, recommended single-pin traction through the tibia combined with knee flexion to adjust final alignment of the distal fragment.[20] He was concerned with the risk of femoral artery perforation that could occur with insertion of a pin in the distal femur. Bohler in 1956 reported on the results of a simi-

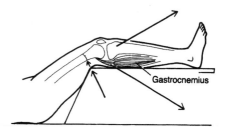

Figure 8–9. Single-pin traction used to treat a distal femoral fracture, with a supporting frame placed with its angle directly under the distal femoral fragment to control alignment.

lar form of treatment.[21] He used a single tibial traction pin, combined with a Braun splint placed under the femoral fracture, to control posterior angulation (Fig. 8–9). He claimed to have been able to successfully control fracture position in 100 cases that he personally treated. Charnley and Smillie subsequently advocated similar forms of closed treatment.[22,23]

Stewart et al in 1966 reported the results of treatment of 442 distal femoral fractures.[24] Of those treated nonoperatively 67% had good results, whereas of those treated with open surgical techniques only 54% had good results. They advocated closed treatment methods using the double-pin skeletal traction technique of Modlin.

Neer et al in 1967 reported their results of treatment of 110 distal femoral fractures.[5] They noted that closed treatment produced results that were 90% good and excellent, but that open treatment results were only 52% good and excellent. They strongly advocated the routine use of closed methods of treatment.

The articles by Stewart and Neer had a strong effect on the treatment approach in North America. One must, however, consider that during the 1950s and 1960s surgical techniques and implants were rudimentary by current standards, and acceptable outcomes for that period would not all be considered good and excellent by today's standards. Also in these two series, the more severe fracture patterns, which were difficult to align in traction, were the ones that predominantly underwent surgical treatment. Therefore, fractures with a poorer prognosis were the ones placed into the surgical treatment group.

In an attempt to shorten traction time, hospitalization, and knee immobilization, cast bracing was advocated for the ambulatory treatment of distal femoral fractures beginning in the 1970s.[25–30] Most authors recommended an initial period of immobilization in traction of 2 to 6 weeks, followed by a hinged cast brace that permitted ambulation on crutches and knee motion.

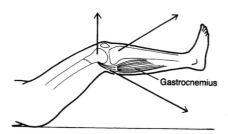

Figure 8–8. Double-pin skeletal traction for treatment of a distal femoral fracture. Longitudinal traction is provided by the pin in the proximal tibia. Anterior traction provided by the distal femoral pin counterbalances the deforming force of the gastrocnemius on the distal fragment.

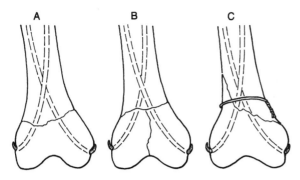

Figure 8-10. Rush nail fixation of distal femoral fractures. **A.** Supracondylar fracture. **B.** Supracondylar-intercondylar fracture. **C.** Spiral supracondylar fracture with additional cerclage wire.

Operative Treatment. Unmansky in 1948 and Altenberg and Shorkey in 1949 presented early reports on the use of open reduction and internal fixation of distal femoral fractures.[31,32] They claimed satisfactory results using a modified Blount plate. White and Russin in 1956 recommended internal fixation, although only 75% of their cases had acceptable results.[33]

Rush and Gelbke in 1957 published an atlas of surgical techniques using Rush nails for the fixation of fractures.[34] Wertzberger and Peltier in 1967 recommended the use of Rush nails based on their surgical experience in 16 supracondylar fracture.[35] Rush in 1968 presented his own series of femoral fractures treated with his intramedullary device.[36] Shelbourne and Brueckmann in 1982 reported their use of Rush nail

fixation of distal femoral fractures, and described techniques to fix even supracondylar-intercondylar fracture patterns (Fig. 8-10).[37]

Zickle et al introduced the Zickle supracondylar nailing system in 1977.[38] Essentially this system is a modification of the Rush nail, customized for the distal femur. The flexible nails are introduced through the medial and lateral condyles and up the intramedullary canal. The nails are then fixed in place with locking screws in the condyles. Zickle and co-workers subsequently reported series of acute fractures[39] and nonunions[40] treated with this device (Fig. 8-11).

In 1965 the Swiss ASIF published its first manual of internal fixation implants and techniques, including their blade plate[41] (Fig. 8-12). Neff and Olerud in 1966 published early articles in the European literature on the use of internal fixation of distal femoral fractures.[42,43] Wenzl et al published the first ASIF report on the internal fixation of distal femoral fractures.[44]

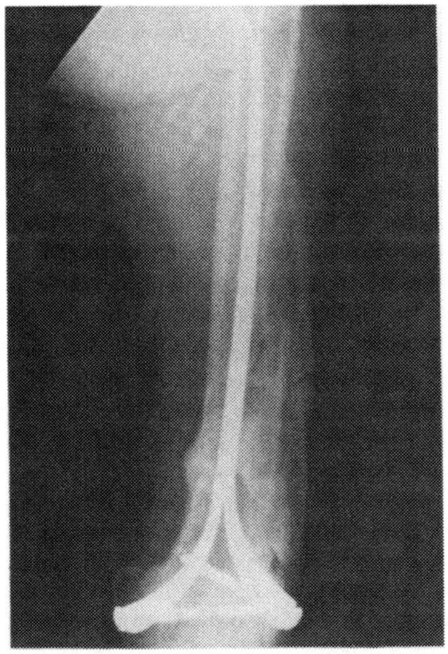

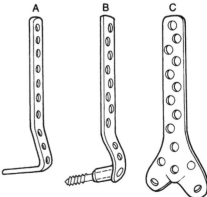

Figure 8-12. Association for the Study of Internal Fixation's internal fixation implants for the distal femur. **A.** 95° Supracondylar blade plate. **B.** 95° Dynamic condylar screw. **C.** Condylar buttress plate.

Figure 8-11. Zickle supracondylar device used to fix a distal femoral nonunion.

They noted 73.5% good and excellent results in 112 cases using stringent rating criteria. Additional support for internal fixation was published in Europe by Slatis et al,[45] Olerud,[46] Chiron et al,[47] and Tscherne et al[48] in the 1970s.

Schatzker and co-workers in 1975 and 1979 were the first to report the use of ASIF techniques and implants in North America.[49,50] Subsequent reports from both Europe and North America recommended the use of ASIF implants and techniques over other forms of closed and open treatment.[51-55]

Attention in the literature began to focus on specific fracture problems. Wade and Okinara in 1959 had identified the supracondylar femoral fracture as more problematic in the elderly than in young patients because of osteoporosis and comorbidity.[56] Brown and D'Arcy in 1971 attributed prior reports of poor results in the elderly to inadequate implant design.[57] They described the use of a fixed-angle nail-plate device with a staple and bolt that were placed from the medial side and locked into the triflanged nail, thereby providing interfragmentary compression of the condyles. Their report does not permit detailed statistical analysis, but noted less final range of motion in their elderly patients. Benum in 1977 recommended the use of bone cement to augment the internal fixation in osteoporotic femurs.[58] Tscherne et al recommended impaction of comminuted metaphyseal segments in osteoporotic bone as a technique to improve the initial biomechanical stability of the fracture (Fig. 8–13).[48] Shortening of 1 to 2 cm in

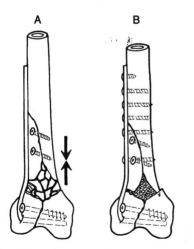

Figure 8–13. Impaction technique for comminuted metaphyseal segment in osteoporotic bone. **A.** The articular fragments are reduced, a blade plate is inserted, and axial alignment is restored. **B.** The metaphyseal region is impacted with manual pressure or dynamic compression prior to plate fixation to the shaft.

the elderly was considered acceptable in exchange for better fixation and quicker healing. Schatzker and Tile expressed caution when attempting to perform internal fixation in osteoporotic bone and considered severe osteoporosis a relative contraindication to surgical treatment.[54] Siliski et al in a series of 52 type C fractures treated with ASIF implants, noted no cases of loss of fixation in the elderly.[4] Most of their fractures in the elderly were treated with the impaction technique of Tscherne and/or bone grafting of the metaphysis. They also noted that the elderly had results as good as those of the younger patients in their series.

Indirect reduction techniques have been advocated by Johnson[59] and Mast et al.[60] The advantage of this technique is that minimal soft tissue striping of metaphyseal fragments is performed, leaving a better blood supply for healing. The articular fragments are anatomically reduced, and the distal fragment is then appropriately aligned to the diaphysis using the fixation device and/or a femoral distractor to achieve the approximate reduction of the intervening metaphyseal fragments (Fig. 8–14).

Condylar screw-plate devices have been developed as an alternative to the blade plate[2,61-65] (see Fig. 8–12B). These devices have several potential advantages over blade plates, including ease of insertion, adjustment of flexion after insertion of the lag screw, and interchange of side plates. A potential disadvantage is the reaming done for the lag screw, which leaves a large defect if a revision internal fixation becomes necessary. Results with these condylar screw-plate devices have been similar to those with the fixed-angle blade plates.

Intramedullary nailing of femoral fractures has the advantage of closed methods that avoid open exposure and striping of soft tissues.[66] Closed intramedullary has become the standard technique for fixation of femoral diaphyseal fractures. The addition of interlocking screws and bolts has extended the portion of the femur amenable to nailing, although problems with implant failure have been reported.[67] Until recently, extraarticular distal femoral fractures as close as 10 cm to the joint were considered treatable by antegrade locked nailing. Now even intraarticular fractures are being considered for antegrade and retrograde locked nailing (Fig. 8–15). Whittle et al reported 75% good and excellent results with no infections in a series of 28 type C fractures using antegrade locked nailing.[68] Twenty-five percent of the fractures were open, and the overall infection rate was 3.6%; however, the reported malunion rate was 10.7% in this series of predominantly type C1 and C2 fractures. Henry et al reported the use of a locked retrograde nail which may be inserted percutaneously through an entry site in the intercondylar notch[69] (Fig. 8–16). They noted a shorter operating time, less blood loss, and fewer implant failures with their intramedullary nail as compared with plate-

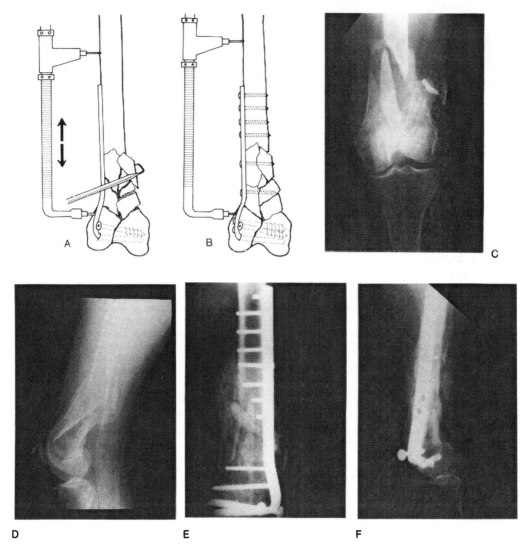

A   B   C

D   E   F

Figure 8–14. Indirect reduction used for distal femoral fractures. **A.** Diagram of a distal femoral fracture with extensive metaphyseal comminution. Articular fragments have been reduced, a blade plate has been inserted, and the femoral distractor has been inserted proximal and distal to the area of comminution. With the fracture pulled out to length and axial alignment restored, intervening fragments can be manipulated into better position with minimal exposure and handling.

B. Diagram of completed internal fixation, with solid fixation of the plate above the fracture and selected screws placed through the middle portion of the plate to fix large fragments. **C.** Type C2 fracture in an osteoporotic elderly woman. Anteroposterior x-ray. **D.** Lateral x-ray. **E.** Postoperative x-ray taken 10 weeks after indirect reduction, cancellous bone grafting, and internal fixation. **F.** Lateral x-ray at 10 weeks.

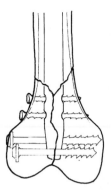

Figure 8–15. Type C1 fracture with interfragmentary compression of the condyles and locked antegrade nailing of the supracondylar fracture line.

screw fixation. The use of locked intramedullary nails for the treatment of intraarticular distal femoral fractures at the current time must be considered experimental until additional reports establish these devices and techniques as safe and effective.

Type C, and especially type C3, fractures may require extensile exposure (see Chapter 5). When 95° plates cannot be used because of frontal plane fracture lines, double plating on the medial and lateral sides of the

femur may be necessary to stabilize the metaphyseal portion of the fracture[70] (Figs. 8–12C and 8–17).

Open fractures may have lower infection rates if the fracture and soft tissues are stabilized by an internal fixation[71]; however, open distal femoral fractures, as all open fractures, have a higher rate of sepsis than do closed fractures.[4] Although open distal femoral fractures are at risk for the development of infection, immediate debridement and internal fixation have their merits. Helpenstell and Hansen reported a series of 51 open distal femoral fractures treated with immediate open reduction and internal fixation.[72] The infection rate was 7%, and the nonunion rate was 2%. At final follow-up 77% had good and excellent results, and there were no poor results. External fixation has also been reported as a treatment option for open distal femoral fractures[73,74] (see Chapter 6).

Treatment Goals

The basic goals of treatment are the following: (1) to minimize the complications of treatment, (2) to minimize the period of convalescence and rehabilitation, (3) to minimize the risk of posttraumatic arthritis, and (4) to restore the patient to prefracture functional status. The historic review described many options for treatment that have been used in the past century. Most of these options still have appropriate indications for use at present.

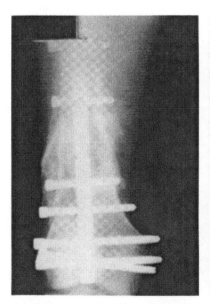
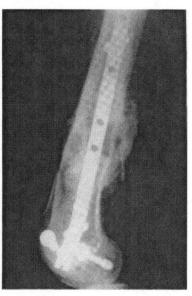

A
B

Figure 8–16. Retrograde locked nailing of a type C2 fracture, using interfragmentary screws to fix the condylar fractures and a locked nail to fix the supracondylar fracture. **A.** Anteroposterior x-ray. **B.** Lateral x-ray.

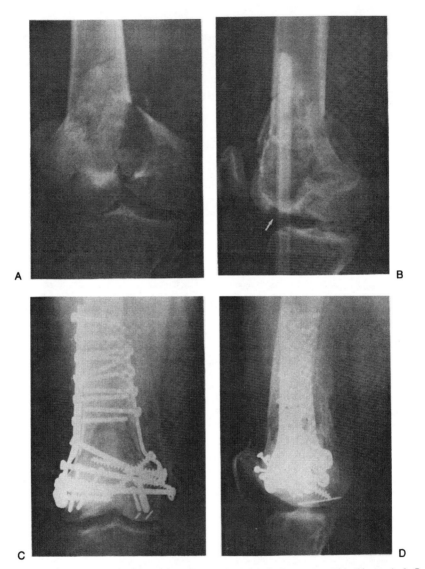

Figure 8-17. Double plating of type C3 fracture (see Fig. 5-1 for extensile exposure used in this case). **A.** Preoperative anteroposterior x-ray. **B.** Preoperative lateral x-ray showing frontal plane fracture lines (arrow). **C.** Postoperative anteroposterior x-ray. **D.** Postoperative lateral x-ray.

Currently, however, most distal femoral fractures are treated by established methods of internal fixation. If treated surgically, the specific goals are (1) anatomic reduction of the joint surface; (2) repair of the associated joint injuries; (3) restoration of bone length, rotation, and alignment; and (4) stable internal fixation that permits (5) early knee motion and functional rehabilitation. These fractures may include very complex injuries, and a fixation implant on the operating table does not automatically make the surgery easy or the result excellent.

The rest of this chapter focuses on nonoperative and operative techniques of treatment for distal femoral fractures.

Indications for Surgery

Absolute Indications. Absolute indications include the following:

1. Extraarticular fractures not controllable by closed methods
2. Displaced intraarticular fractures (types B and C)
3. Open fractures
4. Fractures with associated vascular injury
5. Fractures with associated tibial fractures (floating knee)
6. Fractures with associated displaced patellar and tibial plateau fractures
7. Pathologic fractures
8. Contralateral lower extremity fractures
9. Polytrauma

Relative Indications. Relative indications require a thoughtful decision made by the surgeon, patient, and family:

1. Young patients with a satisfactory reduction by closed methods but a wish to avoid prolonged bedrest
2. Elderly patients with a satisfactory reduction by closed methods but predicted poor tolerance of prolonged traction, bedrest, or casting

Contraindications. Several situations may be contraindications to internal fixation:

1. Polytrauma patients who are hemodynamically unstable
2. Very high risk medical patients
3. Contaminated open wounds, burns, and severe soft tissue loss
4. A severely comminuted joint surface that cannot be reconstructed
5. Severe osteopenia, such as seen in paraplegia

Medical Treatment

Nondisplaced, extraarticular (type A1) supracondylar fractures can be satisfactorily treated in a cast or brace with the knee in slight flexion. Once the patient is comfortable, a hinged functional brace can be applied so that motion can be started. Within 4 weeks partial weight bearing can be started. Within 8 to 12 weeks the bracing can be discontinued, and the patient advanced as tolerated to full weight bearing as comfort, strength, and motion permit. Fractures that are impacted can be advanced the most quickly.

Skeletal traction may be used in unstable type A1 and multiple-fragment type A2 and A3 fractures. A large Steinmann pin is inserted across the tibia below the tibial tubercle, approximately 10 cm below the joint line.

The pin is inserted far enough from the joint so that pin site contamination would have a minimal risk of causing infection of the joint and fracture, especially if open reduction is subsequently chosen. With a single tibial traction pin, length rotation and varus–valgus alignment can usually be controlled; however, the pull of the gastrocnemius muscle on the distal fragment tends to pull the fracture alignment into recurvatum. To counterbalance this force, multiple options exist, including (1) placing the hip and knee into more flexion, (2) placing a Bohler–Braun frame under the extremity with the frame angle under the fracture site, and (3) placing a second traction pin in the distal femoral fragment to apply anterior traction. Traction may be continued until the fracture is solidly united at 8 to 12 weeks. As an alternative, traction may be discontinued and a functional hinged brace applied once callus formation begins and there is some inherent stability in the fracture site, which usually takes 3 to 6 weeks.

Surgical Techniques

Preoperative Planning. Planning before surgery is essential to ensure that the necessary implants, instruments, equipment, and personnel are present. Intraarticular distal femoral fractures are often difficult to reduce and fix, and a step-by-step plan for the procedure should be developed and written before surgery begins.[60] Templates are now available for many of the implants that are used for fracture fixation, and these can be used with x-rays and tracings of the fracture and the intact contralateral femur for planning. Before the start of surgery, the surgeon should have a clear plan for the positioning of the patient, the surgical exposure, the provisional reduction, the steps of internal fixation, the implants including each screw, and the use of adjunctive techniques such as bone grafting, impaction, and cement augmentation.

Timing. These injuries are treated emergently for several associated conditions:

1. Open fracture
2. Arterial injury
3. Irreducible fracture dislocation
4. Polytrauma (The patient is taken to the operating room for other reasons, and internal fixation is considered beneficial for mobilization and nursing care.)

Most other cases are taken to the operating room early, at 1 to 3 days, when the patient is medically prepared, the surgical team has completed its planning, and all equipment and implants are available. While awaiting surgery, unstable fractures should be held in single-pin skeletal traction to maintain length and alignment and to lessen pain and medication requirements.

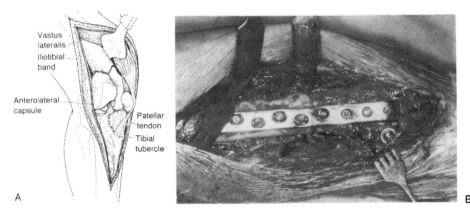

A

B

Figure 8–18. A. Diagram of lateral approach to the distal femur and knee, with elevation of the vastus lateralis muscle from the intermuscular septum and femur. **B.** Clinical example of lateral exposure for internal fixation of a type C1 fracture.

Exposure. The patient is positioned on a radiolucent table if fluoroscopy is to be used to monitor the steps of reduction and internal fixation. A roll under the ipsilateral pelvis and greater trochanter will prevent external rotation of the limb. If the limb is long, and the fracture is confined to the very distal portion of the femur, a tourniquet may be placed about the upper thigh before prepping and draping. If, however, the limb is short, and the fracture extends more proximally, no tourniquet is applied initially. The entire limb is sterilized and draped free. During surgery, if space is available, a sterile tourniquet can be applied; however, many distal femoral fractures cannot be repaired under tourniquet control.

Exposure of the knee is covered in Chapter 5. The reader is referred there for a detailed description of the surgical exposures used for distal femoral fractures.

Most distal femoral fractures are exposed from the lateral (subvastus) approach (Fig. 8–18). This exposure may remain extraarticular for treatment of a type A fracture or may be extended distally through the lateral capsule for intraarticular type B and C fractures. A tibial tubercle osteotomy may be added for extensile exposure for the following indications: (1) comminuted medial condyle, (2) double plating of the distal femur, and (3) late or revision surgery with soft tissue stiffness (Fig. 8–19). The lateral approach is preferable for fractures to be stabilized with fixed-angle implants, whether type A or C.

A select number of fractures may be treated through

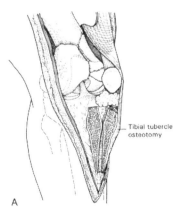

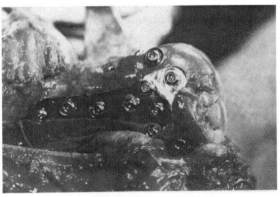

A

B

Figure 8–19. A. Tibial tubercle osteotomy added to a lateral approach, improving access to the medial condyle and medial femur (see Chapter 5 for detailed description). **B.** Intraoperative photograph of exposure of the distal femur achieved with lateral approach and tibial tubercle osteotomy.

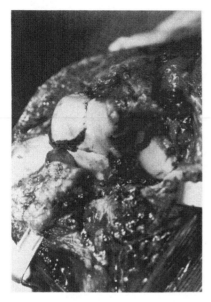

Figure 8-20. Anterior approach to the distal femur through a medial parapatellar incision (same case as in Fig. 8-17).

an anterior approach with a medial parapatellar arthrotomy (Fig. 8-20). These should be fractures with limited proximal extension, but comminuted joint surfaces that require complicated reduction and double plating.

A limited medial subvastus approach may be useful for internal fixation of type B fractures involving the medial condyle. It is also an option for double plating the medial side of the femur when the main exposure has been done laterally and the surgeon wishes to avoid a tibial tubercle osteotomy.

Implants

Screws. Screws alone are sufficient to fix some unicondylar type B fractures (Fig. 8-21). If there is a single fracture line in good bone that reduces with interdigitation of the fragments, interfragmentary cancellous screws alone are sufficient to hold the reduction and begin early motion; however, the surgeon may decide that a buttress plate added to the screw fixation may be necessary to resist shear forces. Type B3 fractures do not present an option for buttress plating, as the posterior condylar fragment is almost entirely covered by articular cartilage. Multiple interfragmentary screws placed predominantly from anterior to posterior are used to fix the fracture. Weight bearing in these fractures must be delayed until union is solid. In most cases, either a plate or intramedullary nailing system is used to fix these fractures.

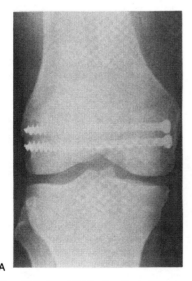
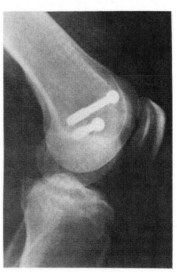

A   B

Figure 8-21. Type B2 (unicondylar) fracture fixed with screws alone. **A.** Anteroposterior x-ray. **B.** Lateral x-ray.

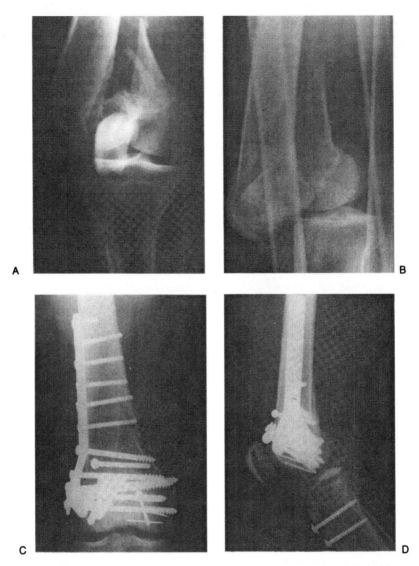

Figure 8–22. Condylar buttress plate used to fix a type 3C fracture with articular comminution. The medial cortex has been reconstructed so that a second medial plate is not necessary. **A.** Preoperative anteroposterior x-ray. **B.** Preoperative lateral x-ray. **C.** Postoperative anteroposterior x-ray. **D.** Postoperative lateral x-ray (same case as in Fig. 8–19B).

Condylar Buttress Plate. The condylar buttress plate has an expanded distal portion that maximizes coverage of the lateral condyle for placement of multiple screws in the distal fragment (see Fig. 12C). This type of plate is the easiest to apply and is the best plating option for type C3 fractures with comminution of the articular fragments (Fig. 8–22). This plate does not, however, resist progressive varus deformity if a stable medial cortex cannot be reestablished during the reduction. Consequently, a second (usual smaller) plate on the medial side of the femur may be required to maintain varus–valgus alignment (see Fig. 8–17). In a small femur, or one that has a knee prosthesis in place, the new ASIF tibial plateau plates may be used as an alternative. These plates are reversed in orientation to place the expanded end distally (see Fig. 24–2).

Blade Plate and Screw Plate. The 95° angled blade plate (see Fig. 8–12A) has been a commonly used implant for over 20 years. It has been made in blade lengths of 50, 60, 70, and 80 mm. Various side-plate lengths are available in two-hole increments. A newer variation of this blade plate is the 95° condylar screw plate (see Fig. 8–12B). The ASIF version has lag screws in 5-mm increments and separate interchangeable side plates in two-hole increments. Both of these related implants share several characteristics. The intraosseous portion (blade or lag screw) is inserted parallel to the subchondral surface of the distal femur, so that the side plate is parallel to the lateral cortex. They are typically used in fractures that have supracondylar components, which need a fixed-angle device to maintain alignment of the articular portion to the diaphysis. These implants are therefore used in type A and C fractures except type C3, which has fracture lines in the frontal plane.

Both 95° fixed-angle devices require a thorough understanding of the three dimensional anatomy of the distal femur. If a type C1 or C2 fracture exists, the condylar fragments must first be anatomically reduced and fixed with one to three (usually two) interfragmentary cancellous screws which will not interfere with placement of the 95° device. Typically, these screws are inserted proximal to the blade or lag screw position, with one screw anterior and the other posterior to the plate (Figs. 8–23 and 8–24). Once these interfragmentary screws are in place and the condyles are reunited, a guidewire is placed. This guidewire must be inserted into the distal fragment for proper placement of a chisel (for the blade) or reamer (for the lag screw). A three-step technique is used to place the final guidewire (see Fig. 8–23). Wire 1 is placed along the distal articular surface of the femur. Wire 2 is placed over the anterior articular surface of the femur. Wire 3 is placed parallel to wire 1 as viewed anteriorly and parallel to wire 2 as viewed from end on. (If wire 3 is inserted 5 to 10° diver-

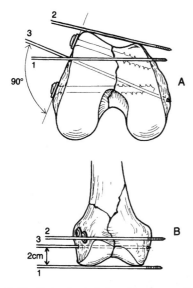

Figure 8–23. Three-wire technique for placement of lag screw in distal femur. Wire 1 is placed parallel to the distal femoral articular surface. Wire 2 is placed parallel to the anterior articular surface. Wire 3 is a summation wire, which on the anterior view is placed parallel to wire 1 two centimeters proximal to the joint line. Wire 3 may be placed parallel to or slightly divergent from wire 2 when viewed from end on. If wire 3 is placed at 90° to the surface through which it is inserted on the lateral condyle, the plate will ultimately lie flush with the lateral cortex. A. End-on view of distal femur. B. Anterior view of the distal femur.

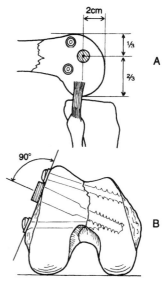

Figure 8–24. Placement of interfragmentary screws and lag screw in the distal femur. A. Lateral view of the distal femur, with lag screw inserted 2 cm proximal to the distal articular surface and one third of the distance back from the anterior articular margin using the longest diameter of the distal femur. The interfragmentary screws are placed just proximal to the lag screw insertion site, and anteriorly and posteriorly to avoid interference with plate position over the lateral cortex. B. End-on view of the distal femur showing final placement of interfragmentary screws and lag screw in the distal femur. The trochlear groove and femoral notch have been avoided by proper angulation of these screws to remain within the bone. The lag screw ends within the bone without perforation of the medial cortex.

gent from wire 2, the plate will usually come to rest
with a better fit along the femoral shaft.) Wire 3 is
drilled into the femur starting one third of the distance
from the anterior to the posterior surfaces, which places
the wire in line with the center of the medullary canal
of the distal femur. Wire 3 is drilled into the bone 1 cm
proximal to the articular surface if a blade plate is being
used, or 2 cm if a condylar screw plate is being used.
Placement of wire 3 should be confirmed by x-ray or
fluoroscopy prior to proceeding, as the remainder of the
reduction and fixation is dependent on proper placement of the blade or lag screw. If the metaphyseal fracture line is a simple one that can be reduced and pro-
visionally fixed, it is also possible to check guidewire
placement with 95° guide placed along the lateral cortex
of the femur. Once the final guidewire position is
achieved, the length of the intraosseous portion of the
wire is determined so that a blade or lag screw of
appropriate length is chosen. It is important to recall
that the medial border of the distal femur as seen on
an anterior view is approximately 10 mm more medial than that portion of the bone that is potentially in
contact with the blade or lag screw (Figs. 8–22 and 8–
24). If wire 3 is inserted until it just enters the medial
cortex, it is properly positioned for length measurement, although it will appear approximately 10 mm
"short" on an anterior radiographic view. The goal in
selection of blade or lag screw length is to choose the
maximum length that does not penetrate the medial
cortex and cause soft tissue impingement and pain. If a
blade plate is to be used, a small rectangular window is
cut in the lateral cortex just above the guidewire, so
that the chisel will be inserted 1.5 to 2.0 cm proximal to
the distal articular surface. The seating chisel is then inserted with a mallet to the desired depth in the bone,
remaining parallel to wire 3 (see Fig. 8–24A). Rotational control during chisel insertion must also be maintained, as adjustment of the flexion–extension position
is not possible with the single-piece blade plate. Careful
inspection of the lateral surface of the femur is needed
to properly position the seating chisel if the metaphysis
is not already reduced and available as an additional
guide. If a screw plate device is being used, the reamer
is set for the desired length and is advanced over the
guidewire inserted 2.0 cm proximal to the distal articular surface (see Fig. 8–24B).

The implant is then inserted. An osteotome may be
used to remove a small piece of bone just proximal to
the blade or lag screw site so that the final implant can
rest snugly against the lateral cortex (Fig. 8–25). With a
blade plate, an implant with the desired blade length
and plate length is chosen. It is inserted with a holding
device. With a screw plate, the track for the lag screw is
tapped, and the lag screw is inserted with a special holder. These lag screws are keyed to fit the side plate, and
on its final insertion, the lag screw must be in a rota-

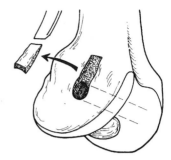

Figure 8–25. Curved osteotome used to remove a small
piece of bone just proximal to the lag screw insertion site, so
that the side plate can be set against the lateral cortex unim-
peded.

tional orientation to result in appropriate reduction of
the fracture and alignment of the plate along the femoral shaft. The lag screw can be readjusted until this goal
is achieved. Also, the interchangeability of the side
plates allows the surgeon to exchange plate lengths if
needed prior to fixing the plate to the femoral diaphysis. A set screw placed through the plate and into
the lag screw can be tightened to generate additional
impaction forces between the condyles if desired (Fig.
8–26).

If the metaphyseal fracture has already been reduced
prior to plate insertion, fixation is simply completed
with appropriate-length cortical and cancellous screws.
These screws may also be used for dynamic compression of the supracondylar fracture line, or interfragmentary compression, as the fracture pattern permits;
however, if the metaphyseal region is comminuted and
anatomic reduction of the multiple fragments is not
being attempted, the side plate is used to guide reduction of the distal fragment to the diaphysis. To restore
length and facilitate indirect reduction of the intervening fragments, a femoral distractor can be applied with

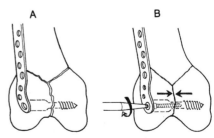

Figure 8–26. Set screw inserted through the side plate into
the lag screw to generate additional impaction force between
the two condyles in addition to the previously placed interfragmentary cancellous screws.

pins drilled into the diaphysis proximally and through a distal screw hole of the plate distally (see Fig. 8–14). The distractor is used to bring the fracture out to length. With limited handling, the intervening frag- ments can be manipulated into the best positions possi- ble. The plate is then fixed to the diaphysis with several screws, although some of the central screw holes may be left unfilled (see Fig. 8–14). If there is a short seg- ment of comminution in the metaphysis in osteoporotic bone of an elderly patient, distraction to normal femo- ral length may be less desirable than impaction of 1 to 2 cm to improve the stability of the fracture construct (see Fig. 8–13).

Flexible nails, such as Rush nails and the Zickle supracondylar system, are inserted from both sides of the femur just above the articular surfaces. For many type A fractures, the procedure can be done percutane- ously with fluoroscopic assistance; however, open re- duction and internal fixation may be required to add cerclage wires for supracondylar butterfly fragments or interfragmentary screws for intercondylar fractures (see Fig. 8–10).

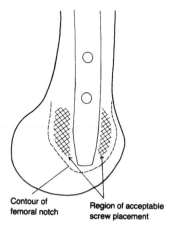

Figure 8–27. The space available to insert screws across the condyles is limited to small areas anterior and posterior to the intramedullary device.

Contour of femoral notch

Region of acceptable screw placement

Antegrade Interlocked Intramedullary Nails. Antegrade interlocked intramedullary nails are inserted through the proximal femur and advanced under fluoroscopic control into the distal femur. The surgeon choosing this technique should be experienced with intramedullary nailing and distal femoral fractures, as this type of im- plant has only recently been used in type A and C frac- tures. At least one and preferably two crossing screws are inserted in the distal fragment to control alignment (see Fig. 8–15). Attention should be paid to the metaphyseal reduction, as insertion of the nail for a fracture at this level will not automatically restore axial alignment because of the flare of the medullary canal. The nail should be locked proximally if the metaphysis is comminuted and may shorten postoperatively. Type C fractures require internal fixation of the intercondylar fracture line(s). Nondisplaced single fracture lines can be fixed percutaneously with cancellous screws, but the space available in the distal femur is very limited (Fig. 8–27). Displaced and more complicated fractures re- quire open reduction and internal fixation before ante- grade nailing.

Retrograde Interlocked Intramedullary Nails. Retrograde interlocked intramedullary nailing shares many similar- ities with antegrade nailing. The main difference is that retrograde nailing is performed with insertion of the nail through the distal femur with an entry site just anterior to the posterior cruciate ligament attachment. This can be accomplished percutaneously. Devices cur- rently in development and trial have several holes in the nail so that crossing screws can be inserted into the bone above and below the metaphyseal fracture. An

open reduction and internal fixation may be necessary for type C fractures.

External Fixators. External fixators have a limited role in the treatment of distal femoral fractures. They may be used in selected open fractures with complicated soft tissue injuries when the surgeon does not wish to use in- ternal fixation, but needs stabilization of the bone and access to the soft tissues. If an external fixator is used, interfragmentary fixation of the articular fragments with a few screws may restore the joint surface and provide a distal fragment that can accept pins or wires for a fixator. The reader is referred to Chapter 6 for a com- prehensive review of external fixation about the knee.

Specific Fractures. The different fracture patterns re- quire different exposures and implants. Table 8–1 pre- sents common surgical approaches to each of the nine main categories of distal femoral fractures. Associated

Table 8–1

Type	Exposure	Implant
A1	Lateral	Blade plate or screw plate; Nails
A2	Lateral	Blade plate or screw plate; Nails
A3	Lateral	Blade plate or screw plate; Nails
B1	Lateral	Screws ± buttress plate
B2	Medial	Screws ± buttress plate
B3	Lateral	Screws
C1	Lateral	Blade plate or screw plate; Nails
C2	Lateral	Blade plate or screw plate; Nails
C3	Lateral ± tibial tubercle osteotomy	Condylar buttress plate ± medial plate
	Anterior	
	Lateral and medial	

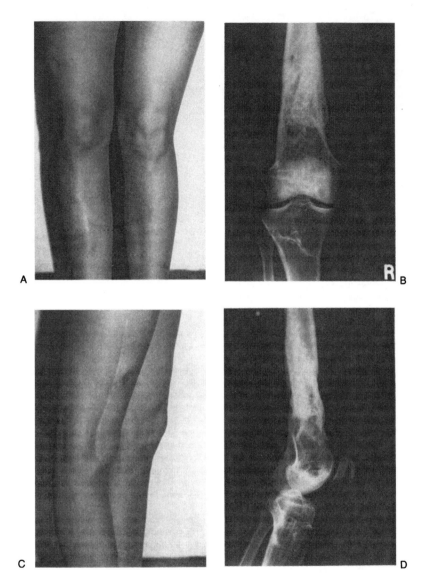

Figure 8–28. The most common malreduction position of distal femoral fractures is varus and recurvatum. Shown is a right distal femoral fracture treated by internal fixation with subsequent hardware removal. **A**. Clinical varus alignment of right lower extremity. **B**. Final anteroposterior x-ray showing 90° alignment of the joint line with the femoral shaft. **C**. Clinical recurvatum of the right distal femur. **D**. Lateral x-ray of distal femur showing recurvatum of the distal femoral fragment.

---▷

Figure 8–29. Type C3 distal femoral fracture with an open wound after high-energy injury. **A**. Initial anteroposterior x-ray. **B**. Anteroposterior x-ray showing initial internal fixation with screw plate device, with supracondylar nonunion. **C**. Lateral x-ray of the femur showing proximal displacement of posterior portion of the lateral condyle with lag screw placed through the fracture line (arrow). **D**. Lateral approach to the distal femur with hardware removal, residual large defect from the lag screw and barrel site, and reduction of the posterior lateral condyle (arrow) with interfragmentary fixation from anterior to posterior. **E**. Completed internal fixation with bone grafting of tract of the screw in the distal femoral fragments and lateral plating with a condylar buttress plate. The supracondylar nonunion was also bone grafted. **F**. Postoperative x-rays showing internal fixation of the supracondylar fracture which healed uneventfully. **G**. Postoperative lateral x-ray showing anatomic reduction of the frontal plane fracture of the lateral condyle, fixed with cancellous screws placed from anterior to posterior.

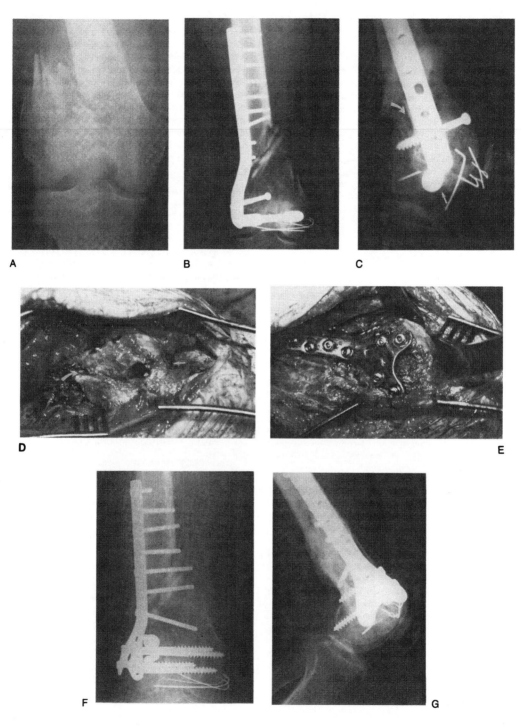

A

B

C

D

E

F

G

injuries, such as patellar fractures, tibial plateau fractures, ligament tears and avulsions, and open wounds, may alter the surgical treatment.

Adjunctive Techniques. Bone grafting should be considered in addition to internal fixation when there is bone loss, diminished vascularity, comminution, or osteoporosis. There are no controlled studies that clearly define when bone grafting should be performed, although bone grafting has been performed in large percentages in some series.

Polymethylmethacrylate cement may be used to augment the purchase of screws in osteoporotic bone. After internal fixation is performed, chilled cement is mixed and loaded into a syringe with the tip bored out with a 3.2-mm drill bit. Screws are removed from the holes to be augmented with cement, the holes are injected, and the screws quickly reinserted while the cement is hardening. Cement should not be inserted at sites where it may fill fracture lines and prevent fracture healing.

The impaction technique of Tscherne may be used in osteoporotic bone with comminution of the metaphyseal region. Shortening of the femur by 1 to 2 cm is acceptable in the elderly in exchange for the added fracture stability achieved intraoperatively.

Complications

Malreduction, Loss of Fixation, and Nonunion

Malreduction can occur in many sites in the distal femur, including the following: (1) intraarticular step-off, (2) malrotation of intercondylar fracture line, (3) varus–valgus malalignment, (4) flexion–extension malalignment, (5) rotational malalignment, (6) inadvertent shortening.

The most common sources of malreduction are the following technical depths: (1) missed intraarticular fracture line, (2) inability to control a fracture by closed methods, (3) inability to correctly achieve a satisfactory reduction by open means, (4) loss of fixation because of osteoporotic bone, (5) loss of fixation as a result of inadequate internal fixation, (6) loss of fixation as a result of drift of a C3 fracture into varus. The most common repositioning errors are recurvatum and varus (Fig. 8–28). Loss of fixation may result in a malunion as the fracture goes on to heal, with the option of late corrective osteotomy. If the loss of fixation is substantial then a decision may be made to operate early to re-reduce and internally fix the fracture. Loss of fixation may also result in nonunion if the fracture is not controlled (Fig. 8–29). The reader is referred to Chapter 21 for a detailed review of the treatment of malunion and nonunions about the knee.

Stiffness

Distal femoral fractures can be expected to produce some loss of knee motion. The worse the articular involvement, the less motion is expected. Type C3 fractures have been reported to recover an average of 99° of flexion.[4] The loss of motion in this group of injuries may have several sources, including the following: (1) bony blocks, (2) extensor mechanism stiffness, (3) intraarticular adhesions, (4) posttraumatic arthritis. The reader is referred to Chapter 20 for review of the evaluation and treatment of the stiff knee after trauma.

Infection

As noted in the historic review, infection rates in recent decades have ranged up to 7%. Series with substantial numbers of open fractures have had a higher infection rate, as would be expected. Treatment of deep wound infections can be extremely difficult, especially if the joint as well as the fracture lines is involved with sepsis. Treatment options include serial debridements, hardware removal, prolonged antibiotic treatment, and temporary fracture stabilization with traction or external fixation. Once the infection has been eradicated, subsequent reconstructive procedures are likely to be required to treat nonunions, stiffness, and other structural problems that remain.

References

1. Kolmert L., Wulff K. Epidemiology and treatment of distal femoral fractures in adults. *Acta Orthop Scand.* 1982;53:957–962.
2. Regazzoni P, Leutenegger A, Ruedi T, Staehelin F. Erste erfahrungen mit der dynamishen kondylenschraube (dcs) bei distalen femurfrakturen. *Helv Chir Acta.* 1986;53:61–64.
3. Arneson TJ, Melton LJ III, Lewallen DG, O'Fallon WM. Epidemiology of diaphyseal and distal femoral fractures in Rochester, Minnesota, 1965–1984. *Clin Orthop.* 1988;234:188–1894.
4. Siliski JM, Mahring M, Hofer HP. Supracondylar–intercondylar fractures of the femur. Treatment by internal fixation. *J Bone Joint Surg Am.* 1989;71:94–104.
5. Neer CS II, Grantham SJ, Shelton ML. Supracondylar fracture of the adult femur. *J Bone Joint Am.* 1967;49:591–613.
6. Seinsheimer F. Fractures of the distal femur. *Clin Orthop.* 1980;153:169–179.
7. Müller ME, Nazarian S, Koch P, Schatzker J. *The Comprehensive Classification of Fractures of Long Bones.* Berlin/Heidelberg: Springer-Verlag; 1990.
8. Walling AK, Seradge H, Spiegel PG. Injuries to the knee ligaments with fractures of the femur. *J Bone Joint Surg Am.* 1982;64:1324–1327.
9. Peltier LF. A brief history of traction. *J Bone Joint Surg Am.* 1972;54:1015–1032.
10. Thomas HO. *The Treatment of Deformities, Fractures and Diseases of Bones in the Lower Extremities.* London: HK Lewis; 1890.

11. Buck G. An improved method of treating fractures of the thigh illustrated by cases and a drawing. *Trans NY Acad Med.* 1961;2:232–250.
12. Russell RH. Theory and method of extension of the thigh. *Br Med J.* 1921;2:637–638.
13. Steinmann FR. Eine neve extensionsmethode in der Frakturenbehandlung. *Zentralbl Chir.* 1907;34:938–942.
14. Kirschner M. Ueber nagelextension. *Beitr Klin Chir.* 1909;64:266–279.
15. Mahorner HR, Bradburn M. Fractures of the femur. Report of 308 cases. *Surg Gynecol Obstet.* 1933;56:1066–1079.
16. Tees JD. Fracture of the lower end of the femur. *Am J Surg.* 1937;38:656–659.
17. Modlin J. Double skeletal traction in battle fractures of the lower femur. *Bull US Army Med Dept.* 1945;4:119–120.
18. Hampton OP. *Wounds of the Extremities in Military Surgery.* St. Louis: CV Mosby; 1951.
19. Wiggins HE. Vertical traction in open fractures of the femur. *US Armed Forces Med J.* 1953;4:1633–1636.
20. Watson-Jones R. *Fractures and Joint Injuries.* 4th ed. Baltimore: Williams & Wilkins; 1956.
21. Bohler L. *Treatment of Fractures.* New York: Grune and Stratton; 1956
22. Charnley J. *The Closed Treatment of Common Fractures.* 3rd ed. Edinburgh: E & S Livingstone; 1961.
23. Smillie IS. *Injuries of the Knee Joints.* 4th ed. Baltimore: Williams & Wilkins; 1971.
24. Stewart MJ, Sisk TD, Wallace SL. Fractures of the distal third of the femur. *J Bone Joint Surg Am.* 1966;48:784–807.
25. Borgan D, sprague BL. Treatment of distal femur fractures with early weight bearing. *Clin Orthop.* 1975;111:156–162.
26. Connolly JF, Dehne E. Closed reduction and early cast-brace ambulation in the treatment of femoral fractures. *J Bone Joint Surg Am.* 1973;55:1581–1599.
27. Connolly JF. Closed management of distal femoral fractures. *Instr Course Lect.* 1987;36:428–437.
28. Moll J. The cast brace walking treatment of open and closed femur fractures. *South Med J.* 1973;66:345–352.
29. Mooney V. Fractures of the distal femur. *Instr Course Lect.* 1987;36:427.
30. Rockwood CA Jr, Ryan VL, Richards JA. Experience with quadrilateral cast brace. *J Bone Joint Surg Am.* 1973;55:421. Abstract.
31. Unmansky AL. Blade-plate internal fixation for fracture of the distal end of the femur. *Bull Hosp Joint Dis.* 1948;9:18–21.
32. Altenberg AR, Shorkey RL. Blade-plate fixation in nonunion and in complicated fractures of the supracondylar region of the femur. *J Bone Joint Surg Am.* 1949;31:312–316.
33. White EH, Russin LA. Supracondylar fractures of the femur treated by internal fixation with immediate knee motion. *Am J Surg* 1956;22:801–820.
34. Rush LV, Gelbke H. *Atlas der intramedullaren frakturfixation nach Rush.* Munich: JA Barth; 1957.
35. Wertzberger JJ, Peltier LF. Supracondylar fractures. *Kans Med Soc.* 1967;68:328–332.
36. Rush LV. Dynamic intramedullary fracture fixation of the femur. *Clin Orthop.* 1968;60:21–27.
37. Shelbourne KD, Brueckmann FR. Rush-pin fixation of supracondylar and intercondylar fractures of the femur. *J Bone Joint Surg Am.* 1982;64:161–169.

38. Zickle RE, Fietti VG Jr, Lawsing JF III, Cochran GV. A new intramedullary fixation device for the distal third of the femur. *Clin Orthop.* 1977;125:185–191.
39. Zickle RE, Hobeika P, Robbins DS. Zickle supracondylar nails for fractures of the distal end of the femur. *Clin Orthop.* 1986;212:79–88.
40. Zickle RE. Nonunions of fractures of the proximal and distal thirds of the shaft of the femur. *Instr Course Lect.* 1988;37:173–179.
41. Müller ME, Allgower M, Wilenegger H. *Technique of Internal Fixation of Fractures.* Berlin: Springer-Verlag; 1965.
42. Neff G. Zur Behandlung der Supracondylaren und tiefen oberschenkelfrakturen. *Monatsschr Unfallheilk.* 1966;69:151–159.
43. Olerud S. Operative treatment of supracondylar–condylar fractures of the femur. Technique and results in fifteen cases. *J Bone Joint Surg Am.* 1972;54:1015–1032.
44. Wenzl H, Casey PA, Herbert P, Belin J. Die operative behandlung der distalen Femurfraktur. *AO Bull.* Dec 1970.
45. Slatis P, Ryoppy S, Huttinen V. AO osteosynthesis of fractures of the distal third of the femur. *Acta Orthop Scand.* 1971;42:162–172.
46. Olerud S. Reconstruktion av distala femur vid komminut frakur. *Svensk Kir For Forh.* 1966;24:93–94.
47. Chiron HS, Tremoulet J, Casey P, Muller M. Fractures of the distal third of the femur treated by internal fixation. *Clin Orthop.* 1974;100:160–170.
48. Tscherne H, Ostern HJ, Trentz O. Spatergebnisse der distalen femurfraktur und irhe besonderen probleme. *Zentralbl Chir.* 1977;102:897–904.
49. Schatzker J, Horne G, Waddell J. The Toronto experience with the supracondylar fracture of the femur, 1966–1977. *Injury.* 1975;6:113–128.
50. Schatzker J, Lambert DC. Supracondylar fractures of the femur. *Clin Orthop.* 1979;138:77–83.
51. Della Torre P, Aglietti P, Altissimi M. Results of rigid fixation of 54 supracondylar fractures of the femur. *Arch Orthop Traumat Surg.* 1980;97:177–183.
52. Mize RD, Bucholz RW, Grogan DP. Surgical treatment of displaced, comminuted fractures of the distal end of the femur. *J Bone Joint Surg Am.* 1982;64:871–879.
53. Healy WL, Brooker AF. Distal femoral fractures. Comparison of open and closed methods of treatment. *Clin Orthop.* 1983;174:166–171.
54. Schatzker J, Tile M. *The Rationale of Operative Fracture Care.* New York: Springer-Verlag; 1987.
55. Johnson KD. Internal fixation of distal femoral fractures. *Instr Course Lect.* 1989;38:437–448.
56. Wade PA, Okinara AJ. The problem of the supracondylar fracture of the femur in the aged person. *Am J Surg.* 1959;97:499–512.
57. Brown A, D'Arcy JC. Internal fixation for supracondylar fractures of the femur in the elderly patient. *J Bone Joint Surg Br.* 1971;53:420–424.
58. Benum P. The use of bone cement as an adjunct to internal fixation of supracondylar fractures of osteoporotic femurs. *Acta Orthop Scand.* 1977;48:52–56.
59. Johnson EE. Combined direct and indirect reduction of comminuted four-part intraarticular T-type fractures of the distal femur. *Clin Orthop.* 1988;231:154–162.
60. Mast J, Jakob R, Ganz R. *Planning and Reduction Techniques in Fracture Surgery.* New York: Springer-Verlag; 1989.
61. Hall MF. Two-plane fixation of acute supracondylar and

intracondylar fractures of the femur. *South Med J.* 1978;71:1474–1479.

62. Giles JB, DeLee JC, Heckman JD, Keever JE. Supracondylar–intercondylar fractures of the femur treated with a supracondylar plate and lag screw. *J Bone Joint Surg Am.* 64:864–870.

63. Pritchett JW. Supracondylar fractures of the femur. *Clin Orthop.* 1984;184:173–177.

64. Schatzker J, Mahomed N, Schiffman K, Kellam J. Dynamic condylar screw. A new device. *J Orthop Trauma.* 1989;3:124–132.

65. Sanders R, Regazzoni P, Reudi T. Treatment of supracondylar–intraarticular fractures of the femur using the dynamic condylar screw. *J Orthop Trauma.* 1989; 3:214–222.

66. Winquist RA, Hansen ST, Clawson DK. Closed intramedullary nailing of femoral fractures. *J Bone Joint Surg Am.* 1984;66:529–539.

67. Bucholz RW, Ross SE, Lawrence KL. Fatigue fracture of the interlocking nail in the treatment of fractures of the distal part of the femoral shaft. *J Bone Joint Surg Am.* 1987;69:1391–1399.

68. Whittle AT, Russell TA, Taylor JC, Tagert BE. Interlocking interfragmentary nailing of distal intraarticular femoral fractures. Posterior Exhibit No. 4, Orthopedic Trauma Association, 1992 Annual Meeting, Minneapolis.

69. Henry SL, Seligson D, Trager S. Management of supracondylar fractures with the GSH intramedullary nail. In: *American Academy of Orthopedic Surgeons, Annual Meeting*; 1991: Paper 279.

70. Sanders RW, Swiontkowski M, Rosen H, Helfet D. Complex fractures and malunions of the distal femur: Results of treatment with double plates. *J Bone Joint Surg Am.* 1991;73:341–346.

71. Matter P, Rittman W. *The Open Fracture.* Bern: Huber; 1978.

72. Helpenstell TS, Hansen ST. Review of 51 open distal femoral fractures treated with imediate open reduction and internal fixation. In: *American Academy of Orthopedic Surgeons, Annual Meeting*; 1991: Paper 274.

73. Seligson D, Kristiansen TK. Use of the Wagner apparatus in complicated fractures of the distal femur. *J Trauma.* 1978;18:795–799.

74. Stein H, Makin M. Use of the Wagner apparatus in fractures of the lower limb. *Orthop Rev.* 1980;9:96–99.

9
Tibial Plateau Fractures

Kenneth J. Koval and Roy Sanders

Introduction

Tibial plateau fractures result from (1) indirect coronal and/or (2) direct axial compressive forces.[1] These forces drive the femoral condyle into the tibial plateau, producing a spectrum of fracture patterns. According to recent series, tibial plateau fractures are most commonly the result of falls or motor vehicle accidents.[2-4]

Fracture fragment size, location, and displacement are determined by the direction, magnitude, and location of the generated force, as well as the bone quality and the degree of knee flexion at the moment of impact.[2,5,6] The combination of compression and valgus produces a lateral plateau fracture, whereas compression coupled with varus results in a medial fracture pattern (Fig. 9–1).[6] The prevalence of lateral plateau fractures is related to the valgus inclination of the anatomic axis and the usual lateral direction of the applied force[7-10].

Patient age and bone quality influence the resultant fracture pattern and associated ligamentous injury.[9,10] Young patients, whose strong subchondral bone resists depression, typically develop split fractures. These patients are at the highest risk for collateral or cruciate ligament rupture. With advancing age, the subchondral bone is less able to resist axial loading and typically depression or split-depression fractures occur. As the bone compresses, the force is dissipated and protects the opposite collateral ligament from injury.

Diagnosis and Associated Injuries

A tibial plateau fracture should be considered whenever a patient presents with pain and tenderness about the knee following injury. A hemarthrosis is often present; however, with significant capsular or bony disruption,

leakage of the hemarthrosis into the surrounding soft tissue will occur.[1]

The neurovascular status of the extremity, degree of swelling, and skin condition must be noted. Popliteal, posterior tibial, and dorsal pedis pulses must be palpated, and if absent, Doppler studies should be performed. The examining physician must be aware of any obvious deformity causing vascular kinking. Using gentle straight-line traction, the physician should restore limb alignment before committing to a diagnosis of vascular injury.

If the patient is responsive, sensory and motor examination of the extremity is completed. At this time the limb should be examined for the possibility of a

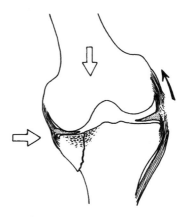

Figure 9–1. A combination of compression and valgus force produces lateral plateau fractures. Medial collateral ligament sprains may also occur during the same injury.

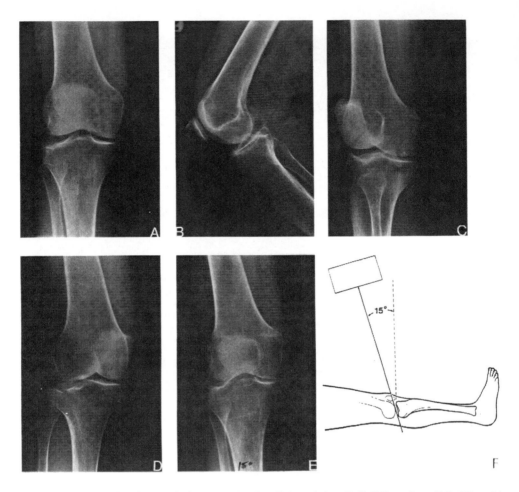

Figure 9–2. Knee trauma series of x-rays. **A.** Anteroposterior view. **B.** Lateral view. **C, D.** Oblique views. **E, F.** 15° caudal view.

compartment syndrome. These patients will present with pain out of proportion to the injury, swelling, pain to passive stretch, pallor, pulselessness, hypesthesia, and motor weakness. Clinical assessment is not entirely reliable, and accurate assessment may be impossible without direct measurement of intracompartmental pressure.

Any open wound must be evaluated for the possibility of an open joint injury. If not obvious, the physician should perform a saline load test by injecting at least 50 mL of saline into the knee away from the wound. Any leakage of fluid from the wound confirms the diagnosis of an open joint.

The wound should be examined for evidence of ligamentous instability. Tenderness and swelling over the medial collateral ligament suggest collateral sprain. Coronal plane stress testing (varus/valgus) can aid in the determination of associated ligamentous disruption, but should be performed after radiographic evaluation. Testing cannot be accurately performed if a hemarthrosis or excessive pain exists. After arthrocentesis, intraarticular lidocaine injection may allow a more accurate exam. If this is not possible, the patient is tested under anesthesia. Despite this, clinical examination may not distinguish fracture instability from ligamentous disruption.

Initial radiographs should include anteroposterior, lateral, two obliques, and the 15° caudal plateau

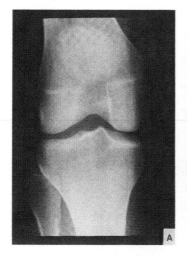
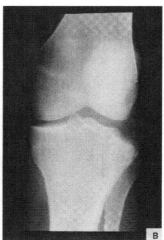
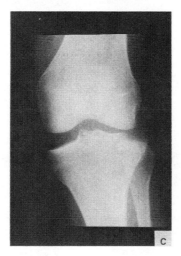

Figure 9–3. Radiographs taken with valgus stress provide a comparison of the width of the medial joint space in the injured and uninjured knee. Widening suggests significant injury to the medial collateral ligament. **A.** Stress views of normal right knee. **B.** Anteroposterior x-ray of left knee. **C.** Stress view of left knee revealing laxity of medial collateral ligament. At surgery, the avulsed MCL was reattached to the tibia.

view.[5,9–11] These five x-rays are known as the knee trauma series (Fig. 9–2). These films should be analyzed for rim widening, articular depression, shaft extension, and bony avulsions.[9,10,12] The amount of condylar depression can be measured from the remaining intact articular surface on the 15° caudal plateau or lateral radiographs.[5,9–11]

Stress radiographs of the knee can be useful for the detection of collateral ligament ruptures[12,13] (Fig. 9–3). Significant widening of the opposite joint line will not occur with an isolated plateau injury.[13] Greater than 1-mm increase of the medial or lateral clear space, compared with the contralateral limb stressed in the same degree of flexion, is suggestive of a collateral ligament disruption.[13]

Comparison radiographs of the uninvolved knee are

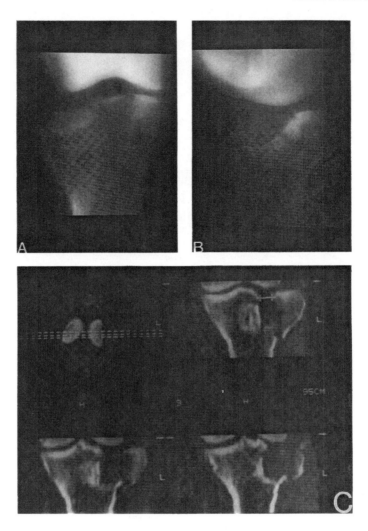

Figure 9–4. Split fragment and depression of central plateau. **A.** Anteroposterior tomogram. **B.** Lateral tomogram. **C.** CT scan frontal plane reconstruction.

useful for preoperative planning. Trispiral and computer tomography (CT) coupled with sagittal reconstructions are helpful in evaluating the degree of articular displacement[5,14] (Fig. 9–4). The tibial spines are well visualized and bony avulsion of the cruciate ligaments can be identified by either technique. Computer tomography is most useful, however, when viewed in the horizontal (transverse) plane (Fig. 9–5). This permits analysis of the entire periphery of the plateau for rim avulsions that are associated with fracture dislocations.

Additionally, these studies are an excellent adjunct to plain films in the preoperative planning of lag screw placement, particularly when contemplating percutaneous fixation. Magnetic resonance imaging (MRI) may play a role in the future in the evaluation of meniscal and ligamentous injuries associated with these fractures. At present, however, no definitive studies to determine its usefulness exist. Finally, if clinical or radiographic evaluation raises the suspicion of a vascular injury, an arteriogram is indicated.

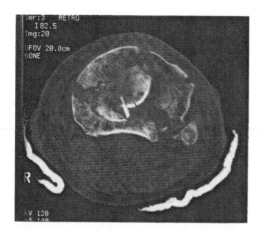

Figure 9–5. CT scan through the subchondral region of the tibial plateau. Information on the number, size, and location of fragments may assist in planning surgical exposure and fixation.

Classification

The most widely accepted classification has been that proposed by Schatzker[9,10,15] (Fig. 9–6). Type I is a wedge (split) fracture of the lateral tibial plateau. Type II is a split-depression fracture of the lateral plateau. In this fracture, the femoral condyle first splits the condyle and then depresses the medial edge of the remaining plateau. Type III is a pure central depression fracture of the lateral plateau without an associated split. It is usually the result of a lower-energy injury occurring in the older-age population. The type IV fracture is a fracture of the medial tibial plateau usually involving the entire condyle. As the medial plateau requires a greater force to fracture than the lateral plateau, this fracture is often the result of a high-energy injury and may be associated with a traction lesion of the peroneal nerve. Type V is a bicondylar fracture and typically consists of split fractures of the medial and lateral plateaus without articular depression. Finally, type VI is a tibial plateau fracture with an associated proximal shaft fracture. This fracture is the result of a high-energy injury, is often highly comminuted, and may be associated with popliteal artery disruption. Traction tends to displace the metaphyseal/diaphyseal fracture, rather than produce articular reduction.

Fracture dislocations are distinguished by the fact that they are associated with instability, because of either the soft tissue injury or the pattern of osseous involvement. These fractures usually require operative management and have been classified by Moore as either split, entire condylar, rim avulsion, rim compression, or four-part fracture[16] (Fig. 9–7). Split fractures are restricted to the medial plateau. The fracture line is coronal and involves the posterior half of the articular surface. The fragment is usually unstable and displaces with knee flexion, allowing subluxation of the medial femoral condyle. In entire condylar fractures, the fracture line extends beyond the intercondylar eminence, thereby involving both cruciate ligaments. Rim avulsion fractures, identified by the "lateral capsular sign," indicate significant capsular and ligamentous injury. Rim compression fractures signify rupture of the opposite collateral and both cruciate ligaments. In four-part fractures, the medial eminence (with the cruciate ligaments) is a separate fragment, separated from the shaft.

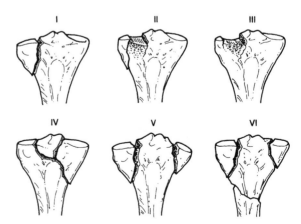

Figure 9–6. Schatzker classification of tibial plateau fractures. **I.** Wedge (split). **II.** Split depression. **III.** Central depression. **IV.** Medial condyle. **V.** Bicondylar. **VI.** Bicondylar with shaft involvement.

A. Split fracture   **B.** Entire condyle

C. Rim avulsion   **D.** Rim compression

E. Four part

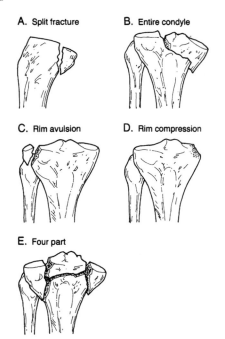

Figure 9–7. Fracture patterns of the tibial plateau associated with fracture dislocation of the knee. **A.** Split. **B.** Entire condylar. **C.** Rim avulsion. **D.** Rim compression. **E.** Four part.

Immediate Care

Once the diagnosis has been made, the leg is wrapped in a toe-to-groin bulky Jones dressing and immobilized. The knee should be splinted in approximately 15° of flexion for comfort. If the fracture does not require operative intervention and only minor swelling exists, the patient may be discharged with toe-touch weight bearing in a long leg cast or brace. Otherwise the patient should be admitted, the limb elevated above the level of the heart, ice applied, and frequent neurovascular evaluations performed.

Surgical Indications

Controversy still exists regarding the specific indications for open versus closed management of tibial plateau fractures.[3,9,10,17–19] Some authors advocate nonoperative treatment for fractures with up to 1 cm of depression.[3] Others accept only minimal displacement of the articular surface.[9,10,17] There is general agreement that instability of greater than 10° (as compared with the uninvolved knee) of the nearly extended knee is an indication for operative intervention.[8,20]

The amount of articular displacement resulting in in-

stability is unknown; it is dependent on the fracture type, location, and associated ligamentous disruption. Split fractures, in addition to disrupting the articular surface, involve the rim of the tibial plateau and are likely to be unstable to axial loading.[9] Split fracture reduction can be achieved through ligamentotaxis; however, maintenance of reduction requires prolonged traction unless operatively stabilized.[2] Split-depression fractures are at a higher risk of instability secondary to the depressed surface adjacent to the split component.[9] Although the split fragment can be reduced through ligamentotaxis, traction will not effect a reduction of the depressed central surface.[9] Pure central depression fractures are usually stable unless the depression involves the entire plateau; the intact cortical rim provides varus/valgus stability.[9] Plateau fractures that are associated with a tibial shaft fracture are usually not amenable to closed treatment, as traction often results in separation of the shaft components rather than reduction of the articular surface.[9] Finally, open tibial plateau fractures or those associated with a compartment syndrome or vascular insult require emergent care.

Treatment Plan

Closed Treatment

Protected mobilization (hinged cast brace) should be used for tibial plateau fractures with minimal articular displacement and ligamentous stability.[1,3,8] Patients should begin both immediate isometric quadriceps exercises and progressive active and active-assisted range of motion. Weight bearing should be limited to toe touch until radiographic evidence of healing, usually at 8 to 12 weeks. At that time range of motion should be full, and progression to full weight bearing may be pursued.

Surgical Intervention

Preoperative Planning. The exact nature of the fracture should be understood before attempts at any form of surgical intervention are made. Although useful for simpler fractures, preoperative planning is critical for more complex injuries. It forces the surgeon to understand the "personality of the fracture" and mentally prepare an operative plan. Radiographs of the opposite, normal extremity serve as templates. The entire operation, from incision to closure, should be listed in a logical stepwise manner. All aspects of the reduction and fixation must be drawn out to avoid technical pitfalls and ensure that all the needed equipment is available. If this is done, not only will surgical time decrease, but the technical aspects of the surgery will be easier. It is hoped this will improve the surgical outcome.

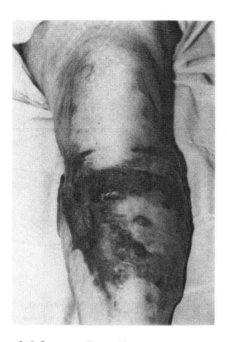

Figure 9–8. Severe swelling and fracture blisters after a high-energy comminuted tibial plateau fracture. Internal fixation in such a case must be either delayed or even avoided. Alternative treatment forms such as traction, percutaneous reduction and fixation, or external fixation may be necessary because of the soft tissue envelope.

Timing of Surgery.   The timing of surgery is dependent on the soft tissue conditions.[10] Early postinjury swelling represents fracture hematoma. Within 8 to 12 hours, however, the soft tissues become edematous and definitive surgery should be delayed to allow swelling to subside and local skin conditions to improve. High-energy tibial plateau fractures, especially those that result from an anterior blow to the tibia, often require a minimum of 3 to 5 days to allow the soft tissues to normalize. Early surgical intervention requiring incisions through compromised soft tissues is inadvisable as this may be associated with a higher incidence of wound complications (Fig. 9–8).

Limited Open Reduction.   There have been excellent results with the use of indirect methods to achieve a limited open reduction.[21-25] As proposed by Mast et al, this allows a more "biologic" approach, preserving soft tissue vascularity while still allowing adequate bony stabilization, early motion, and functional recovery.[26]

As an alternative to direct visualization of the joint, fluoroscopy may be used to assess articular con-

gruence.[21,24] Image intensification can accurately evaluate split fracture reduction; however, it is less sensitive in the assessment of depressed central fracture reduction.[24] The reason for this lies in the fact that radiographically a split fracture fragment can clearly be seen on image, whereas a depressed fragment is buried within the remaining plateau, creating a confluence of shadows. Furthermore, image intensification does not reveal associated intraarticular pathology.

Arthroscopy has recently been reported as an effective method of assessing fracture reduction.[22,23,25] Certain authors advocate arthroscopic evaluation of even minimally displaced split fractures, as theoretically the meniscus may become trapped in the fracture line.[9,10] Although sensitive for the evaluation of central depression and intraarticular pathology, arthroscopy does not adequately evaluate rim pathology or metaphyseal alignment.

These limited open techniques are most useful in the treatment of pure split- or central depression fractures.[24] Split-depression fractures (Schatzker type II) are less amenable to these limited techniques as the amount of depression and articular incongruity is more severe than that of either split- or central depression fractures.[24] Part of the difficulty arises in trying to percutaneously position a tamp under the severely depressed fragments. The degree of difficulty is increased with the amount of comminution. For split-depression tibial plateau fractures, the authors believe that an open reduction is the only reliable method to restore articular congruity.

Surgical Technique for Limited Open Reduction

Patients are placed on a radiolucent operating table in the supine position with a tourniquet and the ipsilateral anterior iliac crest prepared for possible graft. If arthroscopy is to be used, the end of the table should be flexed. The use of the tourniquet is optional.

Pure Split Fractures (Schatzker Types I, IV, and V).   In fractures where a split fragment is displaced only medially or laterally, a tenaculum clamp can be used to achieve reduction. If the split fragment is also depressed, reduction can be accomplished using ligamentotaxis with the aid of a femoral distractor placed on the same side as the fracture (Fig. 9–9).

In fractures without articular impaction, bone grafting is not needed, as reduction is maintained using compression alone. In these situations, bone graft may actually prevent accurate interdigitation of the fracture fragments and preclude an anatomic reduction. Once reduced, the fracture is stabilized with two or more percutaneously placed 6.5- or 7.0-mm cancellous lag screws with washers inserted parallel to the tibial joint surface. An antiglide screw with a washer may be placed at the

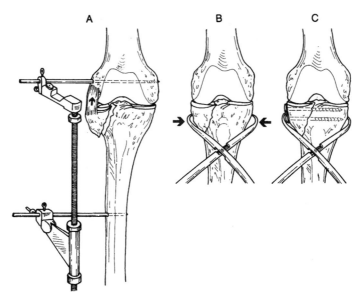

Figure 9–9. A. Reduction of a wedge fracture using ligamentotaxis (manual or by femoral distractor) for elevation. **B.** Bone tenaculum used for final reduction and compression. Reduction is assessed by fluoroscopy and x-ray. **C.** Internal fixation is achieved using percutaneous screws.

distal apex of the fracture. This serves to buttress the fragment against collapse. Care should be taken to use screws whose threads do not cross the fracture line, or the lag effect will be lost.

Pure Depression (Schatzker Type III).   In fractures with central depression, the metaphyseal cortex should be fenestrated and the depressed fragment elevated from below, using a bone tamp. The placement of the cortical window and the tamp is best seen using fluoroscopy. The elevation of depressed central fracture fragments creates a metaphyseal defect which should be filled with a spacer to prevent articular collapse. Cancellous iliac bone grafting has been used for this purpose; cancellous bone compacts into the shape of the defect, offers structural support, rapidly revascularizes, and retains its inductive and conductive properties.[10] Corticocancellous blocks are useful when greater structural support is required.

One disadvantage of iliac crest bone graft harvesting is that it adds considerable morbidity to the procedure.

Recent reports have indicated that allografts and synthetic bone substitutes can be used instead as effective spacers in the treatment of tibial plateau fractures.[9,10] As a minimally invasive procedure is one of the advantages and goals of limited open reduction, these alternatives should be considered. Once grafted, percutaneously placed 6.5- or 7.0-mm cancellous lag screws are inserted parallel to the joint surface immediately below the graft to act as a supporting beam.

Open Reduction.   Open reduction should be considered for the treatment of split-depression (Schatzker type II) fractures and those with metaphyseal–diaphyseal dissociation (Schatzker type VI). This offers the best chance for both an anatomic joint reduction with axial alignment and stable fixation allowing early functional range of motion. If the soft tissue envelope does not permit formal open reduction, limited open reduction as described earlier may be necessary, accepting the limitations of those techniques for more complicated fracture patterns. A circular frame external

Figure 9–10. A. Photograph of leg with marked swelling and fracture blisters over proximal tibia. **B, C.** X-ray showing type VI fracture pattern. **D, E.** Elevation of depressed segment of lateral tibial plateau using percutaneous technique under fluoroscopy. **F.** Packing bone graft under lateral plateau. **G, H.** Fixation achieved with percutaneous screws, cancellous bone graft, and circular frame external fixator.

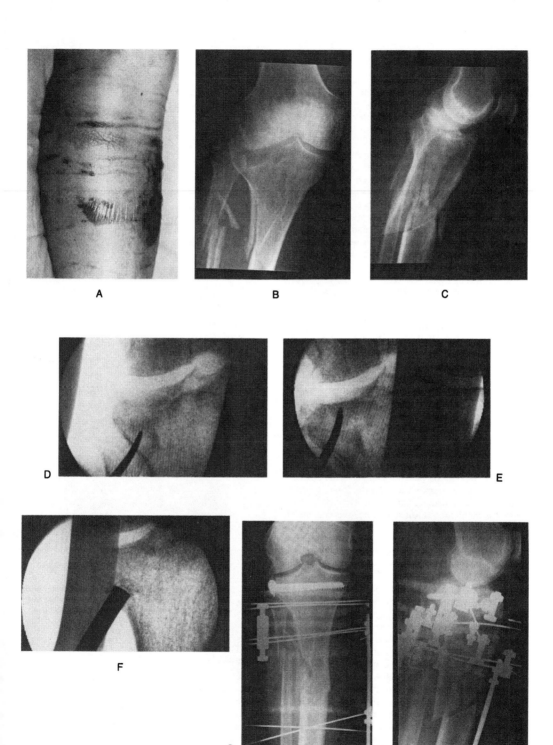

fixator may be used to support the metaphyseal and
diaphyseal portions of the fracture (Fig. 9–10).

The operative procedure should be performed under
tourniquet on a radiolucent operating table with image
intensification. Fracture reduction is aided by ligamentotaxis, using a femoral distractor. This should be
placed on the ipsilateral side of the tibial plateau fracture, extending across the knee joint, with one pin in
the femoral condyle and the other pin in the mid- to
distal tibia, well away from the anticipated distal end
of the implant(s). Furthermore, these Schanz screws
should be inserted *before* exsanguination to maximize
tourniquet time. In the event of bicondylar or type VI
fractures, bilateral femoral distractors may be required.
One large centrally threaded Steinman pin may be
placed through the distal femur parallel to the joint
under fluoroscopic control. Distally, two half-pins are
recommended to avoid thermal necrosis associated
with transfixion pin insertion in this cortical diaphyseal
region.

Before inflation of the tourniquet the knee should be
flexed to allow the quadriceps muscle to stretch distally.
The plateau should be approached through a midline
incision in anticipation of possible future reconstructive
surgery. A full-thickness skin flap extending to the fascial and retinacular expansions is then raised on the side
of the injury, usually the lateral plateau. The other flap
is lifted only if open reduction of that condyle is
needed. The crural fascia over the tibia and the iliotibial
band are then split vertically and retracted. An arthrotomy is made horizontally through the coronary ligament, taking care to preserve the meniscus and sufficient ligament on the tibia for later repair. All clot and
blood should be irrigated out and the joint should be
distracted. A "Z" knee retractor can then be placed
under the meniscus to lift it superiorly, exposing the entire joint surface (Fig. 9–11). The joint must be examined for evidence of meniscal pathology. Meniscal
tears have been reported in as many as 50% of tibial
plateau fractures.[6,27,28] Lesions that are not appropriate
for repair should be excised at this time. Peripheral
tears should have a suture repair at closure.

In our experience, incision of the anterior horn of the
meniscus as described by Perry et al does not offer any
advantage and, instead, may prevent early postoperative motion because of its necessary repair[29] (Fig. 9–12).
If visualization of the joint is not adequate, extending
the limits of the incision, including partial sectioning of
the iliotibial band, is usually all that is required. If the
view is still less than optimal, a Z-plasty of the patella
tendon should be contemplated[9,10] (see Chapter 5).
This is usually needed only in type VI fractures. The
physician must first ascertain, however, that a fracture
of the tibial tubercle does not already exist. In this
case, the fractured tubercle should be lifted to afford
visualization instead.

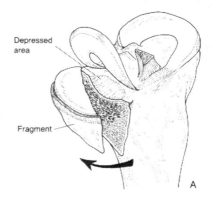

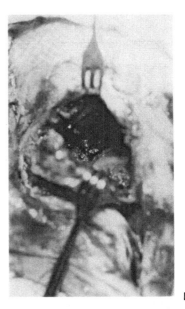

Figure 9–11. A. Diagram of exposure of the lateral tibial
plateau with a type II fracture, elevating the meniscus and
rolling open the wedge fragment. **B.** Intraoperative exposure.

Open Reduction Internal Fixation of Schatzker Type II Fractures

The split fracture line is identified. Exposure of the depressed articular fragment is then accomplished by
opening up the metaphysis like a book at the split fracture line and hinging the peripheral fragments outward,
thus preserving their soft tissue attachment. Reduction
of the depressed articular surface fragment should start
with recognition of the area of uninvolved articular surface. Depressed articular fragments should be elevated

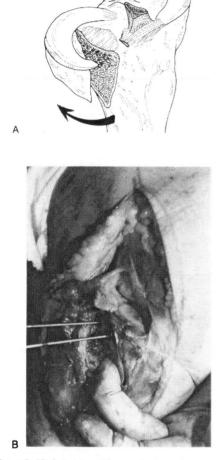

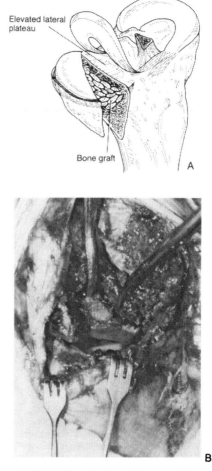

Figure 9–12. A. Incision of the anterior horn of the meniscus. (Adapted with permission from Perry et al.[29]) **B.** Intraoperative exposure.

Figure 9–13. A. After elevation of the central depression, bone grafting of the underlying void is done with cancellous and corticocancellous strips. **B.** Intraoperative packing of bone graft under elevated plateau (same case as in Figs 9–11 and 9–15).

from below, en masse, as large cancellous blocks to prevent articular surface fragmentation.[9,10] This can be achieved with the use of a bone tamp or elevator working through the split component.

Once the fragment(s) is elevated, provisional stabilization of the articular fragments to the medial condyle using K-wires is performed. These K-wires should be placed in an anterior-to-posterior direction to avoid interfering with reduction of the split fragment. At this point the surgeon has two choices: (1) bone grafting of the metaphyseal defect followed by reduction and pro-

visional stabilization of the split component, or (2) reduction and provisional stabilization of the split fragment followed by bone grafting (Fig. 9–13). The latter approach requires that the graft be inserted through a separate metaphyseal window.

Definitive stabilization requires the insertion of two 6.5- or 7.0-mm cancellous lag screws parallel to the joint followed by metaphyseal buttress plating (Fig. 9–14). This buttress must be located at the distal extent of the fracture line and serves to prevent shear forces from causing late collapse. The choice of plates is dependent

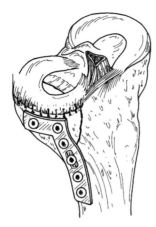

Figure 9–14. The split fragment is rotated back into position over the central fragment and bone graft. An appropriate plate is contoured and used to buttress the fracture. The most proximal screws are placed just under the subchondral bone to help support the elevated central fragment.

on the degree of cortical comminution, and may be as simple as a washer (one-hole plate), two-hole plate, T or L buttress plate, or Burri plate. The surgeon should select that plate that offers stable fixation yet minimizes bulk to prevent complications with wound closure. If a large plate is selected, the cancellous lag screws should be inserted through its proximal holes (Fig. 9–15).

Schatzker Type VI Fractures

Most type VI fractures can be reduced and stabilized without the creation of large medial and lateral soft tissue flaps. The medial plateau fragment is usually large and extraarticular, and it should be used as a building block on which to attach the lateral fragments and shaft. When the fracture extends into the articular surface of the medial plateau, however, reduction and stabilization of this fragment may require a medial exposure. The authors have found that it is usually not necessary to raise a large medial flap as limited reduction techniques usually suffice.

After articular reconstruction Schatzker type VI fractures require shaft stabilization. This can be accomplished depending on fracture configuration by either (1) a single plate, (2) double plates, (3) one plate and a contralateral two pin external fixator, or (4) a small wire circular fixator (Figs. 9.16 and 9.17).

When plates are used, fracture pattern determines implant choice. If the fracture line exiting the cortex opposite the plate is transverse, then a single plate will suffice. Oblique fracture lines exiting the cortex opposite the plate require the use of an additional small anti-

glide plate or a two-pin external fixator to neutralize shearing forces. If a second plate is needed, a thin plate (1/2 or 1/3 tubular) should be inserted with a minimal dissection. Care should be taken that the two plates do not end at the same level to avoid creating a stress riser. If a two-pin frame is used as an adjunct, one pin is placed parallel to the joint in the metaphysis, and one pin is placed in the shaft distal to the end of the plate.[30] Finally, if the shaft component is extremely proximal, a small wire circular fixator should be considered.

Wound closure is performed over suction drains. If the wound cannot be closed without tension, it is preferable to leave the incision partially open and covered with a sterile dressing. Wound closure may then be performed at a later date.

Postoperative Care. Postoperatively, the knee should be protected in a hinged knee brace and started on continuous passive motion, with a range of motion of 0° to 30° and advanced as tolerated. The machine is kept on as much as possible during waking hours; early motion has been clearly demonstrated to promote cartilage healing.[31] When the extensor mechanism is compromised by the fracture or approach, flexion must be limited by the surgeon. Physical therapy for active-assisted range of motion and touch-down weight bearing is begun on postoperative day 3 and continued until the patient is independent with ambulatory aids. Polytrauma and multiply fractured patients are treated according to their concomitant injuries with the aforementioned therapeutic regimen as the goal. Full weight bearing is permitted by 12 weeks based on radiographic evidence of consolidation. In cases with two-pin external fixators, the frame may be removed after 6 to 8 weeks. Similarly in patients with small wire circular fixators, dynamization and/or progressive weight bearing may be started at 6 to 8 weeks.

Ligamentous Injury

The significance of associated ligamentous disruption and the need for repair remain controversial.[3,8–10, 12,19,32–34] Up to 30% of tibial plateau fractures have an associated ligamentous disruption.[3,35,36] It is not known which, if any, associated knee ligament injuries will result in postoperative instability. Proponents for the operative treatment of ligamentous disruptions argue that the collateral ligaments are essential for maximal joint function.[3,9,10,12,33] There is less enthusiasm for acute operative treatment of associated cruciate disruptions. We agree with the proponents for the nonoperative treatment of associated ligamentous disruptions who argue that collateral ligament repair requires additional soft tissue dissection and that large series of tibial plateau fractures treated without collateral ligamentous repair resulted in no significant collateral instability.[8] In

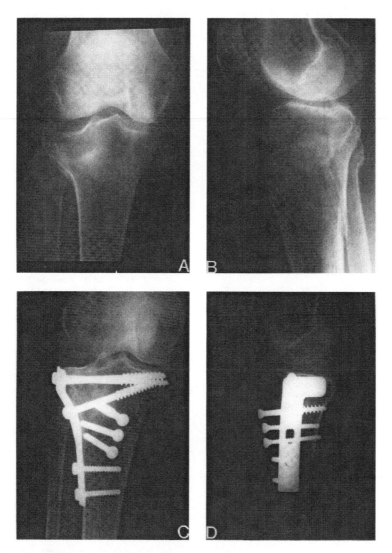

Figure 9–15. A, B. Preoperative x-ray of a type II fracture. **C, D.** Postoperative x-ray after open reduction, bone grafting, and internal fixation (same case as in Figs 9–11 and 9–13). **A, C.** Anteroposterior. **B, D.** Lateral.

addition, there is overwhelming evidence that an isolated medial collateral ligament injury heals satisfactorily without surgical intervention.[37] Avulsion fractures involving the intercondylar eminence should be stabilized; reattachment of the cruciate ligaments with a piece of bone will allow early range of motion.

Open Fractures

At the time of initial irrigation and debridement, limited internal fixation of the articular surface using lag screw fixation may be performed. This protects the joint from the consequences of an articular malunion if asso-

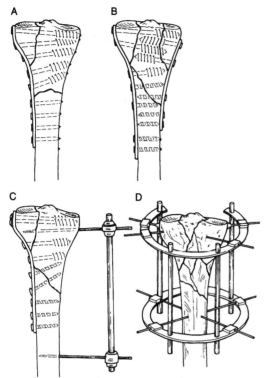

Figure 9–16. Fixation options for type VI fractures. **A.** Single plate. **B.** Double plate. **C.** Single plate with external fixator. **D.** External fixation with small wire circular fixator.

ciated injuries or infection precludes further surgery before fracture healing. If additional stability is required, temporary external fixation can be placed across the knee and exchanged for internal fixation at a later date. Alternatively a definitive small wire circular frame may be applied. Cast treatment or traction may complicate the postoperative care of an extremity that has an extensive soft tissue injury and the authors do not recommend this approach.

Complications

Infection following tibial plateau fracture occurs in up to 12% of cases[6] and may be related to either the initial fracture status or subsequent surgical intervention. Skin slough, a risk factor for later infection, is a particular concern in the proximal leg secondary to poor soft tissue coverage. The major predisposing factors for skin slough include (1) poor surgical timing; (2) inappropriate incisions, especially the triradiate; and (3) improper

soft tissue handling, particularly when associated with the use of bicondylar implants. Once wound compromise has occurred, debridement and soft tissue reconstruction will be required. This may be as simple as split-thickness skin grafting or may require a gastrocnemius or free tissue transfer.

Loss of fixation may be prevented by proper preoperative planning. Stabilization of tibial plateau fractures with lag screws alone should be attempted only in pure split or central depression fractures. Split-depression fractures, those with metaphyseal–diaphyseal dissociation, and fractures occurring in osteopenic bone require buttress plate fixation. Bone grafting should be performed in all depressed fractures.

Posttraumatic arthrosis may occur as a result of cartilage damage from the initial injury or can be related to residual joint incongruity. Preservation of the menisci is important to prevent excessive load bearing by the underlying plateau.[38] Some loss of joint motion is to be expected secondary to periarticular soft tissue injury and is compounded by prolonged immobilization. Rare complications include popliteal artery laceration, avascular necrosis, peroneal neuropathy (following either surgery or casting), nonunion, and malunion.[6]

Results

Most authors agree that minimally displaced tibial plateau fractures do well with nonoperative treatment; most series report about a 90% acceptable result rate.[1,3,8] It is difficult to evaluate the results of treatment of displaced tibial plateau fractures as there is no universally accepted classification scheme, indication for surgery, or grading system for follow-up results. It has been noted that patients who have an abnormal radiologic appearance may have a good clinical result.[8,39] This may be related to the fact that almost the entire load carried by the lateral plateau is borne by the lateral meniscus.[38] Conversely, patients may have complaints of pain associated with degenerative joint disease without radiologic changes.

Schatzker reported on 70 tibial plateau fractures followed for an average of 28 months.[15] Those fractures treated with open reduction and internal fixation, including elevation of the plateau en masse with bone grafting and early motion, had an 89% acceptable result rate. In a series of 52 operatively treated tibial plateau fractures, Savoie et al reported an 87% satisfactory result rate at an average of 24 months of follow-up.[19] Porter reported a 96% acceptable result rate in fractures with less than 10-mm depression treated with early motion.[3] Fractures with greater than 10-mm depression had a 47% acceptable result rate when treated with early motion and an 80% acceptable result rate with open reduction, internal fixation, and bone grafting. Lansinger et al, using clinical instability of the ex-

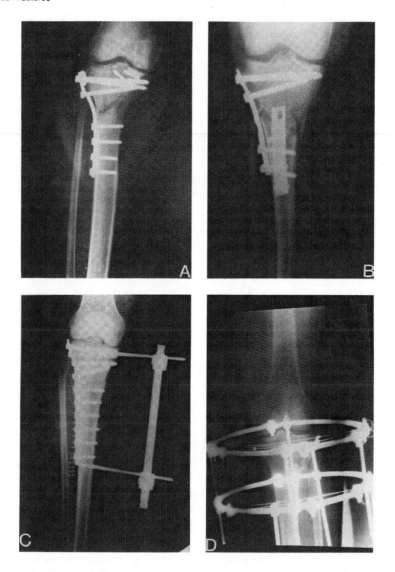

Figure 9–17. Clinical examples of internal fixation for type VI fractures. **A.** Single plate with supplemental interfragmentary screws. **B.** Double plating. **C.** Single plate with medial external fixation. **D.** Interfragmentary screw and small wire circular fixator, using olive wires for compression.

tended knee joint as the main indication for surgical treatment, found a 90% good to excellent result rate in 102 patients examined at a mean follow-up of 20 years.[20] Jennings treated 21 tibial plateau fractures with arthroscopic-assisted reduction.[23] Eighty-five percent had good results at 1 to 5 years of follow-up.

A retrospective review of 20 tibial plateau fractures treated with indirect reduction and percutaneous screw fixation at Tampa General Hospital was performed.[24] Fracture type was classified according to Schatzker: I (seven), II (eight), III (one), IV (two), V (two). Follow-up averaged 9.3 months (range, 6–18 months).

All fractures united by 12 weeks. In no case was settling of the articular surface noted. There were no infections. Overall, there were six excellent (33%), ten good (56%), and two fair (11%) results.

Conclusion

The goal in the treatment of any intraarticular fracture is to achieve a stable, aligned, and congruous joint, with a painless restoration of motion and function. Surgical reduction and stabilization mandate careful evaluation of both the fracture "personality" and its soft tissue envelope. There is no question that the timing of surgery as well as the handling of the soft tissue in this region is critical to successful treatment outcome. Following restoration of a congruous joint surface, bone grafting and buttress plating may be needed to allow early aggressive range of motion. By adhering to these principles, the physician can optimize the results in these fractures.

References

1. Hohl M, Larson RL, Jones DC. Fractures and dislocations about the knee. Part I: Fractures about the knee. In: Rockwood CA Jr, Green DP, eds. *Fractures in Adults.* Philadelphia: JB Lippincott; 1984:1429–1479.
2. Apley AG. Fractures of the lateral tibial condyle treated by skeletal traction and early mobilization. *J Bone Joint Surg Br.* 1956;38:699–708.
3. Porter BB. Crush fractures of the lateral tibial table. Factors influencing the prognosis. *J Bone Joint Surg Br.* 1970;52:676–687.
4. Roberts J. Fractures of the condyles of the tibia. *J Bone Joint Surg Am.* 1968;50:1505.
5. Newberg AH, Greenstein R. Radiographic evaluation of tibial plateau fractures. *Radiology.* 1978;126:319–323.
6. Schulak DJ, Gunn DR. Fractures of the tibial plateau. A review of the literature. *Clin Orthop.* 1975;109:166–177.
7. Courvoisier E. Les fractures des plateaux tibiaux. *Bern AO Bull.* 1973.
8. Rasmussen PS. Tibial condyle fractures. Impairment of knee joint stability as an indication for surgical treatment. *J Bone Joint Surg Am.* 1973;55:1331–1350.
9. Schatzker J. Fractures of the tibial plateau. In: Schatzker J, Tile M, eds. *The Rationale of Operative Orthopaedic Care.* Berlin/Heidelberg/New York: Springer-Verlag; 1988:279–295.
10. Schatzker J. Fractures of the tibial plateau. In: Chapman MW, ed. *Operative Orthopaedics.* Philadelphia: JB Lippincott; 1988:421–434.
11. Moore TM, Harvey P. Roentgenographic measurement of tibial-plateau depression due to fracture. *J Bone Joint Surg Am.* 1974;56:155–160.
12. Delamarter RB, Hohl M, Hopp E Jr. Ligament injuries associated with tibial plateau. *Clin Orthop.* 1990;250:226–233.
13. Martin AF. The pathomechanics of the knee joint. 1. The medial collateral ligament and lateral tibial plateau fractures. *J Bone Joint Surg Am.* 1960;42:13–22.
14. Elstrom J, Pankovich Am, Sassoon H, Rodriguez J. The use of tomography in the assessment of fractures of the tibial plateau. *J Bone Joint Surg Am.* 1976;58:551–555.
15. Schatzker J, McBroom R, Bruce D. The tibial plateau fracture. The Toronto experience 1968–1975. *Clin Orthop.* 1979;138:94–104.
16. Moore TM. Fracture-dislocations of the knee. *Clin Orthop.* 1981;156:128–140.
17. Burri C, Bartzke G, Coldewey J, Muggler E. Fractures of the tibial plateau. *Clin Orthop.* 1979;138:84–93.
18. Knight R. Treatment of fractures of the tibial condyles. *South Med J.* 1945;38:246.
19. Savoie FH, Vander Griend RA, Ward EF, Hughes JL. Tibial plateau fractures. A review of operative treatment using AO technique. *Orthopaedics.* 1987;10(5):745–750.
20. Lansinger O, Bergman B, Korner L, Andersson GBJ. Tibial condyle fractures. A twenty-year follow-up. *J Bone Joint Surg Am.* 1986;68:13–19.
21. Buchanan WJ, Lenihan M, Dossick P. Percutaneous reduction and stabilization of tibial plateau fractures: A new method of articular fracture management. Presented at the fifty-seventh annual meeting of the American Academy of Orthopaedic Surgeons, New Orleans, Louisiana, February 1990.
22. Caspari RB, Hullon PMJ, Whipple TL, Meyers JF. Arthroscopy in the management of tibial plateau fractures. *Arthroscopy.* 1985;1(2):76–82.
23. Jennings JE. Arthroscopic management of tibial plateau fractures. *Arthroscopy.* 1985;1(3):160–168.
24. Koval K, Borelli J, Sanders R, Dipasquale T, Helfet D. Indirect reduction and percutaneous screw fixation of displaced tibial plateau fractures. Presented at the sixth annual meeting of the Orthopaedic Trauma Association, Toronto, Ontario, November 1990.
25. Lemon RA, Bartlett DH. Arthroscopic assisted internal fixation of certain fractures about the knee. *J Trauma.* 1985;15(4):355–358.
26. Mast J, Jakob R, Ganz R. *Planning and Reduction Technique in Fracture Surgery.* Berlin/Heidelberg/New York: Springer-Verlag; 1989.
27. Anger LC, Saunders JB, Bost FC, Anderson CE. Etude critique du traitement des fractures articulaires de l'extremite superieure du tibia. *Rev Chir Orthop.* 1944;54:259.
28. Reibel D, Wade P. Fractures of the tibial plateau. *J Trauma.* 1962;2:337.
29. Perry CR, Evans LG, Rice S, Fogarty J, Burdge RE. A new surgical approach to fractures of the lateral tibial plateau. *J Bone Joint Surg Am.* 1984;66A:1236–1240.
30. Christensen KP, Powell JN, Bucholz RW, Sills M. Early results of a new technique for the treatment of high grade tibial plateau fractures. Presented at the fifth annual meeting of the Orthopaedic Trauma Association, Philadelphia, Pennsylvania, October 1989.
31. Salter RB, Dimonds DF, Malcolm BW, Rumble EJ, MacMichael D, Clements ND. The biological effect of continuous passive motion on the healing of full-thickness defects in articular cartilage. An experimental investigation in the rabbit. *J Bone Joint Surg Am.* 1980;62:1232.
32. Hallen LG, Lindhal O. The lateral stability of the knee-joint. *Acta Orthop.* 1965;36:179–191.
33. Hohl M. Tibial condyle fractures. *J Bone Joint Surg Am.* 1967;49:1455–1467.
34. Hohl M, Luck JV. Fractures of the tibial condyle. A clinical and experimental study. *J Bone Joint Surg Am.* 1956;38:1001–1018.
35. Foster E, Mole L, Coblenz J. Etude des lesions ligamentaires dans les fractures du plateau tibial. *Ned Tijdschr Geneesdk.* 1961;105:2175.

36. Solonen K. Fractures of the tibial condyles. *Acta Orthop Scand Suppl*. 1963: No. 63.
37. Indelicato PA. Non-operative treatment of complete tears of the medial collateral ligament of the knee. *J Bone Joint Surg Am*. 1983;65:323–329.
38. Walker PS, Erkman MJ. The role of menisci in force transmission across the knee. *Clin Orthop*. 1975;109:184.
39. Duwelius PJ, Connolly JF. Closed reduction of tibial plateau fractures. A comparison of functional and roentgenographic end results. *Clin Orthop*. 1988;230:116–126.

10

Arthroscopic Treatment of Fractures of the Proximal Tibia

Charles Carr

Introduction

Historically, methods of treating intraarticular fractures of the proximal tibia have been controversial. This chapter discusses the therapeutic options that arthroscopy provides for the treatment of plateau fractures and intercondylar eminence fractures of the proximal tibia.

Therapeutic options for treating tibial plateau fractures range from closed reduction and immobilization[1-3] to open arthrotomy with anatomic reduction and rigid internal fixation.[4-8] No one treatment appears to be superior, however, as most studies reported similar results with the various methods of treating plateau fractures of the proximal tibia. Numerous factors cause poor results in tibial plateau fractures. The instability caused by joint depression and/or ligamentous injury results in an axial malalignment of the limb.[4] This malalignment combined with joint incongruity[7] produces the morbidity seen following tibial plateau fractures, including decreased range of motion, pain, and posttraumatic osteoarthritis.

The best method to manage these difficult fractures is one that demands the least soft tissue dissection, permits the restoration of articular congruity, and uses adequate internal fixation to allow for early motion and subsequent recovery of function. Arthroscopically assisted management of selected fractures of the tibial plateau can achieve these goals.

There is controversy about the best treatment for the complete separation of the intercondylar eminence of the proximal tibia. This uncommon fracture, seen most frequently in children, has been the subject of many recent studies. Intercondylar eminence avulsions in children are considered to be the equivalent of anterior cruciate ligament (ACL) ruptures in adults[9] because the tibial spine serves as the attachment for the ACL.

Several studies have questioned the effectiveness of any treatment for displaced tibial spine fractures in children, as anatomic reduction does not always prevent laxity or loss of full knee extension.[9-12] It has been hypothesized that the ACL stretches prior to failing at its tibial attachment site.[11] Despite these studies, most authors still recommend the anatomic reduction of completely displaced anterior tibial spine fractures.[9,11-15] Because of the anterior tibial spine's intraarticular position, displaced fractures of this anatomic structure can be successfully evaluated and treated arthroscopically.[13,16]

Evaluation

As described in the previous chapter, routine anteroposterior (AP) and lateral knee x-rays will demonstrate a fracture in the proximal tibia but are not adequate for assessing the complexity of the bony injury.[17] Two oblique views and a 10° caudal plateau view provide an excellent initial evaluation of most fracture patterns.[2,4,17] The AP and lateral tomograms are a useful adjunctive radiographic study.[18] Plain radiographs and linear tomography, in addition, improve our ability to preoperatively classify these fractures correctly.[17,18] Three-dimensional computed tomography scan imaging may become the adjunctive study of choice for defining the extent of the osseous injury.

It is often difficult to evaluate the associated soft tissue injuries involving menisci and ligamentous structures with an acute injury. Generally, most patients require an examination under anesthesia to determine if there is any ligamentous injury. The AP instability associated with tibial eminence avulsions is easily detected, but the medial/lateral instability associated with plateau fractures makes it difficult to distinguish fracture instability from ligamentous injury. In these cases, the use of fluoroscopy, arthroscopy, and a physical examination under anesthesia can aid in the diagnosis.

Classification

Two classification systems have been widely used for tibial plateau fractures. The first system was described by Hohl in 1956 and was modified approximately a decade later.[7,8] The second system, described by Schatzker, is more widely accepted today.[4,5] The six fracture patterns in Schatzker's classification are described in detail in the previous chapter (Fig. 10–1).

Meyers and McKeever's classification of intercondylar eminence fractures is the most simple and useful system.[14,19] Their system divides these fractures into three main types. The type I fracture is minimally displaced with only a slight elevation of the anterior aspect of the intercondylar eminence. The type II fracture occurs when only the anterior third or half of the eminence is elevated, producing a beaklike appearance on the lateral roentgenogram. The type III fracture involves the complete separation of the tibial intercondylar eminence from its osseous bed. The type III fracture can be further subdivided into types IIIA and IIIB to delineate whether the displaced fragment is malrotated. Zaricznyj added type IIIC to describe displaced, comminuted fractures because it was the most common fracture pattern seen in his series (Fig. 10–2).[15]

Schatzker's classification scheme for plateau fractures and Meyers and McKeever's classification for eminence fractures will be referred to throughout the remainder of this chapter.

Principles of Treatment

Surgical Indications

Tibial Plateau Fractures. The indications for the surgical treatment of tibial plateau fractures are unclear. As acute pain limits the physical examination of plateau fractures for ligamentous or meniscal pathology, arthroscopy is an effective diagnostic and therapeutic method for evaluating these fractures. Arthroscopy has been advocated by several authors[20-26] as a means to assess the fracture and concomitant soft tissue injuries. Arthroscopic examination and treatment of tibial plateau fractures should be used when a patient has the following: borderline fractures that are difficult to define by roentgenographic examination,[21] fractures associated with ligamentous or meniscal pathology, and selected fractures that can be treated with arthroscopic reduction and percutaneous or limited open reduction techniques. Severely comminuted and displaced fractures requiring arthrotomy and open reduction should not be treated by arthroscopic methods.[20,21]

Tibial Intercondylar Eminence Fractures. The management of intercondylar eminence fractures of the tibia for nondisplaced (type I) and minimally displaced (type II) fractures is conservative.[13-15,19] The treatment of displaced (type III) fractures is, however, more controversial. Most authors recommend reduction by closed, open, or arthroscopic means to avoid malunion. If the fracture is allowed to heal with residual displacement, a mechanical block to full extension will ensue. This will result in a relative shortening of the ACL and

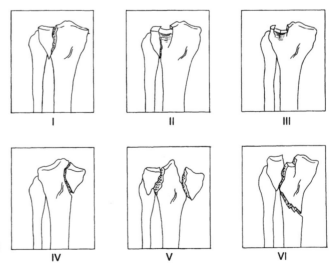

Figure 10–1. Schatzker's classification of tibial plateau fractures.[4]

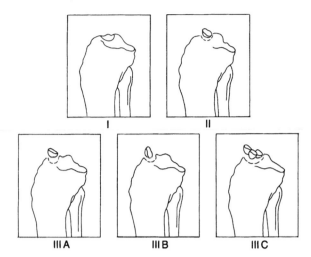

I   II

III A   III B   III C

Figure 10–2. Meyers and McKeever's classification of intercondylar eminence fractures[14] with Zaricznyj's modification.[15]

subsequent instability secondary to insufficiency of the ACL.[15] If the displaced eminence fragment cannot be adequately reduced by extension of the knee, then operative reduction of the fracture is recommended. Arthroscopic surgery provides an alternative to open arthrotomy as a treatment for these injuries. Arthroscopy can also be used to evaluate and treat associated meniscal pathology, which is seen in a large percentage of cases.[13,15,27]

Operative Technique

Tibial Plateau Fractures. The patient is placed in the supine position on a standard operative table with a tourniquet applied. Placing the limb in a thigh holder allows for varus and valgus manipulation. The end of the operating table is flexed so that the knee can be brought freely to at least 100° of flexion. The anterior iliac crest is prepared for possible cancellous bone graft. Fluoroscopy is used to aid the placement of the percutaneous screw fixation (Fig. 10–3).

The knee is examined under anesthesia to ascertain the integrity of the ligamentous structures. An inflow cannula is placed into the suprapatellar pouch. Gravity insufflation is used to irrigate out the hemarthrosis and intraarticular debris. An infusion pump can be used but is not recommended because of the risk of compartment syndrome from fluid extravasation through the fracture

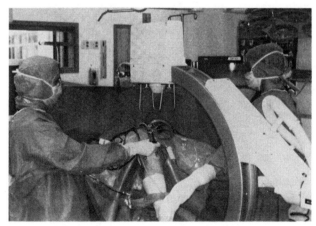

Figure 10–3. Operating room setup.

and into the calf. Although this complication has not been reported, it remains a possibility. The arthroscopic cannula is introduced in the anteromedial or anterolateral portal opposite the fractured compartment. Once a clear field of vision is established using continuous saline inflow and suction outflow, all the compartments of the knee can be surveyed. As maintaining a clear field of vision can often be difficult because of bleeding from the cancellous surfaces, suction and irrigation must be used intermittently. A hook probe is inserted through an anterior portal on the same side as the fracture. While examining the knee compartments, it is important to look for associated injuries. The menisci, collateral ligaments, cruciate ligaments, and articular surfaces are palpated carefully with the calibrated probe. Any necessary repairs of associated peripheral meniscal tears or ligamentous tears are done after the tibial plateau fracture has been reduced and stabilized. Subsequent reduction and fixation techniques are determined by the specific fracture pattern.

Split or Wedge Plateau Fractures (Schatzker Types I, IV, and V)

A simple split fracture, either medial or lateral, with no associated depression, is the fracture type most easily repaired by arthroscopic techniques. Once any small bone fragment or entrapped meniscus is removed from the fracture site, then the split fragment can be arthroscopically reduced.

Several methods can be used to achieve reduction of a split fracture. One method is to manipulate a fragment with manual pressure while simultaneously using a probe or curette intraarticularly. Another method is to place a smooth pin into the fragment percutaneously to use as a "joystick" to manipulate the fragment while viewing arthroscopically (Fig. 10–4). A third method is to use an intraarticular bone hook placed from an anterior portal opposite the fracture (Fig. 10–5). The hook is placed over the rim of the affected plateau and the split fracture fragment and is used to lever the fragment into position. Once reduction is achieved, one or two cannulated 6.5- or 7.0-mm screws, with or without a washer, are placed across the fracture in a subchondral position and parallel to the joint surface (Fig. 10–6). Fluoroscopy is used to help place these screws, as it is difficult to determine the appropriate level of insertion with arthroscopy. Bone grafting is not required in the pure split or wedge fracture types (Fig. 10–7).

Split Depression or Central Depression Plateau Fractures (Schatzker Types II and III)

Lateral tibial plateau fractures with articular depression are treated by reducing the lateral rim fragments and elevating the central depression. It is more difficult to perform arthroscopic reduction and fixation on these

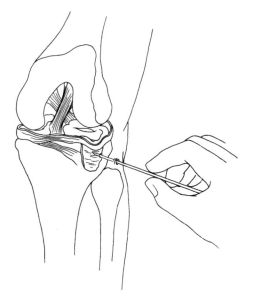

Figure 10–4. Manipulation of a fracture fragment percutaneously with a K-wire "joystick." (Adapted with permission from *Technique for Arthroscopic Fracture Management System*. Mansfield, MA: Acufex Microsurgical, Inc; 1991.)

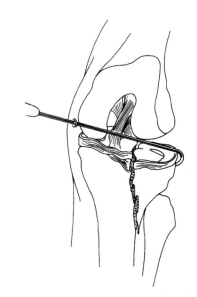

Figure 10–5. Intraarticular hook to aid the reduction of a split fracture fragment. (Adapted with permission from *Technique for Arthroscopic Fracture Management System*. Mansfield, MA: Acufex Microsurgical, Inc; 1991.)

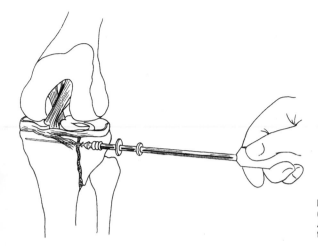

Figure 10-6. Cannulated screw placement. (Adapted with permission from *Technique for Arthroscopic Fracture Management System*. Mansfield, MA: Acufex Microsurgical, Inc; 1991.)

fracture types than on the split fracture patterns. Thus, if a surgeon chooses to treat a depressed plateau fracture arthroscopically, he or she should be quite skilled in both fracture management and arthroscopy. When greater than 3 mm of depression is seen arthroscopically, then the depressed segment should be elevated from below. Inserting an intraarticular guide through the standard anterior working portal on the side of the fracture is the first step to achieving articular reduction. This guide can be any standard ACL tibial tunnel guide that allows for placement of a guide pin for various cannulated drills. Inserted below the flare of the tibia, the guide pin exits intraarticularly at the posterior aspect of the depression (Fig. 10-8). Drilling over the guide pin with an 8- or 9-mm cannulated drill up to the fragment creates a window below the fragment (Fig. 10-9). Fluoroscopy can help place the guide pin and determine the proper depth to drill with the cannulated drill. Various instruments can be used to elevate the depressed segment. Cannulated tamps can be fitted directly over the guide pin or a simple noncannulated bone tamp or curette can be used to aid in reduction through the predrilled hole (Fig. 10-10). It is useful to overelevate the fragments and to allow the femoral condyle to mold the adjacent tibial plateau.[24] Once the fragments are reduced, a cancellous bone graft taken from the iliac crest is placed under the fracture through the window to support the tibial plateau. Internal fixation with at least two cannulated screws in a subchondral position is needed to support the elevated fragment. Several authors believe that a buttress plate is necessary for adequate fixation of a split depression fracture and that subchondral screws alone provide insufficient fixation.[4-6]

Meniscal tears are excised or repaired arthroscopical-ly and ligamentous tears are repaired through open incisions at the surgeon's discretion.

Tibial Intercondylar Eminence Fractures.   Types I and II tibial eminence fractures, as described by Meyers and McKeever,[14,19] are successfully treated by closed methods. A long leg cast applied with the knee in a comfortable, slightly flexed position is adequate. Immobilization should continue for approximately 8 to 10 weeks until there is roentgenographic evidence of bone healing.

Most surgeons agree that the reduction of displaced type III intercondylar eminence fractures should be performed. The setup for arthroscopic evaluation and treatment of these fractures is the same as for tibial plateau fractures. The patient is placed supine on a standard operating table with the thigh supported in a leg holder. The end of the operating table is folded down to provide room for the knee to flex without restriction. A tourniquet is used, and fluoroscopy should be available to assist in the placement of fixation devices.

The knee is examined for associated ligamentous injuries and these are repaired or treated nonoperatively, according to the surgeon's preference. Recently, the author has not been openly repairing medial collateral ligament tears in isolation[28] or in combined injuries undergoing ACL reconstruction or anterior tibial spine reattachment. Inflow is established through the suprapatellar pouch, and gravity irrigation washes out blood and intraarticular debris through a cannula introduced anterolaterally. With the knee flexed 90°, a curved curette or a hook probe is introduced through an anterolateral portal. The fracture site is visualized arthroscopically and fibrous tissue and small osteochondral

Charles Carr

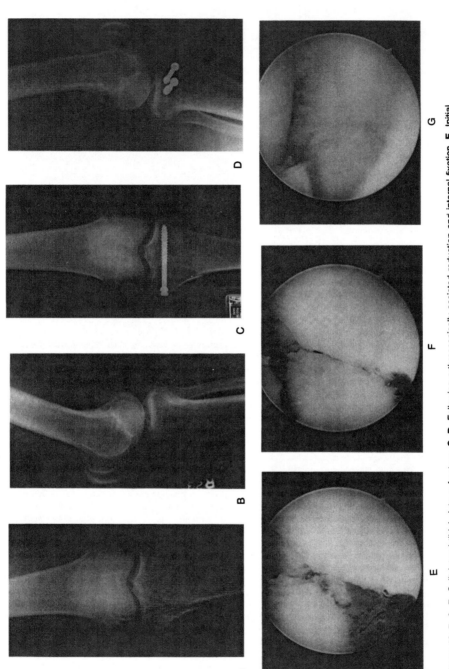

Figure 10–7. A, B. Split lateral tibial plateau fracture. **C, D.** Following arthroscopically assisted reduction and internal fixation. **E.** Initial displacement seen arthroscopically. **F.** Following arthroscopically assisted reduction. **G.** After reduction and compression with 7.0-mm cannulated screws.

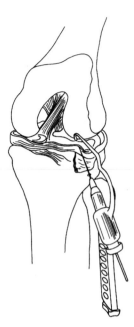

Figure 10–8. Intraarticular guide for pin placement to be used with a cannulated drill. (Adapted with permission from *Technique for Arthroscopic Fracture Management System.* Mansfield, MA: Acufex Microsurgical, Inc; 1991.)

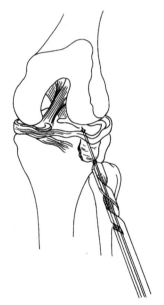

Figure 10–9. Window created with cannulated drill beneath depressed fragment. (Adapted with permission from *Technique for Arthroscopic Fracture Management System.* Mansfield, MA: Acufex Microsurgical, Inc; 1991.)

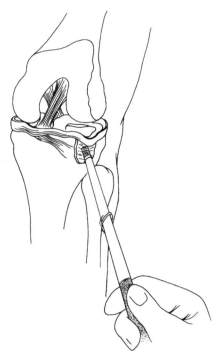

Figure 10–10. Tamp used through window to elevate depressed fragment. (Adapted with permission from *Technique for Arthroscopic Fracture Management System.* Mansfield, MA: Acufex Microsurgical, Inc; 1991.)

fragments are removed. The fracture is reduced by depressing the fragment back into its bed. The knee is extended and the reduction verified by arthroscopy, lateral fluoroscopy, and/or radiography. If the reduction is satisfactory and can be maintained in extension, then a long leg cylinder cast is applied for 4 weeks. The patient is immobilized for 4 weeks in full extension and is then placed in a cast with 20° of flexion for 4 additional weeks.

If the fragment cannot be held reduced in an extended position, then fixation of the fracture is required. Two methods can be used to maintain reduction. McLennan describes the use of smooth Kirschner wires (K-wires) introduced retrograde from proximal to the tibial tuberosity into the reduced fragment.[13] The K-wires are placed percutaneously in a crossed fashion proximal to the tibial tuberosity and on each side of the patellar tendon (Fig. 10–11). Arthroscopy and fluoroscopy are used to verify that the wires are placed correctly. All the wires are withdrawn until they are just beneath the articular surface of the fragment. Cannulated screws are more aesthetic than K-wires but we have found that the spine fragments are so small that it is difficult to get adequate fixation with a screw.

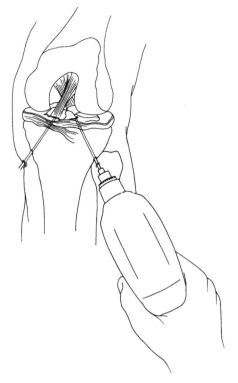

Postoperative Management

Tibial Plateau Fractures

Postoperatively, patients are placed into a hinged knee brace. Allowable motion in the brace is determined by the fracture pattern and the adequacy of fixation. Ideally, a patient should be placed on a continuous passive motion (CPM) machine immediately after surgery. Early motion has been shown by Salter to clearly enhance cartilage healing[29] and may also help mold plateau fragments that are not ideally fixed, as seen with comminuted fractures. The CPM machine is progressed from 30° of flexion to 80° or 90° of flexion before it is discontinued. Physical therapy is started on the first postoperative day for active assisted range of motion and non-weight-bearing crutch training. The patient is not allowed to fully support his or her weight on the knee until 3 months postoperatively.

Tibial Intercondylar Eminence Fractures

Patients treated for tibial intercondylar eminence fractures should also have their postoperative management tailored to the injury and the type of fixation used. Patients are treated differently if crossed wires are used for fixation rather than a wire loop. If crossed wires are used, as described by McLennan,[13] the knee is placed in

Figure 10-11. Placement of crossed K-wires for fixation of type III intercondylar eminence fractures.

Another method of fixation employs a loop of suture or wire to maintain reduction (Mayor, personal communication, 1992). Again, a reduction is achieved by depressing the fragment with a hook probe or curette. Two small-diameter drill bits with "eyes" at the end are passed retrograde from proximal to the tibial tuberosity to the medial and lateral margins of the eminence fracture. A tibial guide used for ACL surgery can assist in proper orientation and placement of the eyed drill bits or K-wires. A 20-gauge wire, or a No. 5 nonabsorbable suture, is passed through the anteromedial portal with an arthroscopic forceps instrument. The wire or suture is passed through one eye, around or through the base of the ACL attachment site, and through the eye of the second drill bit. The drill bits are pulled antegrade with the attached wire or suture out the anterior tibia and are tied snugly over the anterior tibial cortex (Figs. 10-12 and 10-13). Subsequent removal of the wire or suture is unnecessary in adults but is recommended if the physeal plate is violated in a growing child.

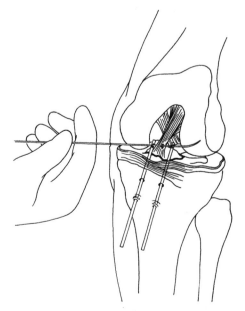

Figure 10-12. Loop technique for fixation of intercondylar eminence fractures.

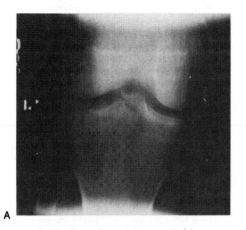

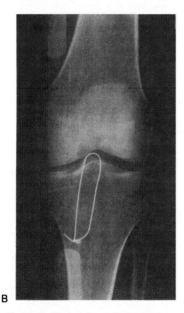

Figure 10-13. A. Displaced type III tibial intercondylar eminence fracture. **B.** After arthroscopically assisted reduction and fixation with a 20-gauge wire loop.

a locked hinged brace or in a cast at 20° to 30° of flexion for 6 weeks. Because the K-wires may pull out, motion is not allowed during the initial phase. The patient is encouraged to perform isometric quadriceps exercises and straight leg raising soon after surgery. At 6 to 8 weeks postoperatively, the pins are removed and physical therapy is begun, including active assisted

range of motion and passive stretching. The loop technique allows motion to begin earlier. As pullout strength is not as great a concern, the patient can be placed into a hinged knee brace with range of motion from 0° to 60°. At 4 to 6 weeks, the brace is unlocked completely and further active and active assisted range of motion exercise continues. The brace is removed at 8 weeks and further passive stretching and active exercises are continued.

Because these postoperative regimens are based on isolated injuries, they must be modified if concomitant ligamentous or meniscal repairs are performed.

Complications and Pitfalls

The immediate postoperative complications of skin slough and infection are decreased when plateau fractures are treated arthroscopically rather than with open management; however, the long-term sequelae can be made worse if these methods are used in inappropriate situations. Arthroscopic management of these difficult fractures has its limitations and complications will arise when attempts are made to arthroscopically treat fractures that cannot realistically be managed by arthroscopic techniques. Simple split and locally depressed tibial plateau fractures, as well as minimally displaced anterior tibial spine fractures, are excellent choices for arthroscopic treatment. Complex fractures, split depression-type plateau fractures, rim compression fractures, and fractures occurring in osteopenic bone usually require buttress plate fixation; the use of percutaneous, cannulated screws alone through limited incisions will invariably result in loss of fixation for most of these fracture patterns.

The shortcomings of arthroscopic treatment of tibial plateau fractures have been discussed.[30] The arthroscopic reduction of severely depressed and incarcerated fragments is limited. Rim fragments are not only difficult to visualize arthroscopically because of their position beneath the meniscus, but they require buttress plating for adequate fixation. Bone grafting is often recommended under reduced, depressed fragments to prevent settling and the arthroscopic placement of bone graft is limited by the position of the blind tunnel created beneath those depressed fragments.

The arthroscopic fixation of tibial eminence fractures creates similar concerns. If an adequate reduction cannot be obtained by arthroscopic manipulation, then a surgeon should open the fracture and treat it more conventionally. Recent papers have suggested that the reduction and fixation of displaced tibial eminence fracture are unnecessary because results are not improved[9-12]; however, many believe that reduction should be achieved if possible.[13-15] There have been no reports of growth plate or apophyseal arrest, but the author recommends that fixation devices be removed 2 to 3 months postoperatively if they cross the physis in a growing child.

Compartment syndromes from fluid extravasation have not been identified as a problem and no infections related to the arthroscopic surgery have been reported in any series to date. Peroneal neuropraxias have been reported[24] and this author has experienced a case of postoperative arthrofibrosis requiring manipulation under anesthesia to regain motion. The long-term complications of posttraumatic arthrosis are not yet known but the rate of occurrence will ultimately determine the usefulness of arthroscopy in managing these fractures.

Results

There are few reported outcomes following the use of arthroscopically assisted internal fixation of tibial plateau and eminence fractures. Jennings treated 21 tibial plateau fractures by arthroscopically assisted reduction using both internal and external fixation techniques. Forty-three percent of the fractures treated in his series were Schatzker type II and Jennings reported an overall success rate of 85% at 1 to 5 years follow-up.[22] Caspari et al reported on 20 tibial plateau fractures examined arthroscopically; 15 of these fractures were treated by arthroscopically assisted reduction techniques. Specific results are not reported in this series but the authors felt that arthroscopy helped to precisely define the fracture and the associated soft tissue injuries. They also stated that *selected* fractures could be effectively reduced and stabilized with arthroscopic methods.[24] Carr also described the use of a similar technique in nine cases, of which 33% were Schatzker type II fractures.[20] He achieved a success rate of 90%. Reiner promotes the use of diagnostic arthroscopy in the initial evaluation of selected tibial plateau fractures,[21] and Lemon and Bartlett describe the successful use of arthroscopic fixation techniques in single-fragment, major intraarticular fractures about the knee.[25]

There are even fewer reports on the use of arthroscopy to assist the reduction and fixation of tibial eminence fractures. McLennan reports the only major series on his method of arthroscopic reduction and crossed percutaneous pin fixation.[13] Thirty-five patients were treated for type III displaced avulsion fractures of the tibial spine. Thirty-three patients required arthroscopic reduction and 33% of those patients required the use of percutaneous pins to maintain the reduction. The majority (70%) of eminence fractures were maintained in a reduced position solely by extending the knee. Forty percent of the patients had an associated lateral meniscal tear. McLennan's results showed residual anterior instability in 14% and incomplete extension in 17%.[13] No series has yet reported on the loop technique of fixation of tibial eminence fractures.

Conclusion

Defining the extent of bony and soft tissue injury in fractures of the proximal tibia is a common problem for surgeons. The extent of the injury is often underestimated and arthroscopy can often help with choosing the appropriate course of treatment. Some fracture patterns can be easily treated by arthroscopically assisted methods; however, inappropriate use of these minimally invasive techniques can lead to poor results. Comparison of long-term follow-up results of arthroscopic fracture management about the knee with open techniques is needed before its use can be unconditionally supported.

References

1. Brown GA, Sprague BL. Cast brace treatment of plateau and bicondylar fractures of the proximal tibia. *Clin Orthop.* 1976;119:184–193.
2. Apley AG. Fractures of the lateral tibial condyle treated by skeletal traction and early mobilization. *J Bone Joint Surg Br.* 1956;38:699–707.
3. Drennan DB, Locher FG, Maylahn DJ. Fractures of the tibial plateau. Treatment by closed reduction and spica cast. *J Bone Joint Surg Am.* 1979;61:989–995.
4. Schatzker J. Fractures of the tibial plateau. In: Schatzker J, Tile M, eds. *The Rationale of Operative Orthopaedic Care.* New York: Springer-Verlag; 1988:279–295.
5. Schatzker J, McBroom R. The tibial plateau fracture. The Toronto experience 1968–1975. *Clin Orthop.* 1979;138:94–104.
6. Perry CR, Evans LG, Rice S, et al. A new surgical approach to fractures of the lateral tibial plateau. *J Bone Joint Surg Am.* 1984;66:1236–1240.
7. Hohl M, Luck JV. Fractures of the tibial condyle. A clinical and experimental study. *J Bone Joint Surg Am.* 1956;38:1001–1018.
8. Hohl M. Tibial condylar fractures. *J Bone Joint Surg Am.* 1967;49:1455–1467.
9. Gronkvist H, Hirsch G, Johansson L. Fracture of the anterior tibial spine in children. *J Pediatr Orthop.* 1984;4(4):465–468.
10. Baxter MP, Wiley JJ. Fractures of the tibial spine in children. An evaluation of knee stability. *J Bone Joint Surg Br.* 1988;70:228–230.
11. Smith JB. Knee instability after fractures of the intercondylar eminence of the tibia. *J Pediatr Orthop.* 1984;4(4):462–464.
12. Wiley JJ, Baxter MP. Tibial spine fractures in children. *Clin Orthop.* 1990;255:54–60.
13. McLennan JG. The role of arthroscopic surgery in the treatment of fractures of the intercondylar eminence of the tibia. *J Bone Joint Surg Br.* 1982;64:477–480.
14. Meyers MH, McKeever FM. Fracture of the intercondylar eminence of the tibia. *J Bone Joint Surg Am.* 1959;41:209–222.
15. Zaricznyj B. Avulsion fracture of the tibial eminence: Treatment by open reduction and pinning. *J Bone Joint Surg Am.* 1977;59:1111–1114.
16. Lars E, Hertel P, Goudarzi AM. Arthroscopic management of dislocated ruptures of the intercondylar eminence on children and adolescents. *Unfallchirurgie (Munchen).* 1987;90(10):471–477.

17. Newberg AH, Greenstein R. Radiographic evaluation of tibial plateau fractures. *Radiology.* 1978;126:319–323.
18. Elstrom J, Pankovich AM, Sassoon H, et al. The use of tomography in the assessment of fractures of the tibial plateau. *J Bone Joint Surg Am.* 1976;58:551–555.
19. Meyers MH, McKeever FM. Fracture of the intercondylar eminence of the tibia. *J Bone Joint Surg Am.* 1970;52:1677–1684.
20. Carr DE. Arthroscopically assisted stabilization of tibial plateau fractures. *Techniques Orthop.* 1991;6(2):55–57.
21. Reiner MJ. The arthroscope in tibial plateau fractures: Its use in evaluation of soft tissue and bony injury. *J Am Osteopath Assoc.* 1982;81:704–707.
22. Jennings JE. Arthroscopic management of tibial plateau fractures. *Arthroscopy.* 1985;1(3):160–168.
23. Caspari RB. The techniques for arthroscopic management of tibial plateau fractures. *Arthroscopic Surg Update.* 1985;5:113–119.
24. Caspari RB, Hutton PMJ, Whipple TL, et al. The role of arthroscopy in the management of tibial plateau fractures. *Arthroscopy.* 1985;1(2):76–82.
25. Lemon RA, Bartlett DH. Arthroscopic-assisted internal fixation of certain fractures about the knee. *J Trauma.* 1985;25(4):355–358.
26. Vierhout PAM, Smulders BHN, Hohmann FR, et al. Reconstruction of the tibial plateau fracture under arthroscopic control without arthrotomy. *Ned Tijydschr Geneeskd.* 1991;135(20):893–896.
27. Clanton TO, DeLee JC, Sanders B, et al. Knee ligament injuries in children. *J Bone Joint Surg Am.* 1979;61:1195–1201.
28. Indelicato PA. Nonoperative treatment of complete tears of the medial collateral ligament of the knee. *J Bone Joint Surg Am.* 1983;65:323–329.
29. Salter RB, Dimonds DF, Malcolm BW, et al. The biological effect of continuous passive motion on the healing of full-thickness defects in articular cartilage. An experimental investigation in the rabbit. *J Bone Joint Surg Am.* 1980;62:1232.
30. Pankovich AM. Letters to the editor. *Arthroscopy.* 1986;2(2):132–134.

Part 3
Extensor Mechanism Injuries

11
Fractures of the Patella

David W. Lhowe

Introduction

Fractures of the patella constitute approximately 1% of adult fractures seen acutely and are relatively rarer in children.[1] Although the role of the patella in augmenting extensor force is now well understood, it was not always so. A little over 50 years ago, the patella was felt to be largely vestigial, and efforts to repair it futile. As an example of a poorly designed but widely influential study, Brooke's 1937 report (with a supporting review by Hey-Groves) is worth reading.[2]

The present approach to patellar fractures aims to anatomically restore articular congruity and extensor continuity with sufficient stability to permit early knee motion and weight bearing. Where complete repair of the patella is not possible, salvage of a functional patella may sometimes be possible with a partial patellectomy. In those rarer cases where no significant portion of the patella can be reasonably reconstructed, total patellectomy is undertaken with the understanding that the resulting extensor weakness is preferable to extensor weakness *plus* debilitating patellofemoral pain.

Functional Anatomy

The patella lies in continuity with the extensor mechanism. It is therefore subject to the tensile forces of quadriceps contraction as well as the compressive forces of direct blunt trauma. Lateral patellar dislocations can produce shear forces, fracturing cartilaginous or osteocartilaginous fragments from the patella.

The quadriceps and patellar tendons insert more anteriorly than posteriorly on the patellar poles, a fact that must be kept in mind when partial patellectomy and tendon advancement are performed. The extensor retinaculum adjacent to the patella shares in the transmission of extensor force, and this explains how a minimally displaced patellar fracture may retain sufficient stability to permit straight-leg raising. Retinacular repair performed at the time of fracture fixation can impart significant immediate stability to the construct.

The mechanical function of the patella is to increase the moment of the extensor force. It does so incrementally, with the moment increasing as the knee moves toward full extension.[3,4] This effect counteracts the loss of contractile force that occurs as the quadriceps shortens during extension, and helps to maintain a more constant torque through the full range of knee extension.

Patellofemoral contact varies with flexion of the knee, but the distal pole of the patella does not articulate with the femur. All parts of the articular surface of the patella *do* contact the trochlea at some point during knee motion[5] (Fig. 11–1).

Evaluation

Soft Tissue

As most patellar fractures result from direct compressive force, the overlying skin and subcutaneous tissue are often contused. In high-energy injuries or where no layer of clothing is present, significant abrasions can further compromise the skin. Blood supply may be impaired as a result of soft tissue swelling and further reduced in the presence of a large hemarthrosis producing pressure from below. If surgery is contemplated, the timing and placement of the incision should respect soft tissue integrity.

Extensor Mechanism

Wide displacement of fracture fragments usually denotes disruption of the extensor retinaculum as well as the patella itself. In cases of minimal displacement

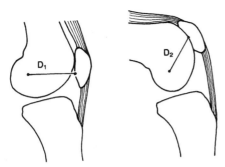

Figure 11-1. Schematic depiction of the changing extensor moment arm during flexion. The moment arm in full extension (D_1) is greater than the moment arm at 90° of knee flexion (D_2). Because the contraction force of the quadriceps is less at full extension than at 90° of flexion, this variation in the moment arm helps maintain a more constant torque throughout the full range of knee extension.

being considered for nonoperative treatment, continuity of the extensor mechanism should be confirmed by asking the patient to perform a straight-leg raise. If the maneuver is too painful, assisted straight-leg raising with progressive removal of support will be more easily tolerated. Inability to initiate or maintain extension implies a disrupted extensor retinaculum. If a determination of retinacular integrity is critical to the therapeutic plan, the knee may be aspirated and simultaneously injected with lidocaine to more effectively test for straight-leg raising.

Associated Injuries

Although unusual, the patellar fracture may not be the only locus of extensor mechanism disruption. Palpation for obvious defects in the quadriceps muscle or infrapatellar tendon should be routinely performed. Gross instability of the knee in the setting of a patellar fracture should suggest that knee dislocation occurred at the time of fracture, even though the knee appears well reduced on x-ray. If the patellar fracture occurred from a dashboard impact, the axial force may have also caused fracture of the proximal femur or acetabulum, possibly including dislocation of the hip joint.

Radiographic Imaging

Standard anteroposterior (AP) and lateral radiographs are sufficient for evaluation of the vast majority of patellar fractures (Fig. 11-2). Where a vertical fracture line is suspected from the routine views, a skyline view may demonstrate the fracture more conclusively (Fig. 11-3). Bipartite patellae may present confusion, but the usual location of the accessory ossicle is superolateral

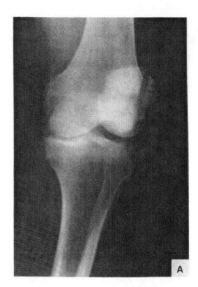

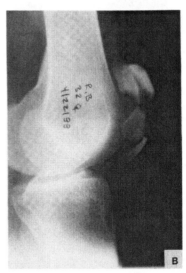

Figure 11-2. Standard anteroposterior (**A**) and lateral (**B**) views are sufficient to image the majority of patellar fractures. Given the presence of the distal femur on the anteroposterior view, x-rays will tend to underestimate the amount of comminution present.

and the condition is typically bilateral (Fig. 11-4). Comparison views of the opposite knee are helpful in such cases. The lateral view should be assessed for evidence of patella alta or baja as well as avulsions from

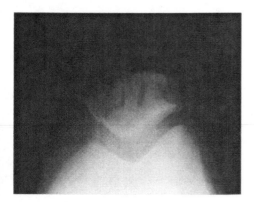

Figure 11–3. A skyline view may help image vertical fracture lines more clearly, although it may be difficult to obtain because of patient discomfort.

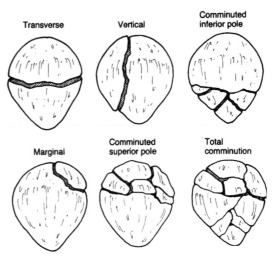

Figure 11–5. Some typical fracture pattern variants. With increasing amounts of energy absorbed, the likelihood of articular surface injury increases, above and beyond the bony injury seen on the anterior surface.

the tibial tubercle. Where patellar position appears abnormal, comparison views of the opposite extremity can clarify its significance. In cases where no fractures are demonstrated on plain films, tomograms may disclose a fracture more clearly[6] and are a justifiable expenditure if the information derived will alter treatment. Computed tomography and magnetic resonance imaging have little role in evaluating these injuries.

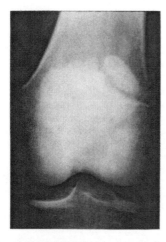

Figure 11–4. Bipartite patellae can be differentiated from acute fractures by the superolateral location of the accessory ossicle and the finding that the margins about the ossicle are typically smooth rather than sharp.

Fracture Patterns

Nondisplaced Fractures

As a general rule, 3 mm of separation and 2 mm of anteroposterior "stepoff" are the upper limits for a nondisplaced fracture definition. These limits are attributed to Boström[7] and are derived from a large retrospective study in which residual displacement of fracture fragments was compared with later function. Small marginal avulsions (not including pole fractures) do not require such rigid standards and may be considered nondisplaced for purposes of treatment planning. Nondisplaced fracture patterns include transverse, proximal/distal pole, vertical, and comminuted variants. The last category includes transverse or polar fractures in which one fragment remains intact and the other exhibits comminution.

Displaced Fractures

Using the 3-mm separation/2-mm stepoff criterion, displaced fractures may be transverse, polar, or comminuted. A purely vertical displaced fracture is quite unusual. Within this group, the transverse pattern is most common (Fig. 11–5).

Recommended Treatment

Nondisplaced Fractures

Nondisplaced fractures with an intact extensor retinaculum are best treated nonoperatively. Compliant patients may be treated in a knee immobilizer or hinged knee brace that is held in full extension for weight bearing but progressively loosened to allow range-of-motion exercises to advance during the 6 weeks of use. Straight-leg raises and isometric quadriceps contractions are begun immediately, followed by active flexion and passive or active-assisted extension exercises. Noncompliant patients may be immobilized with the knee in 10° of flexion in a long leg fiberglass cast for 4 to 6 weeks, weight bearing as tolerated, performing quadriceps contractions and straight-leg raises during the interval.

Displaced Fractures

All displaced fractures of the patella should be considered for operative repair, most often open reduction and internal fixation. Where appropriate, partial and even total patellectomy may be preferable to a doomed internal fixation. Although preoperative planning is always a valuable exercise and helps anticipate the surgical procedure, it is possible that the operative findings will dictate a modification of the preoperative plan as the true extent of comminution, degree of osteopenia, or presence of chondral injuries become more apparent. A worthwhile preoperative plan should include options for such contingencies, so that the plan can be modified should the surgical findings warrant.

For example, based on the radiographic appearance of his fracture and physical examination of his soft tissues, an elderly patient with a moderately comminuted distal pole fracture is appropriately planned for open reduction/internal fixation using a modified tension band. At surgery, however, his lower pole is found to be more comminuted than predicted by his radiographs. In addition, his bone quality is more osteopenic than anticipated. This additional information might cause an alteration of the surgical plan from open reduction/internal fixation to partial patellectomy with excision of the distal pole and advancement of the patellar tendon. If the preoperative plan is developed in this manner, it will anticipate technical problems but allow for appropriate modifications during the procedure in light of the operative findings.

Open Fractures

Open fractures are obvious surgical emergencies and require immediate debridement and stable internal fixation or patellectomy. As for all open fractures, excision of devitalized tissue, avoidance of additional trauma to soft tissues, and articular surface restoration are the applicable principles. As these fractures are usually the result of high-energy trauma, the resulting fracture patterns are typically very comminuted, are widely displaced, and may be more appropriately treated with partial or complete excision of the patella, rather than an unsatisfactory effort at internal fixation.

Incision

Although a transverse incision theoretically approximates the line of fracture and retinacular disruption in many cases, a longitudinal midline incision is preferable for several reasons. First, because the most commonly used forms of internal fixation require access to the proximal and distal patellar poles, a transverse incision will require flaps at least as large as those in a longitudinal approach. Second, a longitudinal incision is easily used for later reconstructive surgery. Third, a longitudinal approach is completely extensile without endangering cutaneous nerves and is not subjected to as much distraction when range of motion is begun in the face of postoperative swelling. The incision should avoid contused, abraded, or contaminated skin where present. Full-thickness skin and subcutaneous flaps are developed medially and laterally, sufficient to provide access to the medial and lateral apices of the retinacular tear. The fracture is inspected and carefully debrided of organized hematoma and any devitalized periosteum or free bony/cartilaginous fragments. The knee is then irrigated and the articular surfaces of the patella and femur are inspected through either the fracture or retinacular tear. Palpation and visual inspection will help determine the extent of articular surface injury. At this point, the fracture is reevaluated relative to the preoperative plan. Can the planned reconstruction be reliably obtained or must the surgical plan be altered in light of the operative findings?

Fixation of the Fracture

In recent biomechanical studies[8,9] of various fixation constructs, no method was found to produce absolute rigidity in cadaveric specimens. The method found most reliably stable to distraction forces was the modified tension band, as developed by the AO (Fig. 11–6).

Modified Tension Band

The modified tension-band method of fixation relies on an anteriorly placed tension band of 18-gauge wire that is anchored by longitudinally directed Kirschner wires that provide alignment of the fracture in the coronal and sagittal planes.[10] The technique is illustrated in Fig. 11–7.

Predrilling of the Kirschner wires in dense bone is helpful but not always necessary in osteopenic bone. Retrograde placement in the proximal fragment is followed by reduction of the fracture, which is then stabilized with an appropriate bone reduction forceps. Purchase of the forceps on the patella can be improved by making a small drill hole in each fragment to accommodate the points of the forceps. Reduction is next assessed by inspection of the anterior cortical fracture line. In cases of comminution or severe osteopenia, this

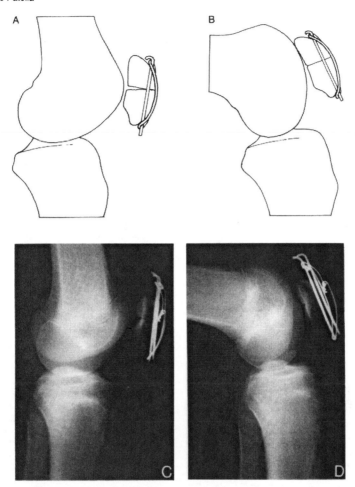

Figure 11-6. A line drawing of an anterior tension band shows application of the tension-band wire anteriorly with the knee in extension (**A**). As the knee moves into flexion, the patella is pulled against the trochlea, and the anterior tension band neutralizes the forces that would otherwise distract the fracture. The result is a compressive rather than distractive force across the fracture line (**B**). Lateral radiographs in extension (C) and flexion (D) show the effect of these forces on a transverse patellar fracture.

may not adequately represent the articular surface alignment. Palpation of the articular surface through the retinacular tear will confirm the adequacy of the reduction. The surgeon should not hesitate to enlarge the retinacular tear somewhat, if the reduction is difficult to assess by palpation. With the reduction confirmed, the knee is flexed and a Kirschner wire is driven antegrade, across the fracture and out the distal pole of the patella. If the wire is kept parallel to the long axis of the patella, in the anterior portion of the bone, its distal tip can be kept accessible for placement of the anterior tension

band. Next, an 18-gauge wire is passed posterior to the Kirschner wire ends and a loop is created directly opposite the twisted ends of the wire. The loop and twisted ends are tightened simultaneously with the fracture under direct vision until compression is seen across the fracture site.

At this time, AP and lateral radiographs are obtained to assess the reduction and hardware placement. If satisfactory, the knee is passively flexed to 90° under direct vision, observing for any distraction of the fracture. Further tightening of the tension band wire may

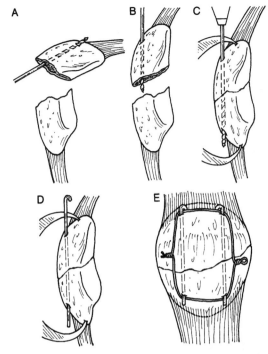

Figure 11–7. Technique of modified tension-band fixation as developed by the AO. **A.** The fracture is distracted sufficiently to permit retrograde drilling of the proximal fragment. The path of the drill should reside well anterior to the middle of the patella. **B.** The drill is then withdrawn and reinserted in an antegrade direction, advancing the tip until it is just visible at the fracture surface of the proximal fragment. **C.** Next, the fracture is reduced and held in place with appropriate bone reduction forceps and the drill is advanced into the distal fragment, exiting alongside the insertion of the patellar tendon. **D.** The drill bit is then withdrawn and a Kirschner wire (0.062 in.) is replaced in the drill tract. Note that steps A to D are all performed with two wires simultaneously. **E.** An 18-gauge wire is then passed behind both ends of each wire and tightened simultaneously on the medial and lateral sides. After sufficient tightening, the excess wire is trimmed and bent posteriorly. The Kirschner wires are bent posteriorly over the 18-gauge wire proximally and left unbent distally. They are then trimmed to an appropriate length. Where the bone is not extremely dense, it may be possible to drive the individual Kirschner wires directly through bone without predrilling. The ability to control the path of the Kirschner wire in this case is less certain, and the wire may exit from the patella at an unintended location.

be necessary. Next, the proximal ends of the Kirschner wires are bent 180° and the bent portions are trimmed to approximately 5 mm. They are then carefully tapped into the proximal pole cortex, trapping the anterior tension-band wire. The distal ends are next cut approximately 1 cm distal to the cerclage wire and are *not*

bent, to facilitate their later extraction, if necessary (see Fig. 11–7E). Finally, the retinaculum is repaired using O absorbable suture, beginning at the apex of the tear and proceeding toward the midline. Drains are placed beneath both flaps and the wound is closed in layers. A knee immobilizer or hinged knee brace locked in full extension is placed.

Alternative Wiring Techniques

A wiring technique originally described by Magnusson[11] has been biomechanically tested by Weber et al[9] and shown to be nearly equivalent to the modified tension band in preventing motion of a cadaveric transverse fracture (Fig. 11–8). In this wiring method, the malleable 18-gauge wire passes *through* the patella, thereby providing both alignment and compressive functions.

Longitudinal anterior band plus cerclage (LAB/C), described by Lotke and Ecker,[12] is a modification of the Magnusson technique in which the wire is subsequently looped and crossed anteriorly to provide a tension band effect (Fig. 11–9). In cadaveric testing, the longitudinal anterior band (without cerclage) was slightly less stable to distraction than the modified tension band.[8]

Screw Fixation

Where fractures are more comminuted and the fracture planes deviate from transverse, lag screw fixation can be used to control fractures not reliably fixed by a wiring technique alone. Partially threaded, 4.0-mm cancellous screws (Synthes No. 207) may be used. Alternatively, if good cortical purchase is possible, a 3.5-mm cortical screw (Synthes No. 204) placed in lag fashion may achieve more reliable fixation. If used, screw fixation should be undertaken initially to reduce the fracture to a two-part configuration with subsequent wire

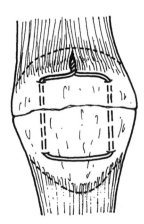

Figure 11–8. Technique of Magnusson wiring.

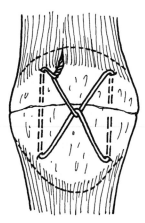

Figure 11-9. Technique of longitudinal anterior band wiring. In cases of more severe comminution, this wiring technique may be augmented with a cerclage wire, placed prior to the definitive fixation.

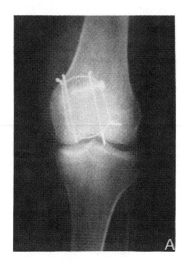

fixation (Fig. 11-10). On occasion, an unstable fragment will be too small to fix reliably with screws yet too large to consider excision. In this setting, one or two smooth Kirschner wires may be used to "lock" the fragment in place prior to compressive wiring. The wire is then trimmed off at the cortex.

Rehabilitation

Quadriceps setting/straight-leg raises are begun as soon as quadriceps function returns. Mobilization is permitted, weight bearing as tolerated, in either a knee immobilizer or hinged knee brace locked in extension. *Active* flexion and *passive* extension are begun to minimize the distractive forces acting across the fracture site (Fig. 11-11). In time, passive extension may be advanced to active-assisted extension. Range of motion at the knee is advanced progressively in this fashion. If x-rays demonstrate progressive healing without distraction at 6 weeks, the brace is removed and progressive resistance exercises are initiated.

Partial Patellectomy

Where the entire patella cannot be reasonably reconstructed using one or more of the preceding methods, excision of the most comminuted segment with salvage of the remaining portion is preferable to a suboptimal internal fixation. If either pole is severely comminuted, the fragments may be excised, preserving the most extreme polar fragment to provide bone/bone apposition when reapproximating tendon to patellar remnant. If the central portion is most comminuted, then the prox-

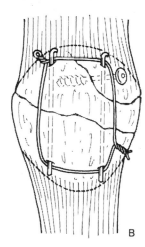

Figure 11-10. In some comminuted patellar fractures, a composite form of fixation using both lag screws and a modified tension band may be employed. In general, an attempt should be made to reduce the fracture to a simpler transverse pattern with lag screws prior to placement of the modified tension band.

imal and distal poles may be brought together after shelling out the comminuted middle portion (Fig. 11-12).

Reattachment of the patellar tendon (or quadriceps tendon), initially described by Thomson,[13] has traditionally been advised at the articular surface, that is, posteriorly.[14] The reason for this has been to avoid the "patellar tilt" that a more anterior point of attachment

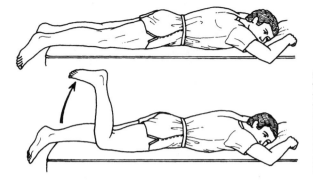

Figure 11-11. In the prone position, active knee flexion can be followed by gravity-assisted knee extension. This method permits the knee to flex without the pull of the quadriceps, as they are subject to reflex inhibition when the hamstrings are active. Extension is performed by the force of gravity, rather than the quadriceps themselves. In the early stages of fracture healing, or when fixation is less than optimal, this method of ranging the knee will minimize the potential for loss of reduction.

would cause, resulting in locally increased contact pressures and more rapid deterioration of articular cartilage. A recent cadaveric study by Marder et al found that increased contact area (and therefore decreased contact pressure) was produced with *anterior* reattachment of the tendon to the patella.[15] Also noted was a reduction in contact area to less than 50% when a 60% patellectomy was performed. They therefore recommended that the tendon be reattached *anteriorly*. Suture of the patellar tendon should be through drill holes in the patellar remnant, to provide more secure fixation (Fig. 11-13).

Protection of a partial patellectomy should be routinely provided by means of an 18-gauge wire[10] (Fig 11-14). The effectiveness of this protection wire has been biomechanically tested by Perry et al.[16] The wire should be tight enough to protect the repair from distraction at up to 90° of knee flexion. Further tightening may lead to patellar tendon contracture and failure to regain flexion.

Rehabilitation is advanced more slowly than for patients undergoing stable open reduction/internal fixation. A hinged knee brace is set to range up to 30° for the initial 6 weeks and progressively opened to full flex-

ion over the next 6 weeks. Progressive weight bearing is permitted with the brace locked in extension. Quadriceps exercises are limited to isometric contractions and straight-leg raises for 6 weeks, after which time active-assisted extension (gravity removed) may be added. Purely active and subsequent progressive resistance exercises are started no earlier than 12 weeks postoperatively.

Total Patellectomy

When the patellar remnant constitutes less than 50% of the articular surface, long-term patellofemoral function deteriorates. This was observed by Böstman, who found poor clinical outcomes in patients whose partial patellectomies resulted in more than 40% loss of the patella.[17] A more recent study by Saltzman et al found that outcome from partial patellectomy varied only with the initial fracture configuration and *not* with the size of the retained patellar fragment.[18] In addition, they found progressive enlargement of the patellar remnant over time by as much as 30% as measured from serial radiographs.

The resulting loss of quadriceps strength following

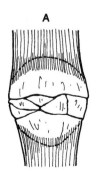 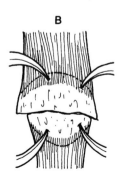 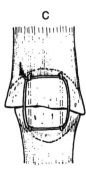

Figure 11-12. In most cases of comminuted patellar fractures, either the proximal or distal pole is the most involved locus. In some cases, however, it is the middle of the patella that must be excised. In such a case (A), the intervening comminuted fragments are excised and the proximal and distal poles are reduced as anatomically as possible, palpating the articular surface to achieve the best possible reduction (B). A modified tension-band fixation is then placed (C).

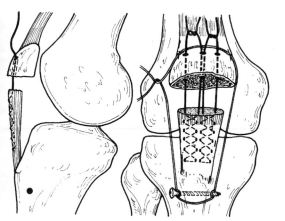

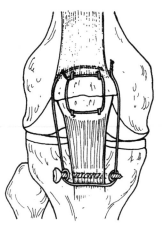

Figure 11–13. The method of partial patellectomy described by Marder et al[15] emphasizes anterior reattachment of the patellar tendon to the retained proximal pole. Drill holes are used and oriented in such a way as to draw the patella tendon anteriorly in continuity with the anterior cortex of the proximal pole. The anteroposterior view shows placement of a patellar protection wire, anchored over a cortical screw.

Figure 11–14. A protection wire may help reduce distraction of the fracture in cases where bone quality is poor, fixation is tenuous, or bone/tendon healing must occur. The wire may be anchored by looping it about a cortical screw placed near the tibial tubercle or it may be passed through bone itself. Proximally, the wire is passed through the quadriceps tendon; a sharp cannula, such as a 12- or 14-gauge intravenous catheter, is useful for this purpose.

total patellectomy has been well described,[19–21] and in general, patients undergoing patellectomy report permanent difficulty in such activities as stair climbing, running, and rising from a chair but retain a functional range of knee motion. Pain is variably reported, but usually less than prior to patellectomy in cases of patellofemoral arthritis. Complete relief of pain is the exception, however.

Indications for acute primary patellectomy are relatively few. In most cases of patellar fracture, at least 50% of the articular surface can be reliably reconstructed and early rehabilitation begun. If patellofemoral pain and/or knee stiffness become severe, a subsequent patellectomy can be performed.

Techniques of patellectomy are numerous and not all

are applicable to patellar fracture where simultaneous soft tissue trauma is the rule. A cadaveric study by Kaufer did not disclose any particular method to be superior, but such testing may not truly approximate the living extensor mechanism where viable muscles act at certain points on their length/tension curves to produce extensor forces.[3]

In acute cases, primary attention should be directed at restoring continuity of the extensor mechanism and maintaining normal quadriceps length. Where primary closure of the defect cannot be obtained, a "turndown" of the quadriceps tendon to bridge the unclosable defect may be performed[22,23] (Fig. 11–15). Baker and Hughston advocate further modification of this proce-

Figure 11–15. Where the extensor mechanism cannot be directly repaired without undue tension, a turndown flap as previously described by Murphy[22] and Shorbe and Dobson[23] may be used. First, the flap is created by incising through the rectus tendon as shown. The defect is closed medially and laterally as the flap of rectus tendon is folded down over the defect and sutured in place. The donor site is then reapproximated as illustrated.

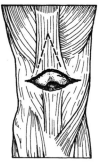

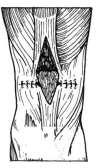

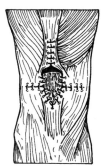

dure by advancing both medialis and lateralis tendons toward the midline to reestablish ideal length.[24] As an alternative to turndown of the quadriceps tendon, a large defect may be bridged by fascial autograft or allograft. The fascia lata may be used for this purpose by tubularizing an appropriate length and weaving it through distal quadriceps and proximal patellar tendons.

Rehabilitation is greatly facilitated by the presence of a protection wire as fascial healing is harder to predict and serially assess than bone healing. The program outlined earlier for partial patellectomy will be applicable in most cases, with modifications as dictated by the security of the repair obtained.

References

1. Ray JM, Hendrik J. Incidence, mechanism of injury, and treatment of fractures of the patella in children. *J Trauma*. 1992;32:464–467.
2. Brooke R. Treatment of fractured patella by excision *Br J Surg*. 1937;24:733–747.
3. Kaufer H. Mechanical function of the patella. *J Bone Joint Surg Am*. 1971;53:1551–1560.
4. Perry J, Antonelli D, Ford W. Analysis of knee joint forces during flexed knee stance. *J Bone Joint Surg Am*. 1975;57:966–967.
5. Huberti HH, Hayes WC. Patellofemoral contact pressures. The influence of Q angle and tendofemoral contact pressures. *J Bone Joint Surg Am*. 1984;66:715–724.
6. Apple JS, Martinez S, Allan NB. Occult fractures of the knee—Tomographic evaluation. *Radiology*. 1983;148:383–387.
7. Boström A. Fracture of the patella. *Acta Orthop. Scand*. 1972;143(suppl):1–80.
8. Benjamin JA, Bried J, Dohm M, McMurty M. Biomechanical evaluation of various forms of fixation of transverse patella fractures. *Trauma*. 1987;1:219–222.
9. Weber MJ, Janecki CJ, McLeod P, Nelson CL, Thompson JA. The effect of various forms of internal fixation in patella fractures. *J Bone Joint Surg Am*. 1980;62:215–220.
10. Müller ME, Allgower M, Schneider R, Willenneger H. *Manual of Internal Fixation*. 3rd ed. Berlin: Springer-Verlag; 1991:564–567.
11. Magnusson PB. *Fractures*. 2nd ed. Philadelphia: JB Lippincott; 1936: Ch 18.
12. Lotke PA, Ecker ML. Transverse fractures of the patella. *Clin Orthop*. 1981;158:180–184.
13. Thomson JEM. Comminuted fractures of the patella. *J Bone Joint Surg Am*. 1935;17:431–434.
14. Andrews JR, Hughston JC. Treatment of patella fractures by partial patellectomy. *South Med J*. 1977;70:809–813.
15. Marder RA, Swanson TV, Sharkey NA, Duwelius PJ. Effects of partial patellectomy and reattachment of the patellar tendon. *J Bone Joint Surg Am*. 1993;75:35–45.
16. Perry CR, McCarthy JA, Kain CC, Pearson RL. Patellar fixation protected by a load sharing cable: A mechanical and clinical study. *J Orthop Trauma*. 1988;2:234–240.
17. Böstman O. Comminuted displaced fractures of the patella. *Injury*. 1981;13:196–202.
18. Saltzman CL, Goulet JA, McClellan RT, Schnieder LA, Matthews LS. Results of treatment of displaced patellar fractures by partial patellectomy. *J Bone Joint Surg Am*. 1990;72:1279–1285.
19. Sutton FS, Thompson CH, Lipke J, Kettlekamp D. The effects of patellectomy on knee function. *J Bone Joint Surg Am*. 1976;58:537–540.
20. Watkins MP, Harris BA, Wender S, Zarins B, Rowe CR. Effect of patellectomy on the function of the quadriceps and hamstrings. *J Bone Joint Surg Am*. 1983;65:390–395.
21. Wilkinson J. Fracture of the patella treated by total excision. *J Bone Joint Surg Br*. 1977;59:352–354.
22. Murphy JB. Tuberculosis of the patella. *Surg Gynecol Obstet*. 1908;6:262–273.
23. Shorbe HB, Dobson CH. Patellectomy. *J Bone Joint Surg Am*. 1958;40:1281–1284.
24. Baker CL, Hughston JC. Miyakawa patellectomy. *J Bone Joint Surg Am*. 1988;70:1489–1494.

12

Extensor Mechanism Disruptions

David W. Lhowe

Introduction

The essential function of knee extension against gravity contributes to nearly all activities involving the lower extremity. Although less critical to the functions of standing and walking on level surfaces, significant extensor power is required to walk on inclined surfaces, ascend/descend stairs, run, and jump.

The mechanism responsible for knee extension is a muscle, tendon, and bone composite beginning with the quadriceps muscles at their origins on the pelvis and femur. The force of muscular contraction is then transmitted through the quadriceps tendon to the patella, which acts as a larger lever to increase the moment arm of the extension force. This results in as much as a 50% increase in extensor power.[1] The final link in this mechanism is the patellar tendon which provides force transmission to the tibial tubercle. Tensile forces generated within this mechanism are substantial and occasionally sufficient to rupture either muscle, tendon, or bony insertion site. (The patella, in contrast, typically fails in *compression*, usually as the result of blunt trauma. This specific type of extensor mechanism injury is addressed in Chapter 11.)

Excluding patellar fractures, extensor mechanism disruptions all occur as the result of quadriceps contraction against a flexing knee. Typically, this occurs as an individual struggles to prevent a fall. As the knee buckles, a powerful contraction of the quadriceps occurs and the resultant forces literally tear the extensor mechanism apart.

The location of the rupture and the force required to produce it depend on the quality of tissue present. In healthy individuals, midsubstance tendon ruptures are unusual. In this group failure is more likely to occur at the bone–tendon junctions or, perhaps, within the mus-

cle itself. In older or more debilitated individuals, failure of the quadriceps or patellar tendons in midsubstance is more common. An exception to this appears to be the well-documented incidence of extensor disruptions seen in patients with chronic renal failure and secondary hyperparathyroidism. Recently, a small series of renal dialysis patients was studied. Pathologic examination of their injured tissues showed consistent failure at the tendon insertion as a result of bony resorption.[2] In each case, the avulsed tendon contained bony fragments and none failed in its midsubstance, although significant tendon degeneration was seen in each case studied.

Another increasingly frequent cause of extensor mechanism failure is reconstructive knee surgery. Total knee arthroplasty[3] and anterior cruciate ligament reconstruction[4,5] (using the middle third of the patella tendon) may devascularize or directly injure the patella tendon or patella, resulting in late failure through tendon rupture/avulsion or patella fracture.

Diagnosis

It is virtually impossible to miss the diagnosis of extensor mechanism disruption if the examiner tests for continuity by asking the patient to extend the knee against gravity. If pain prevents this maneuver, then the knee can be placed at or near full extension, and the patient asked to maintain the position against gravity. All other elements of the history and physical examination are less reliable.

A history of fall or near fall with a flexed knee is frequently found, but degenerative tears can occur without significant trauma. Local injection of corticosteroid, particularly if repetitive, predisposes to tendon degeneration. Pain and swelling may be localized to the disruption but may be diffuse and minimal. In late presentations, pain may be absent. Palpable defects can usually be detected early, but may be obscured by acute hematoma within 24 hours or organized hematoma and early scarring thereafter.

Imaging studies are rarely needed in diagnosing the acute rupture. Plain films will typically show proximal migration of the patella with patellar tendon rupture and distal migration with a quadriceps tendon rupture. Bony avulsions can be seen from the proximal/distal patella, tibial tubercle, or anterior iliac spines. In late presentations, computed tomography (CT) and magnetic resonance (MR) scanning can show disruption and spare the need for exploratory surgery in equivocal cases.[6]

Specific Extensor Disruptions and Their Treatment

Avulsion of Rectus/Sartorius Origins

These are unusual injuries and involve primarily the direct head of the rectus muscle from the anterior inferior iliac spine. Although not a knee extensor, avulsions of the sartorius origin from the anterior superior iliac spine are treated in similar fashion. Pain can be elicited by extending the hip while simultaneously flexing the knee. Local tenderness may or may not be found. X-rays will show an avulsed bony fragment, if present (Fig. 12–1).

Treatment. Symptomatic treatment is usually sufficient, as the extensor mechanism can continue to function quite well without the sartorius or rectus femoris at normal length. Activity is advanced progressively as pain permits, with application of ice and nonsteroidal anti-inflammatory medication helpful during the acute period. Repair of a rectus bony avulsion in the competitive athlete can be considered, although the basis for this is more theoretical than clinically proven. If surgical repair is performed, it must be protected a minimum of 6 weeks against resisted hip flexion and another 6 weeks against full-strength competitive contractions.

Midsubstance Quadriceps Muscle Ruptures

Midsubstance quadriceps muscle ruptures may be mistaken for contusions of the quadriceps muscle. As Albright points out, rupture typically occurs through the rectus femoris and vastus medialis.[7] As a substantial portion of the quadriceps remains in continuity, knee extension may be well preserved. A defect may be palpable or not, depending on the extent of hematoma and the amount of subcutaneous fat present.

Treatment. In most cases, sufficient function will return without operative treatment, which is technically

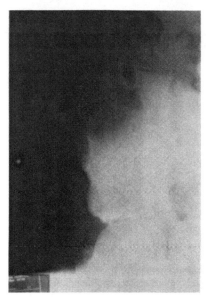

Figure 12–1. X-ray showing avulsion of sartorius origin from the anterior superior iliac spine. An iliac oblique view shows this fragment most clearly.

difficult as direct suture of muscle to muscle is impossible. Further, attempted repair can increase the amount of muscle damage, delay restoration of motion, and potentially shorten the extensor mechanism, predisposing to patellofemoral dysfunction. Nonoperative treatment involves placement of a knee immobilizer for 2 to 3 weeks with protected weight bearing, quadriceps setting, and active knee flexion exercises, followed later by straight leg raising and progressive resistance quadriceps exercises. In rarer cases, where (1) extension is substantially weakened in the presence of a significant defect, (2) functional expectations are high, and (3) surgery can be performed within several days of rupture, a direct repair may be attempted as described by Albright.[7] He recommends use of iliotibial band graft or Dacron tape if the defect that remains after evacuation of hematoma and resection of devitalized muscle exceeds 3 cm. Further, he emphasizes the need to suture to fascial tissue of either the vastus intermedius or rectus femoris. Patients presenting later than 5 days should *not* be treated operatively.

Quadriceps Tendon Rupture

In their 1981 review of the orthopedic literature, Siwek and Rao found that 88% of these ruptures occurred in patients over 40 years of age.[8] In contrast, they found

80% of patellar ligament ruptures occurred in patients under age 40. The quadriceps tendon and its bony insertion seem to be the most common locus for rupture in patients with either chronic renal failure/secondary hyperparathyroidism or diabetes.

The quadriceps tendon tears most often at its insertion onto the patella, but may tear more proximally. Rarely, a discrete avulsion of the superior patellar pole will occur. Early exam will usually show a palpable defect, and a hemarthrosis will be present if the tear extends through the synovium of the knee joint. The patella may be displaced distally and will not move proximally with a quadriceps contraction. As with other extensor mechanism disruptions, the essential test is attempted quadriceps contraction, looking for abnormal contour and failure to extend the knee against gravity. As pain can inhibit contraction, it is important to place a hand proximally on the thigh to assess the extent of the muscular effort. X-rays may or may not show patella baja. Avulsed fragments, if present, will usually be obvious. Late presentation may be clarified by CT or MR scan.

Treatment. Operative treatment is recommended. In acute presentations, when a sufficient distal stump of tendon remains, repair can usually be effected by end-to-end mattress sutures using No. 2 or heavier material. In healthy tissue, absorbable material is satisfactory; I prefer nonabsorbable suture in cases where prolonged healing is anticipated. In the majority of the cases, the distal stump itself will be inadequate in amount or quality to provide suture fixation sufficient for early range-of-motion exercises.

A tourniquet should be placed very proximally or avoided entirely to not inhibit quadriceps excursion. Begin by evacuation of hematoma and careful debridement of devitalized muscle and tendon. Identify synovium at the depth of the tear, and proceed to more superficial layers through the vastus intermedius, the vastus medialis/lateralis, and, most superficially, the rectus femoris. The various layers may be torn at different locations and it is worthwhile to take the time to identify both ends for each layer involved. It is my preference to suture the rectus tendon to the patella through 2.5-mm drill holes in the superior pole (Fig. 12–2). These should be made prior to closure of the defect in an oblique direction to avoid violating the articular cartilage. Confirmation of the position of each drill hole can be made visually or by palpation. If necessary, additional reinforcement can be provided by passing an 18-gauge wire through a transverse drill hole in the patella or tibial tubercle and looping it through the quadriceps tendon, proximal to the repair, as previously described by McLaughlin[9] and Muller et al[10] (Fig. 12–3). The wire should be tightened sufficiently to completely relieve tension on the repair with the knee

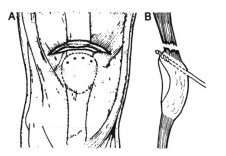
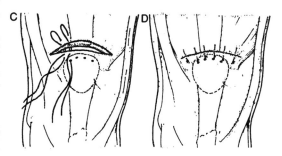

Figure 12–2. A. The patella is prepared by making several 2.5-mm drill holes to provide a more reliable distal anchorage for the repair. **B.** Passing the drill bit obliquely as shown will avoid damage to articular cartilage. **C.** Vertical mattress sutures are placed sequentially. **D.** The completed repair.

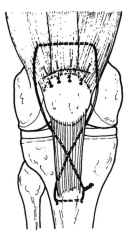

Figure 12–3. Reinforcement of quadriceps tendon repair is accomplished by means of an 18-gauge wire passed through the quadriceps tendon proximally and the tibial tubercle distally.

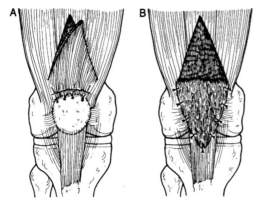

Figure 12–4. A. A distally based flap of quadriceps tendon is created proximal to the repair. **B.** The flap is turned down over the repair and sutured to the patellar retinaculum and patellar tendon.

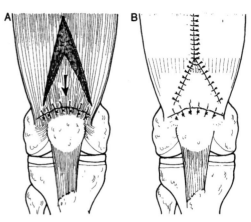

Figure 12–6. A. A V-Y flap is created to permit adequate mobilization of the proximal side of the tear. **B.** Closure of the V-Y flap.

flexed to 90°. This should provide an adequate safety margin to permit progressive range of motion up to 120° during the initial postoperative period. Rehabilitation is begun with active flexion and passive extension of the knee, progressing to active-assisted and then active extension against gravity at approximately 6 weeks. Ambulation is begun, weight bearing as tolerated, in a brace locked in extension with subsequent increase to a range 0° to 30°.

In late presentations, repair is considerably complicated. The proximal end will usually have retracted at least several centimeters. If the proximal side of the dis-

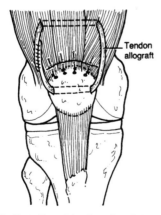

Figure 12–5. Illustration of tendon allograft to reinforce a quadriceps repair. The tendon allograft is passed through the quadriceps tendon proximally and a transverse tunnel through the patella distally. It is then sutured to itself.

ruption can be gently mobilized into apposition with the distal side, then treatment is as for acute tears described earlier. Reinforcement of the repair with a Scuderi flap[11] and/or protection wire is recommended (Fig. 12–4). In another method, allograft tendon performs the same function as the reflected flap of quadriceps tendon augmenting a tenuous reapproximation (Fig. 12–5). In cases where the ruptured tendon cannot be reapproximated to within several centimeters, it is futile to attempt simple or even protected primary repairs. One approach is to lengthen the quadriceps tendon by means of a V-Y advancement flap, attaching the lengthened segment to the patella through drill holes (Fig. 12–6). A Scuderi flap may then be reflected over the suture line for further reinforcement, or the repair can be protected with a protection wire or allograft tendon. Intraoperative assessment is made of the "safe" initial postoperative range of motion. Physical therapy is begun with active knee flexion and passive extension, progressing to active-assisted and then purely active extension as the healing repair permits. A hinged, long leg brace is used, initially locked in full extension and removed only for exercises and bathing. The protection wire should remain in place for 8 weeks, possibly longer if the repair is tenuous or the patient shows reduced healing potential.

Patellar Tendon Ruptures

The most distal of the extensor disruptions, patellar tendon rupture, occurs typically in individuals under 40 and is not often seen in association with chronic illness. The most common location is an avulsion injury at the inferior patellar pole. Diagnosis is seldom missed, as

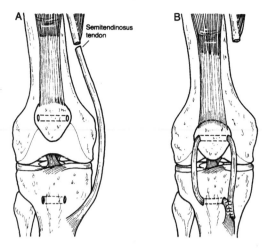

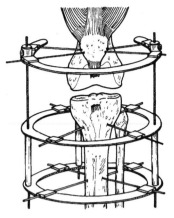

Figure 12-7. A. Method of patellar tendon substitution described by Kelikian et al.[12] The semitendinosus is divided far enough proximally to provide adequate length for the repair. B. The semitendinosus is passed through a transverse tunnel beneath the tibial tubercle and then through a transverse tunnel in the patella before being sutured to itself at its insertion.

Figure 12-9. A retracted extensor mechanism may be progressively advanced by means of a ring fixator. In this configuration, the proximal 5/8 ring controls the patella and is distally advanced in sequential fashion. Repair of the patellar tendon may then be performed by means of direct suture, allograft reinforcement, or autograft substitution.

there is little soft tissue to obscure the ruptured tendon. As with other extensor tendon disruptions, assessment of extensor continuity is the essential diagnostic test. X-rays will usually show patella alta when the tendon *and* the distal retinacular attachments have all been disrupted.

Treatment. Nonoperative treatment may be considered where continuity of the extensor mechanism remains intact through the retinaculum, but the majority of these tears should be surgically repaired, particularly when x-rays show proximal migration of the patella.

Acute tears are best repaired with end-to-end approximation using No. 2 absorbable mattress sutures; nonabsorbable material is preferred when delayed healing is anticipated. In most cases, there will be inadequate tendon on one side for direct tendon-to-tendon repair, and drill holes through the inferior patellar pole or tibial tubercle should routinely be used. The inferior patellar pole does not articulate with the femur, giving greater latitude in the placement of these drill holes than at the superior pole. As for quadriceps tendon ruptures, protection of the repair can be provided by a wire.

Delayed tears can be treated by attempting distal mobilization using a Steinman pin through the patella. A V-Y lengthening of the quadriceps tendon may be necessary to bring the patella distally into its normal location. If this permits an end-to-end repair, then the suture line should be protected with a protection wire; rehabilitation is advanced slowly, as for late repairs of the quadriceps tendon.

In cases where good primary apposition of healthy tendon cannot be obtained, an augmentation or substitution using the semitendinosus has been described by Kelikian et al[12] (Fig. 12–7); the use of both the semitendinosus *and* gracilis has been described by Ecker et al[13] (Fig. 12–8). Allograft tendon may also be woven through the drill holes in place of autograft.

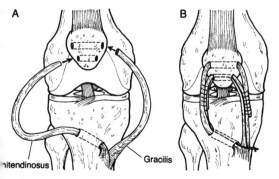

Figure 12-8. A. Alternative method of patellar tendon substitution described by Ecker et al.[13] The semitendinosus is used as in the method of Kelikian et al, but the repair is further augmented by passage of the gracilis tendon through a second bony tunnel in the patella. B. After the tendons are sutured to each other, the repair is protected by means of an 18-gauge wire passed through patella and tibial tubercle as shown.

Another option for treating the delayed tear with proximal retraction of the patella is with a ring fixator. With this device the tibial segment is fixed, while the patella is progressively mobilized in a distal direction by sequential advancement of the 5/8 ring which is secured to the patella by two transfixion wires (Fig. 12–9).

In total knee arthroplasty with patellar tendon failure, a more extensive method of reconstruction has been described by Emerson et al[3] whereby an allograft composite consisting of quadriceps tendon, patella, patellar tendon, and tibial tubercle is substituted en bloc for the ruptured patellar tendon. The authors report good initial results which compare quite favorably to the generally poor outcome of attempted primary repair (See Chapter 25).

References

1. Watkins MP, Harris BA, Wender S, Zarins B, Rowe CR. Effect of patellectomy on the function of the quadriceps and hamstrings. *J Bone Joint Surg Am.*1983;65:390–395.
2. Ryuzaki M, Konishi K, Kasuga A, et al. Spontaneous rupture of the quadriceps tendon in patients on maintenance hemodialysis—Report of 3 cases with clinicopathological observations. *Clin Nephrol.* 1989;32:144–148.
3. Emerson RH, Head WC, Malinin TI. Reconstruction of patellar tendon rupture after total knee arthroplasty with an extensor mechanism allograft. *Clin Orthop.* 1990; 260:154–161.
4. Bonatus TJ, Alexander AH. Patellar fracture and avulsion of the patellar ligament complicating arthroscopic anterior cruciate ligament reconstruction. *Orthop Rev.* 1991;20:770–774.
5. DeLee JC, Craviotto DF. Rupture of the quadriceps tendon after a central third patellar tendon anterior cruciate ligament reconstruction. *Am J Sports Med.* 1991;19:415–416.
6. Kuvila TE, Brems JJ. Diagnosis of acute rupture of the quadriceps tendon by magnetic resonance imaging. A case report. *Clin Orthop.* 1991;262:236–241.
7. Albright JP. Musculotendinous problems about the knee. In: Evarts CMC, ed. *Surgery of the Musculoskeletal System.* 2nd ed. New York: Churchill Livingstone; 1990; 4:3499–3537.
8. Siwek CW, Rao JP. Ruptures of the extensor mechanism of the knee joint. *J Bone Joint Surg Am.* 1981;63:932–937.
9. McLaughlin HL. Repair of major tendon ruptures by buried removable suture. *Am J Surg.* 1947;34:758–764.
10. Müller ME, Allgower M, Schneider R, Willenegger H, ed. *Manual of Internal Fixation.* 3rd ed. Berlin: Springer-Verlag; 1991:564.
11. Scuderi C. Ruptures of the quadriceps tendon. *Am J Surg.* 1958;95:626–635.
12. Kelikian H, Riashi E, Gleason J. Restoration of quadriceps function in neglected tear of the patellar tendon. *Surg Gynecol Obstet.* 1957;104:200–204.
13. Ecker ML, Lotke PA, Glazer RM. Late reconstruction of the patellar tendon. *J Bone Joint Surg Am.* 1979;61:884–886.

13

Patellar Dislocations

George Thabit III and Lyle J. Micheli

> *And I said of medicine, that this is an art which considers the constitution of the patient and has principles of action and reason in each case.*
>
> —*Plato*, Gorgias

Introduction

The words of Plato ring as true today as they did in classical Greece; for as we shall see, patellar instability presents as a spectrum of disease whereby each case must be specifically diagnosed and treated to achieve clinical success. Traditional classifications of instability identify the temporal nature of the event and were listed as acute or recurrent entities. Modern classifications of patellofemoral instability focus on extensor mechanism pathomechanics and include acute dislocations occurring in the anatomically normal and the dysplastic knee; lateral patellar compression syndrome, chronic subluxation patella, recurrent dislocation patella, and chronic dislocation patella, which generally occur in the setting of developmental patellofemoral dysplasia; and congenital dislocations and dislocations associated with genetic syndromes (Table 13–1).

To appreciate the current treatments used to manage patellofemoral instability, a brief historical review will provide the backdrop for a discussion of this complex topic so that we may examine the colorful past of patellar dislocations and thus obtain a finer appreciation for the current treatments which are still evolving.

History

Historically, the treatment of patellar instability has been fraught with frustration. Plagued by inconsistent clinical results, our orthopedic forefathers devised and used an armamentarium of surgical procedures to stabilize the slipping patella, as with more recent surgical treatments which alternated between attempts to correct the dislocation either proximal to the patella or distal to it. The orthopedic community of the 19th century viewed patellar dislocations as a disease afflicting young girls possessing "lax muscular fiber and feeble development."[1] A component of patellofemoral dysplasia was universally present. Patella alta, ligamentous laxity, patellofemoral bony hypoplasia, as well as weakness of the quadriceps muscle, weak feet, and genu recurvatum or valgum, were identified as features that predisposed individuals to patellar instability[2] (Fig. 13–1).

Furthermore, Duchenne, in his monumental work *Physiology of Motion*, focused attention on the dynamic extensor mechanism and hypothesized that pathophysiology of the quadriceps contributed to patellar instability. His method of faradization of the quadriceps muscle unit revealed the role of the vastus medialis and the vastus lateralis in maintaining patellar alignment and that "atrophy of the vastus medialis permits separate contraction of the vastus lateralis with resulting lateral luxation of the patella in rapid walking, jumping, dancing, etc."[2]

In 1850, Heller performed the first documented proximal extensor mechanism realignment procedure.[3] Fifty years later, Hoffa reported the results of a capsular reefing technique to correct instability.[4] Goldthwait in 1904 reported his split patellar tendon transfer[5] (Fig. 13–2). While other authors advocated a variety of soft tissue procedures, other surgeons focused their efforts on the dysplastic lateral femoral condyle, which commonly accompanied the condition. Trendelenburg, Jones, and Albee modified the lateral femoral condyle anatomy through bone grafting, osteotomy, and peg techniques.[6] Thomas promoted new bone formation by inducing a traumatic osteitis by repetitive mallet percussion of the

Table 13–1. Classification of Patellofemoral Instability

A. Acute trauma
   1. Anatomically normal knee
   2. Anatomically normal knee with osteochondral fracture
   3. Anatomically dysplastic knee
   4. Anatomically dysplastic knee with osteochondral fracture
   5. Intraarticular dislocation
B. Development dysplasia
   1. Lateral patellar compression syndrome (LPCS)
   2. Chronic subluxation of the patella (CSP)
   3. Chronic dislocation of the patella (CDP)
C. Congenital dislocation
   1. Reducible
   2. Permanent
D. Instability associated with genetic syndromes
   1. Down's syndrome
   2. Marfan's syndrome
   3. Nail–patella syndrome

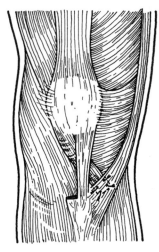

Figure 13–2. Roux–Goldthwait transfer of the lateral half of the patellar tendon, passed under the medial half and sutured to soft tissues.

lateral condyle.[7] The goals of such bony procedures were to elevate the static lateral restraint of the lateral femoral condyle on patellar instability. Despite such diverse procedures, Goldthwait's procedure proved to be the gold standard until 1938 when Hauser reported on the total patellar tendon transplantation for the slipping patella.[8] These two procedures and/or their modifications provide the foundation for modern orthopedic surgical treatment of the unstable extensor mechanism.

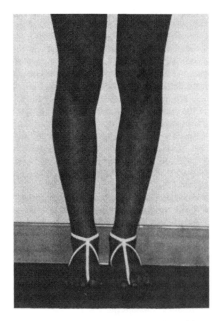

Figure 13–1. Note the degree of internal femoral torsion and external tibial tubercle positioning. Such malalignment often predisposes individuals to symptomatic patellofemoral subluxation.

Yet, just as orthopedists appeared to be on the verge of answering the therapeutic questions pertaining to patellofemoral instability, a curious event occurred; someone changed the question. In 1928, Aleman called attention to the posttraumatic cartilage softening found at operation, thus coining the term *chondromalacia patellae posttraumatica*.[9] In 1936 Owre simplified the term to chondromalacia patella, and the anterior knee pain that had previously been ascribed to extensor mechanism pathomechanics was attributed to the softened cartilage.[10]

Over the next 30 years, the association of chondromalacia with anterior knee pain was so common that the symptom and pathologic tissue changes were equated. Unfortunately, surgical procedures were directed at debriding the softened cartilage and did not address the true underlying pathology contributing to the extensor mechanism pathomechanics. Interestingly and not surprisingly, the failure to recognize and to treat the specific cause of the instability led to many poor clinical outcomes.

In 1968, Hughston changed the perception that patellar dislocations were a disease of young girls. His work demonstrated that males and females had similar rates of patellar dislocation.[11] Treatment modalities were refocused on extensor mechanism pathomechanics rather than secondary pathologic findings. He emphasized the importance of therapeutic exercise as a primary treatment of extensor apparatus instability. Surgical treatment was employed only after the failure of a monitored exercise program and was directed at correcting

Table 13-2. Radiographic Measurements of Patellofemoral Congruence

A. Sulcus angle
 The angle is formed by the condyles and the
 sulcus (Brattstrom).
 Mean = 138°, SD = 6°.
 Correlates well with instability.

B. Congruence angle
 A zero reference line bisects the sulcus angle;
 the angular distance of the articular ridge from
 that line is the congruence angle (Merchant et
 al.).
 Mean = −6°, SD = 6° (Aglietti et al.).
 Measures subluxation.

C. Lateral patellofemoral angle
 The angle between the intercondylar line and the
 lateral facet (Laurin et al.).
 It should open laterally.
 Measures tilt with subluxation.

D. Patellofemoral index
 M = the closest distance between the articular
 ridge and the medial condyle; L = the closest
 distance between the lateral facet and
 condyle.
 Ratio M/L = 1.6 or less (Laurin et al.).
 Measures tilt and subluxation.

Reprinted with permission of John B. McGinty, ed. from *Operative Arthroscopy*, New York: Raven Press; 1990;273.

the major pathoanatomic deficiency contributing to the patellar instability.

Ficat and Hungerford and Merchant refined our appreciation for the spectrum of patellofemoral dysplasia and its relationship to instability and pain.[12,13] Detailed radiographic techniques allowed meaningful and reproducible data to be collected pertaining to patellar instability and patellofemoral pathomechanics and permitted critical analysis of such data (Table 13-2). This information has led to the general belief that chondromalacia is the result of patellar pathomechanics and rarely should be ascribed to intrinsic patellar disease (Fig. 13-3).

During our review of patellar instability, we shall examine the evaluation and treatment of acute primary patellar dislocations, developmental patellofemoral instability and pain syndromes, as well as dislocations present at birth or that arise in the setting of genetic syndromes. Treatment options are reviewed and the authors' preferred method of treatment is provided for each subgroup of instability pattern presented.

Acute Dislocations

Acute patellar dislocations present in a dramatic fashion and result either from direct lateral trauma or indirectly

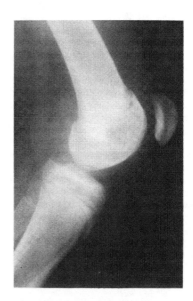

Figure 13-3. Lateral radiograph of patella alta. Note the patellar subchondral sclerosis resulting from subluxation events and chondro-osseous overload.

from a valgus external rotation moment applied to the flexed knee. Acute patellar dislocations have a high incidence of associated anatomic dysplasia of the patellofemoral joint, although dislocations can certainly occur in anatomically normal joints.[11] In addition to dysplasia, congenital, genetic, and neuromuscular conditions may predispose an individual to acute dislocation. The anatomically normal knee appears to be quite resistant to patellar dislocation, and correspondingly the magnitude of force required to elicit an injury correlates inversely with the degree of dysplasia.

The history of a patient possessing an acutely injured knee often focuses the physician's physical examination to the extensor mechanism. "I felt my knee pop out and back into place again" is a common refrain. Although spontaneous or patient-mediated reductions are generally the rule, they often leave the patient with a tender, swollen knee and the physician with a diagnostic dilemma. Occasionally the patella remains laterally dislocated at the time of presentation. In such instances, the patella is atraumatically reduced by gently flexing the hip and gradually relocating the patella by direct lateral pressure.

Careful examination of the acutely injured knee is of tantamount importance, not only in establishing the diagnosis but also in ascertaining the magnitude of soft tissue injury. In addition to an effusion, parapatellar tenderness suggests injury to the extensor retinaculum. In severe cases, a large gap may be palpated along the insertion of the medial retinaculum. Patella alta may be of developmental or traumatic nature and thus the integrity of the extensor mechanism must be tested. Aspiration of the effusion reveals blood but may also include fat droplets, which is highly suggestive of a concomitant osteochondral fracture. Following aspiration of the effusion, the instillation of a local anesthetic can allow the knee to be placed through a range of motion and permits functional testing of the extensor apparatus. An inability to passively move the knee through a full range of motion should alert the examiner to search for an associated intraarticular fracture or a meniscal tear. In addition, careful examination for associated ligamentous disruption, particularly of the anterior cruciate ligament, should be done. We have had a number of cases of anterior cruciate ligament injury in which the patient described an initial dislocation of the patella followed, apparently, by tearing of the unprotected cruciate ligament.

Postreduction radiographs are obtained to evaluate patellar alignment and the presence of osteochondral or marginal fractures (Figs. 13–4 and 13–5). Although some authors state that residual patellar tilt or subluxation on axial radiographs is an indication for acute repair and realignment of the extensor apparatus, others report that good axial patellar views are difficult to

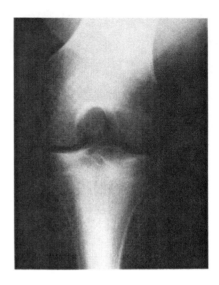

Figure 13–4. Anteroposterior radiograph demonstrating an osteochondral fragment in the intercondylar notch resulting from a patellar dislocation.

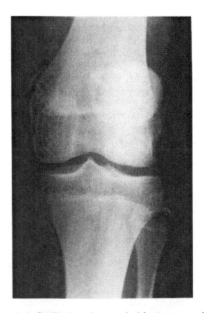

Figure 13–5. Ossification of a marginal fracture occurring at the medial patellar chondro-osseous junction.

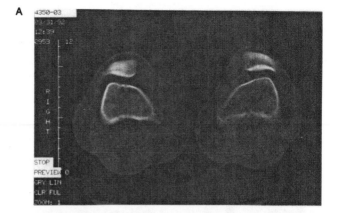

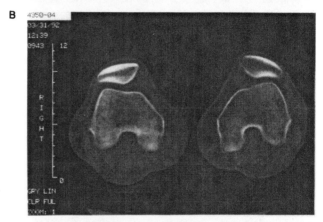

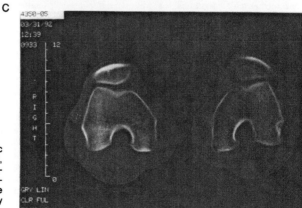

Figure 13–6. Sequential computed tomographic views of the patellofemoral joint taken at 0°**(A)**, 20°**(B)**, and 40°**(C)** of knee flexion. Note the sensitivity of the scan in identifying patellar subluxation at 0° and 20° of flexion as compared with the 40° view. Associated arthrosis is exquisitely defined.

obtain in the acute setting and that the presence of a large effusion may be make radiographic measurements of patellar alignment unreliable.[14] Magnetic resonance imaging (MRI) and computed tomography (CT) are often used as noninvasive means of evaluating the patellofemoral articular surfaces and are especially helpful in identifying associated ligamentous and meniscal injuries[15–17] (Fig. 13–6).

The management of acute patellar dislocations has a history founded on conservative nonoperative care. In the absence of osteochondral fracture, a 3- to 6-week period of immobilization has been recommended to permit soft tissue healing prior to vigorous rehabilitation of the quadriceps muscle group; however, a review of conservatively managed acute dislocations reveals inconsistent clinical results. The recurrent rate of instability approach 52% in some series.[18] On closer review, two distinct patient populations coexist and appear to have differing outcomes with respect to nonsurgical treatment. Cash and Hughston highlighted this difference by comparing the results of conservatively managed acute patellar dislocations in individuals with anatomically normal knees and knees with underlying patellofemoral dysplasia.[19] In a group of patients possessing an anatomic predisposition to patellar instability, only 52% of the patients had good or excellent results compared with 75% of patients with no such predisposing factors. The inconsistent results of nonoperative treatment regimes have led other investigators to primary surgical management of acute patellar dislocations.

Presently, advocates of early surgical intervention find the 15 to 50% recurrence rate of patellar instability obtained by nonoperative treatment to be unacceptable.[18–23] Furthermore, the high incidence of associated intraarticular fractures, as well as ligamentous and meniscal pathology, provides further justification for acute operative evaluation.

In 1971 Sargent and Teipner recommended an early medial capsular reefing.[24] Boring and O'Donoghue reported that 16 of 17 patients were satisfied with the results of acute proximal and/or distal realignment procedures.[25] Cofield and Bryan and Foudren et al recommended strong consideration of primary surgical treatment for patients possessing anatomic features predisposing them to recurrent instability, for athletic individuals, and for dislocations accompanied by intraarticular fractures.[18,26] Hawkins et al recommended consideration of primary surgical intervention based on their study which found that 40 to 70% of conservatively treated patients complained of chronic pain associated with recurrent instability.[20]

Yamamoto reported good results (19/20) achieved by acute arthroscopic medial capsular repair.[27] Dainer et al treated 29 consecutive acute patellar dislocations by arthroscopy, repair, or removal of intraarticular osteochondral fractures, and randomized lateral release.[28] Overall, 83% of patients achieved good and excellent results with a 14% recurrence rate. Of particular interest is that the lateral release group fared worse than the nonrelease cases. Patients treated by lateral release reported 73% good and excellent results and a 27% rate of redislocation, whereas those treated with arthroscopy demonstrated 93% good and excellent results and no recurrent instability. Immediate knee motion was suggested as a factor contributing to the poorer results of lateral release, as a period of immobilization was used for all patients treated without lateral release. Dainer et al recommended that acute patellar dislocation be treated with arthroscopy, appropriate management of osteochondral fractures, and a period of immobilization to enhance soft tissue healing as the treatment of choice.

Ten Thije and Frima in reviewing nine acute dislocations associated with chondral injury found that 50% of the arthroscopically identified intraarticular fractures were unrecognized preoperatively.[29] Arthroscopic fixation or removal of the intraarticular fragments was combined with medial capsular reefing and distal realignment as needed to correct anatomic dysplasia. Postoperatively, immediate motion was permitted for 1 week, followed by 5 weeks of splinting.

Vainionpaa et al reported 80% good and excellent results in 56 consecutive patellar dislocations treated with arthroscopy, removal, or repair of intraarticular fractures and lateral release in conjunction with medial reefing.[30] Postoperative knee flexion was restricted for 2 to 3 weeks to facilitate soft tissue healing.

Although Cash and Hughston recommended conservative management for patellar dislocations, a review of their surgically treated patients revealed that 89% of anatomically normal but acutely injured knees treated by either arthroscopy or other open procedures had good and excellent results.[19] Similarly, 91% of acute dislocations occurring in dysplastic knees treated by open repair had good and excellent results. Arthroscopy alone produced a 50% recurrence rate.

Harilainen and Myllynen reported that only 7 of 56 patellar dislocations treated by surgical stabilization fared poorly.[31] Concomitant major ligamentous or meniscal injuries were noted in 12% of cases.

Although surgical procedures are used primarily to stabilize the patella and thus prevent recurrence, the incidence of significant intraarticular fracture is alarmingly high. Multiple authors state that 40 to 50% of acute dislocations are associated with acute chondral or osteochondral fractures, typically from the medial patellar facet, trochlea, or lateral femoral condyle[14,28–32] (Fig. 13–7). These fractures are often not seen on routine radiographs and often may be missed by CT and MRI scans. Despite the increased use of MRI to evaluate the acutely injured knee, recent evidence suggests that a large number of false-negative scans are identified in patients in whom loose bodies are noted during subsequent arthroscopy.[33] Thus, arthroscopy continues to be most useful in evaluating the knee for the presence of osteocartilaginous and cartilaginous loose bodies. In the future contrast-enhanced MRI may improve the ability to preoperatively identify intraarticular loose bodies and thus contribute significant information in the management of patellar dislocations.

In summary, most surgeons favoring acute surgical evaluation of patellar dislocations distinguish two treatment groups. In patients with anatomically normal knees, arthroscopy and either removal or repair of associated intraarticular fractures, followed by immobilization for 3 to 6 weeks, provide very good results. In patients possessing dysplastic anatomic features that predispose to high rates of recurrence, arthroscopy, intraarticular fracture repair or removal, medial capsular repair, and lateral release yield good results (Fig. 13–8). In cases of severe patellofemoral dysplasia, distal realignments are employed with similar good results. When necessary, extensive surgical realignment of the extensor mechanism must be combined with early motion if posttraumatic arthrofibrosis is to be avoided.

Our patient population tends to be younger than most, and our treatment is thus biased to a conservative bent. In the absence of an irreducible dislocation or osteochondral fracture as noted by plain radiographs, CT scan, or MRI, the knee is immobilized in extension for approximately 3 weeks. Thereafter, a patellar stabilization brace and a static, straight leg raising, progressive resistive quadriceps exercise therapy (PRE) program are employed to rehabilitate the quadriceps mechanism. A goal of three sets of ten repetitions is increased weekly by one-half- to one-pound increments to a total of 12 pounds. Using this format, we have achieved 80 to 90% good and excellent results.[34] Should our patients fail to reach the 12-pound goal or continue to have pain or instability that prevents them from

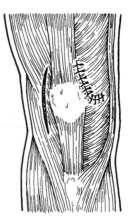

Figure 13–8. Patellar realignment achieved by a combination of lateral release and medial retinacular repair and/or reefing. The extent of the medial quadricepsplasty may be varied to adjust tension on the medial side of the patella.

obtaining the goals of the PRE program, dynamic arthroscopic evaluation of patellofemoral motion and lateral release are used followed by the aforementioned exercise plan. Results mirror those of other authors— 85 to 90% good and excellent results.[35,36] Formal proximal and/or distal realignments are reserved for individuals who fail conservative and arthroscopic treatments and who possess residual patellar tilt subluxation or anatomic dysplasia. All surgical realignments are followed by vigorous quadriceps restrengthening.

Of special note is the rare intraarticular patellar dislocation. Pathoanatomic failure at the chondro-osseous margin enables the superior or inferior pole of the patella to dissociate from the extensor mechanism and lock in the intercondylar notch.[37] Open reduction is recommended to atraumatically reduce the joint and to treat associated osteochondral and soft tissue pathology.

Patellofemoral Dysplasia

Although more frequent in presentation, symptoms resulting from the spectrum of patellofemoral dysplasia are quite subtle when compared with acute dislocation. Anterior knee pain and varying degrees of patellar instability or recurrent dislocation make the dysplastic knee a diagnostic challenge. The presence of dysplasia does not, however, condemn an individual to a dysfunctional existence. The expression of symptomatic disease appears to be multifactorial and results from developmental and environmental predisposing factors. For example, normal mechanisms of growth may produce pathologic conditions when preexisting muscle imbal-

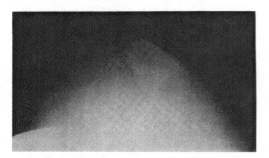

Figure 13–7. Merchant view of a lateral patellar dislocation and associated patellar osteochondral fracture.

ances are accentuated during the adolescent growth spurt.[38] Accelerated growth may create a relative patella alta or lead to the development of tight hamstrings and an iliotibial band which contribute to lateral patellar subluxation. Thus, a continuum of clinical syndromes has been classified.[12,13,39] These syndromes reflect increasing degrees of anatomic dysplasia and are based on the patient's history, physical findings, and 30° axial patellar radiographs.

Lateral Patellar Compression Syndrome

Lateral patellar compression syndrome (LPCS), first described by Ficat and Hungerford in 1977, describes the development of activity-related knee pain in the absence of patellar instability.[12] Symptoms include dull aching anterior knee pain that is exacerbated by prolonged knee flexion. Complaints from prolonged sitting or climbing stairs are frequently volunteered by the patient. The physical examination reveals variable degrees of superolateral and inferomedial retinacular patellar facet tenderness. Effusion is rare and suggests advanced arthrosis. Most importantly, the patellar apprehension sign is negative, and the tight lateral retinaculum and soft tissue patellar restraints prevent passive medial patellar excursion, which normally is 50% of the patellar diameter at 20° of knee flexion.

The production of pain has been postulated to arise

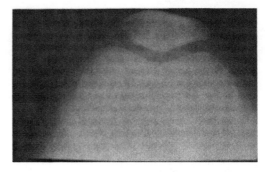

Figure 13–9. Merchant view of lateral patellar compression syndrome (LPCS). Note normal patellofemoral appearance.

from numerous causes, including synovitis resulting from cartilage degradation by-products, elevated subchondral bone pressure, and high peripatellar soft tissue stress with subsequent small nerve injury and fibrosis.[40]

Axial radiographs obtained in 30° of knee flexion reveal patellar tilt, lateral facet sclerosis, or loss of lateral joint space, or may be entirely normal (Figs. 13–9 to 13–11). There is no subluxation of the patella noted on plain radiographs.

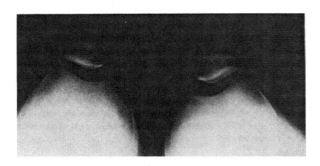

Figure 13–10. Bilateral Merchant views demonstrating lateral patellar compression syndrome (LPCS) and lateral patellar facet subchondral sclerosis. Note associated trochlear hypoplasia.

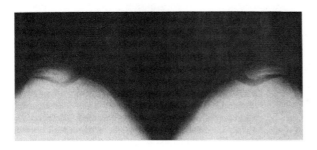

Figure 13–11. Bilateral Merchant views demonstrating lateral patellar compression syndrome (LPCS) and patellar tilt.

Chronic Subluxation of the Patella

Symptoms of chronic subluxation of the patella (CSP) are often similar to those of LPCS but may include mechanical symptoms such as locking or giving way as the knee initially moves from full extension to flexion. The apprehension test is variably present and is not diagnostic of this entity. In addition to demonstrating the presence of patellar subluxation and tilt, 30° axial radiographs provide a means of assessing patellofemoral incongruence by measuring the sulcus angle, congruence angle, lateral patellofemoral angle, and patellofemoral index (Figs. 13–12 and 13–13; see Table 13–2).

Recurrent Dislocation of the Patella

Mechanical symptoms of locking and catching predominate in recurrent dislocation of the patella (RDP). Episodic buckling and recurrent effusion are also commonly observed. Axial radiographs highlight the marked skeletal deficiencies that are the hallmarks of RDP (Fig. 13–14). If one considers the patellofemoral dysplasias as a continuum of increasing musculoskeletal abnormality, the distinction between CSP and RDP is largely one of degree of associated symptoms. Episodes of patellar subluxation are minimally symptomatic, characterized by a transient sense of instability or "giving way" of the knee, whereas episodes of recurrent dislocation are much more commonly associated with residual pain, tenderness, or effusion.

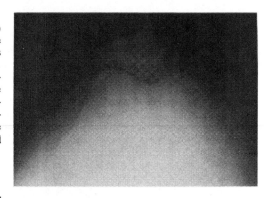

Figure 13–12. Merchant radiograph demonstrating chronic subluxation of the patella (CSP). Note the presence of patellar subluxation and tilt. Trochlear hypoplasia is also present.

Chronic Dislocation of the Patella

Chronic fixed dislocation of the patella (CDP), whether of congenital or acquired etiology, presents with the most severe expression of patellofemoral dysplasia. The acquired form of CDP results most commonly from neglected childhood trauma or progressive quadriceps contracture secondary to repetitive intramuscular injections. The permanently dislocated patella is usually

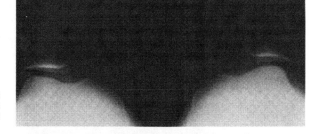

Figure 13–13. Bilateral Merchant radiographs demonstrating chronic subluxation of the patella (CSP). Note the degree of subluxation and the presence of subchondral sclerosis.

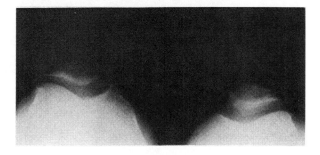

Figure 13–14. Bilateral Merchant radiographs demonstrating untreated end-stage recurrent dislocation of the patella (RDP) of the right patella. Note the patellotrochlear arthrosis with osteophyte formation and patellar lateral facet joint space diminution.

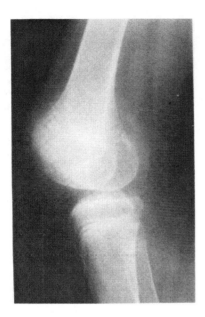

Figure 13-15. Lateral radiograph of chronic dislocation of the patella (CDP). Note absence of patella. Lateral displacement of the patella results in a superimposed image in the lateral view.

found tightly bound to the lateral aspect of the lateral femoral condyle. The knee typically bears a flexed valgus position. The absence of normal patellofemoral modeling forces results in severe patellar and distal femoral hypoplasia. Axial radiographs clearly demonstrate the severity of skeletal dysplasia (Figs. 13–15 to 13–17).

Treatment of Patellofemoral Dysplasias

Under experimental conditions, articular cartilage degradation has been produced by repetitive sheer and compressive forces.[41–43] Adult articular cartilage appears incapable of satisfactory repair once significant injury has occurred.[44] Furthermore, clinical studies have documented the natural history of untreated patellofemoral dysplasia and have found that if left untreated, continued pathomechanics will lead to a high likelihood of knee pain, disability, and progressive arthrosis.[40,45,46] Thus, early treatment of patellofemoral dysplasia aimed at establishing patellofemoral congruency and thus diminishing peak articular contact forces is mandated. Our experience based on hundreds of childhood and adult arthroscopic procedures is that cumulative articular trauma produces two distinct injury patterns. Immature patients rarely develop true articular cartilage degenerative changes. Rather, we hypothesize that the cumulative effect of repetitive traumatic forces acting on immature individuals possessing open physes is the development of osteochondritis dissecans. Clinical observation suggests that the loss of articular cartilage integrity occurs after skeletal maturity has been attained.

A review of conservatively treated dysplasia-related anterior knee pain and instability reveals satisfactory results in approximately 85% of patients.[35,36,47] Exercises, manipulative therapy, and braces constitute the mainstays of nonoperative treatment. Pearson in 1884 first reported the use of a felt orthosis to treat the dislocating patella.[48] Over the years, patellar stabilization orthoses have evolved into the currently employed elastic and Velcro models, which include a lateral pad to block patellar translation.

In 1954, MacAusland and Sargent first promoted combination therapy using a knee brace, as well as patellar manipulation and strengthening exercises.[49]

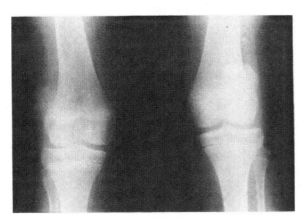

Figure 13-16. Bilateral standing view of chronic dislocation of the patella (CDP). When compared with the normal left knee, the right patella lies along the lateral aspect of the distal femur. The patella is hypoplastic and osteopenic.

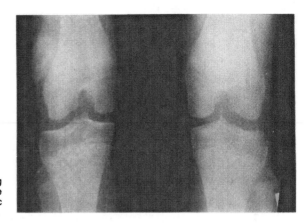

Figure 13–17. Bilateral tunnel views demonstrating right chronic dislocation of the patella (CDP). Note the fixed lateral displacement of the osteopenic patella as well as early patellofemoral joint arthrosis.

The importance of exercise therapy was subsequently emphasized by Hughston, who refined and promoted such therapeutic programs.[50] The goals of manipulative and exercise programs are to mobilize the contractive passive lateral patellar soft tissue restraints and to balance the quadriceps mechanism by strengthening the atrophied vastus medialis muscle. Patellar mobilization techniques, hamstring, iliotibial band, and gastrocnemius stretching and quadriceps strengthening through a static, straight-leg raising progressive resistance exercise program form the foundation of treatment. We have found that 90% of patients able to perform three sets of ten repetitions at 12 pounds of weight achieve resolution of their symptoms.[34,47] Although data suggest the equal efficacy of isokinetic and isometric exercise regimens, we do not allow dynamic resistance exercise until the 12-pound goal has been maintained for 3 months.[51] Furthermore, when compared with a therapist-guided isokinetic program, an isometric exercise program is far more cost effective. Our results for conservative management of LPCS and CSP have been duplicated by other authors and consistently result in 80 to 90% good results.[35,36]

Although 85% of patients respond to exercise programs, 10 to 20% of patients either continue to experience symptoms of pain and instability despite reaching the 12-pound goal or are unable to reach the goal because of disability. When a patient fails such conservative treatment, percutaneous or open lateral release is very successful in achieving clinical success. The best clinical response to lateral release occurs in those patients who present with LPCS or CSP and thus manifest patellar tilt and/or subluxation because of tight lateral soft tissue restraints. Lateral release in the absence of contracted lateral soft tissue restraints often results in poor clinical outcome and may be complicated by medial patellar subluxation.[52]

On closer examination of treatment results, a subset of patients is identified. One should be particularly conservative when treating female patients possessing hypermobile patellae with associated patella alta and generalized ligamentous laxity. They generally do not possess lateral soft tissue contracture and rarely benefit from lateral release. Often their condition is exacerbated by such operative intervention. Although some data suggest the distal transfer of the tibial tubercle may be beneficial in this subset of patients, we have no experience with this procedure.[53] Additionally, a substantial body of information documents the distal and medial transfer of the tibial tuberosity (Hauser procedure) as producing poor long-term results.[54–56] Thus, a protracted course of exercise and bracing is recommended for these patients.

Overall, the results of lateral release are quite encouraging. With properly selected patients, multiple authors consistently quote success rates near 85%.[57–67] After performing open or percutaneous lateral release by either mechanical, electrocautery, or laser techniques, we recommend our quadriceps rehabilitation program to obtain optimal results. We reserve formal extensor mechanism realignment for patients who do not respond to the combination of conservative treatment and lateral release or in whom significant deformity is present distal to the patella.

Contrary to the excellent clinical results of conservatively treated LPCS and CSP, RDP and CDP usually require surgical intervention. Both proximal and/or distal realignment procedures have been employed successfully. When treating the skeletally mature individual, we recommend a tibial tubercle osteotomy of the Elmslie–Trillat variation (Figs. 13–18 and 13–19). We have been quite satisfied with our results, which parallel those reported by Cox and Trillat.[68,69]

The presence of open physeal growth plates prohibits

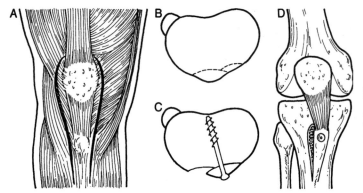

Figure 13–18. Modified Elmslie–Trillat tibial tubercle transfer. **A.** The soft tissues along both sides of the extensor mechanism are released. **B.** A long osteotomy of the tubercle is created, and the adjacent medial bone is contoured. **C, D.** The tubercle is rotated medially, based on a distal periosteal and cortical hinge, and fixed in its new location with a screw.

us from performing an osseous realignment procedure. When surgical means are required to treat the growing child, we have found the proximal quadricepsplasty as recommended by Green to be quite satisfactory[70] (see Fig. 13–8). A recent long-term review of such patients suggests that early treatment is necessary, as the presence of degenerative articular changes at the time of the index procedure frequently demonstrated deterioration of clinical outcome over time.[71]

The Galleazzi semitendinosus transfer provides another reliable means of stabilizing recalcitrant cases of skeletally immature patellar instability[72] (Fig. 13–20). Our indications for using this procedure include the presence of open physes, significant deformity distal to the patella, and patellotrochlear hypoplasia associated with generalized ligamentous laxity. We often combine this procedure with a lateral release and a proximal quadricepsplasty to passively restrain the patella from lateral translation. When performed at an early age, this procedure encourages patellofemoral modeling of plastic articular cartilage to deepen the trochlear sulcus and thus improve the presenting degree of anatomic dysplasia. If symptoms recur or persist into adulthood, a formal osseous realignment procedure is used.

Congenital Dislocation of the Patella

The etiology of patellar dislocations present at birth remains obscure. A number of in utero and perinatal insults, including trauma, muscle ischemia and subsequent fibrosis, and abnormal muscular and fascial attachments, have been implicated. Some evidence suggests that congenital dislocations have a genetic basis of development through an autosomal dominant mode of transmission.[73] The most favored mechanism of congenital patellar dislocation relates to the failure of normal internal rotation of the myotome containing the quadriceps femoris and patella.[74] Despite a high association with concomitant genetic disorders, congenital patellar dislocation does occur in otherwise normal children.[75]

The true incidence of congenital patellar dislocation is unknown because the diagnosis is often delayed until functional deficits or deformity lead the parents to seek orthopedic evaluation of the child.

The clinical presentation of congenital patellar dislocation varies with the age of the child. Stanisavljevic et al suggested that dislocations could be either permanent and irreducible or unstable and capable of being

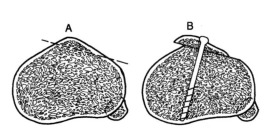

Figure 13–19. An oblique osteotomy of the tibial tubercle transfer permits elevation of the tubercle as it is shifted medially.

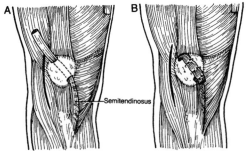

Semitendinosus

Figure 13–20. Semitendinosus transfer is performed through a drill hole in the patella, with tensioning of the free end of the tendon as it is sutured over the patella and back to itself.

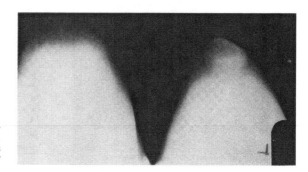

Figure 13–21. Bilateral Merchant radiographs demonstrating a congenital dislocation of the right knee. The patella and trochlea are hypoplastic. The patella is fixed to the lateral aspect of the distal femur. Early trochlear arthrosis is present.

manually reduced.[74] The incidence of bilateral involvement ranges from 10 to 30%.[75,76] In infants and toddlers, the only finding may be an inability to passively fully extend the knee. The hypoplastic patella may be palpated outside the trochlear groove along the lateral femoral condyle but frequently is too small to be manually identified.

As the child ages, secondary musculoskeletal deformities result from the altered biomechanical forces acting on the knee. A flexion contracture, valgus deformity, and external rotation of the tibia develop from the resultant force vector of the quadriceps femoris, which falls posterior and lateral to the axis of knee motion. A painless limp noted at the onset of walking or a deterioration of established gait often heralds the presence of the disease.

Ossification of the patella, which normally occurs at 3 to 5 years of age, may be significantly delayed. Thus, plain radiographs are not diagnostic in young children; however, ultrasound examination has successfully identified unossified patella and is the preferred diagnostic study in this population.[77]

Once ossification has begun, plain radiographs reveal the severe skeletal dysplasia characteristic of this disorder. Patellar displacement and hypoplasia of the patella, lateral femoral condyle, and trochlear sulcus are well visualized (Fig. 13–21). In late-diagnosed cases, MRI defines the degree of associated bony deformity and the presence of degenerative changes in the articular surfaces.

Early surgical treatment of congenital patellar dislocation prior to the development of secondary deformity provides the best chance of achieving normal function. A variety of soft tissue procedures have been successfully used. As a rule, surgery must address the following pathologic tissue changes present in this condition: contracture of the quadriceps femoris and, in particular, the vastus lateralis; contracture of the iliotibial band and lateral retinaculum and capsule; attenuation of the vastus medialis and medial retinaculum

and capsule; and lateralized insertion of the patellar ligament.

Stanisavljevic et al recommended a subperiosteal realignment of the extensor compartment.[74] Gao et al achieved 87.5% satisfactory results by combining a lateral release, medial plication, advancement of the vastus medialis, quadriceps femoris lengthening, and a Goldthwait procedure as needed.[76] A satisfactory result was defined as an asymptomatic patient possessing full knee flexion and no extensor lag.

In our experience, complete lateral release and medial capsular imbrication have been successful. When significant deformity below the patella exists, the proximal quadricepsplasty as described by Green and/or the Galleazzi procedure may be used. We defer formal osseous extensor mechanism realignment until skeletal maturity has been obtained. Following 3 to 6 weeks of immobilization, rehabilitation of the extensor mechanism is crucial in achieving satisfactory results.

In summary, early treatment of congenital dislocation of the patella prior to the development of secondary deformity provides the best opportunity for achieving normal function by restoring patellofemoral biomechanics, by encouraging normal patellotrochlear cartilaginous modeling, and by preventing early articular degenerative change.

Patellar Dislocation Associated With Genetic Syndromes

A variety of genetic syndromes leading to generalized ligamentous laxity have been described.[78] Down's syndrome, in particular, has been frequently associated with patellar instability and dislocation (Fig. 13–22). The incidence of patellar dislocation ranges from 5 to 10% of Down's patients.[79,80] In addition to patellar dislocation, subluxation of the atlantoaxial joint and dislocation of the hip joint are well characterized and are ascribed to abnormal joint laxity and muscle hypotonia. Despite the prevalence of patellar dislocation in

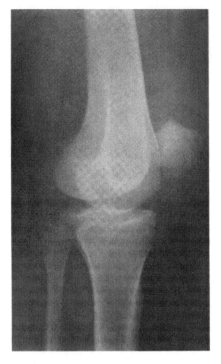

Figure 13–22. Radiograph of a lateral patellar dislocation in a patient with Down's syndrome.

Down's patients, individuals are rarely disabled. There appears to be no correlation between increasing patellofemoral instability and progressive loss of functional status.[81]

Because of problems related to low intelligence, obesity, and soft tissue quality, careful selection of surgical candidates has been stressed by Watanabe et al.[82] Matsusue et al recommended primary orthotic treatment for subluxation or reducible patellar dislocation.[83] Other authors have reported satisfactory results in patients with permanent chronic patellar dislocations and secondary deformity by using double upright knee braces.

Surgical management may be effective when conservative care fails. Mendez et al recommend lateral release and medial soft tissue imbrication for the individual who presents with pain, frequent falls, and an absence of secondary deformities.[81] Eighty-six percent of operated Down's patients with poor or fair preoperative ambulatory status become "good" ambulators after appropriate surgical intervention.

Our experience indicates that the vast majority of patellar instability associated with Down's syndrome

and other genetic syndromes is managed satisfactorily by conservative means. Indications for surgical intervention are similar to those recommended by Mendez et al.[81]

Additionally, we would consider acute repair in a good community ambulator who sustains an acute dislocation complicated by residual patellar tilt or subluxation and in the presence of a displaced intraarticular fracture. We tend to be more aggressive surgically in the acute setting because patient intelligence limits their ability to participate in a rehabilitative exercise program. Thus we recommend anatomic restoration of the disrupted capsular tissues in these selected patients.

Summary

Patellar dislocations represent a diverse spectrum of clinical disease. Acute dislocations affect the normal as well as the dysplastic knee. A classification of patellar instability should reflect varying degrees of anatomic dysplasia, as such features predispose individuals to pain and recurrent disability.

Orthopedic management of the unstable extensor mechanism should be customized to the needs of each patient to restore normal patellofemoral biomechanics. The presence of a highly motivated patient, a supportive physician, and a diagnosis-specific treatment plan will help to ensure the clinical success of nonoperative and surgical modalities alike.

References

1. Bradford EH, Lovett RW. *Treatise on Orthopaedic Surgery*. New York: William Wood & Company; 1905.
2. Duchenne GB; Kaplan EB, trans. *Physiology of Motion*. Philadelphia: JB Lippincott; 1949.
3. Huebscher C. Ueber Operationen bei Habitueller Luxation der Kniescheibe. *Z Orthop Chir*. 1909;24:1.
4. Hoffa A. Zur Behandlung der habitueller Patellarluxation. *Arch F Klin Chir*. 1899;59:543.
5. Goldthwait JE. Slipping or recurrent dislocation of the patella. *Boston Med Surg J*. 1904;150:169.
6. Bick EM. *Source Book of Orthopaedics*. 2nd ed. Baltimore: Williams & Wilkins; 1948:362–363.
7. Jones R. *Orthopaedic Surgery of Injuries*. London: Frowde, Hodder & Stoughton; 1921;321.
8. Hauser ED. Total tendon transplant for slipping patella. A new operation for recurrent dislocation of the patella. *Surg Gynecol Obstet*. 1938;66:199.
9. Aleman O. Chondromalacia post-traumatica patella. *Acta Chir Scand*. 1928;63:149.
10. Owre A. Chondromalacia patellae. *Acta Chir Scand*. 1936;77(Suppl):41.
11. Hughston JC. Subluxation of the patella. *J Bone Joint Surg Am*. 1968;50:1003.
12. Ficat RP, Hungerford DS. *Disorders of the Patellofemoral Joint*. Baltimore: Williams & Wilkins; 1977.
13. Merchant AC. Patellofemoral disorders: Biomechanics, diagnosis, and nonoperative treatment. In: McGinty JB, ed. *Operative Arthroscopy*. New York: Raven Press; 1990;273.

14. Vainionpaa S, Laasonen E, Patiala H, et al. Acute dislocation of the patella: Clinical, radiographic, and operative findings in 64 consecutive cases. *Acta Orthop Scand.* 1986;57:331.
15. Martinez S, Korobkin M, Fondren FB, et al. Diagnosis of patellofemoral malalignment by computed tomography. *J Comput Assist Tomogr.* 1983;7:1050.
16. Inoue M, Shino K, Hirose H, et al. Subluxation of the patella: Computed tomography analysis of patellofemoral congruence. *J Bone Joint Surg Am.* 1988;70:1331.
17. Kujala UM, Osterman K, Kormano M, et al. Patellofemoral relationships in recurrent patellar dislocation. *J Bone Joint Surg Am.* 1989;71:788.
18. Cofield RH, Bryan RS. Acute dislocation of the patella: Results of conservative treatment. *J Trauma.* 1977; 17:526.
19. Cash JD, Hughston JC. Treatment of acute patellar dislocation. *Am J Sports Med.* 1988;16(3):244.
20. Hawkins RJ, Bell RH, Anisette G. Acute patellar dislocations. *Am J Sports Med.* 1986;14(2):117.
21. Henry JH, Crossland JW. Conservative treatment of patellofemoral subluxation. *Am J Sports Med.* 1979; 7(1):12.
22. Hughston JC, Walsh WM. Proximal and distal reconstruction of the extensor mechanism for patellar subluxation. *Clin Orthop.* 1979;144:36.
23. Larsen E, Lauridsen F. Conservative treatment of patellar dislocation. Influence of evident factors on the tendency to redislocation and therapeutic result. *Clin Orthop.* 1982;171:131.
24. Sargent JR, Teipner WA. Medical retinacular repair for acute and recurrent dislocation of the patella: A preliminary report. *J Bone Joint Surg Am.* 1971;53:386.
25. Boring TH, O'Donoghue DH. Acute patellar dislocation: Results of immediate surgical repair. *Clin Orthop.* 1978; 136:182.
26. Fondren FB, Goldner JL, Bassett FH. Recurrent dislocation of the patella treated by modified Roux–Goldthwait procedure. *J Bone Joint Surg Am.* 1985;67:993.
27. Yamamoto RK. Arthroscopic repair of the medial retinaculum and the capsule in acute patellar dislocations. *Arthroscopy.* 1986;2:125.
28. Dainer RD, Barrack RL, et al. Arthroscopic treatment of acute patellar dislocations. *Arthroscopy.* 1988; 4(4):267.
29. Ten Thije JH, Frima AJ. Patellar dislocation and osteochondral fractures. *Neth J Surg.* 1986;38(5):5.
30. Vainionpaa S, Laasonen E, Silvennoinen T, et al. Acute dislocation of the patella: A prospective review of operative treatment. *J Bone Joint Surg Br.* 1990;72:366.
31. Harilainen A, Myllynen P. Operative treatment in acute patellar dislocation. *Am J Knee Surg.* 1988;1:178.
32. Jensen CM, Roosen JU. Acute traumatic dislocations of the patella. *J Trauma.* 1985;25:160.
33. Speer K, Spritzer C, Goldner J, et al. Magnetic resonance imaging of traumatic knee articular cartilage injuries. *Am J Sports Med.* 1991;19:396.
34. Micheli LJ. Special considerations in children's rehabilitation programs. In: Hunter LY, Funk FJ Jr, eds. *Rehabilitation of the injured knee.* St Louis: CV Mosby; 1984;406.
35. DeHaven K, Dolan W, Mayer P. Chondromalacia patellae in athletes. *Am J Sports Med.* 1979;7:5.
36. Henry JH. Conservative treatment of patellofemoral subluxation. *Clin Sports Med.* 1989;8(2):261.
37. Ogden JA. *Skeletal Injury in the Child.* Philadelphia: WB Saunders; 1990;768.
38. Micheli LJ, Slater J, Woods E, et al. Patella alta and the adolescent growth spurt. *Clin Orthop.* 1986;213:159.
39. Ficat RP, Philippe J, Hungerford DS. Chondromalacia patellae: A system of classification. *Clin Orthop* 1979; 144:55.
40. Insall J, Aglietti P, Tria Jr AJ. Patellar pain and incongruence. II. Clinical application. *Clin Orthop.* 1983; 176:225.
41. Radin EL, Paul IL. Response of joints to impact loading, I. In vitro wear. *Arthritis Rheum.* 1971;14:356.
42. Repo RU, Finlay JB. Survival of articular cartilage after controlled impact. *J Bone Joint Surg Am.* 1977;59:1068.
43. Zimmerman NB, Smith DG, Pottenger LA, et al. Mechanical disruption of human patellar cartilage by repetitive loading in vitro. *Clin Orthop.* 1988;229:302.
44. Mankin HJ. The response of articular cartilage of mechanical injury. *J Bone Joint Surg Am.* 1982;64:460.
45. Insall J, Falvo KA, Wise DW. Chondromalacia patellae: a prospective study. *J Bone Joint Surg Am.* 1976;58:1.
46. Maquet P. Mechanics and osteoarthritis of the patellofemoral joint. *Clin Orthop.* 1979;144:70.
47. O'Neill DB, Micheli LJ, Warner JP. Patellofemoral stress. A prospective analysis of exercise treatment in adolescents and adults. *Am J Sports Med.* 1992;20:151.
48. Pearson CY. Aftertreatment of lateral dislocation of the patella by a new form of knee cap. *Lancet.* 1884;1:1.
49. MacAusland WR, Sargent AF. Recurrent dislocation of patella. *Surg Gynecol Obstet.* 1922;35:35.
50. Hughston JC. Patellar subluxation: A recent history. *Clin Sports Med.* 1989;8:153.
51. McMillen W, Roncarati A, Koval P. Static and isokinetic treatments of chondromalacia patella: A comparative investigation. *J Orthop Sport Phys Ther.* 1990;12:256.
52. Hughston JC, Deese M. Medial subluxation of the patella as a complication of lateral retinacular release. *Am J Sports Med.* 1988;16:383.
53. Simmons E Jr, Cameron JC. Patella alta and recurrent dislocation of the patella. *Clin Orthop.* 1992;274:265.
54. Crosy EB, Insall J. Recurrent dislocation of the patella: Relationship to treatment to osteoarthritis. *J Bone Joint Surg Am.* 1976;58:9.
55. DeCesare WF. Late results of Hauser procedure for recurrent dislocation of the patella. *Clin Orthop.* 1979; 140:137.
56. Hampson WG, Hill P. Late results of transfer of the tibial tubercle for recurrent dislocation of the patella. *J Bone Joint Surg Br.* 1975;57:209.
57. Betz RR, Lonergan R, et al. The percutaneous lateral retinacular release. *Orthopaedics.* 1982;5(1):57.
58. Ceder LC, Larson RL. Z-plasty lateral retinacular release for the treatment of patellar compression syndrome. *Clin Orthop.* 1979;144:110.
59. Chen SC, Ramanathan EBS. The treatment of patellar instability by lateral release. *J Bone Joint Surg Br.* 1984; 66:344.
60. Grana WA, Hinkley B, Hollingsworth S. Arthroscopic evaluation and treatment of patellar malalignment. *Clin Orthop.* 1984;186:122.
61. Larsen RL, Cabaud HE, Slocum DB, et al. The patellar compression syndrome: Surgical treatment by lateral retinacular release. *Clin Orthop.* 1978;134:158.
62. McGinty JB, McCarthy JC. Endoscopic lateral retinacular release. A preliminary report. *Clin Orthop.* 1981; 158:120.
63. Merchant AC, Mercer RL. Lateral release of the patella—A preliminary report. *J Bone Joint Surg Am.* 1973;55:422.

64. Merchant AC, Mercer RL. Lateral release of the patella. *Clin Orthop.* 1974;103:40.
65. Metcalf RW. An arthroscopic method for lateral release of the subluxating or dislocating patella. *Clin Orthop.* 1982;167:9.
66. Micheli LJ, Stanitski CL. Lateral patellar retinacular release. *Am J Sports Med.* 1981;9:330.
67. Sherman OH, Fox JM, Sperling H, et al. Patellar instability: Treatment by arthroscopic electrosurgical lateral release. *Arthroscopy.* 1987;3(3):152.
68. Cox JS. Evaluation of the Roux–Elmslie–Trillat procedure for knee extensor realignment. *Am J Sports Med.* 1982;10:303.
69. Trillat A, Dejour H, Coutette A. Diagnostic et traitement des subluxations recideventes de la tule. *Rev Chir Orthop.* 1964;50:813.
70. Green WT. Recurrent dislocation of the patella—Its surgical correction in the growing child. *J Bone Joint Surg Am.* 1965;47:1670.
71. Laurencin CT, Silver SA, Tannenbaum BA, et al. Late results of the Green quadricepsplasty for recurrent dislocation of the knee. *Clin J Sports Med.* 1992; 2(4):244.
72. Hall JE, Micheli LJ, McManama GB Jr. Semitendinosus tenodesis for recurrent subluxation or dislocation of the patella. *Clin Orthop.* 1979;144:31.
73. Borochowitz Z, Soudry M, et al. Familial recurrent dislocation of patella with autosomal dominant mode of inheritance. *Clin Genet.* 1988;33:1.
74. Stanisavljevic S, Zemenick G, Miller D. Congenital, irreducible, permanent lateral dislocation of the patella. *Clin Orthop.* 1976;116:190.
75. McCall RE, Lessenberry HB. Bilateral congenital dislocation of the patella. 1987;7:100.
76. Gao GX, Lee EH, Bose K. Surgical management of congenital and habitual dislocation of the patella. *J Pediatr Orthop.* 1990;10:255.
77. Walker J, Rang M, Daneman A. Ultrasonography of the unossified patella in young children. *J Pediatr Orthop.* 1991;11:100.
78. McKusick VA. *Heritable Disorders of Connective Tissue.* 4th ed. St. Louis: CV Mosby; 1972.
79. Diamond LS, Lynn D, Sigmund B. Orthopaedic disorders in patients with Down's syndrome. *Orthop Clin North Am.* 1981;12(1):57.
80. Dugdale TW, Renshaw TS. Instability of the patellofemoral joint in Down's syndrome. *J Bone Joint Surg Am.* 1986;68:405.
81. Mendez A, Keret D, MacEwen G. Treatment of patellofemoral instability in Down's syndrome. *Clin Orthop.* 1988;234:148.
82. Watanabe R, Akashi K, Morii S. A case of bilateral dislocation associated with Down's syndrome. *Knee.* 1986;12:7.
83. Matsusue Y, Ueno T, Yamamuro T. Effective treatment by orthosis of dislocation of the patella associated with Down's syndrome: A case report. *Arch Jpn Chir.* 1991;60(3):189.

Part 4
Ligaments and Menisci

14

Anterior Cruciate Ligament Injuries

Charles H. Brown, Jr. and Mark E. Steiner

The anterior cruciate ligament (ACL) is the most frequently injured ligament in the knee. In a prospective study involving members of a Southern California Health Maintenance Organization (San Diego Kaiser–Permanente), Miyasaka et al reported an incidence of 60 people per 100,000 members with pathologic knee motion (≥ 3 mm KT-1000 arthrometer side-to-side difference) following an acute injury to the knee.[1] The ACL accounted for approximately 50% of these injuries, making it the most frequently injured knee ligament.

On the basis of these data, there are an estimated 90,000 acute injuries to the ACL each year in the United States. Because of the increased emphasis on and participation in sporting activities of all age groups, the treatment of ACL injuries will continue to challenge the orthopedic surgeon. The goals of this chapter are to discuss the diagnosis, operative management, postoperative rehabilitation, and results of surgical treatment of ACL injuries.

Diagnosis

History

> Please listen to the patient, he's trying to tell you what disease he has.
>
> Michael H. Brooke
> A Clinician's View of Neuromuscular Disease

Today because of increased reliance on sophisticated diagnostic tests, there is often a tendency for the busy clinician to ignore or skip over history taking during the evaluation of a patient suspected of having an acute knee injury. This is a mistake, as much valuable information can be obtained from the history if the clinician bothers to take the time to obtain it. As in other fields of medicine, the diagnosis of a pathologic process first begins by obtaining an accurate history. It is the history that guides the clinician during the physical examination and dictates the selection of diagnostic tests.

For patients suspected of having a knee ligament injury it is important to inquire about the following:

1. Mechanism of injury
2. Pain
3. Feeling or hearing a "pop"
4. Feeling that the knee "gave way" or went "out of place"
5. Ability to continue playing
6. Swelling
7. Loss of knee motion
8. History of previous knee injuries

The history of a patient who has sustained an injury to the ACL is fairly typical. Most "isolated ACL" injuries occur as a result of noncontact, deceleration, hyperextension, twisting, and pivoting mechanisms.[2-8] Patients often describe a feeling of the joint "going out of place," and approximately 40 to 65% feel or hear a "pop" at the time of the injury.[2-4,7] The injury is followed by an inability to continue playing and joint swelling within 24 hours.[2-4,7] Any patient who gives a history similar to the preceding should be suspected of having an ACL injury until proven otherwise.

In many cases the patient will seek treatment at the local emergency room where radiographs of the knee are taken and usually reveal no acute bony injury. In some patients the correct diagnosis is established and the patient is referred to an orthopedic surgeon for further evaluation and treatment. In many cases, however, the patient is told that he or she has a "sprained knee" and is given crutches, an elastic bandage, and knee immobilizer. Following the acute injury, within a few weeks there is usually a significant improvement in pain, swelling, and range of motion of the knee. Many patients attempt to return to athletics only to find that the knee is undependable or unstable. The patient usually seeks orthopedic consultation after repeated episodes of giving way, pain, and swelling. At that time the diagnosis of an ACL tear is usually made.

Physical Examination

The role of physical examination of the injured knee is to establish which structures have been injured and to determine the severity of the injury. It is only after establishing an anatomic diagnosis that the orthopedic surgeon can determine the prognosis of the injury and select appropriate treatment options. Examination of the knee begins first with inspection, followed by palpation, ligamentous examination, and special tests. Following an acute injury to the ACL, or after a reinjury in a patient with a chronic ACL tear, the patient often walks with a limp and holds the knee in a flexed position because of pain, swelling, and hamstring spasm. Examination usually reveals an effusion and a loss of motion, particularly extension. Areas of ecchymosis should be noted, as they can indicate the location of damage to other structures. Areas of tenderness are often associated with patellar dislocations and meniscal and collateral ligament injuries.

Ligamentous examination of the knee is performed next. It is often helpful to examine the uninjured knee first to win the patient's confidence and to determine the motion limits of the normal knee. As it is the function of knee ligaments to limit motion between the tibia and femur, the hallmark of a knee ligament injury is an increase in motion, or abnormal motion, between the tibia and femur.[9-14] The status of the ACL is determined first. Biomechanical studies have established that the ACL is the primary ligamentous restraint to anterior tibial translation.[9,13,14] A tear of the ACL is followed by an increase in anterior translation of the tibia with respect to the femur.[9-15] This increase in anterior tibial translation can be clinically detected by both the Lachman and anterior drawer tests. According to Strobel and Stedtfeld, advantages of the Lachman test over the anterior drawer test include the following[16]:

1. The Lachman test is highly specific for the ACL.
2. The stabilizing affect of the posterior horns of the menisci are minimized.
3. Muscle relaxation is better.
4. A larger amount of anterior tibial translation is produced.

Clinical experience and biomechanical studies have shown that the amount of anterior tibial translation following a tear of the ACL is greatest when the knee is tested between 20° and 30° of flexion, versus 90° of flexion.[13,17] The increased joint motion at 20° to 30° is caused by a decrease in the contribution of the secondary restraints to anterior tibial translation, principally the posterior horns of the menisci.[17] Following an acute knee injury, testing the knee between 20° and 30° of flexion also provides for greater patient comfort and better muscle relaxation. Because of these factors the Lachman test is more sensitive than the anterior drawer test for the diagnosis of an ACL tear.[18-20]

Although the diagnosis of a torn ACL is confirmed by a positive Lachman test it is rotational tests such as the pivot-shift test and the flexion-rotation-drawer (FRD) test[4,7,14,21] that recreate the patient's sensation of giving way. In the acute injury situation it is sometimes difficult to perform a pivot-shift test because of pain and muscle spasm. In these circumstances the FRD test can often be performed and can provide similar information. The results of the pivot-shift test are graded as follows: grade I indicates normal physiologic laxity and no pivot; grade II, a slip or subtle subluxation but no jump, thud, or jerk; grade III, an obvious jerk or jump with gross subluxation and reduction; and finally grade IV, a gross subluxation with impingement of the posterior aspect of the lateral tibial plateau against the femoral condyle.[14] Clinical studies have shown that knees with a grade IV pivot shift have a particularly poor prognosis.[5,22,23]

The status of the collateral ligaments is determined by estimating the amount of joint space opening when varus and valgus rotations are applied to the knee at 0° and 30° of flexion.[24] It is particularly important to determine the status of the posterolateral structures because failure to recognize and treat acute or chronic posterolateral instability can result in failure of the ACL reconstruction.[25,26] Gersoff and Clancy have estimated that associated posterolateral laxity is present in 10 to 15% of chronic ACL-deficient knees.[25] The status of the posterolateral structures is determined by measuring the increase in external tibial rotation with the knee at 30° of flexion as compared with the normal knee[27,28] (Fig. 14–1). The increase in external tibial rotation can be measured by noting the increase in the angle between the thigh and feet or by measuring an increase in the Q-angle. A further increase in external tibial rotation when the knee is flexed to 60° and 90° indicates associated injury to the posterior cruciate ligament (PCL).[27,28] The reverse pivot-shift test can also be used to test the integrity of the posterolateral structures, but like the pivot-shift test, it can be difficult to perform in the acute injury setting.[29]

Special tests such as McMurray's test, which can be useful in the chronic knee to diagnosis a meniscal tear, may be difficult to perform because of pain and spasm in acute knees. As part of the general examination following an acute knee injury it is also important to carefully examine the patellofemoral joint. A patient with a

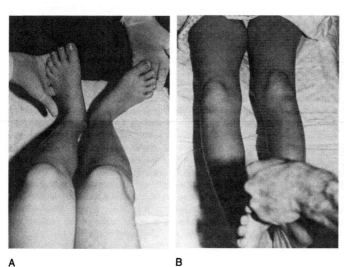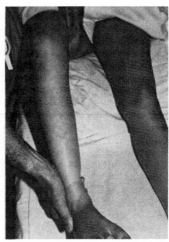

A   B   C

Figure 14–1. A patient with chronic ACL insufficiency and associated chronic posterolateral instability. Reconstruction of the ACL with a patellar tendon graft as well as allograft reconstruction of the fibular collateral ligament and popliteus tendon was required. **A.** Increased external tibial rotation at 30° indicating injury to the posterolateral corner (arcuate ligament complex and popliteus tendon).[27,28] **B.** Positive external rotation recurvatum test (Hughston). Note the external rotation of the tibial tubercle and apparent tibia vara resulting from an increase in external rotation and recurvatum of the tibia. **C.** Increased varus rotation at 30° of flexion indicating injury to the fibular collateral ligament.[24,27,28]

patellar dislocation can often present with a history of a noncontact, valgus external rotation injury, symptoms of giving way, and swelling—a history similar to that of a patient with a torn ACL. Dislocation of the patella is usually followed by ecchymosis and swelling along the medial side of the patella, tenderness over the medial patellar retinaculum, and a positive patellar apprehension test. In a patient with an isolated dislocation of the patella, ligamentous examination should reveal no increase in or pathologic tibiofemoral joint motion.

Although the diagnosis of an ACL tear can usually be made on the basis of the history and physical examination, instrumented knee laxity testing machines can also be used to establish the diagnosis of an ACL tear.[10–12,15,30] The most widely used instrumented knee testing machine is the KT-1000 arthrometer (MedMetric Co, San Diego, CA). The KT-1000 arthrometer allows the examiner to measure anterior and posterior translations of the tibia relative to the femur. Use of the KT-1000 and testing protocols have been well described.[10–12,15] In vivo and in vitro measurements of anterior tibial translation of normal knees and of knees with a torn ACL have also been reported.[10–12,15] Because of the large range of absolute measurements, Daniel et al introduced the concept of side-to-side, injured–uninjured, or left–right differences.[10,11] In 92%

of normal knees using an 89-N (20-lb) force, the side-to-side difference is 2 mm or less.[10] The mean injured–uninjured difference in acute ACL tears with an 89-N force has been reported to be 3.8 mm, with a mean manual maximum difference of 5.2 mm.[11] Clinical studies have also shown that a side-to-side difference of 3 mm or greater, using an 89-N (20-lb) force or a manual maximum test, is diagnostic of an ACL tear.[11] Instrumented laxity measurements have also been used during surgery to document satisfactory graft tension, to monitor anterior–posterior displacement during the early phases of the postoperative rehabilitation program and in reporting the results of knee ligament surgery.[30]

All patients with acute knee injuries should have as a minimum standard plain radiographs including anteroposterior, a lateral, and skyline or Merchant's views of the patella. A careful search on the anteroposterior radiograph should be made for a small avulsion fracture located near the tibial articular surface, at the most lateral point of the lateral tibial plateau, the so-called Segond fracture.[31–33] Woods et al demonstrated that the Segond fracture represents an avulsion of the middle one third of the lateral capsular ligament and is often associated with serious ligamentous injuries to the knee, especially the ACL.[33] Dietz et al reported that 75% of patients with a lateral capsular ligament avulsion had an associated ACL tear.[31] Therefore, the presence of a Segond fracture on a plain anteroposterior radiograph should alert the clinician to the possibility of injury to the ACL.

The routine use of magnetic resonance imaging (MRI) in the evaluation of patients with anterior cruciate ligament injuries is controversial. Magnetic resonance imaging (MRI) can provide information about injury to the menisci, cruciate ligaments, and collateral ligaments and occult osseous lesions. The major disadvantage of MRI is its high cost. The accuracy rate of MRI for the diagnosis of ACL tears has been reported to be between 95 and 100%.[20,34] Lee et al compared MRI with arthroscopy and clinical laxity tests in the evaluation of ACL tears.[20] The sensitivity (percentage of patients with disease = true-positive results divided by the sum of the true-positive and false-negative results) of MRI imaging was 94%, 78% for the anterior drawer test, and 89% for the Lachman test. The specificity (percentage of patients without disease = true-negative results divided by the sum of the true-negative and false-positive results) was 100% for all three. The results of this study are interesting in that they suggest that although MRI can provide very accurate information on the status of the ACL, clinical examination of the knee by an experienced knee surgeon is also quite sensitive.

Magnetic resonance imaging is clearly superior to clinical assessment in the diagnosis of meniscal tears. Fischer et al, in a multicenter study involving 1014 patients, compared MRI diagnosis with arthroscopy.[34] They reported accuracy rates of 89% for the medial meniscus (range 64–95%), 88% for the lateral meniscus (range 83–94%), 93% for the ACL (range 78–97%), and 99% for the PCL.

Treatment

Once the diagnosis of an ACL tear has been made the clinician must then select the optimal treatment plan for that particular patient. To determine the optimal treatment for any disease process, it is helpful to understand the natural history of the disease. The natural history represents the outcome of patients with the disease who receive no treatment. Unfortunately, there has never been a true natural history study of knees with a torn ACL. Most of the existing studies in the literature all have major shortcomings, including differing patient populations, a spectrum of associated injuries, and evaluation using different rating systems.[6] Although the existing studies in the literature are not true natural history studies, they do shed some light on the types of problems that can occur following a tear of the ACL.

Most of these studies have documented that a torn ACL causes a variable disability most often experienced with activities involving jumping, pivoting, and cut-ting.[2,3,5,6,23,35–37] The recent studies of Barrack et al[35] and Daniel et al[36] perhaps come the closest to being true natural history studies of the ACL-deficient knee.

Barrack et al reported on the outcome of a population of military personnel who underwent nonoperative treatment of an "isolated ACL" tear.[35] The study group consisted of 72 patients, average age 25, with greater than 90% being males who were active recreational athletes. All patients had an acute, complete (grade III) tear of the ACL proven by arthroscopy. Fifty-two patients (72%) had an associated meniscal tear diagnosed at the time of their initial arthroscopy. Patients with other associated injuries were excluded from the study group. All patients were treated with a standard rehabilitation program of early protected weight bearing, hamstring strengthening, delayed quadriceps strengthening, and protective bracing for sports. The patients were evaluated with a modification of the scoring system as described by Feagin and Blake.[38]

Nonoperative treatment in this uniform population produced 11% excellent, 20% good, 15% fair, and 54% poor results. Only 5% of the subjects could function at the same activity level as they did prior to injury, 87% had difficulty with cutting, and 72% had difficulty with jumping. Late reconstruction of the ACL was performed on 49% (35 of the 72 patients). The authors concluded that "young adults that return to a vocation requiring strenuous physical activity can expect unsatisfactory results most of the time following nonoperative treatment of an acute complete ACL tear."[38]

Daniel et al reported a prospective study of 294 patients at the Kaiser Hospital in San Diego who presented with an acute traumatic hemarthrosis.[36] The study population was divided into four groups: Group I (55 patients) consisted of patients who were felt to be stable based on their initial KT-1000 arthrometer scores (<3-mm side-to-side difference); this group was treated nonoperatively. Group II (149 patients) consisted of the "coper group," who on initial evaluation had unstable KT-1000 scores (≥3-mm side-to-side difference); this group was also treated nonoperatively. Group III (45 patients) consisted of patients with unstable KT-1000 scores who were treated with early ACL reconstruction. Finally, group IV (45 patients) consisted of patients with both stable and unstable KT-1000 scores who were initially treated nonoperatively but underwent late ACL reconstruction after developing functional instability. The incidence of secondary meniscus tears was reported to be 1.8% in group I, 9.4% in group II, 7.1% in group III, and 62% in group IV. Arthrometer measurements indicated that the reconstructed patients were more stable, with group II patients having a mean manual maximum of 5.0 mm versus 3.9 mm for the reconstructed patients in groups III and IV. Daniel et al concluded that ACL reconstruction decreased joint instability and the incidence of late meniscus tears, but the

Table 14–1 Indications for early ACL surgery Meniscus injury risk factors (MIRF).

MIRF	0	1	2
Age	>40	20–40	<20
Sports hrs/yr levels I and II sports	<50	50–200	>200
KT-1000 manual max injured-normal	<5	5–7.5	>7.5
Reparable meniscus	No		Yes

Level I Sports = Sport with cutting or jumping (football, basketball)
Level II Sports = Sport with lateral motion (racquet sport or baseball)
Early Surgery Recommended for MIRF > 3
Indications for Late ACL Surgery
•Disability Secondary to Anterior Instability
•MIRF > 3

reconstructed patients did not participate in cutting, jumping, or turning sports more than the patients who were not reconstructed. On the basis of their findings they felt that acute ACL surgery should be performed on patients at risk for secondary meniscus tears, and they developed a meniscus injury risk factor algorithm[36] (Table 14–1).

Early ACL surgery was recommended if the patient had a closed physis and a meniscus injury risk factor (MIRF) greater than 3. Indications for late ACL reconstruction included functionally disabling instability or a MIRF greater than 3. Because of the high risk of secondary meniscus tears, Daniel et al also felt that late ACL surgery might be indicated in some patients with open growth plates.

Other studies have also documented that the symptomatic ACL deficient knee is characterized by recurrent episodes of giving way, which occur primarily during athletic activities.[2,3,5,6,22,23,35–37] Repeated giving-way episodes can lead to meniscal and chondral injuries and, ultimately in some cases, to early joint arthrosis.[5,6,22,23] Therefore, the goal of patient selection following a tear of the ACL is to identify the high-risk patient and either to modify the patient's lifestyle by eliminating high-risk activities or to stabilize the knee surgically before significant joint damage occurs.

There are two distinct populations of ACL patients to treat: patients with an acute tear of the ACL and patients with a chronic tear. The management of patients with an acute ACL injury differs from those with chronic ACL tears. A patient with a chronic ACL tear has had an opportunity to experience the disability associated with their knee, while the acute patient has yet to appreciate the extent of disability from their injury. On the basis of data from their studies, Noyes et al have stated that an ACL tear will result in a functional disability in the majority of patients.[5,6,22,23] The disability will be manifested mainly with athletics in the majority of patients, but in some, it will affect activities of daily living. The degree of disability is amplified by certain risk factors. The more risk factors a given patient has, the more likely she or he is to experience functional dis-

ability related to the loss of the ACL. According to Noyes et al, risk factors for future disability related to the ACL include the following[5,6,22,23]:

1. High activity level
2. Participation in jumping, pivoting, or cutting sports
3. Presence of meniscal and chondral injuries
4. Large amount of anterior tibial translation (>15 mm)
5. Poor (lax) secondary restraints

On the basis of their data, Noyes et al proposed "the rule of thirds."[5] They suggested that approximately one third of patients with an acute ACL tear would compensate and be able to pursue recreational sports and would not need surgery. Another third would compensate but would have to give up significant activities involving jumping, pivoting, and cutting. Another third would do poorly, with many developing giving way with activities of daily living, and would probably require late reconstructive surgery. They also felt that the patient's activity level and goals were major factors to consider in the decision to perform acute ACL surgery. For the competitive athlete who "wants the best knee possible," surgery was recommended. For the nonathlete, activity modification and no surgery was recommended. The recreational athlete presented a problem patient. At the time of the study they felt that a wait and see approach, with possible late reconstruction, was justified. Advancements in biomechanics, along with improvements in surgical technique and postoperative rehabilitation, have resulted in higher success rates and have significantly reduced the morbidity of ACL surgery. As a result, many recreational athletes who wish to continue to participate in jumping and cutting sports may now elect to proceed with early reconstruction of the ACL rather than adopt a "wait and see attitude."

Present indications for acute ACL reconstruction include the following:

1. Athletically active patients with high activity levels who wish to continue to participate in cutting, pivoting, or jumping sports
2. Active patients with a complete tear of the ACL, and a complete tear of another primary restraint (ie, medial collateral fibular collateral, posterior cruciate ligament)
3. Athletically active patients with an acute ACL tear and a reparable meniscus

Indications for ACL reconstruction in chronic patients include the following:

1. Patients with functionally disabling giving way, who are unwilling to modify their athletic participation
2. Active patients with functional instability and reparable menisci

3. Patients who experience giving way with activities of daily living

Nonoperative Treatment

Nonoperative treatment does not mean no treatment.
Kenneth E. DeHaven, M. D.

It is not the purpose of this chapter to discuss in detail the nonoperative treatment of ACL injuries, but rather to present a brief description of the goals and methods of nonoperative management. For a more detailed discussion of nonoperative treatment, the reader is referred to articles by Minkoff and Sherman,[39] Nichols and Johnson,[40] Johnson et al,[41] and Shelbourne and Nitz.[42]

The initial goals of nonoperative treatment are to reduce pain, swelling, and inflammation and to restore a normal range of motion and muscle strength to the knee as quickly as possible. A knee immobilizer and crutches are used for comfort. These may be discontinued once the patient has good muscular control of the leg. Cryotherapy (Cryocuff, Aircast Inc, Summit, NJ), and nonsteroidal anti-inflammatory medications are useful to control pain, swelling, and inflammation. Physical therapy exercises are prescribed to restore a normal range of motion as quickly as possible. Muscle strengthening exercises for the quadriceps and hamstring muscles, as well as the other lower extremity muscles, are started as soon as possible. The goal is to restore the strength of the quadriceps and hamstring muscles to within 90% of the normal limb before beginning any athletic activities.

Patients are counseled to avoid high-risk activities involving jumping, cutting, and deceleration following nonoperative treatment. Straight-ahead activities such as jogging, biking, hiking, and swimming are encouraged. The use of a functional brace following nonoperative treatment of an ACL tear is controversial, and its role and effectiveness have not been fully established. Bracing has been shown to provide the patient with a sense of confidence, to prevent hyperextension, and to limit anterior tibial translation at low nonphysiologic loads. At higher physiologic loads, however, bracing has not been shown to be effective in limiting anterior tibial translation.

Operative Treatment

In the past, extraarticular reconstructions of the anterior cruciate ligament were advocated by many surgeons because of the lower surgical morbidity and complication rate compared with intraarticular reconstructions.[43,44] Biomechanical and clinical studies have now established that the ACL plays a major role in the maintenance of normal knee joint kinematics and stability.[9,21,45,46] As a result, most surgeons now feel

that it is important to try to reproduce the intraarticular anatomy and function of the ACL to best restore normal knee joint function.[21,46] A better understanding of the biomechanical requirements for intraarticular replacement of the ACL, along with improvements in surgical technique and postoperative rehabilitation, has significantly increased the success rate and reduced the morbidity and complication rate of intraarticular ACL reconstruction. Because of these advances, most surgeons have abandoned extraarticular reconstructions in favor of intraarticular reconstruction of the ACL.

What does it take to replace the human ACL? Successful intraarticular replacement of the ACL is based on the following principles:

1. Replacement with a high-strength graft
2. Proper graft placement
3. Proper graft tension
4. Elimination of graft impingement
5. Rigid graft fixation
6. Early motion and functional rehabilitation

In the sections that follow we discuss some of the basic science considerations for intraarticular replacement of the ACL.

The Basic Science of ACL Replacement

Biology of ACL Grafts

Biologic tissues used to replace the ACL can be divided into autogenous and allograft tissues. At the present time autogenous tissues are most frequently used. Of the autogenous tissues available the hamstring tendons (semitendinosus and gracilis) and the central one third of the patellar tendon are the most commonly used. Patellar tendon and Achilles tendon allografts are the most frequently used allograft tissues. The ultimate success of any biologic intraarticular ACL replacement depends on the ability of the replacement tissue to survive and maintain its initial biomechanical properties in the intraarticular environment of the knee. Because it is difficult to perform the necessary experiments in humans, animal models have most often been used to study the biology of ACL graft healing.

Animal studies have demonstrated that autograft tissues used to replace the ACL are essentially avascular at the time of their implantation.[47-52] The transformation of the avascular autograft tissues into a viable replacement for the ACL is a complex biologic process consisting of graft necrosis, revascularization, cellular repopulation, collagen deposition, and finally graft remodeling and maturation.[47-52] This complex biologic process has been referred to as *ligamentization*, as it results in a replacement structure that resembles the normal ACL grossly, histologically, and biochemically[48,49] (Fig. 14-2).

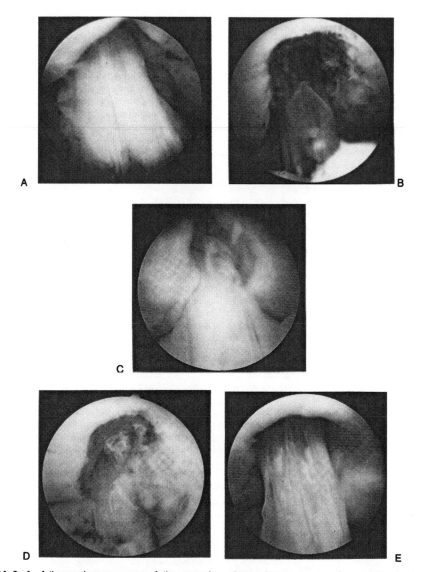

Figure 14–2. A. Arthroscopic appearance of the normal ACL. **B.** Initial arthroscopic appearance of a double-stranded semitendinosus and gracilis ACL graft. **C.** Arthroscopic appearance of the same hamstring graft 1 year postoperatively. The original tendinosus graft now has a ligamentous appearance and closely resembles the normal ACL. **D.** Initial arthroscopic appearance of a patellar tendon graft. **E.** Arthroscopic appearance of the patellar tendon graft 1 year postoperatively. Ligamentization results in a graft that closely resembles the normal ACL irrespective of the initial type of autograft tissue used.

The early phase of the ligamentization process consists of revascularization of the avascular graft. Animal experiments have demonstrated that a transplanted patellar tendon graft is revascularized by vessels that originate from three sources: (1) the fat pad, (2) the synovium, and (3) the drilled endosteal bone tunnels.[47,50–52] A recent human study by Schaefer et al used gadolinium–DPTA-enhanced MRI to evaluate postoperative autogenous patellar tendon ACL reconstructions.[53] Gadolinium–DPTA has been used as a contrast agent with T1-weighted, spin-echo imaging techniques, and results in a marked increase in signal intensity in highly vascularized areas. The authors reported that the maximum MRI enhancement of patellar tendon ACL autografts was present from 3 to 7 months postoperatively, suggesting that revascularization of the graft occurred during this period. The enhancement of the grafts occurred both peripherally about the intra-articular portion of the graft and within the drilled endosteal bone tunnels. These findings suggest that the origin and mechanism of graft revascularization in humans are similar to those seen in experimental animal models.

Following revascularization, the transplanted patellar tendon graft is covered by a synovial sheath, the vascularity being derived from the earlier mentioned sources. This "synovialization" of the graft occurs during the first 4 to 6 weeks following transplantation.[47–52] Based on their studies using a patellar tendon graft in Rhesus monkeys, Clancy et al have speculated that revascularization of human patellar tendon autografts is completed by 8 weeks.[52]

Following graft revascularization, the cell population of the autograft tissue must be reestablished. Amiel et al have shown in a rabbit model that transplanted patellar tendon autografts are repopulated by cells of extrinsic origin.[48,49] On the basis of their studies, they felt that the most likely source of these cells was the synovial membrane (undifferentiated type C synovial cells). Cellular repopulation of the graft was noted to start by 3 weeks and was completed by 4 to 6 weeks. By 30 weeks, histologic examination revealed that the cellular population of the replacement graft had been completely reestablished and the autograft had the appearance of a normal ACL. Based on the results of animal experiments it was postulated that a similar biologic process of graft healing occurs in humans. Recently, Rougraff et al have reported cell viability in human patellar tendon autografts as early as 3 weeks.[54]

The few human studies of ACL graft healing that have been reported have demonstrated that autograft and allograft tissues transplanted into the human knee joint appear to undergo the same biologic process seen in animal models. Alm and Gillquist performed seven open and six arthroscopic biopsies of the ACL in 13 patients who had undergone ACL reconstruction with the medial third of the patellar tendon autograft.[55] The shortest interval between the reconstruction and the biopsy was 3 months, and the longest was 5½ years. They reported that the transplanted patellar tendon autograft resembled normal ligament tissue in a subgroup of patients who had resumed full activity and who also had normal anterior stability following the reconstruction. By gross inspection, the reconstructed ligament was taut and had the appearance of a normal ACL in these patients.

In these patients, histologically there was a parallel arrangement of cells and collagen fibers, with a slight increase in cellularity of the transplant. The femoral attachment site of the ACL graft was placed in a nearly anatomic position, posteriorly and inferiorly, along the inner margin of the lateral femoral condyle. In the patient subgroups that were clinically unstable, the patellar tendon autograft was found to have a variable appearance. Histologically, the collagen fibers appeared to lack the normal parallel alignment, and there were bundles of collagen fibers that appeared to be disintegrating and fragmenting. Some graft specimens showed areas of marked vacuolar degeneration. In this subgroup of patients the location of the femoral attachment site was in a nonanatomic position, most often too anterior in the intercondylar notch.

In summary, the histologic appearance of the transplanted patellar tendon autograft seemed to parallel the clinical result and surgical placement of the graft. Anatomic placement of the autograft resulted in stable knees and histologically the graft seemed to resemble the normal ACL. Nonanatomic placement of the graft resulted in unstable knees and histologically a fragmented disorganized appearance of the graft. This work suggest that graft placement has a profound effect on the healing of the transplanted ACL graft.

The work of Shino et al has provided further experimental evidence that the biologic response of implanted tissues in humans closely parallels that seen in experimental animal models.[56] The authors performed replacement of the ACL in humans with allograft Achilles and anterior and posterior tibial tendons. Arthroscopic evaluation of the transplant was performed in 69 patients, with arthroscopic biopsies being taken in 23 patients. The interval from ACL reconstruction to arthroscopic evaluation ranged from 6 weeks to 55 months. At 6 weeks, histologic examination revealed that the ACL allograft was already covered by a thick hypervascular synovial sheath ("synovialization"). The vascularity seemed to originate from the infrapatellar fat pad. The allografts were noted to remain hypervascular from 3 to 6 months.

Histologic examination at 3 months revealed the allografts to be covered by a thick synovial sheath with viable fibroblasts in the substance of the graft. By 6 months, longitudinally aligned collagen bundles could be identified and the graft was noted to be hypercellular. By 11 to 12 months, the allografts had the gross appearance of a normal ACL. At 1 year, histologic examination revealed that, except for some hypercellularity, the allografts had the appearance of a normal ACL. The authors concluded that transplanted allograft tissue underwent early revascularization, with the vessels being derived from the host (principally the fat pad). Revascularization of the allograft was then followed by cellular repopulation, collagen deposition, and graft remodeling.

Kurosaka et al[57] and Abe et al[58] performed arthroscopic biopsies on 21 patients who had undergone intraarticular reconstruction of the ACL with a patellar tendon autograft. Biopsies of the patellar tendon ACL graft were obtained from patients at intervals ranging from 6 weeks to 15 months postoperatively. Biopsies of the donor patellar tendon as well as the normal ACL were also performed. All specimens were examined by both light and electron microscopy.

The authors reported that by 6 weeks, the patellar tendon autograft was covered by vascular synovial tissue. This "synovialization" of the graft subsided as the graft tissue matured with time. By 1 year, the patellar tendon graft had the gross appearance of a normal ACL. The cell population of the initially avascular patellar tendon autograft was reestablished by a fibroblast-like cell, and the graft was completely repopulated by 6 months. The cellularity of the grafts reached a maximum at around 5 to 8 months and decreased thereafter. By 1 year, the grafts still remained hypercellular compared with the normal ACL.

Light microscopic examination revealed that the collagen fibers of the patellar tendon autograft were longitudinally oriented and interspersed with spindle-shaped fibroblasts. The crimp pattern of the collagen fibers was similar to that of the normal ACL; however, examination of the autograft tissue by electron microscopy demonstrated that the fibroblasts found in the graft tissue were different from those found in the normal donor patellar tendon and the normal ACL. The fibroblasts from the ACL grafts were found to have a larger amount of cytoplasm as compared with fibroblasts found in the normal donor patellar ligament and the normal ACL. The endoplasmic reticulum and Golgi apparatus were especially prominent in the cytoplasm of fibroblasts from the patellar tendon ACL grafts, even at 1 year. The authors concluded that the prominent endoplasmic reticulum and Golgi apparatus in the patellar tendon ACL grafts reflected the active synthesis of extracellular matrix. They felt that this suggested that the patellar tendon ACL autografts were still undergoing cellular remodeling at 1 year.

Cross-sectional electron microscopic analysis of the patellar tendon autografts revealed that the collagen fibrils were densely packed and well organized; how-ever, small-diameter collagen fibrils were noted to be the predominant fiber type, with loss of the larger-diameter collagen fibrils being the most striking feature. This finding has been previously reported by Oakes et al.[59] Kurosaka et al[57] and Abe et al[58] concluded that human autogenous patellar tendon ACL grafts underwent ligamentization, as previously described in the rabbit model[48,49] and by 1 year gross and light microscopy examination revealed the graft to have an appearance similar to that of the normal ACL. Ultrastructural analysis revealed the presence of metabolically active fibroblasts, suggesting that the graft was still undergoing remodeling even at 1 year postoperation.

Rougraff et al reported on the histologic analysis of ACL graft tissue obtained from 23 patients who had undergone reconstruction of the ACL with a nonvascularized autogenous patellar tendon graft.[54] The biopsies were performed at intervals from 3 weeks to 6½ years after ACL reconstruction. All knees were reported to be stable, and there were no signs or symptoms of ligamentous instability before biopsy. Superficial biopsies of the ACL graft were performed in 6 patients and central or core biopsies in 17 patients. Biopsies of the donor patellar tendon were also taken as controls in 11 patients undergoing ACL reconstruction.

The results demonstrated that the transplanted patellar tendon autograft was viable in all specimens except for the central core biopsy of the 3-week specimen; however, the superficial biopsy of the 3-week specimen showed nuclear proliferation, increased metabolic morphology, and increased neovascularity, suggesting partial viability. The authors felt that the partial viability of the 3-week specimen suggested that the cells in the superficial portions of the transplanted graft were able to survive by synovial nutrition, or that these viable cells represented exogenous ingrowth.

The authors also identified four stages of ligamentization of the transplanted grafts. The first stage, repopulation, occurred in the first 2 months following transplantation. This stage was characterized by a modest increase in fibroblast number and metabolic rate and by early neovascular ingrowth. The second stage, rapid remodeling, occurred from around 2 months to 1 year. The fibroblast count, metabolic rate, and neovascularity were noted to rise dramatically compared with controls during this stage. The third stage, maturation, occurred from 1 to 3 years postoperatively. The graft gradually becomes less cellular, less vascular, and less metabolically active. A more mature collagen matrix was present, and the graft tissue was nearly ligamentous by this stage. By 3 years the grafts entered the stage of quiescence and had the appearance of normal ligamentous tissue. There were no significant changes in the graft tissue thereafter. Based on their observations, the authors concluded that patellar tendon autografts underwent revascularization within 3 to 6 weeks, followed by cellular repopulation, but that graft maturation was a much slower process than in rabbits as previously described by Amiel et al.[48,49]

Commensurate with ligamentization there is a change in the biomechanical properties of the ACL autograft. Animal studies have demonstrated that soon after implantation, there is a precipitous drop in tensile strength. This initial drop in tensile strength is followed by a slow gain in strength over time, but no study has shown whether the tensile strength of the graft returns to its initial value.[52,60,61] Clancy et al, in a study on Rhesus monkeys, reported that a transplanted medial-third patellar tendon autograft showed average ultimate tensile strengths (expressed as a percentage of the control patellar tendon) of 53% at 3 months, 52% at 6 months, 81% at 9 months, and 81% at 12 months.[52] The average ultimate failure strength expressed as a percentage of the control ACL was 26% at 3 months, 43% at 6 months, 38% at 9 months, and 52% at 12 months. Importantly, they noted that the Rhesus monkey control medial one-third patellar tendon autograft had an average ultimate failure strength of 300 ± 58 N, whereas the control monkey ACL had an average ultimate failure strength of 600 ± 132 N, indicating that the monkey patellar tendon was only about 50% of the initial ultimate tensile strength of the ACL. The reader should be aware that this situation has been found to exist in other animal models and so caution must be used in interpreting animal data in which graft strength is expressed as a percentage of the control ACL strength.[62] Since the initial strength of the patellar tendon graft at time zero is less than that of the control ACL, the highest tensile strength that the transplanted patellar tendon could ever obtain is its initial strength at time zero. Therefore, Clancy et al felt that a more representative measure of graft healing should compare the strength of the transplanted graft to its initial strength and not to the strength of the ACL.[52] When the authors analyzed the data in this fashion, they reported that the monkey patellar tendon autograft regained 80% of its initial preimplantation tensile strength and speculated that the same would be true for a human patellar tendon autograft. As no biomechanical studies have been performed on transplanted human patellar tendon autografts, it is unknown how the mechanical properties of implanted patellar tendon autografts change with time.

Extrapolation of the results of animal experiments to humans suggests that ACL autografts undergo a marked decrease in initial tensile strength during the first 12 weeks. This initial loss in tensile strength is followed by a gradual increase in strength over the next 9 to 12 months. As animal data have shown that the transplanted tissue never regains its initial tensile strength it is extremely unlikely that this would occur in humans. These findings indicate that any transplanted autograft tissue is strongest at the time of its implantation. It will be seen later that this principle is an extremely important consideration in the postoperative rehabilitation following ACL reconstruction.

In an effort to limit the loss in tensile strength of the ACL autograft and to try to accelerate the healing process, Noyes et al proposed the idea of a vascularized patellar tendon autograft.[62a] They felt that maintaining the blood supply to the patellar tendon graft would result in less necrosis and remodeling of the graft compared with an avascular graft, and this might accelerate the healing of the autograft and might also result in a substitute with a higher tensile strength. Their vascularized patellar tendon autograft was based on vascularity from the inferior medial geniculate artery. Other authors have proposed similar procedures with the vascularity of the graft being based on the lateral geniculate vessel[63,64]; however, experimental studies by Butler et al using a cynomolgus monkey model failed to show any significant time differences in the healing process or improvement in the mechanical properties of vascularized ACL substitutes from those of free grafts.[60] Butler et al also examined the influence of intermittent passive motion on free and vascularized autografts, and again found no significant difference in the mechanical properties with time between the two grafts. These studies led the authors to conclude "that neither intermittent passive motion nor maintaining graft vascularity improved the mechanical properties of the tissues."[60]

What are possible explanations for the loss in tensile strength of biologic grafts after ligamentization? Oakes et al in a study of human ACL autografts have shown that ligamentization results in a change in the original collagen profile of the graft from a structure that initially contains a significant percentage of large-diameter fibrils greater than 100 nm into a structure that contains primarily loosely packed small-diameter collagen fibrils less than 100 nm in diameter (personal communication, July 1993).[59] Ultrastructural determination of the collagen profile of the normal human patellar tendon has revealed that more than 50% of the total cross-sectional area is composed of tightly packed large-diameter collagen fibrils greater than 100 nm in diameter.[59] The semitendinosus also has a collagen fibril profile similar to that of the patellar tendon. The collagen fibril profile of the normal ACL is intermediate between those of the patellar tendon and semitendinosus. There is a bimodal distribution of tightly packed collagen fibrils, with 85% of the cross-sectional area being composed of small (<100-nm-diameter) collagen fibrils and the remaining 15% of the cross-sectional area being composed of large-diameter (>100 nm) fibrils.[59] Oakes et al have hypothesized that it is the tightly packed large-diameter collagen fibrils that are responsible for the high-tensile-failure loads of the patellar tendon and the normal ACL.[59]

The change in the collagen profile of the ACL autograft is thought to result from the inability of the extrinsic fibroblasts to produce large-diameter collagen fibrils. In fact, one measure of the completeness of the remodeling process is the change with time in the collagen profile of the autograft from large-diameter fibrils to small-diameter fibrils. McLean et al evaluated 101 human ACL grafts arthroscopically and histologically using electron microscopy.[65] The patients were 4 months to 20 years postoperative. The authors noted that irrespective of the type of tissue or the surgical technique used, the grafts were replaced by small-diameter collagen fibrils. This small collagen fibril pattern did not change with the passage of time. On the basis of their findings, the authors concluded that intraarticular ACL grafts act purely as scaffolds for synovium-derived fibroblasts to grow into. They felt that the final functional status of the graft was dependent on control of the inflammatory response and the ability of the host to initiate a maximum fibrous response. As the graft acts essentially as a scaffold, the authors felt that as long as the graft was placed so as not to break (isometrically) and securely fixed at both ends, then the final stability was not necessarily related to the initial mechanical properties of the graft. Some recent data (Oakes BW. Personal communication, July 1993) on the fibril size of patellar tendon autografts over time have revealed that the predominance of small fibrils continues out to 5 to 9 years, although in some specimens large-diameter fibrils do persist. Whether these large-diameter fibrils represent persistence of large fibrils from the original patellar tendon that have failed to remodel or re-formation of large fibrils is not yet known (Figs. 14–3 and 14–4).

In summary, ligamentatization of ACL autografts results in a structure composed almost entirely of loosely packed small-diameter collagen fibrils that seem to persist with the passage of time. The loss of the large-diameter collagen fibrils has been hypothesized as one cause of the decreased tensile strength of ACL replacement grafts.

A study by Jackson et al further supports that graft placement and tension may also play a major role in determining the biomechanical properties of an ACL graft following transplantation.[66] Using a goat model, these authors performed a complete kill of the cells of the ACL in situ by freezing. The opposite knee was used as a control. The animals were then rehabilitated, no postoperative immobilization being used. In essence, this model represented an anatomically positioned ACL graft under the correct tension. Animals were sacrificed at time zero, 6 weeks, and 6 months. Evaluation consisted of histology, vascularity, and biomechanical testing.

The results showed no statistically significant differences in anterior–posterior translation at 45° between the operated and control knees at time zero, 6 weeks,

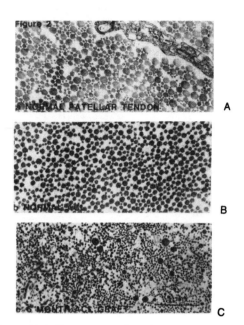

Figure 14–3. Transverse sections through the collagen fibrils of (A) normal young adult patellar tendon (18-year-old man), (B) normal young adult ACL (28-year-old man), and (C) patellar tendon ACL graft 12 months postoperatively. All micrographs ×34,100. The young patellar tendon has a group of large- and small-diameter fibrils (A). The normal young adult ACL (B) has fibrils that are intermediate in size between the patellar tendon (A) and the 12-month-old graft (C). Note the preponderance of small collagen fibrils in the 12-month-old patellar tendon graft (C). Occasional large fibrils are probably remnants of the large fibrils from the original ACL patellar tendon graft (A) that have not undergone remodeling. (Micrographs courtesy of Dr. Barry W. Oakes, Anatomy Department, Monash University, Clayton, Victoria, Australia.)

and 6 months, indicating that the freeze ACL was functioning mechanically as a normal ACL. Biomechanical testing revealed that there was a statistically significant decrease in the maximum load to failure of the ACL between the operated knees and controls at 6 weeks, but not at 6 months: at 6 weeks, freeze = 1915 ± 110 N and controls = 2274 ± 116 N; at 6 months, freeze = 2380 ± 184 N and controls = 2603 ± 213 N. Expressed as a percentage of the control ACL maximum load to failure, at 6 weeks the freeze ACL graft was 84%, and at 6 months, 91%. These values are much higher than previously obtained in the goat model. Tissue culture analysis of the grafts revealed that they were repopulated with fibroblast-like cells. Ultrastructural analysis demonstrated an increase in the relative proportion of small-diameter collagen fibrils between 6 weeks and

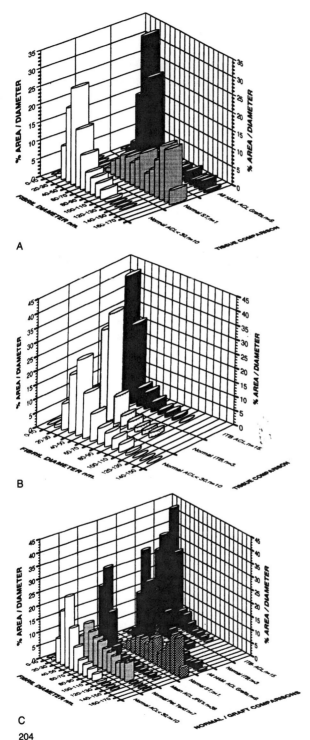

Figure 14–4. Three-dimensional histograms. **A.** Comparison summary of all hamstring ACL autografts greater than 1 year postoperation: hamstring ACL autografts, $n = 9$; Normal semitendinosus tendon, (ST), $n = 3$, now and the profile is the same; normal ACL, $n = 10$, <30 years old. Data are expressed as percent area/fibril diameter group. Note the large percent area (>50% of the total collagen fibril area) occupied by the fibrils larger than 100 nm in the semitendinosus tendon compared with the normal ACL. Also note the great predominance of small fibrils in the hamstring ACL grafts compared with the normal ACL. Almost 80% of the total cross-sectional area of the hamstring tendon ACL grafts is formed by collagen fibrils smaller than 100 nm. The loss of the large-diameter fibrils in the hamstring ACL grafts indicates substantial remodeling of the collagen fibril matrix of the semitendinosus tendon.

B. Comparison summary of iliotibial band ACL autografts greater than 1 year postoperatively (15 months to 6 years): iliotibial band ACL autografts (ITB ACL), $n = 15$; normal iliotibial band (ITB), $n = 3$; normal ACL, $n = 10$, <30 years old. Note the remarkable similarity of the collagen profiles of the normal ACL, normal iliotibial band, and iliotibial band ACL autografts. The significance of this unique observation is as yet uncertain and may be of biologic importance rather than clinical relevance.

C. Grand summary of normal ACL, $n = 10$, <30 years; normal patellar tendon (PT), $n = 7$, 30 years; normal semitendinosus tendon (ST) $n = 3$; normal iliotibial band (ITB, $n = 3$; compared with ACL patellar tendon Jones free autografts (ACL JFGs), $n = 39$; hamstring ACL grafts (HAM ACL), $n = 9$; and iliotibial band ACL grafts (ITB ACL), $n = 15$; expressed as percent area/diameter group. All ACL grafts in this graph were greater than 1 year postoperatively. Note the large area occupied by the large fibrils of the normal patellar tendon (PT) and especially the normal hamstring tendons (ST) (>50% of total area) compared with the normal ACL and all the ACL grafts. *All the grafts have predominantly small fibrils* expressed by the large percent area seen in the small fibril groups (<100 nm in diameter). This is especially so for the hamstring tendon ACL grafts (HAM ACL), in which the large-diameter fibrils are almost totally removed and replaced by small-diameter fibrils (<100 nm). Only a few large-diameter fibrils remain in the patellar tendon ACL autografts (ACL JFGs) at 1 year compared with the normal patellar tendon (PT). Note the remarkably similar fibril profiles of the normal iliotibial band (ITB) and the ITB ACL autografts noted in **B**. (Courtesy of Dr. Barry W. Oakes, Anatomy Department, Monash University, Clayton, Victoria, Australia.)

204

6 months postoperatively, a finding previously reported by Oakes et al,[59] Kurosaka et al,[57] and Abe et al.[58] The authors felt that this relative increase in the proportion of small-diameter collagen fibrils reflected the production of these fibrils by the fibroblast-like cells that had repopulated the graft.

The authors concluded from this experiment that correct isometric graft placement and tension play a major role in the "ligamentization" process, and that these factors, rather than graft vascularity or collagen fibril size, may be more important in determining the ultimate biomechanical properties of the transplanted ACL graft.

In summary, current experimental data suggest that the loss in tensile strength of biologic grafts following transplantation is multifactorial and includes both biologic and biomechanical factors. The data indicate that biologic ACL grafts are repopulated by synovium-derived fibroblasts that synthesize the collagen matrix of the revascularized graft. These extrinsic fibroblasts appear to be incapable of synthesizing or assembling large-diameter collagen fibrils. It is the large percentage of the cross-sectional area occupied by the large-diameter fibrils that is thought to be responsible for the high tensile strength of the patellar tendon, semitendinosus, and normal ACL. The exact reason for the inability of these extrinsic cells to synthesize large-diameter collagen fibrils is not presently known. One theory so far unproven is that the predominance of hyaluronate and other proteoglycans, which are synthesized in large amounts during the repair process, may interfere with collagen fibril assembly to form large-diameter fibrils (Oakes BW. Personnel communication, July 1993).[59] If the extrinsic cells responsible for collagen synthesis could be induced to produce large-diameter fibrils, then perhaps we would have a way to increase the final tensile strength of biologic ACL grafts.

Initial Graft Strength

The ideal ACL replacement graft should be easily accessible. Its removal should result in no donor site morbidity. The ideal graft should reproduce the normal insertion site anatomy of the ACL, allow immediate rigid fixation, and undergo rapid revascularization and healing at the fixation sites. Also, its final mechanical and ultrastructural characteristics should match those of the young human ACL. The ideal ACL replacement graft does not presently exist. At present, selection of an ACL replacement graft involves compromises. To make an intelligent decision about graft selection, the surgeon must consider the following factors:

1. Initial mechanical properties of the replacement graft
2. Healing response of the replacement graft

3. Morbidity of harvesting the graft tissue
4. Morbidity resulting from loss of the graft tissue
5. Initial fixation strength of the graft tissue
6. Biologic incorporation of the graft

Because animal experiments have shown that the final tensile strength of the ACL replacement graft is never greater than its initial tensile strength,[9,52] it is important to understand the structural properties of the normal ACL and tissues used to replace it.

Noyes et al measured the initial mechanical properties of the normal human ACL and autograft tissues commonly used to reconstruct the ACL.[67] The average age of their specimens was 26, similar to the age of patients commonly undergoing ACL reconstruction. In this study, the maximum tensile strength of the normal ACL was 1725 ± 269 N, with a stiffness of 182 ± 33 N/mm. Until recently, these values have been accepted as being representative of the normal young adult ACL.[68]

Noyes et al reported that of the autograft tissues tested, the central one-third bone–patellar tendon–bone unit (13.8 ± 1.4 mm wide) was the single strongest autograft, with an average ultimate failure strength of 2900 ± 260 N, or 168% of their normal ACL value.[67] The stiffness was reported to be 685.2 ± 85.6 N/mm, a value significantly greater than the normal ACL. They reported ultimate failure loads of 1216 ± 50 N for the semitendinosus (70% of their normal ACL value) and 838 ± 30 N for the gracilis (49% of their normal ACL value). The stiffness of the hamstring tendons was close to that of the normal ACL, with values of 186.1 ± 9.2 N/mm for the semitendinosus and 170.9 ± 11 N/mm for the gracilis. Based on the tensile strength values reported in this study, the central one-third patellar–tendon graft has become for many surgeons the "gold standard" for intraarticular replacement of the ACL.[69]

Woo et al, in a similar biomechanical study, have reported significantly higher structural values for the normal ACL.[68] In this study the specimen was tested in an anatomic orientation such that ACL fibers were tensioned in a more uniform manner. They reported that in younger specimens, mean age 29 years (range 22–35 years), the mean ultimate failure load was 2160 ± 157 N, with a mean stiffness value of 242 ± 28 N/mm. Importantly they also noted that the strength of the ACL was very age dependent, with older specimens showing lower values. These new data suggest that the young adult ACL is much stronger and stiffer than previously reported.

A recent study by Cooper et al on the tensile strength of the central-third patellar tendon reported ultimate failure loads of 4389 ± 708 N for a 15-mm-wide graft, 2977 N for a 10-mm-wide graft, and 2238 ± 316 N for a 7-mm-wide graft.[70] Rotating the graft 90° was found to increase the tensile strength by approximately 30%. The results of this new study suggest that central-third patellar tendon grafts commonly used in clinical practice (9–11 mm) may be much stronger than the extrapolated values from the Noyes et al data would suggest.[67]

As a result of Noyes and co-workers' study, many surgeons have questioned whether the initial tensile strength of hamstring tendons is sufficient to achieve predictable postoperative stability. Marder et al[71] and Larson[72] have hypothesized that doubling the semitendinosus and gracilis tendons could double the tensile strength of the combined grafts, at least in the section of the graft with the largest cross-sectional area. This assumes that equal tension is applied and maintained along each limb of the graft. Based on the data of Noyes et al, doubled semitendinosus, gracilis grafts would have an estimated tensile strength of 4108 N or approximately 250% of normal ACL strength.[67]

Although there have been no published biomechanical experiments to document that doubling a soft tissue graft will result in a doubling of the ultimate failure load, the data of Steiner et al[73] demonstrated an increase in the ultimate failure load of double-stranded semitendinosus and gracilis grafts (573 ± 109 N) versus single-stranded semitendinosus and gracilis grafts (335 ± 87 N) in a human cadaver model in which similar fixation techniques were used for both grafts.

In some recent work using human cadavers, Dr. Tim Sitter and Dr. William Grana (personal communication, June 1993) examined the strength and stiffness of double-stranded hamstring grafts. In some preliminary data they reported the average maximum load to failure and stiffness of a single-stranded gracilis graft were 823.8 N and 143.7 N/mm (five specimens, age 50). In one specimen (age 50) a double-stranded gracilis graft had a maximum load to failure of 1326.8 N and a stiffness of 197.4 N/mm. In three specimens (ages 50, 60, and 74) the average maximum failure load and stiffness for a double-stranded semitendinosus graft were 2362.9 N and 409.8 N/mm. These numbers are close to twice the values for a single-stranded semitendinosus graft as reported by Noyes et al (maximum load = 1216 N, stiffness = 186 N/mm).[67] Interestingly these numbers are quite high given the age of the specimens and suggest that the strength of the hamstring tendons may not be as age dependent as is the strength of the ACL.[67,68] They also reported maximum failure loads of 3560.9 and 3395.6 N for a 10-mm central-third patellar tendon graft from a 17-year-old man. These values are similar to those reported by Cooper et al.[70] In a 33-year-old male specimen the strength of a 10-mm central third patellar tendon had decreased to 2569.2 and 2670 N.

The authors felt that their data suggested that a double-stranded hamstring graft does significantly increase the maximum load to failure and stiffness compared with a single-stranded hamstring tendon graft. If further substantiated, these preliminary data would seem to further support that the mechanical properties of double-stranded semitendinosus and gracilis grafts are adequate to provide an acceptable replacement for the human ACL. Clearly, further biomechanical studies are needed to determine the exact effect on the maximum load to failure and stiffness of doubling a graft, as well as the effect of combining grafts with different mechanical properties. (See note added in proofs.)

Because of its cylindrical shape, a hamstring tendon graft has a significantly larger cross-sectional area compared with the commonly used 10-mm-wide patellar tendon graft. A 10-mm-wide patellar tendon graft with a thickness of 5 mm would produce a graft cross-sectional area of 50 mm², versus 63.6 mm² for a 9-mm-diameter double-looped hamstring graft. In fact, it would take a 12.7-mm-wide, 5-mm-thick patellar tendon graft to produce the same cross-sectional area as would a 9-mm hamstring graft. The increased cross-sectional area and tissue volume of hamstring tendon grafts result in a larger number of collagen fibers being placed across the joint compared with a similar-sized patellar tendon graft (Fig. 14–5).

The recent work of Howell et al also suggests that uncorrected graft impingement, irrespective of the graft source, is one of the major causes of graft failure.[74–79] Grafts placed so that they are free of impingement have better extension and instrumented laxity measurements, as well as a lower percentage of positive pivot shifts.[78,79] This work suggests that impingement-free graft placement may be more important than the actual graft source.

Finally, the prospective studies by Marder et al[71] and Aglietti et al,[80] in which both authors reported no statistically significant differences in knee stability or final knee rating between patellar tendon grafts and double-stranded hamstring grafts in chronic ACL-deficient knees, have somewhat negated the question of whether hamstring grafts can provide sufficient initial tensile strength for ACL reconstruction.

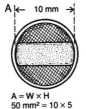 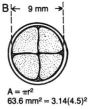

A |← 10 mm →|

$A = W \times H$
$50\ mm^2 = 10 \times 5$

B |← 9 mm →|

$A = \pi r^2$
$63.6\ mm^2 = 3.14(4.5)^2$

Figure 14–5. ACL graft cross-sectional areas. The typical-size hamstring tendon graft (9 mm diameter) has a significantly larger cross-sectional area because of its round nature versus a 10-mm-wide patellar tendon graft.

Donor Site Morbidity

Although one may debate the adequacy of the initial tensile strength and the fixation strength of hamstring tendon grafts versus the patellar tendon grafts, recent studies have suggested that hamstring tendon grafts are associated with fewer donor site complications.[71,80-84] Potential donor site complications of patellar tendon autografts include donor site pain, patellofemoral pain, patellar tendinitis, quadriceps muscle weakness, and the rare but devastating complications of patellar tendon rupture and patellar fracture.[85-97]

One of the major areas of controversy surrounding the issue of graft selection is the relationship of patellofemoral pain to graft source. Sachs et al reported a statistically significant effect of graft source on patellofemoral pain and quadriceps muscle weakness, with patellar tendon grafts having a higher incidence versus hamstring grafts.[83,84]

Recent reports of patellofemoral pain following arthroscopy-assisted ACL reconstruction with a central-third patellar tendon autograft have suggested an incidence of between 15% and 47%,[71,80-82,98-100] as compared with 3 to 21%[71,80-82,101] for hamstring tendon autografts. Aglietti et al, in a prospective randomized study, reported that 16% of patients undergoing arthroscopy-assisted patellar tendon reconstruction experienced patellofemoral pain versus only 3% of patients receiving hamstring tendon grafts.[80] This was the only statistically significant difference between the two graft sources.

Re et al evaluated the incidence of anterior knee pain in a prospective study of 187 patients with documented ACL ruptures.[82] The incidence of anterior knee pain in 50 patients treated nonoperatively was reported to be 22%. Preoperatively, 17% of patients undergoing ACL reconstruction using hamstring tendons were noted to complain of anterior knee pain, compared with 14% postoperatively (not statistically significant). For the allograft group the incidence of anterior knee pain was 22% preoperatively and 26% postoperatively (not statistically significant). The patients undergoing patellar tendon reconstruction were noted to have a 26% incidence of anterior knee pain preoperatively, compared with 47% postoperatively (highly significant, $P = .058$). The authors also reported a statistically significant increase in anterior knee pain between the patellar tendon and hamstring reconstruction groups ($P = .002$). The authors attributed the difference in anterior knee pain between the hamstring tendon reconstructions and the patellar tendon reconstructions to the morbidity associated with the donor site.

Patellar tendinitis also appears to be a more frequent complication following use of a central-third patellar tendon graft. Graf and Uhr reported that 6% of their patients complained of patellar tendinitis following ACL reconstruction with a patellar tendon graft.[90] Patellar tendinitis has been particularly common following use of the patellar tendon in basketball players (Demak R. "One False Move," *Sports Illustrated Magazine*, April 29, 1991). In their prospective study, Marder et al reported that 11% of their patients who underwent reconstruction with a patellar tendon graft experienced tenderness at the inferior pole of the patella with activities versus 0% with hamstring grafts.[71] Rubinstein and Shelbourne have reported an incidence of activity-related patellar tendinitis of 21%.[97] In another study investigating the donor site morbidity of harvest a patellar tendon graft from the opposite knee they reported the incidence to be 55%.[97] They felt that this was rarely a problem after the first year and could be minimized by using closed-chain exercises and activity modification.

Although rare, the devastating complications of extensor mechanism rupture and patellar fracture have been reported following harvest of patellar tendon autograft.[85,86,88-91,93-96] To our knowledge these complications have not been reported following harvest of the hamstring tendons.

The relationship of quadriceps and hamstring muscle weakness to graft source is controversial. For a complete discussion of this issue the reader is referred to the section on Complications.

Allografts have been proposed as an alternative to reduce potential donor site complications and morbidity resulting from the harvest of autograft tissues. For a thorough discussion of the role of allografts in knee ligament surgery, the reader is referred to the work of Jackson et al.[102,103] The proposed advantages of allografts include avoidance of sacrifice of the patient's own tissues, absence of donor site morbidity, and no size limitations. The disadvantages of allografts include the possibility of disease transmission and immunogenicity, alteration of the mechanical properties secondary to the sterilization process, and delayed incorporation compared with autografts.

Jackson et al recently reported a comparison of patellar tendon autograft and allograft ACL reconstruction using a goat model.[62b] Similar-sized patellar tendon autografts and fresh-frozen allografts were used to reconstruct the ACL in 40 female goats. Evaluations of the reconstructed and the contralateral control knees were performed at 6 weeks and 6 months postoperation. At 6 weeks the autografts demonstrated a maximum failure load of 12% of the control value, whereas the allografts were found to have a load 11% of the control ACL value. At 6 months the maximum failure load for the autografts had increased to 62% of the control ACL value, whereas that of the allografts had only increased to 27% of the ACL control value.

Comparison of the initial strength of the patellar tendon graft with that of the replacement ACL patellar tendon revealed that by 6 months, the patellar tendon autografts had approached the initial tensile strength of the donor patellar tendon, whereas the patellar tendon allografts were only approximately 50% as strong as the donor patellar tendon. The autografts were also noted to have a significantly larger cross-sectional area at 6 weeks and 6 months compared with allografts.

The allografts were noted to have more of the original large-diameter collagen fibrils remaining at 6 months compared with the autografts, suggesting a slower time course or incomplete remodeling. Histologic examination of the graft tissue demonstrated an increased and prolonged inflammatory response in the allografts compared with the robust response seen in the autograft. The authors concluded that at 6 months the autografts has significantly less inflammatory response, a more robust production of small-diameter collagen fibrils, and improved mechanical and structural properties compared with similar-sized allografts.

Noyes et al published the results of a large number of patients who had undergone allograft reconstruction of the ACL.[104–106] The first report consisted of 47 patients with acute ACL tears. The surgical procedure consisted of repair of the ruptured ACL and allograft replacement using bone–patellar tendon–bone and fascia lata allografts.[104] Using a very strict knee rating scale (Noyes–Cincinnati knee rating scale), 38% rated excellent, 51% good, and 11% poor. Testing with the KT-1000 arthrometer using an 89-N force revealed the following side-to-side differences:

	Bone–Patellar Tendon–Bone	Fascia Lata
<3 mm	83% (19/23)	53% (10/19)
3–5 mm	13% (3/23)	42% (8/19)
≥6 mm	4% (1/23)	5% (1/19)

The authors were encouraged by the results of the bone–patellar ligament–bone allografts in acute knees, but cautioned against their widespread use. They felt that allografts might be indicated for patients who were at risk for donor site complications, such as patients with preexisting patellofemoral chondrosis, extensor malalignment, narrow-width patellar tendon, and previous failed autografts.

In the second paper Noyes et al reported on 104 patients with chronic ACL-deficient knees.[105] In 64 patients intraarticular ACL reconstruction with an allograft alone was performed, and in 40 patients both intraarticular replacement of the ACL with an allograft and an extraarticular iliotibial band tenodesis were performed. This study demonstrated a significant difference in the overall knee rating score and KT-1000 arthrometer measurements, with the intraarticular allograft-alone group having the worst scores. The KT-1000 values for both groups were as follows:

	Intraarticular Only	Combined Intra- and Extraarticular
<2.5 mm	54%	74%
3–5 mm	34%	22%
≥6 mm	12%	4%

Forty-six percent of the chronic ACL-deficient knees with intraarticular allograft replacement alone had unsatisfactory anteroposterior arthrometer displacements compared with only 17% in their previous acute knee study. In contrast to the results of this study, previous studies involving autografts have reported no major differences between the results of intraarticular reconstruction alone and combined intraarticular and extraarticular reconstruction.[26,107] Because of the higher percentage of unsatisfactory arthrometer displacements the authors cautioned against the use of intraarticular allograft reconstruction alone in chronic knees.

In their third paper on allograft replacement of the ACL, Noyes et al reported the results of a prospective study of 115 chronic ACL-deficient knees.[106] In 66 knees, intraarticular reconstruction with an allograft alone was performed, and in 49 knees an intraarticular allograft and a ligament-augmentation device (LAD) were used. There was no significant difference in knee scores or arthrometer measurements between the two groups. The KT-1000 measurements were as follows:

	Allograft Only	Allograft + LAD
≤2.5 mm	53%	53%
3–5.5 mm	34%	30%
≥6 mm	13%	17%

In this report, 47% of the allografts alone and 47% of the augmented allografts had unacceptable anteroposterior displacements. The authors also reported that increases in anteroposterior displacements could occur as long as 3 years following implantation, suggesting that remodeling of the allograft in chronic ACL-deficient knees might require a long time.

The experience of their three allograft studies, which demonstrated a higher percentage of allograft knees with unacceptable arthrometer displacements compared with previous reports of autografts, and concerns about possible disease transmission have led Noyes et al to recommend use of an autogenous patellar tendon graft in chronic ACL-deficient knees[106]: "we recommend arthroscopically assisted implantation of an autogenous patellar-ligament graft in patients who do not have contraindications to reconstruction with an autogenous graft."[106]

One of the supposed advantages of using allograft tissue to replace the ACL is avoidance of the donor site morbidity associated with autograft tissues; however, a recent study by Lephart et al did not show any significant reduction in donor site morbidity for allografts compared with central-third patellar tendon autografts.[108] This study investigated the effects of graft source on quadriceps strength and power, thigh circumference, and functional tests. The authors reviewed 10 patients who underwent ACL reconstruction with a central-third patellar-ligament autograft and 10 patients who underwent allograft ACL reconstruction. The patients were an average of 18 months postoperative (range 12–24 months). All of the patients underwent a similar postoperative rehabilitation program. At follow-up, all patients were considered fully rehabilitated and had been released from formal rehabilitation. Quadriceps strength was measured using a Cybex isokinetic machine at testing speeds of 60° and 240° per second. The patients also performed four functional tests (hop test, one-leg jump, co-contraction, carioca, and shuttle run test).

The authors reported no significant differences in mean quadriceps peak torque, torque acceleration energy, or average power at both test speeds. The quadriceps index was 92 for the autograft patients and 95 for the allograft group. They also reported no significant differences between the two groups as far as the functional tests were concerned. The hop index was 95 for the autograft patients and 89 for the allograft group. The authors concluded "that harvesting the central one-third patellar tendon for grafting for ACL reconstruction may not compromise the function of the quadriceps mechanism. Thus, the rationale for selecting an allograft reconstruction for the purpose of preserving the quadriceps and its strength and power may be unnecessary."

The work of Jackson et al,[62b] Noyes et al,[104,105,109] and Lephart et al[108] suggests that the use of an allograft for routine uncomplicated ACL reconstructions offers few advantages. In addition to concerns about possible disease transmission and the effects of secondary sterilization on their mechanical properties, the rate of biologic incorporation, the ultimate tensile strength, and the cross-sectional area of allografts appear to be decreased compared with autograft tissues. Postoperative failure rates as determined by anteroposterior arthrometer measurements appear to be higher as well. The work of Lephart et al also suggests that there is no significant difference in donor site morbidity between autografts and allografts in uncomplicated ACL reconstructions.[108] On the basis of these results, allograft tissues are probably not the best initial graft source in patients undergoing routine uncomplicated ACL reconstruction.

Graft Selection

Although the patellar tendon autograft has often been referred to as the "gold standard"[69] for ACL reconstruction, we feel that at the present time there is no true "gold standard" and that graft selection should be individualized. As part of the preoperative evaluation process the surgeon must consider the preoperative status of the knee and the postoperative demands of the patient, and try to select an appropriate graft that will maximize postoperative stability but minimize donor site complications.

The advantages of the central-third patellar tendon graft are its high initial tensile strength, stiffness, and fixation strength. On the basis of these mechanical properties, we favor use of the patellar tendon in patients with chronic ACL-deficient knees and severe stretching of the secondary restraints (a grade IV pivot shift). Because of its greater stiffness we also favor use of the patellar tendon in patients with associated grade III medial or lateral collateral ligament injuries.

Because of the higher incidence of donor site complications, particularly patellofemoral pain and patellar tendinitis,[71,80–97] following use of the patellar tendon, we try to avoid using this graft source in patients whose preoperative status puts them at risk for these complications. Such patients include those with a preoperative history of patellofemoral pain, patellar subluxation or dislocation, or patellar tendinitis and patients who have injury to their dominant jumping leg who plan to return to jumping sports such as basketball and volleyball. Because of donor site pain over the tibial and patellar bone graft sites, patellar tendon grafts are avoided in individuals who must crawl, squat and kneel, such as mechanics, plumbers, and carpenters. A narrow-width patellar tendon is also a contraindication for use of a central-third patellar tendon graft.

The major advantage of hamstring tendon grafts is the lower incidence of donor site complications. We favor use of hamstring tendon grafts in patients at risk for donor site complications. This would include patients with a history of patellofemoral pain, patellar tendinitis, or patellar instability, patients with a narrow patellar tendon (less than 25 mm in width), and patients with injury to their dominant jumping leg who plan to return to jumping sports such as basketball and volleyball. Because of the lower incidence of donor site pain, hamstring tendon grafts are also favored in patients whose occupations require kneeling, crawling, and squatting. Contraindications to use of hamstring tendon grafts include patients who have had previous medial-sided surgery such as medial collateral ligament repairs and pes transfers. In these situations previous dissection and scarring may make it difficult to reliably obtain adequate length grafts.

In summary, hamstring tendon grafts are ideal in the acute setting where the secondary restraints are intact or minimally injured. Because of the lower graft and fixation stiffness values reported by Noyes et al[62] and Steiner et al,[73] we tend to avoid use of hamstring tendon grafts in patients with grade III collateral ligament injuries, particularly patients with injury to posterolateral structures and patients with very loose secondary restraints. This includes patients with generalized ligamentous laxity, patients with severe recurvatum of the knee, and patients with a grade IV pivot shift. We feel that the stiffness of the patellar tendon graft and the stiffness of interference screw fixation may offer an advantage in these cases.

Although the effectiveness of hamstring tendon grafts has been questioned by many surgeons, the recent prospective studies of Marder et al[71] and Aglietti et al[80] both failed to demonstrate any significant differences in stability or clinical outcomes of double-stranded semitendinosus and gracilis grafts versus patellar tendon autografts in patients with chronic ACL-deficient knees. As we have gained clinical experience using hamstring tendon grafts, we have widened our indications for using this graft source to include patients with grade III injuries to the medial collateral ligament (the semitendinosus might be used in some patients to reconstruct the posterolateral structures), as well as some patients with lax secondary restraints. It is our clinical impression that in appropriately selected patients, and if fixed properly, hamstring tendon grafts can produce the same degree of clinical stability as patellar tendon grafts with significantly fewer donor site complications (Table 14–2).

The role of allografts for ACL replacement is controversial, but they appear to offer no advantages in routine uncomplicated cases. At present, the major role for allografts would seem to be in revision ACL surgery and in multiple-ligament reconstruction.

Graft Placement

The objective of intraarticular replacement of the ACL is to replicate the anatomy and function of the normal ACL as closely as possible. Anatomic studies have shown that the human ACL has a complex arrangement of fibers, with each fiber having a unique location, length, and tension.[110-115] Although there is no true anatomic division of the ligament into distinct fiber bundles,[115] functionally the ACL had been divided into two fiber bundles, the anteromedial and the posterolateral bundles[112] (Figs. 14–6 and 14–7).

Experimental studies have shown that the anteromedial fibers of the ACL undergo the smallest length changes through the full range of motion.[110,111,113,114,116-119] (Fig. 14–8). Recent in vivo data from Howe et al using an arthroscopically inserted Hall effect strain transducer demonstrated that the strain of the anteromedial fibers was 4% at 30° flexion with a 150-N load.[118] As a result of these studies, most surgeons feel that the goal of intraarticular replacement of the ACL is to reproduce the anatomy and function of the anteromedial fibers.

Because of the large size and parallel fiber nature of biologic replacements, it is impossible to position the replacement graft so that all of its fibers are isometric.[110,111,114,119] Although it is impossible to achieve truly isometric placement, it is important to position the ACL replacement so that it will not undergo excessive elongation or slackening from its tensioned position.[21,111,113-115,120] Improper graft placement can

Table 14–2 Graft selection algorithm

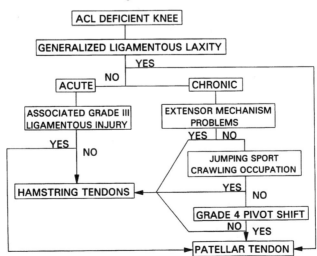

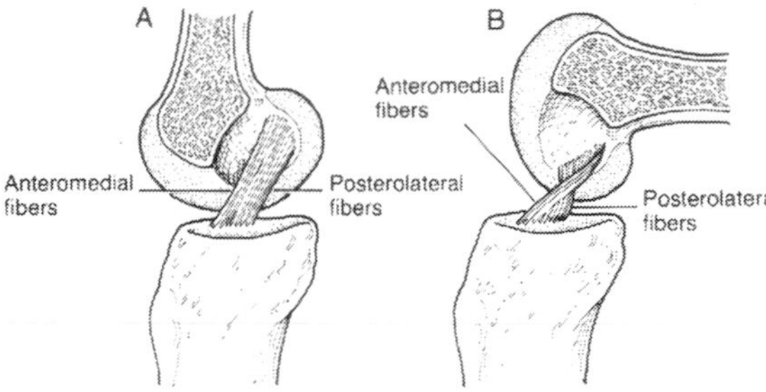

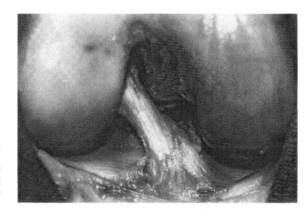

Figure 14–6. Anatomy of the antero-medial and posterolateral bands according to Girgis et al.[112] Both bands are tight in extension. With flexion the posterolateral band loosens.

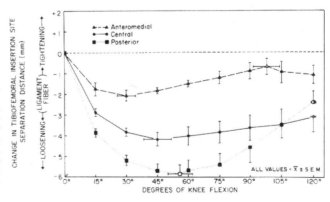

Figure 14–7. Human anatomic specimen demonstrating the complex helical arrangement of the ACL. Each fiber has a unique origin on the inner margin of the lateral femoral condyle and a unique attachment site on the tibia. There is no true anatomic division into bands or bundles.

Figure 14–8. Tibiofemoral insertion site separation distances or anteromedial, central, and posterior tibial fiber locations. Zero degrees of flexion was assigned an arbitrary value of 0. The ACL was intact at the time of testing, and the tibia was unconstrained and allowed to hang free with distraction by gravity. Note that the anteromedial fibers undergo the smallest change in length through the full range of motion. (Reprinted with permission from Sapega et al.[119])

result in a number of complications including loss of motion, graft fixation failure, and failure to eliminate the pathologic laxity.[113,114]

Excessive elongation of the replacement will generate large tissue strains and can cause loss of motion if the replacement fails to elongate. For the knee to regain motion the substitute would have to undergo permanent elongation. Either of these situations leads to failure. It has been estimated that collagen fibers fail at strains of 5 to 6%.[21] If one assumes that the average soft tissue length of a central-third patellar tendon graft is 49 mm,[67] and that of a doubled hamstring tendon graft is

140 mm, then the maximum allowable strain before failure would occur is 3 mm for the patellar tendon graft and 8 mm for the hamstring tendon graft.

Biomechanical studies have demonstrated that ACL fiber length changes in the human knee are most sensitive to the position of the femoral attachment site.[110,111,116,121,122] Changes in the tibial attachment site have significantly less effect on ACL fiber length changes. Fibers positioned anterior to the axis of rotation on the femur exhibit excessive elongation with flexion of the knee, whereas fibers positioned posteriorly exhibit excessive elongation with extension.[110,111,116,121,122]

Current recommendations for femoral tunnel placement vary depending on the nature of the ACL replacement. Clancy et al have shown that ACL substitutes tend to lean toward the edges of the intraarticular bone tunnels.[52,63,123] This produces a shift in the effective fixation point of the graft. To counter this shifting, they proposed that the bone tunnels be placed in an "eccentric" position from the center of the ligament attachment site.

Sapega has also demonstrated that it is the relative size match between the graft and the bone tunnel that determines the eccentric shift of the graft.[124] Round cylindrical grafts such as hamstring tendons placed in snug-fitting bone tunnels produce the smallest eccentric shift, whereas flat ribbonlike substitutes such as the patellar tendon that fail to occupy the entire tunnel produce the largest shifts.

For flat, ribbonlike substitutes such as the patellar tendon the eccentric shift also varies depending on whether the bone block will lie flush with the intraarticular tunnel opening (endoscopic technique) or be recessed up the tunnel (two-incision technique). The shift is greatest for recessed bone blocks and less for bone blocks positioned flush with the intraarticular opening of the tunnel.

Based on this information, the femoral tunnel should be positioned close to the anatomic center of the femoral anatomic attachment site for hamstring grafts and for bone blocks positioned flush with the intraarticular edge of the bone tunnel. A more superior and posterior position from the anatomic center of the ACL should be used for recessed bone blocks.

Brand and Daniel have shown that for recessed bone blocks, the femoral guide pin should be positioned such that there is a 3- to 4-mm length increase with extension.[120] When this eccentric guide-pin position was converted to a bone tunnel the length change was reduced to 1 to 2 mm, which the authors felt was the desired result.

Muller was one of the first to point out the consequences of nonisometric placement of ACL grafts.[21] He demonstrated that if the ACL graft were positioned too anteriorly on the femur, the graft tissue would be subjected to unacceptable tissue strains as the knee was flexed. Either the graft would stretch out and stability decrease, or the joint would be overconstrained and flexion would decrease. Experimental studies by Penner et al and Bylski-Austrow et al have confirmed that if the ACL substitute is placed anterior to the flexion axis of rotation, it will be subjected to large length changes (up to 8.8 mm) and high tensile forces as the knee is flexed.[125,126] These large length changes and tensile forces will result in failure of the substitute (Fig. 14–9).

These experimental data are supported by the clinical work of Melhorn and Henning, who found that an anterior placement of the femoral attachment site led to the largest amount of knee laxity, as measured by the Lachman and anterior drawer tests, and the largest amount of ACL graft strain (20% in a postoperative group of patients who had undergone intraarticular reconstruction of the ACL).[127]

Because the tibial attachment site has less influence on fiber length changes, there has been a tendency to ignore the position of this attachment site. Recent work by Howell et al has shown that the sagittal position of

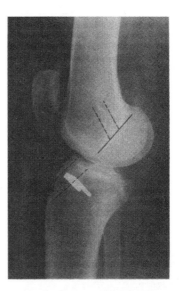

Figure 14–9. Failed ACL reconstruction. Lateral radiograph shows anterior placement of the femoral tunnel; also note the anterior placement of the tibial tunnel. The patient underwent open ACL reconstruction with a patellar tendon graft. Follow-up clinical examination revealed a slight loss of extension and flexion, a +2 Lachman test, and a grossly positive pivot-shift test.

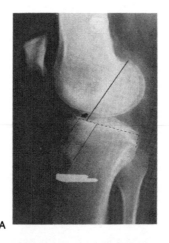

A

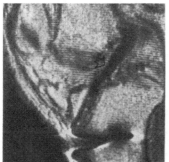

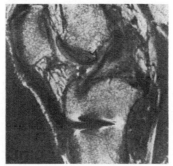

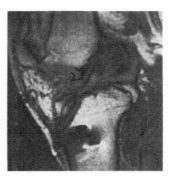

B   C   D

Figure 14–10. Representative radiograph and MRI scans of an impinged ACL graft. Graft impingement is characterized by the tibial tunnel being positioned anterior to the slope of the intercondylar roof with the knee in maximum hyperextension. **A.** Lateral radiograph with the knee in extension demonstrates moderate impingement with an eccentrically positioned tibial tunnel lying 40% in front of the slope of the intercondylar roof (arrow). **B.** The graft signal was normal on the MRI scan at the time of ACL reconstruction. Note there was no space between the graft and the roof of the intercondylar notch with the knee in 10° of flexion (open arrow). **C.** Three months following reconstruction, note the increased signal intensity around the distal two thirds of the graft. The proximal part of the graft remains low in signal intensity. The anterior surface of the graft is seen to be indented by the roof of the intercondylar notch (open arrow). **D.** ACL graft 12 months postoperatively. The magnetic resonance appearance of the graft has not improved. The signal intensity in the distal two thirds of the graft has increased, as has indentation of the anterior surface of the graft. (Reprinted with permission from Howell et al.[76])

the tibial tunnel has an important effect on roof impingement of an ACL replacement.[74-79] Their MRI studies showed that if the tibial tunnel of the ACL replacement is positioned anterior to a line drawn from the femur to the tibia along Blumensaat's line with the knee in maximum hyperextension, roof impingement will result.[78] Roof impingement is characterized clinically by anterior knee pain, swelling, loss of full extension, and increased anteroposterior translation as measured by a KT-1000 arthrometer.[78,79] MRI studies have shown that unimpinged grafts have a homogeneous low signal intensity, whereas impinged grafts show an increase in signal intensity in the distal third of the graft[74-78] (Figs. 14–10 and 14–11).

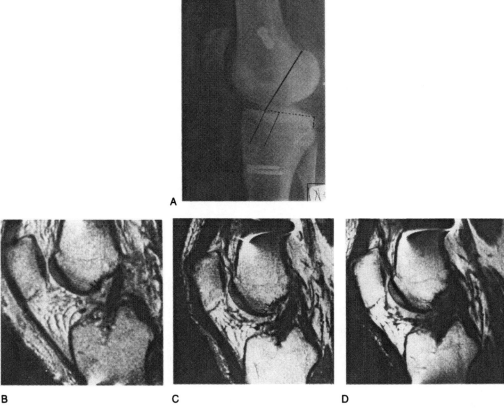

Figure 14–11. Representative radiograph and MRI scans of an unimpinged ACL graft. An unimpinged graft is characterized by the tibial tunnel being positioned parallel and posterior to the slope of the intercondylar roof with the knee in maximum hyperextension. **A.** Lateral radiograph demonstrates that the anterior edge of the tibial tunnel lies parallel to the roof of the intercondylar roof. **B.** The MRI graft signal was normal; signal intensity was low at the time of reconstruction. There is space between the graft and the intercondylar roof (open arrow). **C, D.** The MRI signal of the graft remains black; signal intensity was low at 3 and 12 months postoperatively. A space (open arrow) persists between the graft and the roof of the intercondylar notch. (Reprinted with permission from Howell et al.[76])

Graft Tension

How much tension should be applied to the ACL graft at the time of surgery? As the ACL graft does not tighten with time, undertensioning will result in residual pathologic laxity and surgical failure. What about overtensioning the graft? Yoshiya et al were able to document that overtensioning a patellar tendon ACL graft in a dog model had deleterious effects on the graft.[128] They compared graft pretensions of 1 and 39 N. Microangiography demonstrated improved vascularity in grafts with a preload of 1 N, versus grafts that were pretensioned with 39 N. Histologic examination of the patellar tendon graft pretensioned with 39 N showed focal degeneration within the graft and replacement of the collagen fibers by a myxoid extracellular matrix. By contrast, histology of the grafts pretensioned with 1 N showed no degeneration within the graft. Laxity measurements showed significant differences in the joint laxity between the two different preloads, with the smaller preload showing a larger amount of anteroposterior laxity. By 3 months postoperatively, laxity and mechanical differences between the two preloads were insignificant. They concluded that revascularization of a autogenous patellar tendon graft could be adversely affected by excessive preload, and that the graft should be fixed under the smallest amount of preload necessary to restore normal joint laxity.

Burks and Leland, in a study done on human cadavers, found that the amount of tension required to restore normal preoperative knee laxity after transection of the ACL was highly dependent on the type of replacement tissue used.[129] A 10-mm patellar tendon graft required a mean tension of 3.6 lb (range 2–5 lb). A double-stranded semitendinosus graft required a mean tension of 8.5 lb (range 5–10 lb). The authors speculated that a lower tension was required for a patellar tendon graft because of its greater stiffness and the shorter length of soft tissue compared with a double-stranded semitendinosus graft.

The angle at which the graft is tensioned has also been shown to be important. Bylski-Austrow et al, in a human cadaver model, studied the effects of graft placement, flexion angle at the time of tensioning, and magnitude of the initial tension on the force in an ACL substitute.[126] This study showed that the force in the ACL substitute was most sensitive to femoral attachment site placement, followed by the flexion angle at the time of tensioning, and was least sensitive to the actual tension applied to the graft. The authors found that an anterior placement of the graft resulted in the largest amount of posterior translation of the knee (overconstraint) compared with the intact knee, irrespective of the position of the knee at the time of tensioning or the magnitude of the tension applied to the graft. Grafts with the most isometric placement, tensioned with 44 N (10 lb) at 0°, resulted in the smallest differences in anteroposterior (AP) translation (within 1 mm of the intact knee). Tensioning the substitute at 30° of flexion always resulted in higher forces in the ACL substitute and in an overconstrained joint compared with tensioning the graft at 0° of flexion. In fact, tensioning the grafts at 30° of flexion had a greater effect on AP translation than did doubling the tension applied to the graft from 22 to 44 N. This study again indicates the importance of avoiding anterior placement of the femoral tunnel, and also suggests that overtensioning of the ACL graft and overconstraint of joint motion are more likely to occur if the graft is tensioned at 30° of flexion versus 0° of flexion.

Overconstraint of the joint can result in loss of joint motion or application of excessive compressive loads to the articular surfaces. Schabus et al measured the tibial articular cartilage contact stress under the following conditions[130]:

1. Normal knee
2. Normal knee with the ACL cut
3. After isometric ACL reconstruction with physiologic preload of the ACL replacement graft
4. After isometric ACL reconstruction with a higher graft preload

5. After nonisometric ACL reconstruction
6. After bilateral total meniscectomy

Their results indicated that there was no significant difference in the tibial articular cartilage pressure distribution of normal knees, knees in which the ACL had been cut, and knees that had undergone isometric ACL reconstruction with physiologic graft preload. The highest pressure distributions (even greater than the bilateral meniscectomy knees) were produced in knees with isometric ACL reconstructions and higher graft preload and after nonisometric ACL reconstruction and increased graft preload. The authors concluded that the preload of the ACL graft should not be higher than the physiologic loading of the normal ACL in the hyperextended position to prevent excessive loading of the tibial articular cartilage.

Friederich et al looked at the effects of stress relaxation on the initial preload applied to a patellar tendon graft at the time of ACL reconstruction.[131] This study showed that if preload was applied to the ACL graft and then allowed to drop to zero before the ligament was inserted and retensioned, there was a significant loss of the applied tension with time. A 5-lb preload dropped an average of 43% and a 15-lb preload dropped an average of 35%. When the preload was allowed to drop to zero for 1 minute, the patellar tendon graft had recovered approximately 75% of its viscoelasticity. Of the total average stress relaxation, 40% was felt to be due to the graft, 20% to the sutures, and 40% to other structures in the knee. When the grafts were inserted and overtensioned and then the tension decreased to the desired tension and not allowed to drop to zero, there was a 5 to 25% increase in the applied tension with time.

This work suggests that at the time of graft tensioning the graft should be preloaded and cycled to allow for stress relaxation before the graft is fixed. We feel that this preloading and cycling of the graft prior to fixation are especially important when using multiple-stranded hamstring tendon grafts or endobutton fixation of patellar tendon grafts.

Based on the current studies correct tensioning of ACL replacements is multifactorial and is determined by (1) placement of the femoral tunnel, (2) the position at which the tension is applied, (3) the length and stiffness of the substitute, and (4) stress relaxation of the graft.

At present, we do not have enough information to make specific recommendations for the exact amount of graft tension that should be applied at surgery.

Graft Fixation

Loss of graft fixation can be one of the major causes of surgical failure in the early postoperative period. Holden et al demonstrated in a goat model that ACL graft fixation failure was the major cause of failure in the immediate postoperative period prior to biologic incorporation of the graft at the fixation site.[132] In this study, 11 of 12 specimens failed at the graft fixation site at time zero, but at 2, 4, and 8 weeks after surgery the site of failure moved increasingly to the tissue midsubstance site. This study demonstrates that in the early postoperative period, the graft fixation site is the weak link. Because the ACL autograft is strongest at the time of initial implantation, the limitations of postoperative rehabilitation are based more on graft fixation strength than on the initial tensile strength of the ACL graft.

Ligament graft fixation can be divided into two types, soft tissue-to-bone and bone-to-bone fixation. Kurosaka et al reported on the fixation strength of commonly used ACL grafts and fixation methods.[133] Fixation of patellar tendon bone–tendon–bone units with a 9.0×25-mm custom-designed interference screw was found to provide the highest failure strength and stiffness. The 9.0-mm screw provided an average maximum tensile strength of 475.8 ± 27.5 N, or 47% of the control ACL, and a stiffness value of 57.9 ± 3.9 N/mm in young cadavers. A value of 104 N was reported for a stapled semitendinosus graft. Because of this article, interference screws have become the standard method of graft fixation for patellar tendon grafts.

Robertson et al reported on the fixation strengths of soft tissue to bone for various fixation devices.[134] For tendinous tissue they reported that a screw and plastic ligament washer (180 N) and a screw and metal ligament plate (238 N) provided the highest failure loads. No stiffness values were reported.

Fithian et al in an in vitro study evaluated suture fixation against spiked soft tissue washer fixation using a hamstring tendon left attached at its tibial insertion.[135] The Krackow suture, 8-point plastic and metal spiked washers, and 10-point metal spiked washers were found to provide similar failure loads of approximately 300 N.

A recent study by Matthews et al compared the fixation strength of patellar tendon bone–tendon–bone grafts using interference screws (9×25 mm) and suture screw and postfixation methods (Nos. 2 and 5) in young cadaver specimens.[136] They reported no statistically significant difference between interference screw and suture fixation methods. The mean failure load was 435 ± 33 N for interference screws and 416 ± 40 N for No. 5 nonabsorbable sutures. Although there was no statistically significant difference in the failure loads, stiffness values were not reported.

Two recent studies examining the fixation of soft tissue to bone have reported significantly higher values than previously reported by Robertson et al[134] and Fithian et al.[135] Pyne et al[137] reported a mean maximum failure load of 875 N for bovine tendons that were similar in cross-sectional area to human semitendinosus and gracilis tendons. The tendons were fixed with a belt buckle staple method to the distal femur. Using a figure-eight weave of the tendon around two plastic spiked washers fixed with 6.5-mm bicortical cancellous screws resulted in a mean maximum failure load of 539 N.

Steiner et al, in a biomechanical study using human cadavers, compared different methods of fixation for hamstring tendon grafts and patellar tendon grafts.[73] Suture fixation of single-limbed gracilis and semitendinosus grafts resulted in a maximum failure load of 335 ± 87 N and a stiffness value of 16 N/mm, as compared with a maximum failure load of 573 ± 109 N and a stiffness value of 18 N/mm for doubled grafts. Single-limbed semitendinosus and gracilis grafts were reported to have statistically significant lower maximum failure loads compared with the intact ACL values. There was no statistically significant difference in the maximum failure load of double-limbed grafts versus the intact ACL.

The strongest and stiffest method for fixation of semitendinosus and gracilis grafts was with the grafts doubled and fixed with two 4.5-mm bicortical screws and two 13.5×6.0-mm spiked plastic ligament washers on the femur. The tibial ends of the grafts were fixed by looping three No. 5 nonabsorbable sutures through the axillae of the grafts and tying around a 6.5-mm cancellous screw and metal washer. This fixation method produced a mean maximum load of 821 ± 98 N and a stiffness of 29 ± 3 N/mm.

The strongest and stiffest method for fixation of patellar tendon grafts was interference screw fixation (9×25 mm) at both ends. This method of fixation produced a maximum failure load of 423 ± 175 N and a stiffness of 46 ± 24 N/mm. Patellar tendon grafts fixed with three No. 5 sutures tied around a 6.5-mm cancellous screw and metal washer resulted in a maximum failure load of 396 ± 124 N and a stiffness of 27 ± 13 N/mm. Although there was no statistically significant difference in the maximum failure load between interference screw fixation and suture fixation, suture fixation was noted to produce lower stiffness values. The maximum failure load with interference screws could be further increased by tying three No. 5 nonabsorbable sutures in each bone block around a 6.5-mm cancellous screw and washer on both ends. This method of fixation resulted in a mean failure load of 674 ± 92 N and a stiffness value of 50 ± 9 N/mm.

Comparison of hamstring fixation methods with patellar tendon fixation methods revealed significant differences in stiffness values and in millimeters of displacement to the point of initial graft failure. Patellar tendon grafts fixed with interference screws were found to have stiffness values closer to those of the specimens with intact ACL, whereas hamstring grafts were noted to have significantly lower values. Hamstring grafts were also noted to fail with long displacements, whereas

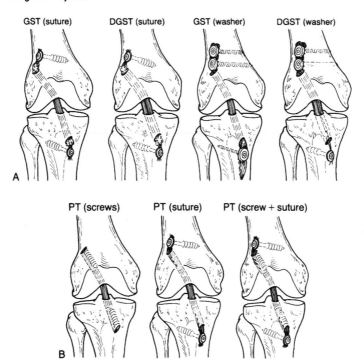

Figure 14–12. A. Hamstring graft fixation techniques.
GST (suture): Single-limb gracilis and semitendinosus free
grafts. A No. 2 Ethibond suture was placed in a whip-stitch
fashion in each end of the grafts. The four suture strands
were tied around a 6.5-mm cancellous screw and metal
washer. *DGST (suture)*: Gracilis and semitendinosus free
grafts bisected to produce four tendon limbs. A No. 2 Ethibond suture was placed in a whip-stitch fashion in the ends of
each graft. Fixation similar to GST (suture). *GST (washer)*:
Single-limb gracilis and semitendinosus grafts were fixed to
the femur by weaving the free ends in a figure-eight fashion
around two 13.5 × 6.0-mm soft tissue washers fixed with 4.5-
mm bicortical screws. The tendons were fixed to the tibia by
their biologic attachments and one 13.5 × 6.0-mm soft tissue
washer fixed with a 4.5-mm bicortical screw. *DGST (washer)*:
The gracilis and semitendinosus tendons were taken as
free grafts and folded to produce two looped ends and four
free ends. The free ends were fixed to the femur by two
13.5 × 6.0-mm soft tissue washers and 4.5-mm bicortical
screws as in the GST (washer) technique. The looped ends
were fixed to the tibia by three No. 5 Ethibond sutures placed
through the looped ends and tied to a 6.5-mm cancellous
screw and washer. **B. Patellar tendon graft fixation techniques.** *PT (screws)*: Femoral and tibial bone blocks fixed
with 9.0 × 25-mm "outside-in" interference screws. *PT (suture)*:
Femoral and tibial bone blocks fixed with three No. 5 Ethibond sutures tied around 6.5-mm cancellous screws and metal washers. *PT (screw + suture)*: Femoral and tibial bone
blocks fixed with 9.0 × 25-mm interference screws and three
No. 5 Ethibond sutures tied around 6.5-mm cancellous
screws and metal washers.

patellar tendon grafts tended to fail abruptly with short
displacements. Both hamstring and patellar tendon
grafts were noted to fail more often on the tibial side
(Figs. 14–12 and 14–13).

The mean failure loads for soft tissue-to-bone fixation
in both of these recent studies[73,137] compare favorably
with values previously reported for interference screw
fixation of patellar tendon grafts.[133] The major difference between hamstring tendon fixation and interference screw fixation of patellar tendon grafts is related to
the stiffness and millimeters of displacement to failure.
Although the increased stiffness of interference screw
fixation may seem to be a major advantage, it can be a
two-edged sword: rigid fixation of a graft that undergoes more than 2 to 3 mm of lengthening may result in
excessive graft forces and early graft failure or "capture
of the joint," leading to an overconstrained joint, and
excessive pressure on the articular cartilage, or loss of
joint motion. In this situation the lower stiffness of
hamstring tendon grafts and soft tissue fixation may be
an advantage.

Because ACL grafts are strongest at the time of implantation, rehabilitation limitations in the immediate
postoperative period are based more on the initial fixation strength of the graft. It has been estimated that the
ACL is subjected to loads of up to 445 N during activi-

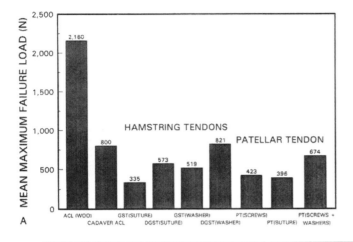

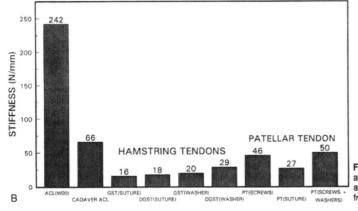

Figure 14–13. Ultimate failure loads (A) and stiffness values (B) of the intact ACL and various ACL fixation techniques. Data from Steiner et al.[73]

ties of daily living.[67,138] Based on this estimated value, interference screw fixation of patellar tendon grafts and the method described by Steiner et al[72] for double-looped hamstring tendons can provide secure enough fixation to allow activities of daily living in the immediate postoperative period prior to biologic incorporation of the graft fixation sites.

Fixation Site Healing

Few investigations have examined the histology or biomechanics of ACL graft healing in bone tunnels. Van Rens et al reported on the histologic changes in the bone tunnels of an iliotibial band ACL replacement graft in a dog model.[139] This study demonstrated the formation of collagen fibers that closely resembled Sharpey's fibers running from the bone tunnels to the soft tissue graft by 4 weeks. By 10 weeks a tideline

marking the border between the bone and the ligamentous tissue was seen. This tideline is present in the normal ACL and marks the transition between the ligamentous tissue of the ACL and the bone of the insertion site. By 12 weeks fibers that closely resembled Sharpey's fibers were noted to continue from the bone into the ligamentous tissue. By 16 weeks the soft tissue bone interface remained unchanged, with fibers closely resembling Sharpey's fibers continuing from the ligament into the bone. Biomechanical testing of the ligament–bone interface was not performed.

Schiavone Panni et al, in a histologic study using New Zealand white rabbits, examined the bone–tendon interface following reconstruction of the ACL with a patellar tendon bone–tendon–bone transplant.[140] The central third of the patellar tendon with attached tibial and patellar bone blocks was harvested and, using a special drill guide, isometric bone tunnels were created and the bone blocks fixed with interference screws. No postoperative immobilization was used. At 2 weeks the tendon was noted to be edematous with clear signs of cellular necrosis. There was degeneration of the connective tissue as well as a distinct lymphocytic and monocytic infiltrate. No form of insertion between the tendon and the bone was evident in the contact zone. After 5 weeks the inflammatory infiltrate had resolved, but the tendon was still separate from the bone tunnel with no signs of junctional tissue present. By 8 weeks a thin layer of fibrocartilage was noted between the bone and the tendon. By 12 weeks a thin layer of calcified fibrocartilage had formed. At 16 weeks this fibrocartilage junction was morphologically similar to the human ACL insertion site, although thinner. This junction was morphologically complete by the 24th week and was indistinguishable from a normal human ACL insertion site. Although no biomechanical studies were performed, the authors speculated that the bone–tendon insertion site would probably have normal strength by 24 weeks because its appearance was normal at that time. The authors concluded that following a tendon reconstruction, a structure with histologic features similar to those, a normal ligament–bone insertion site forms.

Rodeo et al recently reported a histologic and the first biomechanical study of tendon healing in a bone tunnel.[141] Twenty adult mongrel dogs underwent transplantation of the long digital extensor tendon into a drill hole in the proximal tibial metaphysis. Four dogs were sacrificed at 2, 4, 8, 12, and 26 weeks and histologic and biomechanical studies were performed.

Histologic analysis of the 2-week specimens revealed vascular, highly cellular fibrous tissue at the tendon–bone interface with little or no continuity between the tendon and the bone tunnel. No bone remodeling was noted. The 4-week specimens demonstrated a thin seam of new bone lining the bone tunnel. A basophilic ce-

ment line was seen at the junction of the host bone and the newly formed bone. The tendon remained viable with normal-appearing fibroblasts. Occasional continuity of collagen fibers between the fibrous tissue interface and the bone was noted. The 8-week specimens demonstrated occasional collagen fibers spanning the tendon–bone junction, which appeared to be anchored in the bone, but did not always appear continuous with the collagen structure of the bone. The 12- and 26-week specimens demonstrated further maturation and organization of the tendon–bone interface. Collagen fibers oriented at an angle toward the pull of the muscle-tendon unit appeared to connect the tendon to the bone by 12 weeks. These fibers had the appearance of Sharpey's fibers. By 26 weeks a tidemark delineating the zone between the calcified and the noncalcified tissue was present, and there was continuity between the collagen fibers of the tendon and the entire length of the bone tunnel.

Biomechanical testing revealed a progressive increase in fixation strength during the first 12 weeks following transplantation. Specimens at 2, 4, and 8 weeks failed because the tendon pulled out from the bone tunnel. All 12- and 26-week specimens failed at the tendon-clamp junction. There was a statistically significant difference in failure load between the 2- and 4-week specimens, the 4- and 8-week specimens, and the 8- and 12-week specimens. The absolute pullout loads did not significantly increase after 4 weeks; however, when the data were normalized by dividing by the tunnel length there was a significant increase in strength through the 12-week mark. The authors felt that this indicated a significantly greater volume of interface between the tendon and the bone tunnel. Because the normalized data (fixation strength divided by tunnel length) showed a progressive increase with time up to 12 weeks, the longer the bone tunnel the stronger the fixation

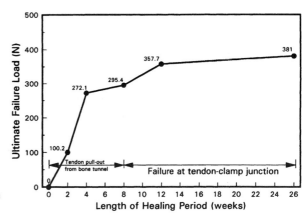

Figure 14–14. Tendon failure strength. Data from Rodeo et al.[141]

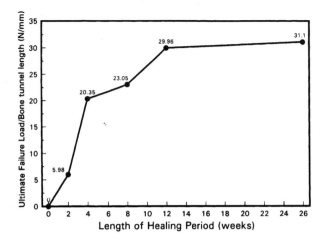

Figure 14–15. Tendon failure strength normalized to bone tunnel length. Data from Rodeo et al.[141]

strength. On the basis of their results the authors recommended that soft tissue-to-bone fixation sites be protected at least 8 weeks (Figs. 14–14 and 14–15).

In summary, there have been few studies investigating bone or soft tissue healing in bone tunnels. Based on the studies of Holden et al[132] and Rodeo et al,[141] it appears that soft tissue grafts take at least 8 weeks before the tendon is firmly attached to bone. Although it has been commonly assumed that the healing of bone blocks in bone tunnels is completed by 6 weeks, we know of no biomechanical studies that prove this point.

Preoperative Planning

Timing of Surgery

Recent studies have shown that the timing of ACL surgery in acute cases has an important effect on the incidence of postoperative knee stiffness.[107,142–144] Strum et al found the incidence of loss of knee motion in acute ACL reconstructions (surgery within 3 weeks of injury) to be 35% versus only 12% in a similar group of patients undergoing chronic ACL reconstruction.[107] Shelbourne et al also reported a statistically significant increase in the incidence of knee stiffness in patients who underwent ACL reconstruction in the first week versus patients who had ACL reconstruction delayed 21 days.[144] Harner et al reported a 37% incidence of loss of motion in patients that had ACL reconstruction acutely (within 4 weeks of injury) versus a 5.5% incidence in chronic reconstructions.[142] They recommended delaying surgery in acute injuries, except for grossly unstable knees.

Shelbourne and Basle,[145] Graf and Uhr,[90] Harner et al,[146] and Aglietti et al[146] also noted that the incidence and magnitude of restricted motion were particularly high with combined injuries in which the ACL and the medial collateral ligament (MCL) were repaired at the same time. Harner et al reported a 44% incidence of stiffness with combined ACL reconstruction and repair of the MCL and/or the posterior oblique ligament.[142] Aglietti et al reported a 29% incidence of loss of motion following combined ACL/MCL surgery, with half of the patients requiring manipulation under anesthesia to regain motion.[146]

On the basis of these studies acute ACL surgery should be delayed for at least 3 weeks, or until the patient has a full range of motion and the acute inflammatory phase has subsided. Exceptions are made for knees with acute lateral and posterolateral injuries, in which case the surgery is performed as soon as feasible.[147,148]

Treatment of Associated Ligamentous Injuries

The treatment of combined ACL/MCL injuries is controversial. Because of the high incidence of stiffness following combined ACL reconstruction and open MCL repair,[90,142,145,146,148,149] there has been a trend toward treating the MCL injury nonoperatively. A recent paper by Shelbourne and Porter documented the success of this approach.[149] They reviewed a series of 84 patients with combined ACL/MCL injuries. The first 16 underwent open ACL reconstruction with a patellar tendon autograft and MCL repair; the subsequent 68 underwent open ACL reconstruction with a patellar tendon autograft, and the MCL injury was treated nonoperatively. The MCL injury was grade II in 78% of the patients and grade III in 22%. Both groups underwent a similar ACL rehabilitation protocol.[42,150,151] No attempt was made to protect the MCL during the postoperative rehabilitation program. The authors reported that nonoperative management of the MCL tear gave excellent stability, with a mean side-to-side KT-1000 measurement of 1.68 mm and 0 to +1 valgus laxity at 30° of flexion, similar to the results of patients who had operative treatment of the MCL injury. There was no significant difference between patients with grade II and grade III injuries. The patients with nonoperative management of the MCL tear were reported to have a greater range of motion (4.5/0/137) compared with patients who had surgical repair of the MCL. Strength values were equal in both groups. The authors concluded that combined ACL/MCL injuries treated with ACL reconstruction using a patellar tendon autograft and nonoperative treatment of the MCL tear can yield an excellent functional outcome and excellent clinical stability.

In acute cases involving combined injury to the ACL and the posterolateral corner, surgical repair of the posterolateral corner and ACL reconstruction are performed as soon as the patient's general condition allows as the results of acute repair appear to be superior to those of chronic reconstructions.[147,148]

Flynn et al recently reported on the results of 12 patients with combined ACL and posterolateral corner injuries.[147] All patients had sustained complete ACL and lateral collateral ligament tears, ten had injury to the popliteus, six had injury to the biceps tendon, and five had sustained injury to the iliotibial band. In four patients there was injury to the peroneal nerve. The average time from injury to surgery was 9 days. Surgical treatment of the ACL consisted of semitendinosus, gracilis augmentation in eight cases and patellar-ligament reconstruction in four cases. The posterolateral corner injuries were primarily repaired with nonabsorbable sutures; avulsions were repaired to a bony bed. Augmentation of the lateral collateral ligament was performed in one case with a split biceps femoris graft. In two patients the popliteus was augmented with a split iliotibial band graft similar to the popliteus bypass described by Muller.[21] In one patient a patellar tendon autograft was used to reconstruct the popliteus.

Using the modified Hospital for Special Surgery (HSS) knee rating scale there were nine excellent to good results and one fair result, for an overall 83% satisfactory results. The average HSS knee score for the group was 87, with the good results averaging 91 points. The poor results occurred in patients with injury to the peroneal nerve. Ten of the 12 patients were able to return to their previous level of activity. Stability testing revealed a 0 to +1 Lachman test in 92% of the patients. All patients had a negative pivot shift. Instrumented laxity testing with a KT-1000 revealed a side-to-side difference of 3 mm or less in 10 of the 12 patients. Four patients had mild +1 varus laxity.

Based on their data, the authors felt that early surgical treatment of combined ACL and posterolateral corner injuries could result in good clinical and functional outcomes provided there was no injury to the peroneal nerve. This study provides support for immediate ACL reconstruction and surgical repair of the posterolateral corner (Fig. 14–16).

Preoperative Rehabilitation

Perioperative rehabilitation considerations are well described in the article by Klootwyk et al.[152] What follows is our present preoperative preparation program. Acute isolated ACL tears and ACL tears associated with grades I and II MCL injuries are protected with a knee immobilizer. Acute ACL tears associated with a grade III MCL sprain are sometimes placed in a hinged knee brace to control valgus rotations and for comfort. Ice or another cold application is used liberally to control pain and swelling. The patient is started on an oral nonsteroidal anti-inflammatory medication for 2 to 3 weeks in an attempt to decrease the inflammatory response to the injury. Weight bearing to tolerance is encouraged. It is important for the patient to regain motion and muscular control of the knee as soon as possible. Active and active-assisted range-of-motion exercises are

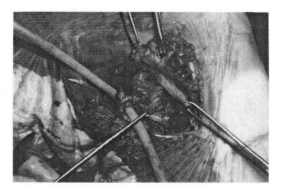

Figure 14–16. Patient with an acute ACL tear as well as associated tears of the fibular collateral, popliteus, and biceps tendons. The Penrose drain identifies the peroneal nerve. The clamp is grasping the fibular collateral ligament which was avulsed from the fibula. The popliteus identified by the nerve hook lies deep to the fibula collateral ligament and was torn at the musculotendinous junction. The patient underwent ACL reconstruction with a patellar tendon graft as well as repair of the fibular collateral ligament and biceps tendon. Number 5 nonabsorbable sutures were placed through the tendinous portion of the popliteus, and a tenodesis was performed passing the tendon through an anterior-to-posterior drill hole.[21]

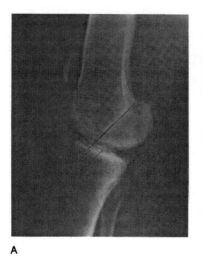

A

B

Figure 14–17. A. Preoperative lateral radiograph in maximum hyperextension. The tibial tunnel (dashed lines) should lie posterior to the roof of the intercondylar notch (solid line) to prevent impingement of the ACL graft in extension. **B.** Patient with marked recurvatum of the knee and a vertical intercondylar shelf (*A*). Because of the recurvatum and vertical intercondylar shelf, the tibial tunnel (*B*) must be placed posteriorly on the sagittal tibial depth line (dashed line) to avoid roof impingement. This placement may result in a graft position out of the zone of the bulk fibers of the ACL. To position the tibial tunnel in a more anatomic position, and to avoid roof impingement of the graft, the slope of the intercondylar shelf must be changed to a more horizontal position (*C*). A more anatomically positioned tibial tunnel (*D*) can then be keyed off this new roof angle.

started as soon as possible with the goal of obtaining a normal range of motion as quickly as possible. If a hinged rehabilitation brace is used for an associated grade III MCL injury, it is important the knee be removed from the brace and full passive hyperextension achieved. Failure to achieve early full passive extension may result in a flexion contracture and further delay of the surgery. Quadriceps and hamstring exercises are started as soon as possible to reduce muscle atrophy and to build strength sufficient for normal gait and activities of daily living. The crutches and brace are discarded when the patient can walk without a limp. Muscular endurance is built with closed-kinetic-chain exercises, such as a stationary bike, stair-climbing machine, ski machine, rowing machine, or swimming program. By 2 to 4 weeks the patient should have minimal swelling, a near-normal range of motion, and good muscular control of the leg. At this point the patient is ready to undergo surgery.

Chronic cases should be started on a preoperative rehabilitation program with the objective of trying to restore normal quadriceps and hamstring function. Prior to surgery, it is also helpful for the patient to receive preoperative instruction on the postoperative ACL rehabilitation program. Knee rating questionnaires can be filled out, and instrumented laxity measurements can also be performed at this time.

Prior to surgery a lateral view with the knee in maximum hyperextension is used to determine the slope of the intercondylar shelf.[78,79] Knees with recurvatum and a more vertical intercondylar shelf require a more extensive roofplasty and a more posterior tibial tunnel position to avoid impingement of the ACL graft in extension[78,79] (Fig. 14–17). This radiograph can also be used to determine the optimal sagittal position for the tibial tunnel. To prevent impingement of the ACL graft the entire width of the tibial tunnel should lie posterior to a line drawn parallel to Blumensaat's line extended across the tibial articular surface.[75–79] A lateral view with the knee in maximum hyperextension and an MRI scan is particularly useful in the preoperative planning for revision ACL surgery in which graft impingement is thought to be the cause of failure (Fig. 14–18).

Surgical Technique

In this section we describe our current technique of ACL reconstruction. As the majority of surgeons will be using autografts, we describe surgical techniques using a central-third patellar tendon graft and double-stranded semitendinosus and gracilis autografts.

Various authors have described two-incision arthroscopy-assisted surgical techniques for the placement of a patellar tendon ACL autograft.[153–155] ACL recon-

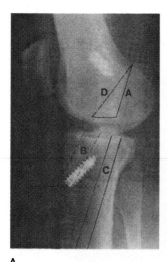
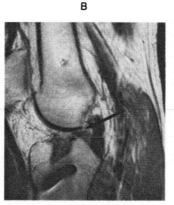

B

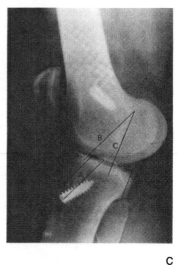

A

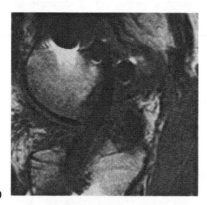

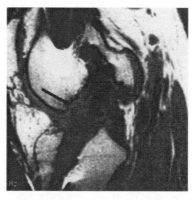

D

C

E

Figure 14–18. **A.** Preoperative planning for a revision of a failed patellar tendon ACL reconstruction. Lateral radiograph with the knee in maximum hyperextension. Note the marked recurvatum of the knee. The solid line *A* on the femur marks the patient's original intercondylar roof. The dashed lines *B* on the tibia outline the old tibial tunnel. The tibial tunnel lies very anterior to the roof of the intercondylar notch, resulting in severe impingement of the ACL graft, the probable cause of graft failure. **B.** Severe impingement was confirmed by a postoperative MRI demonstrating that the graft wraps around the roof of the intercondylar notch distally (arrow). On the MRI there is almost complete absence of the graft distally because of the guillotining effect of the anterior outlet of the intercondylar notch. To avoid impingement of the new graft the surgeon could position the new tibial tunnel posterior to the roof of the intercondylar notch (solid lines *C*), or using the existing tibial tunnel position a large roofplasty (line *D*) would have to be performed. The first situation would result in a nonanatomic position of the tibial tunnel and loss of graft isometry. The second situation would require an excessively large roofplasty, which could interfere with patellar tracking as the knee is flexed. **C.** Preoperative planning can be used to help the surgeon plan the revision operation and avoid either of these undesirable situations. On the lateral radiograph of the knee in maximum hyperextension, the center for the new tibial tunnel is positioned 44% from the anterior edge of the tibia,[75,77,78] solid lines *A*. A new intercondylar roof is then keyed off this tibial tunnel such that the tibial tunnel lies posterior to the roof of the intercondylar notch, solid line *B*. The arc between solid line *B* and solid line *C* (old intercondylar roof) represents the millimeters of bone that will have to be resected from the intercondylar notch. At surgery a calibrated probe or curette can be used to mark the amount of bone to be resected from the roof of the intercondylar roof. An impingement-free tibial guide system (Arthrotek, Inc, San Dimas, CA) can then be used to key off this new intercondylar roof to produce a more posteriorly positioned tibial tunnel. **D.** Postoperative MRI scan 3 months following revision with a doubled gracilis and semitendinosus autograft. Note the new intercondylar roof angle and the more posterior placement of the tibial tunnel. The graft is black with no increased signal intensity distally, indicating the absence of impingement. **E.** MRI scan 9 months postoperatively. The graft is still black with minimal increase in signal activity distally. There is space (arrow) between the roof of the intercondylar notch and the graft. Note the large size of this doubled semitendinosus and gracilis autograft. A lateral radiograph in maximum hyperextension before the original ACL reconstruction would have alerted the surgeon to the severe recurvatum, the vertical roof angle, and the need for a more posterior tibial tunnel placement and more extensive roofplasty.

struction using a doubled semitendinosus autograft performed through an open technique has been described by Mott[156] and Gomes and Marczyk.[157] Arthroscopy-assisted ACL reconstruction using single-stranded semitendinosus and gracilis tendon grafts was first described by Moyer et al.[158] Arthroscopy-assisted ACL reconstruction using a double-stranded semitendinosus and gracilis graft has been described by Friedman,[159] Larson,[172] and Howell.[79]

The advantages of arthroscopy-assisted ACL reconstruction versus open miniarthrotomy or transpatellar tendon approaches include the following:

1. Better illumination and visualization of the femoral attachment site
2. Elimination of capsular incisions, arthrotomy, and patellar dislocation
3. Avoidance of desiccation of the articular cartilage, which could be damaging[160,161]
4. Decrease in trauma to the fat pad, which perhaps decreases postoperative fat-pad scarring and arthrofibrosis
5. Decrease in muscle atrophy compared with open reconstruction[162]
6. Lower incidence of postoperative patellofemoral pain compared with open reconstruction[100,163]

Schoen[100] was able to show a difference in postoperative patellar pain in both acute and chronic cases between ACL reconstructions performed with an arthroscopy-assisted technique and reconstructions performed either through a miniarthrotomy without incision of the vastus medialis or dislocation of the patella[42,164,165] or through a transpatellar tendon approach.[64,93] In a prospective study Schoen reviewed a group of 50 patients with a similar age and sex distribution and associated injuries that were randomly assigned to either open or arthroscopy-assisted ACL reconstruction using a central-third patellar tendon graft. Group A consisted of 6 patients who underwent acute open ACL reconstruction (less than 14 days from injury). Group B comprised 9 patients who underwent acute arthroscopy-assisted ACL reconstruction. Group C consisted of 15 patients who underwent open reconstruction for chronic ACL deficiency. Group D consisted of 20 patients with chronic ACL-deficient knees who were treated with arthroscopy-assisted ACL reconstruction. All the procedures were performed by one surgeon. Intraoperative isometry measurements were made in all cases, and the guide pins were repositioned if there were unacceptable length changes. The postoperative rehabilitation program was the same in all groups and consisted of 2 days of immobilization at 0°, followed by a protected range-of-motion program.

He reported a 33% incidence of patellofemoral pain in group A (acute open) versus a 22% incidence in group B (acute closed). In patients with chronic ACL deficiency, he reported a 33% incidence in group C (chronic open) versus 15% in group D (chronic closed). He also reported that patients that had arthroscopy-assisted reconstructions regained their motion faster, but at 1 year there was no significant difference between the groups. As noted by other authors, the majority of the patients who had motion problems were in the acute surgery groups. He concluded that there was a difference in patellar pain between ACL reconstructions done through a miniarthrotomy or transpatellar tendon approach and those done with an arthroscopy-assisted technique.

Similar findings were also reported by Brown.[163] In a retrospective study he reported a 72.2% incidence of patellofemoral pain during the first 6 postoperative months in 18 patients who underwent ACL reconstruction with a central-third patellar tendon graft performed through a fat-pad splitting technique, versus a 42.9% incidence in 22 patients who underwent an arthroscopy-assisted technique using the same graft source. This difference was said to be statistically significant. Based on these findings the authors concluded that fat-pad splitting techniques appear to produce the greatest patellofemoral dysfunction in the early rehabilitation period.

A single-incision "endoscopic" surgical technique for reconstruction of the ACL has been described by Paulos et al,[166] Olson et al,[167] Hardin et al,[168] Beck et al,[169] and Fu and Olson.[170] The "endoscopic" technique is an attempt to further reduce the morbidity of ACL reconstruction by avoiding a lateral femoral incision and dissection. It has been speculated that by avoiding a lateral incision the endoscopic technique will further decrease postoperative pain and further minimize morbidity to the extensor mechanism. In the endoscopic technique the femoral bone tunnel is drilled in-line through the tibial tunnel and the patellar tendon ACL graft is fixed by inserting an interference screw from inside the joint.

Yates discussed the advantages and disadvantages of the conventional two-incision technique versus the one-incision endoscopic technique.[171] The principal advantages of the endoscopic technique are that it avoids a lateral distal femoral incision and dissection, although as noted by Yates, a conventional two-incision technique can be done with only a 1½-in. incision. He also pointed out that the major morbidity for ACL reconstruction was not the lateral incision, but rather the trauma associated with harvest of the patellar tendon graft, and this is the same in both techniques. The endoscopic technique is said to be faster but there have been no studies to document this fact. The endoscopic technique is also said to produce less postoperative pain than the two-incision technique, allowing for the possibility of outpatient ACL reconstruction. As mentioned earlier, the most painful aspect of ACL reconstruction is not the lateral incision but harvest of the patellar tendon graft. Outpatient ACL reconstruction using a two-incision technique has also been reported.

Another proposed advantage of the endoscopic technique is that the femoral tunnel is drilled in-line with the tibial tunnel, thus decreasing tunnel divergence and graft abrasion as the knee is cycled through a range of motion. The advantage of straight-line tunnels was demonstrated by Graf et al, who analyzed the effect of cyclical loading and femoral tunnel orientation in an animal model.[172] The results of their study showed that graft survival was enhanced for straight-line femoral tunnels (no failure, $n = 5$ after 125,000 cycles) compared with more transversely oriented femoral tunnels (one failure, $n = 5$ after 19,869 cycles).

The disadvantages of the endoscopic technique include the inability in many cases to adequately position the tibial bone block in the tibial tunnel because of a mismatch between the length of the patellar tendon graft and the intraarticular length of the ACL and the length of the tibial bone tunnel. As a result, the tibial bone block protrudes from the tibial tunnel and the surgeon loses the ability to use an interference screw for fixation and bone-to-bone healing in the tibial tunnel. Hardin et al reported that in approximately 25% of their cases alternative fixation had to be used to fix the tibial bone block.[168] One of the major advantages of the patellar tendon graft is the fixation strength and stiffness provided by interference screw fixation. In the endoscopic technique, if the bone block protrudes too far from the tibial tunnel, then alternative (weaker) methods of fixation, usually staples or sutures tied around a screw and washer, have to be used. Such hardware is usually prominent on the tibia, and often a second operation is required for removal.

Another disadvantage of the endoscopic technique is that the femoral tunnel position is somewhat limited as it must be drilled through the tibial tunnel. The femoral tunnel position is also limited by the fact that one must maintain at least 1 to 2 mm of the posterior cortex to fix the graft with an endoscopic screw. In large knees, maintaining this 1- to 2-mm cortex shell is not a problem, but in small knees, maintaining this posterior cortical shell may result in the femoral tunnel being positioned dangerously too anterior (Fig. 14–19).

Difficulties inserting the endoscopic screw so as to ensure placement parallel to the bone block and bone tunnel have also been reported. It does appear that endoscopic screw placement results in larger screw tunnel divergence than in the two-incision technique. The effect of this screw divergence on fixation strength is presently unknown. Damage to the PCL during drilling of the femoral tunnels, damage to the patellar tendon graft by the treads of the interference screw at the time of femoral bone block fixation, and loss of the screw in the joint requiring arthrotomy for removal have been re-

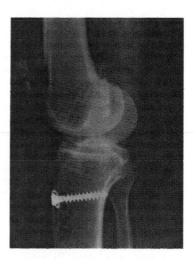

Figure 14–19. Lateral radiograph of failed endoscopic ACL reconstruction resulting from posterior cortical blowout and loss of graft fixation. The bone block from the patellar tendon graft is lying in the over-the-top position and the endoscopic screw is providing little bony fixation. Note also the anterior position of the tibial tunnel. Because of the short horizontal tibial tunnel a graft–tunnel mismatch exists so interference screw fixation could not be used on the tibia. The patient had +2 Lachman and a grossly positive pivot-shift test. If the posterior cortical blowout had been recognized at the time of surgery this case could have been salvaged by conversion to a two-incision technique.

ported with this technique. Finally, if failure of the ACL reconstruction occurs, revision surgery will probably require removal of the screw, which could potentially be very difficult.

Complications of the endoscopic technique are reported in an article by Meade and Dickson.[173] The authors reported 16 complications in their first 40 endoscopic cases. The article suggests that this technique has a steep learning curve and is technically demanding. Hardin et al also cautioned that the endoscopic technique has a steep learning curve and discussed some of the potential pitfalls of the technique in their paper.[168]

Two recent studies, the first by Garfinkel et al, and the second by Sgaglione and Schwartz have compared the results of the one-incision endoscopic technique, to the conventional two-incision technique.[174,175] Both studies failed to show any significant differences in the outcome of the two techniques. However, both authors noted that the one-incision technique was more technically demanding.

In summary, although the endoscopic technique appears to be attractive, the surgeon must be aware that it is a technically demanding procedure. The initial experience of Meade and Dickson suggest that the surgeon who wishes to use the endoscopic technique must be prepared to potentially deal with a host of new complications not usually encountered with the conventional two-incision technique. The only significant advantages of the endoscopic technique at this time seem to be less postoperative pain and cosmesis. Since the clinical outcome of the two techniques appears to be the same, the surgeon must balance these advantages against the greater complexity and steep learning curve inherent in the endoscopic technique. According to Yates, "the only disadvantage of utilizing two incisions is the presence of a 1 to ½-in. incision on the lateral aspect of the thigh. This never seems to be a cosmetic concern to males or females, and does not hinder the normal aggressive postoperative rehabilitation following autogenous patellar tendon ACL reconstructions."[171]

Recently Graf and Rosenberg introduced an "endobutton," which allows for endoscopic fixation of patellar tendon and hamstring tendon grafts.[176] A major advantage of this type of femoral fixation over an endoscopically inserted interference screw is that it allows the femoral bone block to be variably recessed into the femoral tunnel; thus the tibial bone block can be completely contained with the tibial tunnel in all cases. This method of fixation is dependent on No. 5 nonabsorbable sutures placed through drill holes in the patellar bone block. According to the data of Matthews et al[136] and Steiner et al,[73] this method of fixation should provide comparable failure loads, but decreased stiffness values to those of interference screw fixation.

Another advantage of the "endobutton" technique is that because the femoral bone block fixation is not dependent on the integrity of the posterior cortex, one is free to choose the placement of the internal femoral tunnel without the need to maintain a 1- to 2-mm cortical shell. If a more posterior femoral tunnel placement is desired and posterior cortical blowout occurs, the endobutton can still provide rigid fixation as it will be anchored on the lateral femoral cortex. The endobutton also results in the hardware being placed against the lateral femoral cortex instead of inside the joint, thus allowing for easy redrilling of the femoral tunnel and hardware removal if revision surgery becomes necessary. This technique seems to eliminate many of the disadvantages and potential problems of endoscopic interference screw fixation and should yield similar fixation strengths.

Although the endobutton can be used for femoral fixation of hamstring tendon grafts,[176] the tibial end of the graft at present is usually fixed with sutures tied around a screw and washer. This method of fixation has been found to have lower maximum failure and stiffness values compared with fixation of patellar tendon grafts with sutures or interference screws or fixation of doubled hamstring grafts with two spiked ligament washers and No. 5 nonabsorbable sutures.[73] Based on our

studies[73] we would advise caution using an accelerated rehabilitation program if suture fixation is used to secure the tibial end of the graft.

In the section that follows we present a detailed description of the two-incision surgical technique for arthroscopy-assisted placement of autogenous central-third patellar tendon and doubled semitendinosus and gracilis grafts and of endoscopic reconstruction using the "endobutton."

General Setup

For ACL reconstructive surgery to be performed smoothly and efficiently it is important that the operating room personnel be familiar with the equipment and operating room setup necessary for arthroscopy and knee ligament surgery.

Surgery is performed under general or regional anesthesia. For most knee ligament surgery, one of the authors (C.H.B.) prefers epidural anesthesia. Epidural anesthesia is safe and provides excellent intraoperative muscle relaxation. Epidural anesthesia has also been shown to reduce the incidence of postoperative thromboembolic disease. Another major advantage of epidural anesthesia is that the epidural catheter can be left in postoperatively for pain management. If postoperative epidural anesthesia is going to be used, a Foley catheter is inserted into the bladder at the beginning of the case to prevent postoperative urinary retention.

C.H.B. prefers to perform arthroscopy-assisted ACL reconstruction without the use of a circumferential leg holder. A straight padded post is clamped to the operating room table with a Clark ring attachment. If an endoscopic technique is planned the padded post must be positioned so as to allow room for the exit of the passing pin. A padded right-angle foot clamp is secured to the table; a rolled blanket firmly taped to the operating room table may be substituted. The foot rest should be positioned such that when the foot lies on the padded clamp or blanket, the knee is flexed approximately 70° to 90°.

Although leg holders provide many advantages, principally the ease with which the joint compartments can be opened for meniscus surgery, they also have a number of disadvantages:

1. They limit exposure to the posterior compartments of the knee during meniscus repair.
2. They limit flexion during the procedure, which makes it more difficult to check for full motion and stability. It can also make harvest of the hamstring tendons more difficult.
3. They create the potential for venous stasis, compartment syndromes, and nerve injuries to the well leg.

If a leg holder is used, the well leg should be placed in a well-leg holder as recommended by Rosenberg et al.[177]

If an endoscopic technique is planned it is also important to position the leg holder proximally on the thigh, to allow room for the exit of the passing pin.

Diagnostic Arthroscopy

Following examination of the knee under anesthesia, diagnostic arthroscopy is performed prior to graft harvest in acute knee injuries to determine the nature and the degree of injury to the ACL, as well as to identify other intraarticular pathology. In chronic cases, diagnostic and operative arthroscopy is usually performed following graft harvest.

A solution of 0.25% bupivacaine with epinephrine is injected at the site of the arthroscopic portals to decrease bleeding. A large 6-mm inflow cannula is inserted through the superior medial portal if a gravity inflow system is to be used. If an infusion pump is employed, it is often unnecessary to use a separate inflow cannula. Before beginning the arthroscopy, the hemarthrosis is lavaged clear. Standard arthroscopy portals are used for the arthroscope and instrumentation. The arthroscope is inserted into the knee through the anterolateral portal, and an anteromedial portal is created under direct vision for instrumentation. The arthroscopic probe is used to check the status of the articular cartilage, menisci, ACL, and PCL. Partial meniscectomy or meniscus repair is performed as indicated. If the surgeon has elected to perform a hamstring tendon ACL reconstruction, then graft harvest should precede meniscus repair. If the meniscus repair is performed prior to harvesting the hamstring tendons, the repair sutures may be disrupted by the tendon stripper.

For reparable menisci an outside-in technique[178,179] or an inside-out technique[180,181] is used. Whichever technique is used, it is important to protect the neurovascular structures at risk, which are the saphenous vein and nerve on the medial side of the knee and the popliteal artery and peroneal nerve on the lateral side.[181] Transillumination with the arthroscope can often be used to identify the saphenous vein and nerve if an outside-in technique is used.

If the inside-out technique is used a posteromedial incision 3 to 4 cm long is made posterior to the oblique fibers of the MCL at the level of the joint line. Layer 1[182] is then divided. During this step care should be taken to avoid injury to the previously visualized saphenous vein and nerve, which lie in the inferior part of the incision. Blunt dissection is then used to expose layer 3 (the capsule) and the semimembranous tendon.[182] A plane between the tendon of the medial head of the gastrocnemius and layer 3 is established using scissors dissection. The popliteal retractor is inserted between the gastrocnemius tendon and layer 3 and above the direct head of the semitendinous tendon.

For lateral meniscus repairs the peroneal nerve is at risk. Posterolateral exposure is performed by making a 3- to 4-cm-long incision just posterior to the fibers of the lateral collateral ligament (LCL), which is easily palpated with the knee in the figure-four position.[183] Layer 1 on the lateral side is divided at the anterior border of the biceps tendon, at the junction of the muscular fibers of the short head and the tendinous fibers of the long head of the biceps tendon.[184] It is extremely important to avoid dissection along the posterior border of the biceps tendon, as the peroneal nerve lies just below. Scissors dissection is then used to establish a plane between the lateral head of the gastrocnemius and layer 3 and the capsule.[183,184] A popliteal retractor is placed between the gastrocnemius tendon and the capsule, thus protecting the posteriorly positioned neurovascular structures.

Following the completion of the arthroscopy, the arthroscope is removed from the knee and the ACL graft is harvested.

Graft Harvest

Patellar Tendon. Prior to harvesting the patellar tendon graft the skin incision is infiltrated with a solution of 0.25% bupivacaine with epinephrine to decrease bleeding. With the hemostasis provided by the bupivacaine and epinephrine solution, it is usually not necessary to use a tourniquet during graft harvest or during exposure of the distal femur. The patellar tendon graft can be harvested through a straight longitudinal incision 5 to 7 cm long. This incision is placed just medial to the crest of the tibia. A similar-length transverse incision located just above the tibial tubercle can also be used to expose the patellar tendon. I (C.H.B.) favor use of the transverse incision in females and in black patients because of its better cosmetic appearance and decreased tendency for keloid formation (Fig. 14–20).

The skin incision is carried down sharply to the prepatellar bursa. Skin flaps are created at the level of the bursa. A vertical incision centered over the ligament is made through the bursa and peritenon until the vertical fibers of the patellar tendon are exposed. This incision is extended from the tibial tubercle to the superior third of the patella.

Next, the bursa and peritenon are dissected off the patellar tendon. It is important to avoid excessive dissection along the borders of the patellar tendon as troublesome bleeding can be encountered (Fig. 14–21). The dimensions of the patellar tendon are measured and recorded. A 9- to 11-mm-wide section of patellar tendon centered in the middle of the tendon is marked out. Metal templates and graft harvesting knifes are now commercially available to assist the surgeon during this part of the procedure (Acufex Microsurgical Inc, Mansfield, MA; Linvatec, Largo, FL; DePuy, Warsaw, IN). The skin flaps are carefully retracted with two

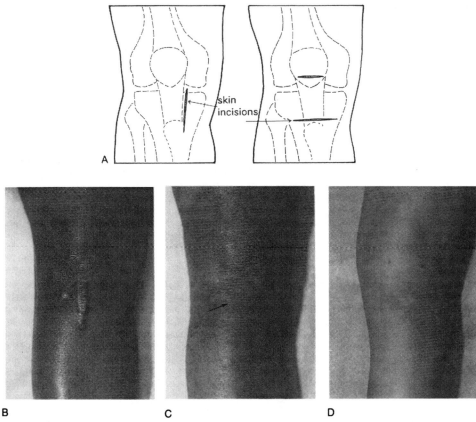

Figure 14-20. A. Incisions used for harvest of the patellar tendon autograft. A straight longitudinal incision just medial to the crest of the tibial tubercle is most commonly used to expose the patellar tendon. A transverse incision at the level of the tibial tubercle can also be used. This incision is most commonly used in females and in patients with a tendency toward keloid formation. The incision should be placed at the level of the tibial tubercle. If the incision is placed too high above the tubercle, then difficulty will be encountered harvesting the tibial bone block and during drilling of the tibial tunnel. If difficulty is encountered during harvest of the patel- lar bone block because of a long patellar tendon, then a small accessory transverse incision just proximal to the inferior pole of the patella can be used. **B.** Photograph of a vertical graft harvest incision in a black patient. This incision resulted in spreading of the scar and keloid formation. **C.** Photograph showing transverse incision (arrow) in a black patient. The transverse incision results in a thin, very cosmetic scar. **D.** Transverse incision in a white female patient. Because of the more limited exposure this incision should be used only after experience has been gained using the conventional vertical incision to harvest the patellar tendon.

small retractors and the appropriate width of the tendon is marked with the electrocautery at the level of the distal pole of the patella, the midportion of the tendon, and at the level of the tibial tubercle. The first cut in the tendon is made through the full thickness of the tendon using a sawing motion. This cut is extended from the inferior pole of the patella to the tibial tubercle (Fig. 14-22). The desired width of the tendon is remarked and a second cut parallel to the first incision is made.

Next, a bone block on the tibial tubercle measuring 25 to 27 mm in length is marked out with the electro- cautery. A microsagittal saw is used to harvest the tibial bone block (Fig. 14-23). The harvested tibial bone block should be trapezoidal in shape. The cuts should extend approximately 8 mm into the bone. It is important that the cuts are deep enough so that all the fibers of the patellar tendon insertion onto the bone block are kept intact. The bone blocks must be large enough to adequately fill the bone tunnels to provide optimal fixation with interference screws. The tibial bone block is carefully levered out from below, using a ¼-in. curved osteotome. The defect in the proximal tibia is packed

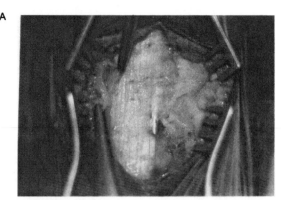

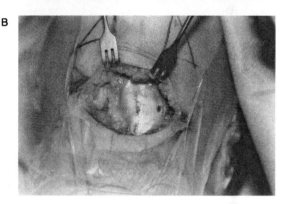

Figure 14–21. A. Exposure of the patella tendon through a vertical incision. The paratenon is being grasped by the forceps. The tissue to the left of the forceps is the prepatellar bursa. During graft harvest the paratenon and the bursa are preserved and closed over the patellar defect. **B.** Exposure of the patellar tendon through a transverse incision. Scissors and blunt finger dissection is used to elevate the superior skin flap. This flap is then gently retracted by lifting upward with small rake retractors to visualize the inferior pole of the patella.

with Gelfoam (Upjohn Co, Kalamazoo, MI) to decrease bleeding from the cancellous bone.

Next, the tibial bone block is grasped with a small pointed AO fracture reduction forceps (Synthes, Paoli, PA). The knee is then placed into extension and tension is placed on the tibial bone block, which pulls the patella inferiorly into the incision. By placing the knee into extension to harvest the tibial bone block the skin incision length can be minimized. The skin edges around the patella are retracted and the patellar bone block, which is 25 mm long, is marked out with the electrocautery. The patellar bone block cuts are made with a microsagittal saw, beveling the side cuts in at about a 45° angle to create a triangular-shaped bone block. The top cut is then completed with the saw. The cuts should be deep enough so that the entire insertion of the patellar tendon into the inferior pole of the patella is removed with the bone block. The patellar bone block is gently lifted out of its bed using a ¼-in. curved osteotome. The graft is given to the assistant for preparation on a separate table.

The patellar bone graft site is packed with Gelfoam

to decrease bleeding. After hemostasis is achieved, the Gelfoam is removed from the patellar defect and bone that has been trimmed from the bone blocks is packed into the defect. Bone grafting of the patellar bone defect is performed in an effort to decrease the risk of a late patellar fracture (Muller W. Personal communication, April 1986).[185–187] Extra bone graft can also be obtained with a small curette from the proximal tibia if needed. The bursa and peritenon are then closed over the ligament defect but the defect in the ligament is left open.

Semitendinosus and Gracilis Tendons. Prior to harvesting the hamstring tendons one should review the anatomy of the pes anserinus tendons. Four excellent sources are the articles by Warren and Marshall,[182] Ferrari and Ferrari,[188] Ivey and Prud'homme,[189] and Pagnani et al.[190] The article by Ivey and Prud'homme is particularly relevant as they describe some of the anatomic variations of the pes anserinus tendons that the surgeon must be aware of in order to avoid damaging the tendons during graft harvest. The course of the

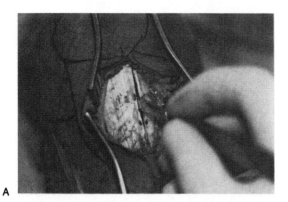

A

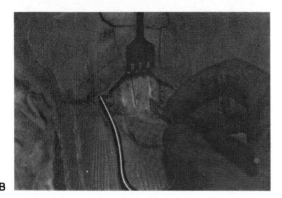

B

Figure 14–22. The patellar tendon is sharply incised from the patella to the tibial tubercle using a scalpel. **A.** Vertical incision. **B.** Transverse incision. The superior skin flap must be gently lifted and the surgeon must stoop down to visualize the inferior pole of the patella. The presized double-blade graft harvesting knives (Defuy, Warsaw, IN) and the dual retrograde cutter (Arthrex, Naples, FL) can help simplify this part of the procedure.

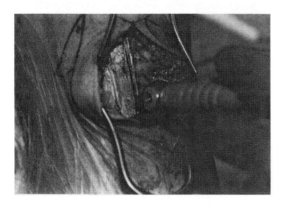

Figure 14–23. A microsagittal saw is used to harvest the tibial bone block.

saphenous nerve which is one of the structures at risk during harvest of the hamstring tendons is beautifully described in the article by Pagnani et al.[190]

Harvest of the hamstring tendons can be performed through either a vertical or an oblique incision over the pes anserinus. Remembering that the top of the sartorius tendon is about one fingerbreadth below the tibial tubercle or three fingerbreadths below the medial joint line helps in placing the incision. The authors prefer an oblique incision at the top of the pes anserinus as it

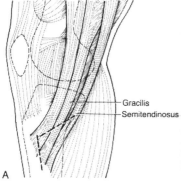
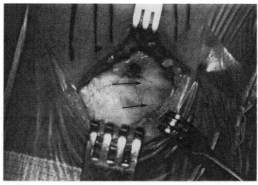

A

B

Figure 14-24. A. The semitendinosus and gracilis tendons can be harvested through a vertical incision or an oblique incision. The authors prefer the oblique incision because it provides better exposure and is more cosmetic. B. Blunt dissection is used to sweep the subcutaneous fat off layer 1, the sartorius fascia. The hamstring tendons can be seen (arrows) and palpated as two small bumps lying under the fascia. It is easier to palpate the tendons as they course across the superficial MCL because they are round at this level. As the tendons near their insertion into the proximal tibia they flatten and are more difficult to feel.

allows the skin to be retracted parallel to the orientation of the tendons, providing better exposure, and produces a more cosmetic scar (Fig. 14–24).

The skin incision is infiltrated with 10 mL of a 0.25% bupivacaine with epinephrine solution. This helps to control skin bleeding and allows graft harvest to be performed without inflating the tourniquet. It also helps to define the plane between the fat and the sartorius fascia. Sharp dissection is carried down until layer 1, the sartorius fascia, is visualized.[182] The subcutaneous fat is bluntly dissected off layer 1 with a sponge and scissors. The gracilis and semitendinosus tendons can then be seen and palpated as two small "speed bumps" lying inferior to the flat tendinous insertion of the sartorius.

The tendons are exposed by making an incision through layer 1 at the top of the gracilis tendon. Care must be taken when making this incision as layer 2, the superficial medial collateral ligament,[182] lies just below and can be injured. Blunt dissection can then be used to sweep the thin filmy fascia between layers 1 and 2 away. The gracilis and semitendinosus can be found on the underside of layer 1. The pes anserinus tendons can be harvested by leaving their biologic insertions intact, in which case a slotted tendon stripper is used, or they may be detached from the tibia first and a closed tendon stripper used (Acufex Microsurgical Inc, Mansfield, MA). CHB has found it easier and faster and the tendons are better visualized by detaching them from their tibial insertions first.

The previous incision in layer 1 at the top of the gracilis tendon is extended to the crest of the tibia using the electrocautery, thus obtaining an extra 10 to 15 mm

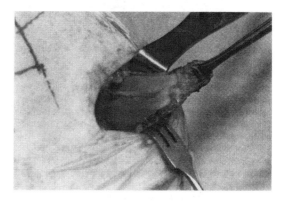

Figure 14-25. The gracilis and semitendinosus tendons lie on the underside of layer 1, between layers 1 and 2. The gracilis is the superior and smaller of the two tendons.

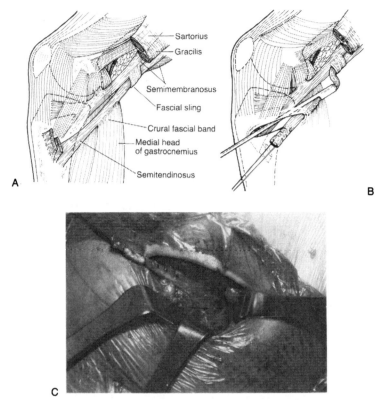

Figure 14–26. A. There are two potential areas of difficulty during harvest of the semitendinosus. The tendinous insertion from the semitendinosus into the crural fascia of the medial head of the gastrocnemius represents the first area of difficulty. This band must be incised with scissors to allow more proximal exposure of the tendon and to prevent premature amputation of the tendon by the tendon stripper. A tight band running from the semimembranosus, which forms a sling for the semitendinosus tendon, represents the second area of potential difficulty. This band can usually be released with blunt finger or scissors dissection. Failure to release this band can result in premature amputation of the tendon and possible injury to the saphenous nerve and vein as the stripper passes outside of the tunnel. **B.** Stripper passing outside of fascial bands can result in premature amputation of the semitendinosus and possible damage to the saphenous nerve and vein. (Redrawn with permission from Ferrari and Ferrari.[188]) **C.** Intraoperative photograph showing the fascial band (solid arrow) connecting the semitendinosus (open arrow) to the medial head of the gastrocnemius. This band must be incised before an attempt is made to harvest the tendon.

of length. A vertical incision starting at the crest of the tibia is extended inferiorly until both of the tendons are freed from the tibia. Traction is then applied to layer 1 and subperiosteal dissection is used to dissect the tendons off the face of the tibia. Excellent exposure of the tendons can be obtained by everting layer 1, and any anatomic variations can be easily identified prior to stripping[189] (Fig. 14–25).

Blunt dissection using a right-angle clamp is used to free first the gracilis and then the semitendinosus tendons from layer 1. By limiting dissection to the underside of layer 1 risk of injury to the saphenous vein and nerve is minimized as these structures lie superficial to

layer 1.[190] After each tendon is released, a running baseball-type whip stitch using a No. 2 nonabsorbable suture is placed in the free end of each tendon.

The stripping of the tendons can be greatly facilitated by flexing the knee, applying traction through the whip stitch, and using finger dissection to bluntly dissect along the course of the tendons toward the posteromedial thigh. Prior to stripping of the tendons, the tendinous insertions from the semitendinosus that blend into the fascia of the medial head of the gastrocnemius must be cut to avoid premature amputation by the stripper.[188,191] According to Ferrari and Ferrari these insertions into the gastrocnemius fascia occur approx-

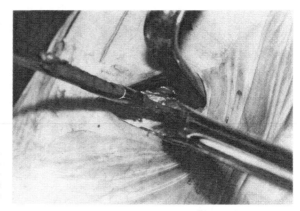

Figure 14–27. Harvesting the semitendinosus tendon with a closed tendon stripper. The skin is retracted with blunt retractors and tension is maintained on the tendon with the previously placed whip stitch. The tendon stripper is slowly advanced parallel to the tendon.

imately 7 cm from the distal tibial attachment site of the semitendinosus.[188] A second potentially troublesome area occurs at a band of thickened fascia that courses inferior and medial to the semimembranosus, providing a sling for the semitendinosus. Ferrari and Ferrari have recommended that if the stripper does not easily pass beyond the 7-cm mark, it should be removed, and longer scissors should be used to release this band to avoid premature amputation of the tendon[188] (Fig. 14–26).

Traction is applied to the tendon, and the tendon stripper is advanced slowly parallel to the direction of the tendon using a slow and steady "back-and-forth" motion (Fig. 14–27). Usually, 25 to 32 cm of length can be obtained. We have noted as have others[192] that examination of the posteromedial thigh months after surgery will reveal the palpable regeneration of these tendons (Fig. 14–28).

Graft Preparation

Patellar Tendon. The patellar tendon graft is prepared on a separate table by the assistant. The graft is wrapped in a moist sponge during its preparation and placed in a flat basin to decrease the risk of accidental dropping. The patellar bone block is trimmed with a bone rongeur until it fits through a 9- or 10-mm metal sizing tube (Acufex Microsurgical Inc, Mansfield, MA). The tip of the patellar bone block is trimmed into a bullet shape to assist in its passage through the bone tunnels. Minimizing the gap between the tunnel and bone block is important to maximize the strength of interference screw fixation.[120] The tibial bone block, which is usually the larger of the two bone blocks, is trimmed into a cylindrical shape to fit through a 9- or 10-mm sizing tube.

As most fixation studies have demonstrated that frac-

ture through a bone block drill hole is a common mode of fixation failure during tensile testing, one drill hole rather than three is made in the patellar bone block. Fewer holes result in fewer stress risers in the bone block. A 2.0-mm pointed drill guide (Synthes, Paoli, PA) is used to place one 2.0-mm drill hole toward the end of the bone block away from the tendon end. One No. 5 nonabsorbable suture is place through the hole in

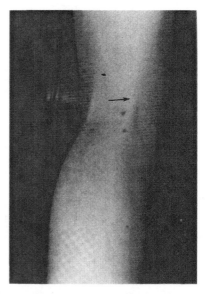

Figure 14–28. Regrowth of medial hamstring tendons (arrow) in a patient 4 months following harvest of the semitendinosus and gracilis tendons.

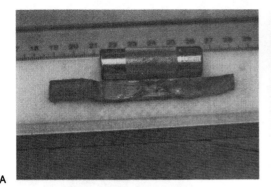

A

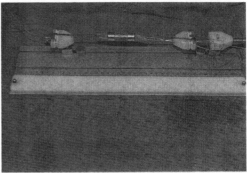

C

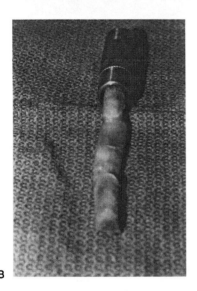

B

Figure 14–29. A. Patellar tendon graft following harvest. **B.** The bone blocks are trimmed to fit through a 9- or 10-mm sizing tube. **C.** Prepared patellar tendon graft is pretensioned to 10 lb.

the patellar bone block. These sutures are then tied together over the tip of the bone block, creating a "leader." This makes graft passage through the joint easier.

Next, two evenly spaced 2.0-mm holes are drilled in the tibial bone block. Two No. 5 nonabsorbable sutures are placed in the hole nearest the patellar tendon attachment and an 18-gauge wire is placed in the last hole furthest from the tendon attachment. The 18-gauge wire can be used to apply tension to the patellar tendon graft should the sutures happen to be cut by the interference screw at the time of graft fixation. This will avoid loss of tension on the bone block and prevent possible advancement of the bone block and subsequent loss of graft tension as the interference screw is tightened[193] (Fig. 14–29).

The prepared graft is wrapped in a blood-soaked sponge and pretensioned to 5 to 10 lb on a tensioning board (Acufex Microsurgical Inc, Mansfield, MA) to preload the graft.

Hamstring Tendons. Preparation of the hamstring tendons is facilitated by use of a graft preparation board (Acufex Microsurgical Inc, Mansfield, MA). The muscle fibers on the proximal ends of the tendons are gently scraped away using a large curette (Fig. 14–30). The musculotendinous end of each tendon is tubularized with a running No. 2 nonabsorbable baseball whip stitch (Fig. 14–31). The ends of three long No. 5 nonabsorbable sutures are then tied together, producing a large composite suture. Each tendon graft is looped around the previously prepared No. 5 composite suture and the lengths of the tendons are equalized (Fig. 14–32). The graft is presized using a sizing tube. The typi-

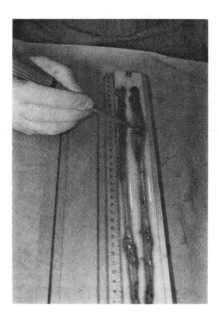

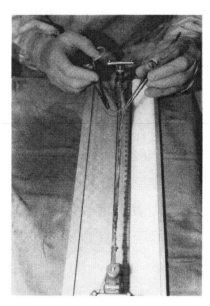

Figure 14–30. A large curette is used to gently strip the muscle fibers from the two hamstring tendons.

Figure 14–31. Whip-stitching of the semitendinosus with a No. 2 nonabsorbable suture. Use of a graft preparation board facilitates preparation of the grafts. (Acufex Microsurgical Inc., Mansfield, MA)

cal diameter of the combined grafts is 8 to 10 mm (average size of 8 mm in females and 9 mm in males).

The No. 2 nonabsorbable sutures on each end of the graft are connected to the tensiometer on the graft preparation board and the composite graft is pretensioned to 10 lb to preload the grafts and to distribute tension equally in all four limbs. The four limbs of the composite graft are then sutured together with an O absorbable suture approximately 2 and 6 cm from the looped end. A circumferential mark 25 mm from the looped end of the graft is made with a marking pen or methylene blue. This mark is used later when the graft is passed to ensure that at least 25 mm of graft material remains in the tibial tunnel (Fig. 14–33).

Exposure of the Distal Femur

The knee is brought back into midflexion and the distal femoral incision is made. Prior to the incision, the skin is infiltrated with 0.25% bupivacaine with epinephrine for hemostasis. The incision is started at the level of the superior pole of the patella and is carried proximally for about 3 to 4 cm. The incision is located about 1 cm above the posterior border of the iliotibial tract (Fig. 14–34). This hides the incision behind the bulge of the vastus lateralis muscle. The incision is carried down sharply to the level of the iliotibial band. Blunt dissection is used to define the posterior border of the band. The iliotibial band is divided at the junction of its thin

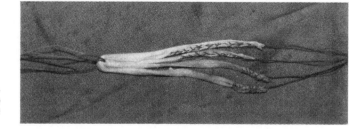

Figure 14–32. The prepared hamstring tendons are looped around three No. 5 nonabsorbable sutures and the tendon lengths equalized.

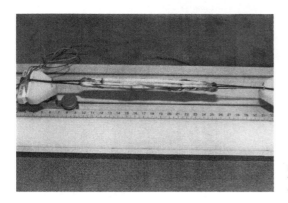

Figure 14–33. The composite graft is then pretensioned to 10 lb on the graft preparation board. Note the large size of the graft, in this case 10 mm in diameter.

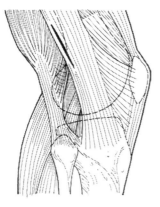

Figure 14–34. The distal femur is exposed through a 3- to 4-cm straight incision placed one fingerbreadth anterior to the posterior border of the iliotibial band.

anterior one third and the thick posterior two thirds, thus preserving the important fibers of the anterolateral femorotibial ligament (ALFTL).[21] This split is extended the length of the incision.

The vastus lateralis is bluntly elevated off the intermuscular septum using digital dissection. Two Z-type retractors or Army–Navy-type retractors are used to retract the vastus lateralis muscle superiorly. The superior lateral geniculate artery and vein are identified and cauterized. The electrocautery is used to reflect the periosteum off the bone just proximal to the flare of the distal femur. This minimizes walkoff of the femoral drill guide when the guide pins are drilled. To avoid potential injury to the peroneal nerve, it is important to avoid dissection below the intermuscular septum. This completes the exposure of the distal femur.

Intercondylar Notch Preparation

Preparation of the intercondylar notch is one of the most important aspects of ACL reconstruction. Proper notch preparation is necessary to allow visualization of the femoral attachment site and to avoid impingement of the ACL substitute.

The knee is placed in approximately 70° of flexion with slight internal rotation of the tibia. The intercondylar notch is exposed by first resecting the ligamentum muscosum. This allows the fat pad to drop away from the notch. Next, a full-radius motorized shaver blade is used to resect the fat pad until the intercondylar notch and the tibial remnant of the ACL are adequately visualized. Excessive resection of the fat pad should be avoided as it can result in troublesome bleeding and increased postoperative scarring.

The ACL remnant is inspected, and the notch size and configuration are studied. The anatomy of the intercondylar notch has been described by various authors[115,194–196] (Fig. 14–35). These authors have noted that intercondylar notch stenosis exists in many knees with chronic ACL deficiency (Fig. 14–36). Notch stenosis makes visualization of the femoral ACL attachment site difficult and may result in bony impingement on the ACL graft. To allow adequate visualization and eliminate bony impingement, a widening or "notchplasty" of the intercondylar notch must be performed.[195]

Howell et al used MRI to predict the amount of bone resection necessary to prevent impingement of the ACL graft in the roof of the intercondylar notch.[75] This study demonstrated that roof impingement of the ACL graft was extremely sensitive to the sagittal position of the tibial tunnel. Using sagittal MRI images, they predicted the degree of roof impingement for three hypothetical tibial positions: the eccentric position as recommended by Clancy et al,[52,63,123] a central position, and a position 3 mm posterior to the center of the ACL insertion in

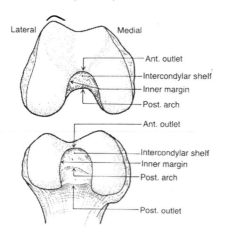

Figure 14–35. Anatomy and nomenclature of the intercondylar notch. (Redrawn with permission from Kieffer et al.[195])

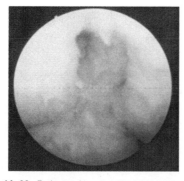

Figure 14–36. Patient with chronic ACL-deficient knee showing the marked narrowing of the intercondylar notch. An extensive notchplasty is required in such a case.

line with the bulk of the ACL fibers. Positioning the center of the ACL graft eccentrically required 4.8 ± 0.6 mm of bone resection from the roof of the intercondylar notch to prevent impingement of the ACL graft in full extension, 1.8 ± 0.8 mm for the central position, and 0.0 ± 0.7 mm for the bulk position.

On the basis of these findings, the authors recommended that a routine "roofplasty" be performed on all acute and chronic ACL reconstructions, and that the tibial tunnel be positioned within the center of the ACL insertion or 3 mm posterior to this position in line with the bulk fibers of the ACL. They felt that the eccentric tibial tunnel position as recommended by Clancy et al[52,63,123] should be avoided as this position would

either lead to roof impingement of the graft or require an excessive roofplasty to prevent impingement (Fig. 14–37).

Once adequate visualization of the intercondylar notch is obtained, the ACL remnant is resected with a motorized shaver. Soft tissue from the roof of the notch and the inner margin of the lateral femoral condyle is removed using a full-radius blade. The soft tissue must be removed from the inner margin of the lateral femoral condyle all the way back to the "over-the-top" drop-off point. The old fibers of the ACL along the inner margin of the posterior aspect of the lateral femoral condyle are resected using the motorized shaver. It is often surprising how much more of the lateral femoral condyle can lie behind this tissue. Failure to remove all of the old femoral stump of the ACL and adequately visualize the posterior outlet of the intercondylar notch is one of the most common errors causing an anterior placement of the graft.

In many knees there is a distinct vertical bony ridge along the inner margin of the lateral femoral condyle that lies approximately 4 to 8 mm anterior to the true over-the-top position. This ridge has been referred to as the *residents* or *fellows ridge* (Fig. 14–38). This ridge must not be confused with the true posterior outlet of the notch because this may lead the surgeon by mistake to position the femoral guide pin too anteriorly. This mistake can be avoided by making sure to resect the soft tissue along the inner margin of the lateral femoral condyle until the back of the condyle is reached and the posterior capsule is clearly visualized.

Following soft tissue debridement of the notch, bony resection is performed. The anterior outlet of the notch is first widened. Bone resection can be performed with a variety of instruments including curettes, osteotomes, and a motorized shaver. The authors prefer to use a small curved arthroscopic gouge to perform the majority of the bony resection (Acufex Microsurgical Inc, Mansfield, MA). The final contouring of the notch is performed using a motorized shaver with an abrader.

If troublesome bleeding is encountered during the notchplasty the inflow cannula should be redirected into the medial or lateral gutter to provide better flow. If this fails to improve the visualization, then the inflow can be switched directly to the arthroscope. As mentioned earlier, with an infusion pump system and the inflow connected directly to the arthroscope, I (C.H.B.) have not encountered excessive bone bleeding during the notchplasty. If either of these adjustments fails to improve visualization then the tourniquet may need to be inflated until the bone tunnels are drilled.

Bone is resected from the inner margin of the lateral femoral condyle ("wallplasty") and the roof of the intercondylar notch ("roofplasty"). During the notchplasty it is important to avoid resecting excessive bone from the

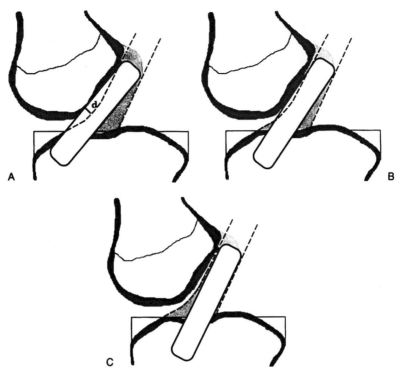

Figure 14–37. A. A 10-mm-wide graft centered on the antero-medial eccentric position, as recommended by Clancy et al,[52,63,123] results in impingement of the graft against the roof of the intercondylar notch in extension. Approximately 5 to 6 mm of bone will need to be resected from the anterior outlet of the intercondylar notch. **B.** If the graft is centered on the center of the ACL, approximately 2 to 3 mm of bone will need to be resected from the anterior outlet of the intercondylar notch to prevent impingement. **C.** If the graft is centered on the bulk portion of the ACL, minimal bone resection is needed. (Reprinted with permission from Howell et al.[75])

posterior attachment site of the old ACL, as this will lateralize the femoral attachment site of the ACL graft and change the axis of the reconstructed ligament. At the completion of the notchplasty, the inner margin of the lateral femoral condyle should be smooth and vertical, and the surgeon should be able to easily visualize the over-the-top dropoff point with the arthroscope in the anterolateral portal (Fig. 14–39).

Tibial Guide-Pin Placement

Although arthroscopy-assisted ACL reconstruction can be performed freehand without the use of a drill guide system, use of a drill guide can make the procedure more accurate and reproducible.[197,198] Currently our drill guide of choice is the Pro-Trac tibial aimer and rear-entry guide system (Acufex Microsurgical Inc, Mansfield, MA).

The external position of the tibial tunnel is varied de-pending on the type of ACL graft used. For the two-incision technique using a patellar tendon autograft, the tibial tunnel is positioned at the top of the pes anserine tendons, just medial to the tibial tubercle. This tibial position combined with the femoral position produced by the rear-entry aimer usually results in an excellent match between the length of the patellar tendon graft and the bone tunnels.

For hamstring tendons the tibial tunnel position on the medial face of the tibia can be varied. Adjusting the Pro-Trac tibial aimer to the "endo" position produces a shorter, more horizontal tunnel closer to the joint line compared with patellar tendon autografts. This shorter tibial tunnel helps to ensure that the hamstring tendon grafts span the entire length of the tibial tunnel, allow-ing for greater bony ingrowth, and reduces the length of the looped sutures between the end of the graft and the fixation screw. As the stiffness of the reconstruction is determined by the length of graft plus the loop sutures

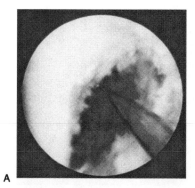

A

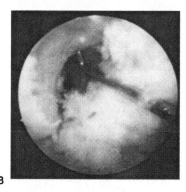

B

Figure 14–38. A. The "residents" or "fellows" ridge is shown by the probe. This ridge can be confused with the true over-the-top position, leading to anterior placement of the femoral guide pin. **B.** Same patient with the probe marking the true over-the-top position. The "residents" ridge can be seen lying anterior to the probe.

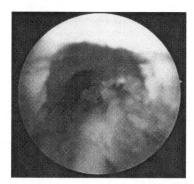

Figure 14–39. Arthroscopic view following notchplasty. At the completion of the notchplasty the surgeon should be able to visualize the posterior capsule and the over-the-top position.

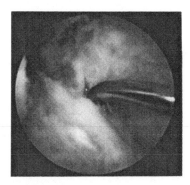

Figure 14–40. Intraoperative photograph showing the position of the tibial guide pin. The tibial guide pin should lie approximately 7 mm anterior to the PCL.

from the femoral fixation to the tibial fixation, a shorter tibial tunnel length will increase the stiffness compared with more vertical and longer tibial tunnels. Because our fixation method allows for recession of the tibial end of the graft, the Pro-Trac aimer can also be adjusted to produce a more conventional tibial tunnel just superior to the sartorius tendon.

In preparation for drilling the tibial guide pin, the electrocautery is used to reflect a flap of periosteum from the tibia at the selected position of the guide pin. The Pro-Trac tibial aiming guide is inserted through the anteromedial portal. The tip of the guide is positioned in the center of the middle third of the tibial remanent, just lateral to the medial intercondylar eminence (Fig. 14–40). The guide is adjusted so that the bullet will lie against the previously prepared site on the medial face of the tibia. A 2.4-mm guide pin is then drilled into the tibia until the tip of the pin is just visible.

Femoral Guide-Pin Position

To position the femoral aimer more accurately a pilot hole for the tip of the aimer is made with a 3-mm closed-angle curette. A small penetration point is made posterior and superior to the center of the old ACL femoral attachment site along the inner wall of the lateral femoral condyle. This point should be approximately 2 to 3 mm anterior to the over-the-top dropoff point, at the 11 o'clock position in a right knee or the 1 o'clock position in a left knee.

The arthroscope is then switched to the anteromedial portal. The curved rear-entry passer is inserted through the anterolateral portal and passed over the top of the lateral femoral condyle under direct vision. During passage of the curved rear-entry passer, it is important that the tip of the passer hug the bone of the lateral femoral condyle and not deviate posteriorly or medially, as this might lead to neurovascular injury. The tip of the surgeon's finger is inserted through the lateral femoral incision above the intermuscular septum at the flare of the distal femur. The surgeon should be able to feel the tip of the passer as it is passed up through the lateral intermuscular septum into the lateral incision.

The appropriate right or left rear-entry femoral aimer is engaged into the eyelet of the passer. The passer and the tip of the rear-entry aimer are pulled into the knee joint under direct vision. The passer is then disengaged and removed from the knee.

The scope is switched back to the anterolateral portal. The tip of the rear-entry femoral aimer is placed in the previously prepared pilot hole. The tripoint bullet is inserted into the guide and pushed down until it contacts the cortex of the distal femur. The handle of the guide is rotated from a horizontal position to a more vertical position. This helps to ensure that the guide pin will be inserted above the intermuscular septum and as far proximal on the femur as possible. The more proximal the femoral guide pin is placed, the less the tunnel divergence and bending moment on the ACL graft. To avoid injury to the posterior neurovascular structures it is extremely important to make sure that the tip of the tripoint bullet is above the intermuscular septum before drilling the guide pin.

A 2.4-mm guide pin is then drilled through the femoral condyle into the knee under direct vision. The tip of the guide pin should enter the intercondylar notch at the site of the previously prepared penetration point (Fig. 14–41). The femoral aimer is then removed from the knee. With the knee between 70° and 90° of flexion the two guide pins should be roughly parallel.

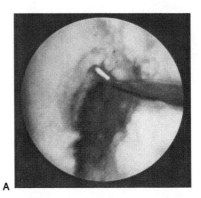

A

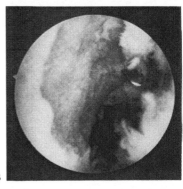

B

Figure 14–41. A. Arthroscopic view following completion of the notchplasty. The correct position for the trial femoral guide pin is marked by the probe. **B.** Femoral guide-pin position. Note the close proximity to the over-the-top position.

Guide-Pin Assessment

At this point in the procedure, the bone tunnels can be drilled if the surgeon is satisfied with the guide-pin placement, or the guide-pin placement can be checked prior to drilling the bone tunnels. To check the guide-pin placement the tibial guide pin is first removed, and a suture retriever (Acufex Microsurgical Inc, Mansfield, MA) is passed through the guide-pin hole into the knee. Next, the femoral guide pin is removed, and a No. 5 Ethibond suture is loaded on a suture pusher (Synthes, Paoli, PA), and pushed through the femoral guide-pin hole into the intercondylar notch. A small arthroscopic grasping clamp is passed through the anteromedial portal and is used to retrieve the suture. With the grasping clamp, the suture is passed through the loop of the suture retriever and the retriever is pulled out of the tibial guide-pin hole. A button is tied to the femoral end of the suture and pulled flush against the bone of the distal femur. The tibial end of the suture is passed through the Graf isometer (Acufex Microsurgical Inc, Mansfield, MA), and the

nose of the isometer is engaged in the tibial guide-pin hole. With the knee at 30° of flexion, slack is removed from the suture and the suture is wrapped around the barrel of the isometer. The spring on the isometer is released and length measurements are made.

Experimental studies indicate that the anteromedial fibers of the ACL undergo the smallest changes in length through the full range of motion.[110–113,114, 116–118,122,124] It is these fibers that we attempt to replace during intraarticular ACL reconstruction. With the knee at 90° this reading on the isometer is taken as zero. The knee is then slowly extended and readings are taken at 60°, 30°, 15°, 0°, and full hyperextension. The knee is flexed back to 90° and the isometer should return to its initial reading. Readings are then obtained as the knee is flexed to 120°. The anteromedial fibers of the human ACL lengthen 2 to 2.5 mm as the knee is extended from 90° into full extension, with most of the lengthening occurring in the last 30° of extension.[113,116–119] There should be no more than 1 to 2 mm of lengthening as the knee is extended from 90° to 120°.

Because the patellar tendon graft will lean along the anterior part of the femoral tunnel, the femoral guide pin must be positioned posterior and superior to the ideal isometric point on the femur.[52,113,114,120,123] Drilling of this eccentric bone tunnel will ensure that the majority of the fibers of the patellar tendon graft come to lie near the most isometric region on the femur, minimizing the number of fibers that lie anterior to the flexion axis of rotation. To prevent a too anterior placement of the femoral tunnel, the femoral guide pin should be positioned so that the isometer indicates at least 2 to 3 mm of lengthening as the knee is extended from 30° to full extension. Brand and Daniel, in a prospective study of 90 patients, found that a mean pilot hole length change of 2.9 ± 1.3 mm of lengthening was decreased to 1.6 ± 1.1 mm of lengthening when the bone tunnels were drilled.[120] They concluded that converting pilot holes to bone tunnels does cause the femoral axis of the graft to come to lie in a more anterior position. They recommended that pilot holes should be selected such that there would be 3 to 4 mm of lengthening when the knee was extended from 90° to full extension. Drilling of the bone tunnels would then decrease this to 1 to 2 mm of lengthening, which they felt was the desired result.

Because round grafts like the hamstring tendons will fill the entire bone tunnel and demonstrate less eccentric shifting, the femoral guide pin need not be positioned so eccentrically. With the use of doubled hamstring tendons, an acceptable guide-pin position should indicate 2 to 3 mm of lengthening with extension from 90° to full extension. This lengthening pattern of the graft with extension indicates that the femoral pilot hole position is posterior to the axis of rotation. If the femoral guide pin is positioned too far anterior to the flexion axis the isometer will indicate a shortening pattern with extension. If the isometer indicates a shortening pattern with extension, the femoral guide pin will need to be repositioned more posteriorly. The 3- and 5-mm parallel drill guides (Acufex Microsurgical Inc, Mansfield, MA) can be used to reposition the guide pin, avoiding the need to reinsert the rear-entry guide. The new guide-pin position can then be rechecked with the isometer.

Once the surgeon is satisfied with the guide-pin position, smooth guide pins are inserted by hand into the previously drilled guide-pin holes. A large curette is inserted into the joint and placed over the tip of the guide pin, to prevent guide-pin migration into the joint during drilling. The bone tunnels are drilled with the appropriate 9- or 10-mm cannulated drill bit. The graft sizing tubes can be used to protect the soft tissues during the drilling of the bone tunnels. The reamings from the

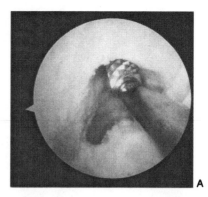

A

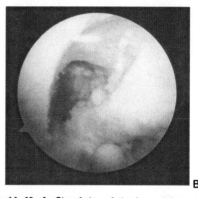

B

Figure 14–42. A. Chamfering of the femoral bone tunnel with a half-round rasp. It is especially important to remove any sharp bony edges to avoid graft abrasion. Graf et al, in an animal experiment, showed that graft survival was enhanced in chamfered versus nonchamfered tunnels.[172] **B.** Final arthroscopic appearance of the bone tunnels.

bone tunnels are saved and used to bone graft the defect in the tibial tubercle.

After the bone tunnels have been drilled, cannulated bone plugs (Linvatec Inc, Largo, FL) are inserted into the bone tunnels to maintain fluid distension. The sharp internal openings of the bone tunnels into the joint are smoothed with a half-round or an ACL chamfering rasp (Acufex Microsurgical Inc, Mansfield, MA) to prevent abrasion of the graft (Fig. 14–42).

It is particularly important to remove all the ACL soft tissue remnants and bony fragments from around and inside the tibial tunnel to prevent the formation of a "cyclops lesion."[199,200] A motorized shaver can be used to remove any further soft tissue and bony debris from inside the tibial tunnel by removing the tunnel plug and inserting the shaver blade directly up the tunnel. Bony debris and the ACL soft tissue remnants have

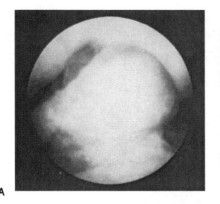
A

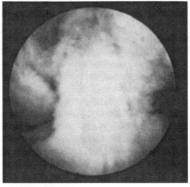
B

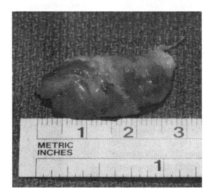
C

Figure 14–43. A. Arthroscopic view of a large "cyclops lesion." Three months following ACL reconstruction with a patellar tendon graft, patient noted the sudden onset of pain and loss of extension. Plain radiographs revealed the tibial tunnel to be positioned posterior to the roof of the intercon- dylar notch with the knee in maximum hyperextension. An MRI scan reveals no evidence of graft impingement. **B.** Arthro- scopic view showing the graft following resection of the "cyclops lesion." Arthroscopic excision eliminated the pain and restored full extension. **C.** Gross specimen.

been implicated by Jackson and Schaefer[199] and Marzo et al[200] as a possible cause of extension loss and an au- dible and palpable clunk with terminal knee extension, the so-called "cyclops syndrome" (Fig. 14–43). Once the bony tunnels have been debrided and chamfered, the ACL graft is ready to be passed.

Graft Passage

The fluid inflow is shut off and the tunnel plugs are re- moved. An 18-gauge wire bent in a loop is passed blind- ly up the tibial tunnel with the knee at around 70° of flexion. If the tunnel divergence is minimal, the wire will easily pass blindly through the joint and exit through the femoral tunnel. If difficulty is encountered in passing the wire, the knee flexion angle may need to be changed. For a double-looped hamstring tendon, the three No. 5 Ethibond sutures looped through the

axilla of the folded grafts are placed in the loop of the 18-gauge wire and pulled across the joint and out of the tibial tunnel.

Under arthroscopic visualization the hamstring ten- don graft is pulled down from the femur. It is important to ensure that the mark that was placed earlier, 25 mm from the looped end of the tendon, is advanced until it lies below the tibial surface. This ensures that at least 25 mm of graft lies in the tibial tunnel for healing.

For patellar tendon grafts a second 18-gauge wire is passed through the loop of the first wire and pulled back across the joint and out of the tibial tunnel. The sutures from the patellar bone block are then passed through the loop in the wire. The wire is passed across the joint, pulling the sutures out of the femoral tunnel. The cancellous surface of the graft is oriented anterior- ly, forcing the flat patellar tendon to lie as posteriorly in the bone tunnel as possible. The graft is then passed with a back-and-forth motion. Once the bone block in the femoral tunnel is seated, the tibial end of the graft is internally rotated 180°. This internal rotation more evenly distributes the tension in the fiber bundles and decreases the size of the graft, decreasing the potential for notch impingement. Cooper et al in the laboratory were also able to show that this twisting of the graft increased the ultimate failure load by 30% over grafts that were not twisted.[70]

If difficulty is encountered in passing the graft, excessive force should not be used as this may damage it. In these circumstances the graft should be passed under arthroscopic control. The ends of the bone blocks are centered in both bone tunnels and the arthroscope is inserted back into the joint to check that the bone blocks do not protrude into the joint.

Femoral Graft Fixation

For patellar tendon grafts, graft fixation is performed using 7.0- or 9.0-mm interference screws. The femoral end of the graft is fixed first. In the average-sized patient we prefer to use a 9.0-mm interference screw, as the data of Kurosaka et al indicate that it will provide superior fixation strength.[134] In small patients, a 7.0-mm screw can be used. The length of the screw is determined by the length of the bone blocks. For optimal fixation strength the screw should engage the bone block along its entire length, but the tip of the screw should not protrude beyond the bone block. If the tip of the screw protrudes beyond the bone block the sharp tip could lacerate the graft.[201] It is also important that when the screw is fully inserted, it be slightly recessed under the cortex to prevent painful impingement against the soft tissues, possibly necessitating early removal. In general a screw the same length as the bone block is selected. The femoral screw is inserted in the anterior part of the tunnel along the cancellous side of the graft. This will help translocate the bone block to the posterior aspect of the femoral bone tunnel. The sutures are pulled away from the side of the graft where the interference screw will be inserted to prevent suture laceration. Tension is maintained on the sutures as the screw is inserted to prevent possible advancement of the bone block into the joint. During the insertion of the interference screw, it is important to insert the screw parallel to the bone tunnel to minimize divergence of the screw from the bone tunnel. The introduction of cannulated interference screws has helped to minimize this complication. The interference screw is tightened down until it lies just under the cortex.

Reznik et al have recently presented data that can be used to help optimize interference screw fixation.[201] They studied the effects of bone density, gap size, and insertion torque on the strength of interference screw fixation in a pig model. They concluded that the fixation

strength was higher in more dense bone and that a gap size of 4 mm or less between the bone block and the bone tunnel provided the strongest fixation. They also measured the insertion torque required to insert the interference screw and determined that an insertion torque greater than 12 in.-lb would provide a fixation strength of greater than 150 lb (668 N) in pig bone during static testing.

Brown et al have performed a similar study using human cadavers.[202] Their data showed that there was a weak positive correlation ($R^2 = 0.45$) between interference screw insertion torque and screw pullout force. Based on their data, a screw insertion torque of 12 in.-lb correlates with a pullout force of 98.5 lb (438 N). With further data screw insertion torque might provide the surgeon with an intraoperative estimate of initial fixation strength.

For double-looped hamstring tendon grafts, femoral fixation is accomplished with two 4.5-mm bicortical screws and two 13.5×4.0-mm or 13.5×6.0-mm plastic spiked washers (Synthes Ltd, Paoli, PA) placed proximal to the femoral drill hole.

The holes are drilled through both cortices with a 3.2-mm drill bit. A spiked plastic washer is placed on the depth gauge so that the thickness of the washer will be taken into account. The holes are then tapped with a 4.5-mm tap. It is extremely important to make sure that both cortices are tapped. The plastic spiked ligament washer is placed on the appropriate-length 4.5-mm cortical screw and the screw is tightened down, thus making sure that the screw length is long enough to engage the second cortex. The screw is then backed out and the tendons are passed under the ligament washers.

The length of the graft is adjusted such that all four arms of the graft will be compressed under both washers. As a result the tibial end of the graft may be recessed up into the tibial tunnel. It is our feeling that at least 25 mm of tendon should remain in the tibial tunnel for bony ingrowth. This can be verified by inserting the arthroscope into the joint and checking for the previously placed 25-mm mark on the tendon. If the mark is not visible, at least 25 mm of graft remains in the tibial tunnel.

Once the length of the graft is adjusted, the two limbs of the graft are wound in opposite directions in an "S" fashion around the two screws and washers. It is extremely important to make sure that the tendons lie under the spiked washers. The proximal screw is tightened first, and in so doing, some of the graft may be extruded from the periphery of the washer as a result of the bulk of the graft. A small hemostat can often be used to keep the grafts under the washers while the screw is being tightened. Traction is then placed on the tibial end of the graft and the screw closest to the femoral hole is tightened down. All four limbs usually fit tightly under this washer. Care must be taken to avoid overtightening the screws as in young bone the bicortical screws can provide enough compression to split the plastic washer. One technique to avoid this is to place an AO metal washer over the plastic spiked ligament washer, in effect, metal backing it.

The length change of the graft is tested by placing the knee through a full range of motion while applying tension on the graft. A change in length of the graft can be detected by pistoning of the graft at the tibial tunnel site.

Graft Tensioning

As mentioned earlier we do not know the correct amount of tension that should be applied to ACL replacements. Burks and Leland showed in a human cadaver model that tension was highly tissue dependent.[129] Stiffer shorter grafts, such as the patellar tendon, required less preload than less stiff longer grafts, such as hamstring tendons.

Before the tibial side of the graft is secured, tension is applied to the graft and the knee is cycled through a range of motion in an attempt to remove any creep from the graft and to distribute the tension equally among the limbs of the hamstring graft. Because the hamstring graft is a composite graft and is less stiff than the patellar tendon, it is particularly important to cycle the knee through a full range of motion, with tension applied to the graft, 20 to 30 times. We believe this "cycling" of the hamstring tendon graft to be a critical part of the procedure. As the knee is being cycled, the surgeon can assess the change in length of the graft

with flexion and extension. In ideal circumstances, the tibial end of the graft should pull into the tibial tunnel approximately 2 mm as the knee is extended from 90° to full hyperextension, indicating lengthening with extension.

For patellar tendon grafts the 18-gauge wire is used to apply tension to the graft, and a second 9-mm interference screw is inserted into the tibial tunnel lateral to the bone block. This helps to translocate the bone block and ACL graft medially, decreasing impingement of the graft against the lateral femoral condyle. The interference screw is tightened down just under the medial cortex of the tibia.

Because of the softer metaphyseal bone in the proximal tibia, there is a greater tendency for the interference screw to diverge from the bone block and bone tunnel, so care must be taken to ensure that the screw is inserted parallel to the bone tunnel. The use of cannulated interference screws can help minimize this problem. The position of the interference screws can be checked by obtaining intraoperative radiographs if necessary (Fig. 14-44).

Our studies have shown that the most common site of fixation failure during mechanical testing is on the tibial side, so if there is any question about the adequacy of the tibial interference screw fixation, the graft can be augmented by tying the No. 5 nonabsorbable sutures around a 6.5-mm cancellous screw and metal washer.

For hamstring tendon grafts, a 6.5-mm cancellous screw and metal washer are inserted below the tibial tunnel. Based on the data of Burks and Leland, we try to apply approximately 8 to 10 lb of tension to the ham-

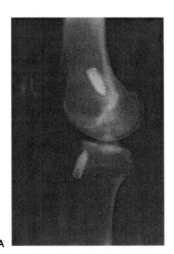
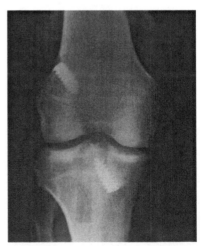

A   B

Figure 14-44. Postoperative radiographs demonstrating proper placement of the interference screws. **A.** Lateral radiograph **B.** AP radiograph.

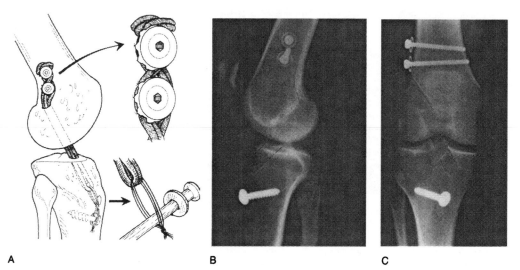

Figure 14–45. A. Our preferred method for fixation of hamstring tendon grafts. **B.** Six-week postoperative lateral radiograph demonstrating correct placement of the fixation hardware. The dashed lines outline the drilled bone tunnels. **C.** AP radiograph.

string tendon graft.[129] With the knee at 0° the No. 5 sutures are tied securely around the 6.5-mm cancellous screw and washer (Fig. 14–45).

We have found the strength and fixation of this graft are such that similar to patellar tendon grafts one must be careful to avoid overtensioning the graft and "capturing" the joint. In our laboratory tests of this fixation method we did not find elongation or failure at either fixation site; rather, the entire graft elongated to failure.[73]

The knee is taken through a full range of motion and stability checked. If pathologic laxity is still present or if the range of motion of the knee is limited, the cause of these problems should be identified and corrected before leaving the operating room. Causes of pathologic laxity and loss of motion include the following:

1. Improper graft placement
   a. Femoral tunnel too anterior = loss of flexion, and failure to eliminate the pivot shift (vertical graft)
   b. Tibial tunnel too anterior = roof impingement and a loss of extension
2. Graft impingement secondary to inadequate notchplasty
3. Inadequate graft tension
4. Excessive graft tension

A common cause for a loss of full extension is impingement of the ACL graft against the roof of the intercondylar notch. Because it is difficult to visualize arthroscopically the ACL graft in the intercondylar

notch in full extension, a true lateral radiograph in full hyperextension can be used to document the position of the tibial tunnel. The anterior part of the tibial tunnel should lie posterior to the slope of the intercondylar notch to avoid graft impingement. If the tibial tunnel is positioned too anteriorly there are two options to correct this problem. The first is to resect more bone from the roof of the intercondylar notch. The second is to chamfer the posterior edge of the tibial tunnel so that the graft comes to lie in a more posterior position. Once these corrections have been made an impingement rod can be used to check for roof impingement with the knee in full hyperextension.[77-79]

If the patient demonstrates a loss of extension and the tibial tunnel is correctly positioned, most likely the femoral tunnel is positioned too posteriorly in the intercondylar notch (over-the-top position). As a result of the posterior femoral tunnel position, the ACL graft will tighten (lengthen) with extension, with maximum tightening occurring in full extension. If the graft were tensioned with the knee in a flexed position, then as the knee was extended the graft would have to tighten (lengthen) further and full extension could be blocked. There are two possible solutions to this problem. The first is to remove the tibial interference fixation screw and retension the graft with the knee in full extension. This ensures a tight graft in the range 0° to 30° (a negative Lachman test) and the knee will be able to achieve full extension. As the knee flexes, the graft loosens, so there is a little more laxity at 90° than at 20°. Because the pivot-shift phenomenon occurs between 30° to 40° and not at 90° of flexion, the knee will be functionally stable.

The second solution is to remove the graft and to use a motorized arthroplasty burr or an ACL chamfering rasp to chamfer the anterior edge of the femoral drill hole. This allows the ACL graft to lie in a more anterior position and should result in a more isometric graft position. After the femoral tunnel position has been corrected, the graft can be repassed and retensioned as described earlier.

If the patient demonstrates a loss of flexion or pathologic laxity, the most common cause is positioning of the femoral drill hole too far anteriorly in the intercondylar notch. Anterior placement of the femoral tunnel will result in a vertically oriented graft and pathologic laxity because of the inability of the graft to control anteroposterior translation of the joint. Muller,[21] Arms et al,[117] Graf,[113] and Penner et al[126] have also shown that if the femoral drill hole is positioned too anteriorly the ACL substitute will lengthen (tighten) excessively as the knee is flexed. This will generate high tensile forces in the ACL graft. One of two things will happen: if a stiff high-strength graft such as the patellar tendon has been used, the graft will overconstrain and "capture the joint," resulting in a loss of flexion; or excessive graft tension will cause the autograft to slowly stretch with time, resulting in a return of pathologic laxity in the postoperative period. Either of these situations will cause a surgical failure.

If flexion is limited or pathologic laxity is still present after the graft is tensioned, then a lateral radiograph of the knee should be obtained. On the true lateral radiograph the femoral bone tunnel location can be easily visualized. The ideal location for the femoral bone tunnel is at the intersection of Blumensaat's line and the roof of the intercondylar notch. If the femoral tunnel is found to be too anterior, the femoral end of the graft will need to be repositioned. If the original femoral drill is very anterior, it is possible to use a rear-entry guide to drill a guide pin and new femoral tunnel posterior to the original tunnel and still maintain a bony bridge between the two tunnels (Fig. 14–46). Because of the large drill hole in the lateral femoral condyle, if it is not possible to redrill a new femoral tunnel behind the original tunnel and maintain a bony bridge between the two, it is probably best to reposition the graft in the over-the-top position. The surgical technique for passing the bone block into the over-the-top position is well described by Burger and Larson.[203] If enough bone remains behind the original drill hole, it is possible to make the over-the-top position more isometric by creating a trough in the back of the femoral condyle. Melhorn and Henning[127] and Penner et al[125] have shown that this grooved over-the-top position provides a nearly isometric position and excellent clinical stability. Karlson et al have also shown that there was essentially no difference in the results of hamstring tendons positioned isometrically through a femoral drill hole and grafts positioned in the over-the-top position.[204] If

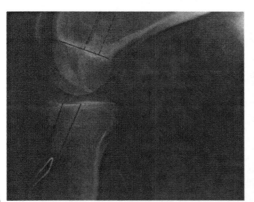 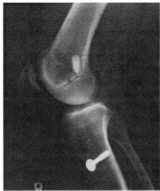

A   B

Figure 14–46. Attempted endoscopic reconstruction of the ACL resulted in placement of the femoral tunnel too anterior in the intercondylar notch. After tensioning of the graft the patient still had a markedly positive pivot-shift sign. **A.** Intraoperative lateral radiograph of the knee demonstrates the anterior position of the femoral tunnel (dashed lines). **B.** The endoscopic technique was converted into a two-incision technique. Because of the anterior position of the femoral drill hole as well as the vertical orientation of the drill hole (dashed lines), it was possible to use a rear-entry aimer to drill a new femoral drill tunnel posterior to the original and still maintain a bony bridge between the two. The femoral bone block was positioned at the cortical edge of the femoral bone tunnel so that interference screw fixation could be used. Because of the recession of the tibial bone block, No. 5 sutures tied around a 6.5-mm cancellous screw and metal washer were used for the tibial fixation. The patient had full range of motion, a negative Lachman, and a negative pivot-shift test.

the over-the-top position is used, a cannulated 4.0-mm cancellous screw is employed to fix the bone block to the distal femur.[203] The No. 5 nonabsorbable sutures are tied around a 6.5-mm unicortical screw and metal washer for additional fixation. The tibial end of the graft is then retensioned and fixed with an interference screw with the knee in full extension.

Endoscopic Reconstruction With Patellar Tendon Graft and Endobutton Fixation

The initial steps for endoscopic reconstruction with a patellar tendon graft are similar to those of the previously described two-incision technique.[8,153–155] Graft harvest, diagnostic arthroscopy, and intercondylar notch preparation proceed as previously described for the two-incision technique. The major differences with the endobutton technique relate to graft preparation, preparation of the femoral socket, and graft fixation. Sizing and preparation of the tibial bone block are performed in the routine fashion as described earlier. The patellar bone block is trimmed 1 mm smaller than the tibial bone block to ease passage across the knee joint. Three 2-mm drill holes are evenly spaced in the patellar block followed by three No. 5 nonabsorbable sutures inserted in a double-looped fashion.[134,135] This method of bone block suture fixation has been shown to be the strongest.[134,135] The tibial end of the patellar tendon graft is then secured to the graft preparation board (Acufex Microsurgical Inc, Mansfield, MA). The endobutton is inserted into the endobutton holder and the three No. 5 nonabsorbable sutures from the patellar

bone block are passed through the two central holes of the endobutton (Acufex Microsurgical Inc). Each individual pair of sutures are clamped together; further preparation of the patellar bone block is delayed until the femoral socket has been drilled.

The graft length, G_{length}, which is the length of the tibial bone block plus the length of the patellar tendon is measured and recorded. G_{length} must be equal to or less than the intraarticular distance of the ACL plus the length of the tibial tunnel, so that the graft is not too long and the tibial bone block does not protrude from the tibial tunnel (Fig. 14–47).

During the drilling of the tibial tunnel the Pro-Trac aimer is set at 55°, resulting in a longer more vertically oriented tunnel typically in the range of 45–50 mm (Fig. 14–48). This longer tibial tunnel results in a longer span for the patellar tendon and thus minimizes the amount of femoral bone block recession needed to contain the tibial bone block completely within the tibial tunnel. During the drilling of the tibial tunnel it is important that the external starting point be halfway between the apex of the tibial tubercle and the most medial portion of the tibia as recommended by Olson et al.[167,170] This position is more medial than previously described.[8,153–155] Placement of the tibial tunnel too close to the tibial tubercle results in the femoral guide pin angle being too parallel to the shaft and lateral cortex of the femur. This can cause several problems: (1) difficulty and possible breakage of the guide pin when drilling across the femur as the pin tends to skive off the lateral femoral cortex, (2) emergence of the guide pin too proximal from the lateral thigh, and (3) a long

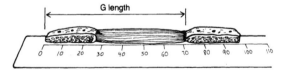

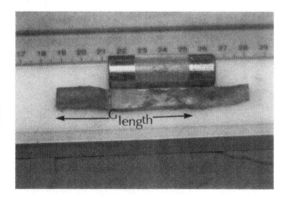

Figure 14–47. G_{length}, which is the length of the tibial bone block plus the length of the patellar tendon, is measured. To avoid graft–tunnel mismatch this length must be less than $T_{tibial+ACL}$, the length of the tibial tunnel plus the intraarticular length of the ACL. If G_{length} is greater than $T_{tibial+ACL}$, then the femoral bone block must be recessed into the femoral tunnel. $T_{tibial+ACL} - G_{length}$ represents the amount of femoral recession needed to avoid a graft–tunnel mismatch. (Bottom portion) Intraoperative photograph showing G_{length}.

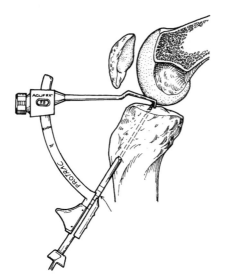

Figure 14–48. The Pro-Trac tibial aimer is used to drill a longer, more vertical tibial tunnel typically in the range 45 to 50 mm.

suture span between the endobutton and the femoral bone block because of the long parallel femoral tunnel. A long suture span will reduce the stiffness of the composite structure because it increases the distance to the point of graft fixation. After the tibial tunnel is drilled, the soft tissue remnants of the ACL are debrided with a motorized shaver, and the posterior edge of the tunnel is chamfered with a rasp. At this point in the procedure it may be necessary to inflate the tourniquet (typical tourniquet time is 10–15 minutes) for the drilling of the closed femoral socket.

With the knee flexed 90°, a pilot hole for the femoral tunnel is established using a small curette. The femoral pilot hole placement can then be checked prior to drilling the guide pin with an Isotac (Acufex Microsurgical Inc, Mansfield, MA).[166,169] The pilot hole position is moved until an acceptable strain pattern has been obtained.[113,120,166,169] After "isometry" is confirmed, the calibrated depth probe is used to measure the intraarticular length of the ACL plus the tibial tunnel length, $T_{tibial+ACL}$. $T_{tibial+ACL}$ is subtracted from G_{length}, previously measured. If positive, this number represents the number of millimeters that the femoral bone block will need to be recessed into the femoral socket for the tibial bone block to be completely contained with the tibial tunnel. If this number is zero or negative, the femoral bone block can be inserted flush with the femoral socket and the tibial tunnel will be long enough to completely contain the tibial bone block.

The knee is flexed to 90° and a 2.4-mm drill-tipped guidewire is drilled through the tibial tunnel into the previously selected site on the femur (Fig. 14–49). The femoral socket is drilled with endoscopic drill bit to avoid injury to the PCL (Acufex Microsurgical Inc, Mansfield, MA). The endoscopic drill bit is manually pushed through the tibial tunnel over the drill-tipped guidewire and past the PCL before drilling. A closed-end socket for the femoral tunnel is then drilled into the lateral femoral condyle. A motorized shaver with the blade window left open can be used to help suction the drilling debris from the back of the knee, allowing improved visualization of the calibrated endoscopic drill bit. Calibrations on the endoscopic drill bit denote the depth of the socket. The femoral socket depth must allow for the length of the patellar bone block (25 mm) plus any needed recession of the bone block plus an extra 6 mm for the turning radius of the endobutton.

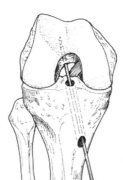 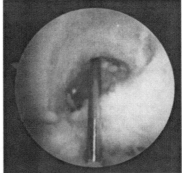

Figure 14–49. A 2.4-mm drill-tipped guide pin advanced through the tibial tunnel and drilled into the preselected site along the inner margin of the lateral femoral condyle. **A.** Schematic overview. **B.** Arthroscopic view of guide pin insertion into the femur.

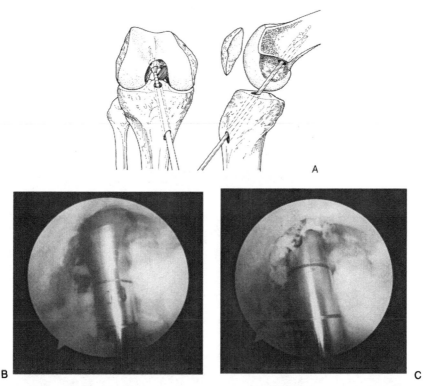

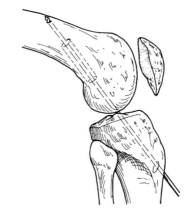

Figure 14–50. A. An endoscopic drill bit is used to ream the closed-end femoral socket. Calibrations on the drill bit denote the depth of the femoral socket. **B.** The endoscopic drill bit is pushed past the PCL before the drill is started. **C.** The femoral socket is drilled to a depth that allows the desired amount of insertion of the femoral bone block plus 6 mm deeper to provide a turning radius for the endobutton.

For a 25-mm patellar bone block with no recession required, this tunnel would equal 25 mm + 6 mm (turning radius of the endobutton) + 4 mm (fudge factor) = 35 mm (Fig. 14–50).

Once the closed-end femoral socket is drilled, the drill-tipped guide pin is removed and a 2.4-mm drill-tipped passing pin is introduced into the tibial tunnel. The knee is flexed to 90° and the passing pin is drilled out through the lateral femoral cortex and skin. The exit position of the passing pin along the lateral thigh can be altered by manipulating the passing pin in the tibial tunnel prior to drilling (Fig. 14–51).

A 4.5-mm endobutton drill bit is then used to over-drill the passing pin. The tunnel length at the moment of breakthrough of the lateral femoral cortex is noted on the drill bit (Fig. 14–52). A more accurate measurement is made by using a calibrated depth probe to measure precisely the femoral tunnel length, T_{femoral} (Fig. 14–53).

Figure 14–51. A drill-tipped passing pin is advanced through the tibial tunnel, the femoral socket, and out through the lateral cortex.

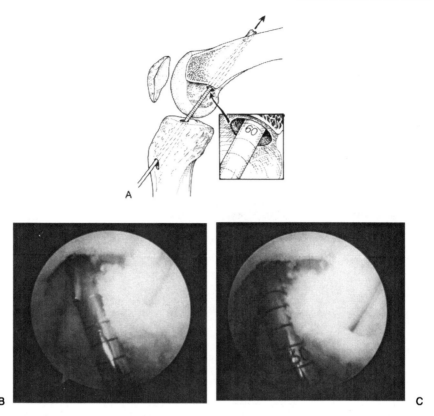

Figure 14–52. A. 4.5-mm endobutton drill bit is used to drill through the lateral femoral cortex, creating a channel for the endobutton. **A.** Schematic overview. **B.** Drill bit starting into the femur seen arthroscopically. **C.** Drill bit advanced further into femur with depth indicated by marks on the reamer.

The desired length of graft insertion, which is measured from the end of the patellar bone block away from the patellar tendon insertion (=length of the patellar bone block + the millimeters of recession), is marked on the graft. This mark is positioned at the length of the femoral tunnel, T_{femoral}, on the calibrated scale of the endobutton holder. This automatically sets the suture span so that when the endobutton lies against the lateral femoral cortex, the desired insertion point will lie flush with the opening of the femoral tunnel. The No. 5 sutures are securely tied together, thus connecting the endobutton to the patellar tendon graft. Prior to insertion, the graft should be pretensioned to 10 to 15 lb for a few minutes to remove any slip in the knots.[134,135] A marking pen is used to make a second mark 6 mm (the turning radius for the endobutton) from the previously marked desired insertion length of the graft. This mark is viewed arthroscopically and used to help determine when to "flip" the endobutton (Fig. 14–54).

EXAMPLE: Let us assume that $G_{\text{length}} = 78$ mm. After the tibial tunnel is reamed, the calibrated depth probe is used to measure $T_{\text{tibial+ACL}}$, which is 75 mm. As $G_{\text{length}} - T_{\text{tibial+ACL}} = 3$ mm, the end of the femoral bone will need to be recessed at least 3 mm up the femoral tunnel. A point 3 mm from the end of the patellar bone is marked on the patellar tendon (desired length of graft insertion). The length of the closed femoral socket = 25 mm (length of the patellar bone block) + 3 mm (recession factor) + 6 mm (turning radius of the endobutton) + 4 mm (fudge factor) = 38 mm. The calibrated depth probe is used to measure T_{femoral}, which is 60 mm.

The endobutton holder is used to set the correct suture span by positioning the desired insertion length previously marked on the graft at 60 mm on the endobutton holder while tying the sutures. A second mark is then placed on the graft 6 mm from the previously marked, desired insertion length. This mark represents the turning radius for the endobutton and is visualized arthroscopically, indicating that the endobutton is free of the lateral femoral cortex and can be flipped.

A No. 5 nonabsorbable suture is passed through the lead hole of the endobutton and a No. 2 nonabsorbable suture through the trailing hole. The No. 5 suture is

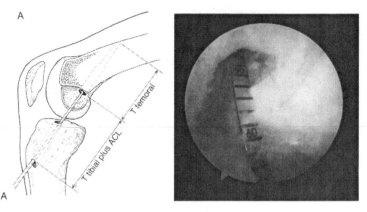

Figure 14–53. A. The calibrated depth probe is used to measure the femoral tunnel length, $T_{femoral}$, and the intraarticular length of the ACL plus the tibial tunnel length, $T_{tibial+ACL}$. B. Intraoperative photograph demonstrating measurement of the femoral tunnel length, $T_{femoral}$.

used to pass the endobutton and the graft across the joint, and the No. 2 suture is used to flip the endobutton once it clears the lateral femoral cortex, similar to the strings working a marionette (Fig. 14–55). The No. 5 and 2 sutures are then loaded into the slotted end of the passing pin, and the graft is passed into the femoral tunnel under arthroscopic visualization using the lead No. 5 suture. The No. 2 suture is used to turn the endobutton once the flipping mark is visualized. Usually

the surgeon can feel the button as it emerges from the femoral tunnel. The No. 2 suture is then used to turn the endobutton (Figs. 14–56 and 14–57). The tibial end of the graft is tensioned, thus engaging the endobutton against the lateral femoral cortex. Intraoperative radiographs can be used to confirm proper deployment of the endobutton prior to fixation of the tibial bone block. Prior to graft fixation the knee should be cycled 20 to 30 times to allow for any further slippage of the knots, to

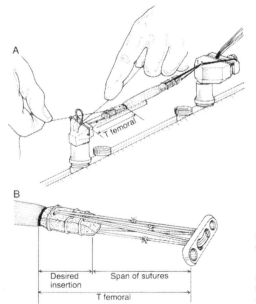

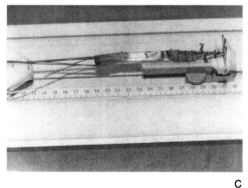

Figure 14–54. A. By use of the graft preparation board the graft is attached to the two central holes of the endobutton. B. No. 5 nonabsorbable sutures are used to connect the endobutton to the patellar bone plug. The desired length of graft insertion (previously determined) is placed at the femoral tunnel length, $T_{femoral}$, on the endobutton holder while the sutures are tied. C. Intraoperative photograph demonstrating graft attachment to the endobutton.

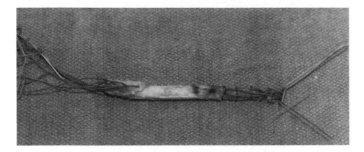

Figure 14–55. A No. 5 nonabsorbable suture is used to lead and pass the endobutton across the joint, and a No. 2 nonabsorbable suture is used as the trailing suture to flip the endobutton as it exits the femoral cortex.

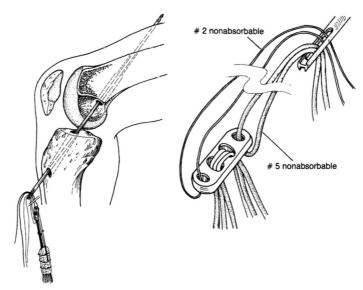

2 nonabsorbable

5 nonabsorbable

Figure 14–56. A drill-tipped passing pin is used to pierce the muscle and skin anterolaterally. The sutures for the endobutton are then loaded into the hole in the passing pin, and the passing pin and sutures are pulled out through the skin anterolaterally.

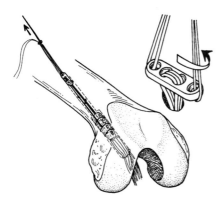

Figure 14–57. A No. 5 suture is used to pass the endobutton and the patellar bone block into the femoral socket. The flipping marker line, which is located 6 mm from the desired amount of graft insertion, is visualized arthroscopically, and when flush with the femoral tunnel, the endobutton is turned by pulling on the No. 2 suture. The endobutton then locks into place as tension is applied to the tibial end of the graft.

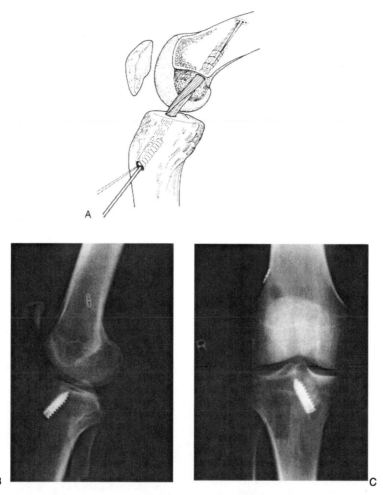

Figure 14–58. A. The tibial end of the graft is tensioned and fixed with a 9 × 25-mm interference screw. **B, C.** Postoperative radiographs of a patellar tendon graft fixed with an endobutton on the femoral side and a 9 × 25-mm interference screw on the tibial side. The femoral bone block and step-cut femoral tunnel can be seen on the anteroposterior radiograph. Anterior view shown in **B**, and lateral view in **C**.

allow for stress relaxation of the graft, and as a check on the fixation of the endobutton. The knee is then placed at 0°, the graft is appropriately tensioned, and the tibial bone block is fixed with a 9 × 25-mm interference screw. The anterior incision is closed in routine fashion (Fig. 14–58).

Closure

Once the surgeon is satisfied with the stability and range of motion of the knee, the arthroscope is rein-serted back into the knee, and a final check is made for evidence of graft impingement. As the knee is flexed, the graft is checked for impingement along the inner margin of the lateral femoral condyle. The knee is then brought into full extension and graft impingement is checked in the roof of the intercondylar notch. If evidence of impingement is found, it is safest to remove the offending bone with a curette rather than risk possible damage to the tensioned graft with a motorized shaver. The tibial end of the graft is checked for any bony, cartilaginous, or soft tissue debris, which could

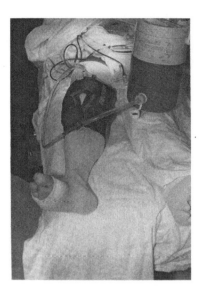

Figure 14–59. A light dressing is applied in the operating room and is held in place by a TED stocking. A Cryocuff (Aircast, Summit, NJ) is then applied to control swelling and pain.

organize and cause a "cyclops lesion." This debris is carefully removed with a motorized shaver.

Finally, the meniscal repair sutures are tied against the capsule with the knee in full extension to avoid overtightening the posterior capsule, possibly limiting extension. Closed-suction drains are placed in the anterior and lateral incisions. One drainage tube is inserted into the joint through the arthroscopic cannula.

The iliotibial tract is closed with interrupted sutures and the skin is closed with a running pullout 3-O nylon subcuticular stitch. Four-inch gauze sponges are placed over the incisions and sterile 4-in. cotton cast padding is used to secure the gauze sponges. A large long TED stocking is applied over the dressing followed by a Cryocuff (Aircast, Summit, NJ) (Fig. 14–59). The Cryocuff is a valuable adjunct for controlling pain and swelling. The patient is taken to the recovery room and if desired is placed in a CPM machine with the range of motion adjusted to 0 to 70°.

Postoperative Rehabilitation

One of the major advances in knee surgery in the past decade has been the acceptance of early motion following knee ligament surgery. For a detailed discussion of the rationale of early motion following knee ligament

surgery the reader is referred to the work of Noyes et al[162] and Paulos et al.[138, 205] Before an early motion program can be safely started certain intraoperative goals must be achieved at the time of surgery.[138,162,206] These goals include the following:

1. Use of a high-strength graft
2. Proper graft placement
3. Elimination of graft impingement
4. Correct graft tension
5. Rigid graft fixation

Paulos et al,[138,205] Noyes et al,[104,162,207] Silverskiold et al,[208] Seto et al,[209] Steadman et al,[210] Shelbourne et al,[42,150,151] DeMaio et al,[206,211] Mangine et al,[212] and Klootwyk et al[152] have all published detailed protocols of postoperative ACL rehabilitation programs. The reader is also referred to the extensive review of rehabilitation strategies for the nonoperative and postoperative management of the ACL-deficient knee by Minkoff and Sherman.[39]

Before we present our present postoperative rehabilitation program, we remind the reader that knee rehabilitation must be individualized and a "cookbook" approach should not be used. It is also important to remember that not all patients proceed through the rehabilitation program at the same pace and appropriate adjustments may have to be made in the program. The postoperative rehabilitation program that follows is a general outline and attempts to provide some structure and give some guidelines to the patient and therapist.

Immediate Postoperative Phase

The goals of the immediate postoperative phase are to (1) control pain and swelling, (2) initiate and maintain full extension, (3) prevent muscle shutdown, and (4) institute gait training.

The epidural catheter, closed-suction drains, and Foley catheter are removed the morning after surgery. An intramuscular oral pain medication or patient-controlled anesthesia (PCA) is used for pain control. During the hospital stay, which is typically 36 hours, CPM is used and the patient is encouraged to increase the flexion setting as quickly as tolerated. Use of CPM following ACL reconstruction is controversial. Mangine et al have discussed the use of CPM following ACL reconstruction and feel that it was useful in the following situation[212]:

1. To prevent anticipated motion problems
   a. Concomitant meniscus repair
   b. Concomitant collateral ligament repair
   c. Cartilage abnormality
   d. Increased pain and swelling (prodromal stage of the infrapatellar contracture syndrome)
   e. Inability to perform active range of motion
   f. History or presence of excessive scar formation

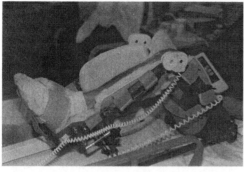
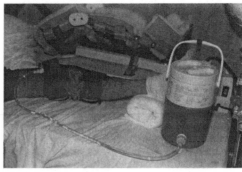

A   B

Figure 14–60. A. A CPM machine can be used postoperatively. **B.** The CPM machine does not allow the knee to achieve full hyperextension; to achieve extension equal to that of the opposite knee the leg must be removed from the CPM machine and a lift placed under the heel. The Cryocuff is an invaluable aid in controlling pain and swelling.

g. History of decreased range of motion following previous intraarticular surgery
2. To motivate the patient to achieve an earlier range of motion

Drez et al have shown that proper calf placement in the CPM machine is important in preventing excessive anterior tibial translation of the knee.[213] In their study, they found that with the calf supported by the CPM machine, the anterior tibial translation was 6.8 mm as compared with 1.5 mm with the calf unsupported. Based on these findings if CPM is going to be used, it is important to select a machine with an adjustable, non-rigid calf support. The calf straps should be loosened to allow the tibia to sag in the machine. These factors can help reduce anterior translational forces on the ACL graft and graft fixation sites.

A Cryocuff (Aircast, Summit, NJ) is used to reduce pain and swelling. The leg is removed from the CPM machine and full passive extension with a pillow or rolled blanket under the heel is performed four or five times a day for 10 to 15 minutes to avoid a flexion contracture. The Cryocuff is applied while the leg is out of the CPM machine to control pain and swelling (Fig. 14–60). Active extension is performed in the range 90° to 45°. Active-assisted extension using the opposite leg is performed from 45° to full extension for the first 4 to 6 weeks to limit quadriceps-induced anterior tibial translation[117] (Fig. 14–61). Early active flexion and hamstring isometrics are encouraged. Renstrom et al

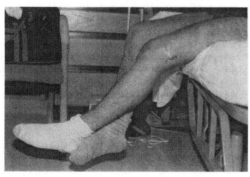
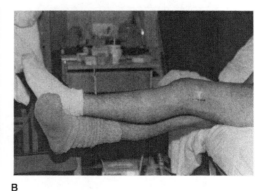

A   B

Figure 14–61. Patient performing active-assisted extension using the opposite leg. Active extension is allowed up to 45°, and then active-assisted extension is performed from **A.** 45° to **B.** full hyperextension.

have shown that hamstring isometrics and isotonics decrease the strain on the anteromedial fibers of the ACL at all knee flexion positions.[214] Because of the low strain produced in the ACL, hamstring isotonics can be started as soon as possible and at all knee flexion angles following ACL surgery. Multiple-angle quadriceps isometrics are started with the knee positioned at 0° and between 45° and 90°.

Once the patient can initiate and maintain a good quadriceps contraction, straight-leg raises can be started. The patient is instructed to contract the quadriceps muscle and lock the knee before lifting it up. It is important that the patient avoid a quadriceps lag (less than 10°) during the straight-leg raise exercise as this can produce large anterior translational forces in the ACL graft. Drez et al have shown that contracting the quadriceps muscle before lifting the leg results in a significant reduction in anterior tibial translation.[214]

Patellar mobilization (slides and tilts) is performed three to four times a day to prevent entrapment of the patella. Maintenance of normal patellar mobility is important to help avoid contracture of the patellar retinaculum, which can result in the development of a patella infera syndrome.[109,142,207,215,216] The knee is placed into full extension, and the patient is taught to perform medial, lateral, and superior patellar glides. Medial and lateral patellar tilts are done to break up scar tissue in the suprapatellar pouch. Vigorous isometric quadriceps contractions done in full extension will pull the patella superiorly and prevent inferior entrapment of the patella (Fig. 14–62).

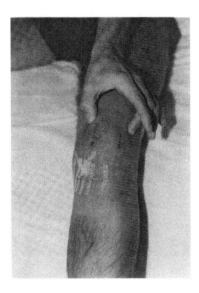

Figure 14–62. Patellar mobilization.

A knee immobilizer or similar type of brace that holds the knee in extension is worn until the patient has adequate muscular control of the leg. Patients are allowed to bear weight as tolerated. If a meniscus repair has been performed, then 25% body weight is initially allowed and patients are advanced 25% body weight per week. Patients can discard their crutches when they have good muscular control of the leg.

Early Rehabilitative Phase

The goals of the early rehabilitative phase are to (1) maintain full extension, (2) maintain normal patellar mobility, (3) increase range of motion, and (4) develop muscle strength sufficient for activities of daily living.

The early rehabilitative phase starts from the time of discharge from the hospital and continues for the first 6 to 8 weeks. Patients are encouraged to gradually increase their knee motion. Flexion is performed in the seated position by pulling the leg back with the hamstring muscles. Flexion can be assisted by using the opposite leg or by gravity with wall slides. The goal is to achieve full flexion by 4 to 6 weeks. Active extension is limited to 45° for the first 4 to 6 weeks to limit quadriceps-induced anterior tibial translation. Active-assisted extension using the opposite leg is performed from 45° to full extension.

One of the major goals of this phase is to build muscular endurance so that the patient may come off crutches and safely return to activities of daily living. Quadriceps isometrics and straight-leg raises at 0° are continued. Hamstring isotonics with ankle weights are started in the standing and prone positions. Toe raises and hip extension and hip flexion exercises are added to the program. Many patients can discontinue crutches by the second to fourth week if there is minimal pain and swelling and they have good muscular control of the leg. The immobilizer or brace is discontinued when the patient has good muscular control over the leg.

During this phase it is very important to maintain full extension and normal patellar mobility to prevent the development of a flexion contracture and an infrapatellar contracture syndrome. If either of these become limiting then aggressive early treatment is indicated. Prone hanging-leg extensions or supine weighted extensions should be started if the patient has difficulty maintaining full extension (Fig. 14–63). Normal patellar mobility must be maintained and carefully monitored. Patellar mobilization should be continued and increased to an hourly basis if the patient shows any signs of decreased patellar mobility.

In the past, most postoperative ACL rehabilitation programs have emphasized open-kinetic-chain exercise programs. Open-kinetic-chain exercises are exercises done with the end segment, the foot, in a free or nonstationary position. A classic example of an open-

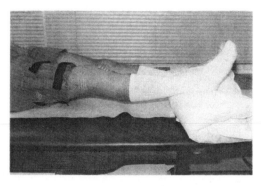 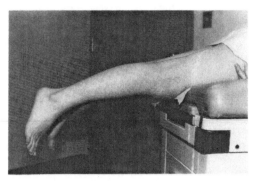

A   B

Figure 14–63. A. Supine weighted knee extension. **B.** Prone hanging-leg extension.

kinetic-chain exercise is the knee extension exercises done on Nautilus, Cybex, and bench machines. Paulos et al[205] and Grood et al[217] have reported that open-kinetic-chain exercises such as resistive knee extensions can place high anterior tibial translational forces and high patellofemoral forces on the knee.

Recent articles have discussed the advantages of closed-kinetic-chain exercise programs.[150,151,208,210–212,218] Closed-kinetic-chain exercises are exercises done with the end segment, the foot, in a stationary or fixed position. Typical closed-kinetic-chain exercises include those done on a stair-climber, leg press machine, and rowing machine. Closed-kinetic-chain exercises decrease anterior tibial translational forces on the knee by providing physiologic compressive loading of the joint. Compressive joint loading results in loading of the menisci and other restraining ligaments about the knee and increases the bony congruency of the joint; all these factors decrease the amount of anterior joint translation. Additionally, closed-kinetic-chain exercises promote co-contraction of the quadriceps and hamstring muscles, further reducing anterior joint translation.[218] Closed-kinetic-chain exercises also decrease the contact pressures on the patellofemoral joint and promote functional training of the vastus medialis obliquus. A further advantage of closed-kinetic-chain exercises is that they load the knee joint with normal physiologic loads and permit the muscles to exercise at speeds and in a manner similar to those they will encounter in everyday life. This prepares the patient for an early and safe return to activities of daily living. Proprioception is also facilitated by closed-kinetic-chain exercises since the joint mechanoreceptors are loaded with physiologic loads.

The biomechanical validity of closed-chain exercise has been established in a recent study by Lutz et al.[219]

This study used a two-dimensional mathematical model to analyze the tibiofemoral shear and compressive forces during open- and closed-kinetic chain exercises in five healthy subjects. Electromyographic activity of the quadriceps and the hamstring muscles was also recorded.

The results of this study showed that during open-chain extension exercise, a maximum posterior shear force (stress on the ACL) of 285 ± 120 N occurred at 30° of flexion. During open-chain extension exercise, knee flexion angles of less than 60° produced significant shear forces on the ACL. This finding had been previously reported by Arms et al[117] in a cadaver study in which strain gauges were used to measure the strain pattern in the anteromedial fibers of the ACL during simulated exercises. Open-chain flexion exercises were reported to produce anterior shear forces (stress on the PCL) at all flexion angles, with the force reaching a maximum at 90° of flexion. These results again confirm the findings of a previous study by Renstrom et al.[214]

In contrast to open-chain extension exercises, closed-chain extension exercises at 30° of flexion produced an anterior shear force (stress on the PCL) of 516 ± 392 N. Unlike the open-chain extension exercises, this force remained fairly uniform as the flexion angle of the knee was increased from 30° to 90°. Closed-chain exercises were also found to produce significantly higher compressive joint forces at the same flexion angles at which the open-chain exercises produced maximum shear forces.

Analysis of the electromyographic data indicated that co-contraction of the quadriceps and the hamstring muscles occurred only during closed-chain exercise. The authors concluded that an isometric closed-chain exercise produces significantly less shear forces on the ACL compared with open-chain exercise. The reduction in shear force was felt to be the result of a more axial orientation of the applied force and muscular co-contraction of the quadriceps and hamstring muscles.

Once the patient has achieved at least 100° of flexion, usually around the second postoperative week, a stationary bicycle program is started. The goal is to cycle at least 20 minutes per day. The resistance on the bike is increased as tolerated. Ericson and Nisell have shown that the stationary bike applies minimal anterior translational and compressional loads to the knee.[220] In their study they found that cycling at 60 rpm with a workload of 120 W, the seat at middle saddle position, and an anterior pedal foot position produced a mean peak tibiofemoral compressive load of 812 N (1.2 × body weight). The maximum anteriorly directed tibiofemoral shear force was only 37 N. The authors noted that the anteriorly directed shear force on the knee, during maximum isokinetic knee extension, was approximately 20 times greater than during cycling. In a previous article, Ericson et al also reported that the muscle activity in the vastus medialis and lateralis during cycling was approximately four to five times that of walking.[221] Because of the low loads applied to the knee and the high level of vastus medialis and lateralis activity with cycling, the authors concluded that cycling is a good exercise in the early postoperative period following ACL surgery (Fig. 14–64).

By the fourth postoperative week the patient can start other closed-chain exercises such as a Nordic ski machine, stair-climber, or rowing machine. Extension is limited to 30° on these machines to decrease the anterior tibial translation forces. If these machines are unavailable, then step-up exercises or resistive exercises using elastic tubing may be substituted.[208,210] A swimming program can also be started at around the third to fourth week. Swimming exercises include flutter kick with a kick board (no whip kicks), water bicycle, and water walking and jogging (Fig. 14–65).

During the first 6 weeks the patient's range of motion and patellar mobility must be monitored closely. Loss of motion is one of the most common and disabling complications following intraarticular ACL reconstruction.[90,142,162,207] Harner et al have discussed the etiology of the stiff knee and have concluded that it is multifactorial[142]:

1. Intercondylar notch scarring
2. Capsulitis (stage 3 = patella infera contracture syndrome)
3. Nonisometric graft placement
4. Extraarticular surgery, especially MCL and PCL repairs
5. Infection
6. Reflex sympathetic dystrophy

According to Harner et al regardless of the etiology, loss of extension results in a flexion contracture which leads to quadriceps weakness and patellofemoral pain.[142] They reported that intercondylar notch scarring and capsulitis were the two most common causes of loss of motion. With early recognition and treatment, they were able to reduce the incidence of loss of extension from 11% in 1986–1989 to 1.7% in 1993.

Patellar mobilization and quadriceps isometrics can help prevent the early stages of capsulitis. The early stages of capsulitis are characterized by a loss of knee motion, usually some degree of both flexion and extension, a decrease in patellar mobility, quadriceps weakness, redness and warmth around the knee, and pain.[142] Patients exhibiting a loss of motion should be started on a restricted motion program.[207] If these measures fail to restore normal patellar mobility and motion, then early surgical intervention may be necessary to prevent permanent disability. Surgical intervention for capsulitis or intercondylar notch scarring usually consists of arthroscopic debridement with lysis of the fat pad and suprapatella adhesions, as well as medial and lateral

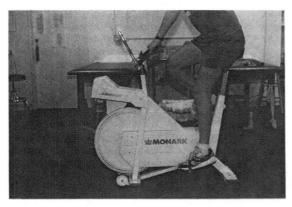

Figure 14–64. Stationary bike. The seat position is adjusted high to decrease the amount of knee flexion required and to decrease patellofemoral forces. (Photograph courtesy of Kennedy Brothers Physical Therapy, Boston, MA.)

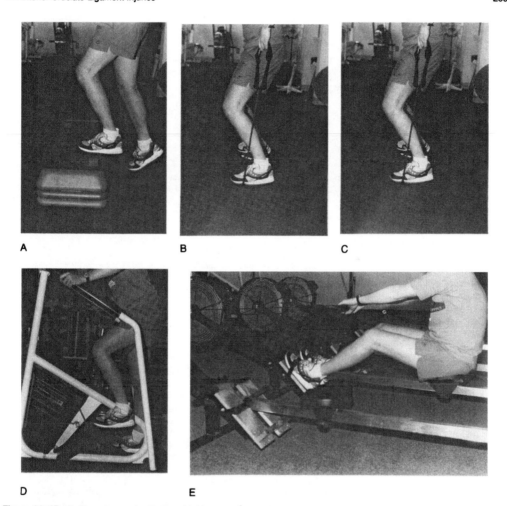

Figure 14–65. A. Step-up exercise **B.** One-third knee dips using Sport Cord (Sport Cord, Inc, Chico, CA). This exercise has been popularized by Dr. Richard Steadman, Vail, Colorado.[208,210] **C.** Closed-kinetic-chain extension exercise using elastic tubing. **D.** Stair-climber. **E.** Rowing machine. (Photograph courtesy of Kennedy Brothers Physical Therapy, Boston, MA.)

retinacular releases.[142,207,222–226] For a more through discussion of the management of the stiff knee, the reader is referred to Chapter 20.

Intermediate Phase

The intermediate rehabilitation phase starts at around 8 weeks and continues until 4 months. During this phase the goals are to (1) continue to build muscular endurance and strength, (2) protect the ACL graft from large anterior translational forces, (3) protect the patello-

femoral joint from high loads, and (4) start proprioceptive training.

The stationary bike, NordicTrack, rowing machine, stair-climbing machine, and Sport Cord program are continued. Isotonic exercises for the hamstrings are continued and a leg curl machine for hamstring strengthening can be started (Fig. 14–66). The patient is instructed to work on increasing the time spent exercising rather than rapidly increasing the resistance. The exercise program should be increased to 20 to 30 minutes twice a day.

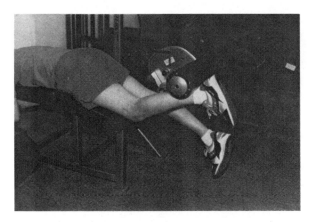

Figure 14–66. A leg curl machine can be used for hamstring strengthening. Early aggressive use of the leg curl machine is cautioned following ACL reconstruction with the semitendinosus and gracilis tendons as this can result in pain and hamstring spasm. In these patients early hamstring strengthening is performed by using closed-chain exercises.

Experimental animal studies have shown that the transplanted ACL autograft is weakest in the period 6 to 12 weeks, so it is important to avoid subjecting the ACL graft to large anterior tibial translational forces during this phase.[52,60] A leg press exercise program using elastic tubing or an inclined leg press machine can be started. It should be noted that the leg press exercise is different from a leg extension exercise. Knee extension exercises result in joint isolation and do not take advantage of the stabilizing effects provided by other muscles in the lower extremity. Grood et al have shown that the knee extension exercise also produces large patellofemoral joint forces as well as high anterior translational forces in the ACL.[217]

The leg press is a closed-chain exercise that recruits other muscle groups in the lower extremity to provide a stabilizing effect against the anterior tibial translation force produced by the quadriceps muscle. The leg press promotes co-contraction of the hamstring muscles, which decreases the anterior shear forces on the ACL.[218] Recent work by Drez et al shows that the leg press exercise causes significantly less anterior tibial translation than the knee extension exercise.[213] Using a computerized arthrometer (KSS, Acufex Microsurgical Inc, Mansfield, MA), they compared the amount of anterior tibial translation produced by a knee extension machine and that produced by a leg press machine in 19 patients with known ACL deficiency. For the knee extension exercise with a 10-lb load and a range of motion from 20° to 90°, they found that the average amount of anterior tibial translation was 9.3 mm in the normal knees versus 13.0 mm in the ACL-deficient knee. For the leg press exercise, with a load of 66 lb and a range of motion from 0° to 90°, they reported the average anterior tibial translation to be 5.3 mm in the normal knees versus 5.4 mm in the ACL-deficient knees. They concluded that the leg press exercise was a far safer

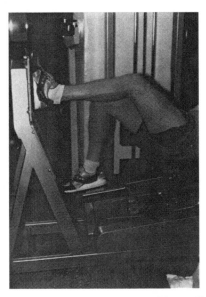

Figure 14–67. A leg press machine is used for quadriceps strengthening.

form of exercise throughout a full range of motion than the knee extension exercise (Fig. 14–67).

It is important to control patellofemoral joint forces during the postoperative rehabilitation program to prevent patellofemoral pain. Although patellofemoral pain is a frequent complication following ACL reconstruction (see Complications), it is important to try to minimize its occurrence for a number of reasons. First, Sachs et al[83,84] and Aglietti et al[81,98] have noted a highly positive correlation between patellofemoral pain and quadriceps weakness. Second, in many series patellofemoral pain is the most common cause of an unacceptable clinical result in the face of a stable knee.[227] Finally, patellar pain is one of the most common reasons for failing to progress through the rehabilitation program.

Although the exact causes of patellofemoral pain have not been fully determined, knee extension exercises, deep squats, and other exercises that result in high patellofemoral contact pressures have been implicated. In an effort to maintain a healthy patellofemoral joint, the closed-kinetic-chain exercise program is continued, and isokinetic and leg extension exercise programs are used sparingly. In general, Nautilus and isokinetic equipment is used only for hamstring strengthening; quadriceps strengthening is performed with closed-kinetic-chain functional exercises.

Proprioceptive training is facilitated by using a balance board, bouncing on a minitrampoline, and doing double- and single-leg one-third knee dips using elastic tubing. By 16 weeks most patients should be ready to advance to the next rehabilitation phase.

Final Phase

The goals of the final phase are to (1) continue muscular strengthening, (2) continue proprioception training, (3) start a running program, (4) institute agility training, and (5) return to sports.

The patient should continue with the strengthening program of the intermediate phase. If the patient has no pain or swelling, full range of motion, and no limp, a straight-ahead jogging program is begun. The patient first begins with a fast walking program outdoors or on a treadmill or a water jogging program. Initially, the patient exercises on alternate days. During off-days the muscular strengthening program is continued. Once the patient can fast walk 1 to 2 miles or water jog for 20 minutes, he or she is ready to advance to jogging outdoors or on a treadmill. Only straight-ahead jogging on a level, soft surface is allowed. Both forward jogging, which emphasizes quadriceps function, and backward jogging, which emphasizes hamstring muscle function, are performed. The goal is to jog every other day, slowly increasing the distance about 10% each outing. The jogging program is advanced to include straight-ahead running (no hills). The patient must be monitored closely for the development of pain and swelling. Rope jumping, which develops both muscular endurance and joint proprioception, is added to the program. This exercise is usually done on the off-days of the running program. The patient should be able to complete the running program without pain or swelling before advancing to agility drills.

By 16 to 20 weeks most patients are ready to begin agility drills. Prior to beginning agility drills the patient is fitted with an ACL functional brace. Although there is no documentation of the efficacy of postsurgical bracing, the brace does seem to provide some psychologic support for many patients. Agility drills such as lateral running, backward running, carioca, and figure-eight running are started. The ACL functional brace should be worn during the drills. Sport-specific drills can be started once the patient can complete the agility drills without pain and swelling.

At 6 months an isokinetic test is run at 120°, 180°, and 300° per second. Wilk et al reported on the results of isokinetic strength testing in 100 male recreational athletes 6 months after arthroscopy-assisted ACL reconstruction using an autogenous patellar tendon graft.[228] All patients were treated using an accelerated postoperative rehabilitation program similar to that described by Shelbourne and Nitz.[42,150] They found that at 6 months the mean quadriceps index (mean peak torque of the operated knee divided by the mean peak torque of the unoperated knee multiplied by 100) was 73 at 180°/s and 81 at 300°/s.

The hamstring index (defined similarly as the quadriceps index) was 97 at 180°/s and 100 at 300°/s. The authors concluded that 6 months following an ACL reconstruction with a patellar tendon graft, most recreational athletes have normal hamstring muscle strength; however, the quadriceps muscle exhibited a 20 to 25% deficit.

Failure to achieve satisfactory quadriceps strength in many patients can be attributed to the development of patellofemoral pain during the rehabilitation program. Patellofemoral pain, quadriceps weakness, and loss of extension have been shown by Sachs et al to be interrelated.[83,84] If quadriceps strength is less than 70% of the normal leg at 6 months, the patient should continue with the closed-chain strengthening program. Any exercises that produce patellofemoral pain should be modified or discontinued. In our experience, the most common cause of postoperative patellofemoral pain has been the aggressive use of knee extension exercises. Most patients with patellofemoral pain can tolerate the stationary bicycle (seat position high), NordicTrack, swimming, and the treadmill. The stair-climbing machine is an excellent rehabilitation tool but may exacerbate patellofemoral symptoms in some patients. If the stair-climber is used the patient is instructed to take short quick steps. If, despite these modifications, the patient continues to have patellofemoral pain the stair-climbing exercise should be stopped. The stationary bike, Nordic ski machine, and swimming programs are continued. The patient is retested in 4 to 6 weeks.

Once the patient has at least 70% to 75% quadriceps strength and at least 95% hamstring strength they can usually return to individual turning, nonjumping sports such as tennis, racquetball, and squash. Jumping and cutting sports are not resumed until 6 to 9 months post-operatively. At present we recommend that patients wear an ACL functional brace for the first year after returning to sports. After 1 year, continued use of the brace is left up to the patient.

Results

Evaluating the results of knee ligament surgery has been a difficult task for a number of reasons.[6] First, there has been no universally accepted knee rating scale. In most of the reported series different rating scales have been used so it has been difficult to compare the results of series. In addition, most rating systems involve weighted subjective evaluation of patient symptoms, yet there has not been any agreement as to what constitutes a significant symptom, what symptoms should be documented, and how much weight that symptom should be given when evaluating the final result.

Another major area of difficulty has been that until recently there were no simple objective methods to evaluate the result following surgery. The introduction of instrumented laxity testing,[10–12,15,30,229] isokinetic strength testing,[229] and the one-leg hop test[229,230] has provided some objective data.

The third major area of difficulty has been the use of "return to sport" as a measurement of the success of the surgical procedure. As Noyes et al pointed out, return to sport is a very ambiguous term, and a more detailed analysis of activity level is needed if this factor is going to be used to evaluate the success of knee ligament surgery.[6] Tegner and Lysholm[231] and Noyes et al[6] have proposed more detailed activity level scales, but so far there is no universally accepted activity rating scale.

In an attempt to solve some of these problems, the International Knee Documentation Committee (IKDC) has introduced a new international knee rating scale. The hope is that surgeons all over the world will use this new rating format, thus allowing results to be compared. The IKDC rating system is still in the development stage, however, and has not been widely used to report the results of knee ligament surgery.

With that introduction, let us look at some of the reported results of ACL reconstructions performed with patellar tendon and hamstring tendon autografts.

Patellar Tendon

Alm and Gillquist reported the results of 123 patients with a minimum 2-year follow-up who had undergone reconstruction of the ACL with the medial one third of the patellar tendon through a medial arthrotomy.[55] In their technique the ACL substitute consisted of the medial one third of the patellar tendon left attached to the tibial tuberosity. Tibial and femoral bone tunnels were used to position the graft in a more anatomic position.

Postoperatively, the patients were placed in a cast for 4 weeks.

They used a numerical rating system that evaluated the patient's subjective symptoms and the surgeon's objective assessment of the anterior drawer sign. Preoperatively, the patient's mean subjective score was 2.8. A score of 2 indicated that the patient had frequent episodes of instability and could not participate in competitive sports. A score of 3 indicated giving way with activities of daily living. After surgery the patients' mean subjective score was reported to be 0.7, indicating that the majority of patients were able to participate in vigorous physical activities with only minor complaints. The patients' preoperative objective assessment revealed a mean score of 2.7, indicating a significant anterior drawer sign. Postoperatively the mean objective score was reduced to 0.8, indicating that the majority of patients still had some anterior laxity. Following surgery, 66% of the patients were reported to have resumed competitive sports to the same extent as before their injury, and 30% were reported to be able to manage without severe complaints during work and low-level activities.

Clancy et al reported on 50 patients with a minimum 2-year follow-up who underwent ACL reconstruction for chronic functional instability using the medial one third of the patellar tendon, augmented by transfer of the pes tendons medially and transfer of the long head of the biceps tendon under the fibular collateral ligament laterally.[123] All patients were reported to experience functional instability with normal activities, and all had a positive pivot-shift test. All patients had failed an aggressive physical therapy program before being considered surgical candidates. The average age of the patients at the time of surgery was 23 (range 17–31 years). The majority of the patients (88%) had sustained the initial injury to the knee in a sporting event. Football and basketball were the most frequently involved sports. Twenty-one of the patients (42%) had a meniscectomy after the initial injury but before the ACL reconstruction. At the time of surgery 30 patients were noted to have torn menisci. Degenerative changes involving the tibiofemoral joint were noted in 27 of the 50 patients, and degenerative changes in the patellofemoral joint were present in 14 of the 50 patients.

Following the procedure none of the 50 patients were reported to have any instability with activities of daily living or recreational sports. Forty-four of the fifty patients (88%) were reported as having a full return to all desired sports. Objective evaluation revealed that 6 patients (12%) had a loss of 5° to 10° of extension, and 14 patients (28%) had a loss of some flexion. The Lachman test was mildly positive (5 mm of anterior translation) in 30 of the patients (60%). The pivot-shift test was negative in 41 patients (82%), trace in 8 (16%), and mildly positive in 1 (2%).

The overall results were graded using a subjective

grading scale. An excellent result implied that the patient had returned to all previous activities without instability or swelling and no or rare pain. A good result was defined as a return to all previous activities with no instability or swelling and occasional pain with strenuous activities. A fair result indicated no instability or swelling, significant pain with sports, but no or rare pain with normal activities. A failure was defined as any episode of instability, swelling, or pain with normal activities. Clancy et al reported 30 patients as having an excellent result (60%), 17 patients a good result (34%), and 1 patient a fair result (2%); 2 patients were considered failures (4%). One failure resulted from severe patellofemoral pain, and one failure resulted from a painful neuroma. Clancy et al were cautiously optimistic about the potential of their procedure to allow a return to recreational sports, but felt that more patients and longer follow-up were needed.

Johnson et al reported long-term follow-up on 87 patients who had undergone open ACL reconstruction using the medial one third of the patellar tendon.[227] The mean follow-up was 7.9 years (range 5–10 years). The mean age of the patients was 26.3 years (range 17–48 years). The initial injury to the ACL occurred during soccer in 56 of the 87 patients (64%). Preoperatively, 85% complained of reinjury episodes, 84% experienced giving-way episodes, and 92% experienced episodes of swelling.

At follow-up examination, subpatellar crepitus was reported in 57 of 87 patients (66%). The subpatellar crepitus was noted to be mild in 43 knees (49%) and severe in 14 patients (16%). Mild patellar crepitus did not affect the clinical result, but severe crepitus did, and was the cause of failure in 11 of 27 cases (40%).

The authors performed objective laxity tests on 59 patients using a specially designed machine. They reported the mean anterior laxity during an instrumented anterior drawer test to be 5.4 ± 2.6 mm in the reconstructed knees and 3.2 ± 1.2 mm in the control knees. The instrumented Lachman test revealed the mean anterior laxity to be 6.8 ± 2.7 mm in the reconstructed knees and 4.8 ± 1.7 mm in the control knees. The authors correlated the mean involved knee minus noninvolved knee anterior laxity difference with the subjective function results, and noted that the presence of less anterior laxity correlated with a better subjective result. The pivot-shift test was negative in 59 of 87 patients (68%), mildly positive in 15 of 87 (17%), and moderate to markedly positive in 8 (9%). The authors noted that a mildly positive pivot shift was not associated with a poor outcome, but that a moderate or markedly positive pivot shift was. In 68% of the patients there was some loss of extension, and 77% had some loss of flexion compared with the control knee. Using a subjective rating system they reported that 60 of 87 patients (69%) had an excellent or good result, and 27 of 87 (31%) had a fair or poor result.

When the causes of failure in the 27 patients were analyzed, only 10 cases were associated with complete failure of the ACL graft. In 11 cases, joint arthrosis was the cause, and in 11 other cases patellar pain was the cause of failure. The authors concluded that intraarticular reconstruction of the ACL using the medial one third of the patellar tendon was a technically demanding procedure and required a prolonged rehabilitation.

Arendt et al reported on 42 patients who had undergone ACL reconstruction through a medial arthrotomy using a vascularized patellar tendon autograft.[232] All patients had a minimum 2-year follow-up (range 24–54 months). The average age of the patients at the time of reconstruction was 24.7 years. Associated meniscal injuries were common, with 89% of the patients having some meniscal damage. Only 11% of the patients were noted to have normal menisci at the time of surgery.

The patients were evaluated and separate results were reported for subjective symptoms, functional ability, and objective stability using a 100-point system. Subjective results rated pain, swelling, crepitus, catching, locking, and instability. At follow-up 36% of the patients were rated very good, 24% good, 9% fair, and 31% poor. The most common symptoms causing a poor result were stiffness, pain, crepitus, and swelling. When pain was analyzed, 55% of the patients had anterior knee pain. When further analysis of the fair and poor results was performed, there was a significant association with meniscectomy. In patients with intact menisci, 72% had a very good or excellent result, versus 57% fair or poor results in patients with a meniscectomy.

Functional results were evaluated using a 100-point rating scale; activities assessed included running, cutting, jumping, and stair climbing. Twenty-eight percent of the patients were rated as very good, 24% as good, 5% as fair, and 43% as poor. As was true in the subjective evaluations, fair and poor results were associated with meniscectomy.

Objective evaluation revealed that the average extension was 1.5°. A loss of more than 5° extension was present in 14% of the patients. Flexion averaged 138°, with 8% of the patients having less than 125° of flexion. Patellofemoral crepitus was noted in 69% of the patients. The pivot-shift test was reported to be negative in 81% of the patients. Instrumented laxity testing using a KT-1000 arthrometer showed that 60% had 0- to 3-mm side-to-side difference at 25° of flexion with a 20-lb anterior force. The objective results were graded using a 100-point system and 59% rated very good, 24% good, 3% fair, and 14% poor.

The authors concluded on the basis of their objective results that it was possible to restore stability to ACL-deficient knees using a vascularized patellar tendon autograft, but there was a significant discrepancy between the patient's objective and subjective results and the functional outcome of the surgery. They felt that the major factors responsible for this discrepancy were prior meniscectomy and postoperative patellofemoral pain and crepitus.

Aglietti et al reviewed 69 patients who had undergone arthroscopy-assisted ACL reconstruction using a central-third patellar-ligament autograft.[98] The average age of the patients was 23 years (range 15–40 years). The average time to follow-up was 2 years (range 1–3 years). The surgical procedure was performed under arthroscopic control, without arthrotomy. Intraoperative isometry measurements were performed using an isometer in all cases. Up to 3 mm of lengthening as the knee was brought into full extension was accepted. The ACL graft consisted of an 8- to 10-mm portion of the central patellar tendon with attached tibial and patellar bone blocks. Associated surgery performed at the time of ACL reconstruction consisted of 17 medial and 25 lateral meniscectomies and 16 medial and 2 lateral meniscus repairs. The first 16 patients (23%) had a concomitant extraarticular reconstruction. Postoperatively, minimal immobilization and an early range of motion program were used.

The postoperative evaluation consisted of a questionnaire, physical examination, KT-1000 arthrometer measurements, and radiographs. The results were graded using the 100-point Italian Knee Surgery Club rating scale. This scale is similar to the 100-point Hospital for Special Surgery Knee Ligament rating scale. Preoperatively, 68 patients (99%) reported giving way with daily activities or recreational activities. Postoperatively, 67 patients (98%) reported no giving way with vigorous activities. The authors reported that 41 patients (60%) were able to return to full participation in vigorous activities, and 20 patients (29%) exercised some caution with jumping and pivoting. When the data were analyzed for sports participation, 71% of patients who had participated in soccer, 77% who had participated in volleyball and basketball, and 91% who had participated in skiing and tennis were able to return to their sports at the same level.

Range-of-motion measurements revealed that five knees (7%) had an extension loss up to 5° compared with the normal knee. Ten knees (15%) lost more than 10° of flexion. Patellofemoral problems were classified as mild if only a slight crepitus was felt by the examiner with knee extension against resistance but was not noted by the patient. Moderate denoted definite crepitus during knee extension, but no pain or swelling during knee flexion activities. Severe signified definite patellar crepitus and retropatellar pain and/or swelling during flexion activities. Patellar crepitus was absent in 30 knees (44%), mild in 24 (35%), moderate in 12 (18%), and severe in 3 (4%). Eleven patients (16%) were noted to have mild patellofemoral crepitus in their operated knee preoperatively. Postoperatively, these patients had an increased incidence of moderate to severe patellar symptoms compared with patients with a normal patellofemoral joint.

Laxity testing revealed that in 93% of the patients the Lachman test was negative or +1 (1- to 5-mm side-to-side difference). Postoperatively, 60 knees (87%) had a negative pivot shift, 7 knees (10%) had a +1 pivot shift (glide), and 2 knees (3%) had a +2 pivot shift. Instrumented laxity measurements with a KT-1000 revealed the following:

	0–3 mm	3.5–5 mm	>5 mm
20 lb			
Preoperative	8 (13%)	11 (18%)	43 (69%)
Postoperative	43 (66%)	16 (24%)	7 (11%)
Manual maximum			
Preoperative	1 (1.6%)	4 (6%)	57 (92%)
Postoperative	37 (56%)	21 (32%)	8 (12%)

The authors noted a correlation between KT-1000 instrumented laxity measurements and the pivot-shift test. Sixty-two percent of knees with a negative pivot shift had a 3-mm or smaller manual maximum test. Only 22% of the knees with a +1 or +2 pivot shift were noted to have a 3 mm or smaller manual maximum test.

The average knee score increased from 63 points preoperatively to 92 points postoperatively. Fifty-two patients (75%) had an excellent result (90–100 points), 13 patients (19%) had a good result (80–89 points), and 4 patients (6%) had a fair result (70–79 points).

The authors also analyzed their results using very strict criteria to determine a satisfactory result. To achieve a satisfactory result the patient had to meet all of the following criteria:

1. No or minimal pain, swelling, and giving way for vigorous activities
2. Less than 5° loss of extension and less than 15° loss of flexion
3. A negative or +1 pivot shift and a Lachman test +1 or less
4. A manual maximum test 5 mm or less

Using these criteria they found that 13 patients (19%) had an unsatisfactory result. Only 1 of the 13 unsatisfactory results was due to instability; pain, swelling, and an unacceptable manual maximum test (>5 mm) were the most common causes of failure.

In an attempt to determine the advantages of arthroscopy-assisted ACL reconstruction, the authors compared the results of this series of patients with those of a series patients who had undergone open ACL reconstruction previously at their institution (Table 14–3). Although it was not possible to make a rigorous scientific comparison between the two series because of significant differences in surgical technique and postoperative rehabilitation, certain trends were apparent. The arthroscopic group had fewer patellofemoral problems, less loss of motion, and fewer unsatisfactory results compared with the open group.

Feagin et al presented a 2- to 10-year follow-up of patients who had undergone intraarticular ACL recon-

Table 14–3 ACL reconstruction with the central third patellar tendon
Comparison between arthrotomy and arthroscopic series.

	Arthrotomy	Arthroscopic
Number of knees	76	69
Average follow-up	5	2
Motion problems	9%	8%
Pain	14%	4%
Swelling	5%	4%
Giving way	4%	1%
Extension loss >5°	4%	0
Flexion loss >15°	5%	0
Pivot Shift		
(−)	93%	87%
Glide (+1)	4%	10%
Jerk (+2)	2%	3%
KT 1000 manual maximum		
0–3 mm	63%	56%
3.5–5 mm	20%	32%
>5 mm	17%	12%
Severe patellar problems	8%	4%
Percent unsatsifactory results	30%	19%

Reprinted with permission from Aglietti P., Buzzi R., D'Andria S., and Zaccherotti G.: Arthroscopic anterior cruciate ligament reconstruction with patellar tendon. Arthroscopy, 8:510–516, 1992.

struction with a semitendinosus anatomic reconstruction and a central-third patellar-ligament autograft without extraarticular augmentation.[233] The authors reported the results of 137 ACL reconstructions in 128 patients, done between 1979 and 1987, with a minimum 3-year follow-up. The mean follow-up was 53 months (range 3–10 years). The average age of the patients was 31. Skiing was the mechanism of injury in 40% of the patients. Sixty of the patients had acute injuries (under 2 weeks), and 77 were chronic cases. Associated injuries were common. The medial meniscus was torn in 30%, the lateral meniscus in 12%, and both menisci in 8%. In the acute cases, 3% of the knees had condylar lesions, and 25% had a tear of the medial collateral ligament.

The surgical procedure consisted of semitendinosus reconstruction in 58% and patellar-ligament reconstruction in 42% of the knees. Twenty-one percent of the patients required arthroscopic partial meniscectomy, 5% meniscus repair, and 20% medial collateral ligament repair. Initial patients were placed in a cast for 4 to 6 weeks, but during the last 6 years early motion and weight bearing to comfort were allowed.

Subjective evaluation of the patients revealed that 30% noted moderate knee pain at follow-up (although the authors did not specify it in their article, we suspect that most of this pain was patellofemoral). Mild swelling was reported in 32% of the patients, occasional giving way was reported in 22%, and 72% reported no problems with stairs. The sports activity level was reported to be unchanged in 37%, 30% participated in the same sport but at a lower activity level, and 23% changed sports because of the knee.

Objective results revealed that 88% had less than a 5-mm right–left difference during the Lachman test; and

the proportion was 92% for the anterior drawer test. The pivot-shift test was negative in 42%, a pivot glide was noted in 33%, and a positive pivot shift was present in 20%. Instrumented laxity testing with a KT-1000 demonstrated that 75% of the knees had less than a 3-mm side-to-side difference during a manual maximum test, 15% had a 3- to 5-mm difference, and 10% had greater than a 5-mm difference. The instrumented laxity measurements were reported not to have deteriorated with time.

Complications included a retear of the ACL graft in 4 patients, a fracture of the patella in 1 patient, and a flexion contracture in 17 patients. Ten percent of the patients were reported to have undergone surgery for arthrofibrosis.

Subgroup analysis revealed that (1) the patients who had patellar-ligament reconstructions were slightly more satisfied with their final result than were patients who had a semitendinosus reconstruction, and (2) the semitendinosus reconstructions had a higher percentage of failure (17%) by instrumented laxity testing (>5-mm manual maximum test) than the patellar-ligament reconstructions (11%). The most common cause for failure by instrumented laxity evaluation was placement of the femoral drill hole too far anteriorly as judged on the lateral radiograph.

On the basis of their results the authors felt that (1) immediate weight bearing and early range of motion did not affect the stability of the reconstruction and resulted in a decrease in postoperative morbidity; (2) extraarticular augmentation was not necessary as reinjury and deterioration of laxity results were rare; and (3) it is particularly important to avoid a too anterior placement of the femoral drill hole.

O'Brien et al reported the results of 79 patients (80 ACL reconstructions) done at the Hospital for Special Surgery in New York from 1980 to 1985.[26] The minimum follow-up for the patients was 2 years, with an average of 4 years (range 2–7 years). The indication for surgery in this patient population was instability defined by repeated episodes of giving way. Surgical reconstruction of the ACL was performed with a central-third patellar-ligament autograft performed through a medial parapatellar arthrotomy. In 48 of the patients (60%) the patellar-ligament intraarticular reconstruction was augmented with a lateral extraarticular "sling," employing a strip of the iliotibial band. Medial collateral ligament reconstructions were performed in 6 patients (7%). Meniscus tears in this patient population were common; 54 knees (67%) had a meniscectomy prior to or at the time of reconstruction. There were 47 medial and 21 lateral meniscus tears, for a ratio of 2.3/1. Postoperatively, the patients were placed in a long leg cast with the knee at 30° of flexion. Evaluation consisted of a subjective questionnaire, physical examination, instrumented laxity measurements using a KT-1000, and radiographs. The patient's final result was rated on a revised Hospital for Special Surgery 100-point ligament rating scale.

The authors reported that postoperatively 94% of the knees had a negative rating or +1 on the Lachman test (59% negative). The anterior drawer was negative or +1 in 98% of the patients. The pivot-shift test was negative in 84% of the patients; 14% had a +1 pivot shift. Giving way was reported by only four patients (5%), all of whom had other associated ligamentous laxities, posterolateral laxity being the most common associated laxity.

Instrumented laxity measurements were performed with a KT-1000 using a manual maximum test at 30° of flexion. A successful result was defined as a side-to-side difference of 3 mm or less. Sixty patients (76%) had a side-to-side difference of 3 mm or less, and 73 patients (92%) had a difference of 4 mm or less. Seventeen of the nineteen patients (89%) who had a side-to-side difference of more than 3 mm had another associated ligamentous laxity that had not been recognized or treated at the time of the ACL reconstruction. Eleven of the seventeen patients (65%) were found to have varying degrees of posterolateral laxity as determined by an increase in external tibial rotation at 30° of flexion. The authors reported a statistically significant linear relationship between increased external tibial rotation at 30° and increased anterior tibial displacements. The mean side-to-side anterior tibial displacement in patients with 10° or more of external tibial rotation was 3.3 mm, as compared with 1.2 mm in the patients who had less than 10° difference in external tibial rotation.

The average score on the Hospital for Special Surgery 100-point ligament rating scale was 93. The most common cause for deduction of points was patellar pain, which was a complaint in 30 knees (37%). Twenty-five of the thirty knees (83%) with patellofemoral pain had more than 1 cm of quadriceps atrophy. The authors did not find a correlation between patellar pain and loss of extension as had previously been reported by Sachs et al.[83,84] Sixty-nine percent of the patients were able to return to the same activity level following the reconstruction. The most common reasons for a postoperative change in activity level were fear of reinjury, patellar pain, muscle weakness, and instability.

In general, the authors felt that the procedure provided excellent results, but they cautioned against ignoring other associated ligamentous laxities, especially posterolateral laxity. They recommended that posterolateral laxity be addressed at the time of ACL reconstruction if external tibial rotation at 30° of flexion was increased 10° over the normal knee. They recommended concurrent reconstruction of the medial collateral ligament if there was more than 5 mm of medial compartment opening and an associated increase in external tibial rotation. Because they were unable to show any significant differences in the Lachman test, the pivot-shift test, the incidence of giving way, and arthrometer measurements in the 48 knees (60%) that had an extraarticular reconstruction, the authors concluded that it did not provide any advantage and was not necessary.

Buss et al, also from the Hospital for Special Surgery, reported on the results of 68 arthroscopy-assisted ACL reconstructions in 67 patients.[99] This study represented their institution's initial experience with arthroscopy-assisted ACL surgery, and was performed between December 1985 and May 1987. The average age of the patients was 24 years. The minimum follow-up time was 24 months, with an average of 32 months. All patients had symptoms of giving-way from a chronic ACL injury. Approximately 50% of the patients had an associated meniscus injury, and 4% had some associated medial collateral ligament laxity which was felt to be clinically unimportant and was not treated. Patients with lateral and posterolateral instability were excluded from the study. Early on in the study, an extra-articular augmentation using a lateral iliotibial sling procedure was performed in 10 knees (15%)

The surgical procedure consisted of intra-articular reconstruction of the ACL with a central one-third patellar-ligament autograft, performed with arthroscopy assistance. Immediate postoperative range of motion exercises were begun in the recovery room in the early patients in the series with a CPM from 10°–90°, and from 0°–90° in later patients.

Postoperative evaluation consisted of a standardized questionnaire, routine physical examination of the knee, and KT-1000 arthrometer measurements. The results were scored with the Hospital for Special Surgery 100 point ligament rating scale. The average Hospital for Special Surgery Ligament score increased from a preoperative score of 55 points to 93 points postoperative. Sixty-five percent of the knees had an excellent score, 22% good, 9% fair, and 4 percent poor. The most common reason for a lower knee rating was pain. The most common postoperative subjective complaint was patellofemoral pain (26%). Two-thirds of the patients returned to their preinjury level of activity.

Eighty-nine percent of the patients had a negative pivot-shift postoperatively. Ninety-two percent of the patients reported no subsequent episodes of instability following surgery. Eighty-four percent of the patients had a 3 mm or less side-to-side difference on the manual maximum test using a KT-1000 arthrometer, and 93% had a 4 mm or less side-to-side difference.

The authors compared the results of this series of patients with a similar group of patients at their institution who had undergone open ACL reconstruction using the central one-third of the patellar tendon.[174] The comparison data is listed below:

	Arthroscopic	Open
H.S.S. Score	90	93
Percent Manipulations	3%	8%
Patellofemoral Pain	26%	37%
Percent Negative Pivot Shift	89%	84%
KT-1000 Manual Max less than 4 mm	93%	88%

The authors noted that the arthroscopy-assisted group had a lower incidence of manipulations for loss of motion, and patellofemoral pain was less compared to the open group.

Shelbourne and Nitz reported on a large group of patients who had undergone open ACL reconstruction using a central-third patellar-ligament autograft done through a miniarthrotomy.[150] Two groups of patients were evaluated. Group 1 consisted of 138 patients who were operated on between 1984 and 1985. Patients in group 1 were treated with a postoperative rehabilitation protocol in which the knee was splinted in slight flexion, and range of motion and weight bearing were limited during the first 6 weeks. Traditional open-kinetic-chain muscle strengthening exercises were largely used, agility exercises were delayed until 7 to 8 months postoperation, and a return to full activities was delayed until 9 months postoperative. Group 2 consisted of 247 patients who underwent ACL reconstruction from 1987 to 1988. Patients in group 2 were treated with an accelerated postoperative rehabilitation program in which immobilization was not used, and full extension, CPM, and weight bearing were started immediately after surgery. A closed-kinetic-chain muscle strengthening program was begun 2 to 3 weeks postoperatively, and patients were allowed full athletic participation at 4 to 6 months.

Follow-up evaluation of the two groups of patients included range-of-motion measurements, stability tests, KT-1000 instrumented laxity measurements, and Cybex isokinetic strength measurements. A subjective evaluation of the knee was done using a modified Noyes 100-point knee rating scale. The range-of-motion measurements indicated that patients in group 2 achieved earlier and more complete extension versus group 1 patients, and maintained this difference throughout the follow-up period. Group 2 patients also achieved final flexion earlier than group 1 patients, but at 2 years there was no statistically significant difference in the final flexion value between the two groups. At greater than 2 years follow-up, the average range of motion for group 1 was 0° to 136°; for group 2 the average range of motion was 5° hyperextension and 135° flexion. Quadriceps strength was measured with a Cybex isokinetic machine at 180°/s. The Cybex measurements indicate that early on, group 2 patients had a faster recovery of quadriceps strength versus group 1 patients, but there was no difference in the final values. Anteroposterior laxity measurements were measured using a KT-1000 arthrometer with the knee at 30° of flexion and a 20-lb force.

The instrumented laxity measurements indicated that group 2 patients had average values as good as or better than those of group 1. There was no tendency for the laxity values to deteriorate with increasing length of follow-up. The final subjective knee rating score was similar in both groups: 91 in group 1 and 93 in group 2. The authors reported that 12% of the patients in group 1 required scar resection to regain full motion versus only 4% in group 2.

The authors concluded that an accelerated postoperative ACL rehabilitation program emphasizing early full extension, early weight bearing, and early closed-kinetic-chain exercises (1) does not cause early or late graft failure, (2) results in fewer motion problems, (3) decreases the incidence of patellofemoral symptoms, and (4) allows an earlier return to normal and athletic activities without compromising graft strength or stability. The authors were careful to caution that this accelerated program has only been proven safe in patients who undergo ACL replacement with a central-third patellar-ligament autograft, and they did not know if it could be successfully used with other autografts.

Our own results from a small group of patients followed in the Harvard Community Health Plan Knee Clinic for a minimum of 2 years following arthroscopy-assisted ACL reconstruction with a central-third patellar tendon autograft revealed average knee ratings of 87 using the Lysholm rating scale and 88 using the Hospital for Special Surgery knee rating scale. The most common reasons for point deductions were patellofemoral pain and pain in patients with chronic ACL deficiency who had preexisting degenerative changes in the knee at the time of reconstruction. Follow-up evaluation revealed that 38% of the patients had mild patellofemoral crepitus and 8% moderate crepitus in the normal unoperated knee. Mild patellofemoral crepitus was noted in 38%, moderate crepitus in 31%, and severe crepitus in 8% of the operated knees. The incidence of patellofemoral pain following surgery was 21%. The average preinjury Tegner activity level was 7.4, the average postoperative activity level was 7.2, and the patient's desired activity level was 7.8.

Clinical examination revealed that 77% had a negative Lachman test and 23% a +1 Lachman test (0- to 5-mm increase from the normal knee). Ninety-two percent had a negative anterior drawer test, and 8 percent were rated as +1. The pivot-shift test was negative in 85%, whereas 15% had a grade II pivot shift (pivot glide).

Objective testing revealed the average hop index was 95 (range 81–100). The quadriceps index at 60°/s was 87 (range 71–100). At 180°/s the average quadriceps index was 98 (range 73–133). Hamstring strength measurements revealed an average hamstring index at 60°/s of 96 (range 68–139); at 180°/s the average hamstring index was 102 (range 77–147). Instrumented laxity testing using a KT-1000 with a 20-lb anterior force revealed the average side-to-side difference to be 2.0 mm. With a 30-lb anterior force the average side-to-side difference was 2.5 mm (range 0.5–4 mm).

Bach et al, have recently reported on their initial experience using a free, autogenous central-third patellar tendon graft without extraarticular augmentation for ACL reconstruction.[234] At the time of follow-up, 62 of the 75 patients were available for clinical review. All patients were a minimum of 2 years postoperative (mean 37 months, range 27–51 months). The patients were operated on by the senior authors between March 1987 and May 1989.

The procedure consisted of a two-incision arthroscopy assisted technique previously described by the senior author.[153] A free, autogenous central-third patellar-tendon graft (10–12 mm) fixed with 9 mm interference screws was used. Postoperatively a CPM, range −10 to 90° was used in the hospital. Active quadriceps exercises in the 0–35° range were limited during the early postoperative period. Patients were weaned from crutches at six weeks. A closed chain rehabilitation program was used following the early postoperative period. Patients were allowed to return to sports at 20 weeks if they met the rehabilitation criteria.

Clinical assessment was performed using the Noyes, modified HSS, Lysholm, and Tegner knee rating scales. Functional assessment were performed using a Cybex dynamometer, KT-1000 knee arthrometer, and the one-leg hop test. The authors reported that 92% had a negative pivot shift at the time of follow-up. Then mean Cybex extension deficit was 12% at 60°, 9% at 180° and 7% at 240° per second. The authors reported an 18% incidence of patellofemoral pain. The mean HSS score was 88 (range 65–99), Noyes score was 86 (range 30–100), and the Lysholm score was 88 (range 52–100). The mean single leg hop test was 88%. KT-1000 data revealed a mean manual maximum difference of 0.3 mm. Ninety-two of the patients were reported to have a manual maximum difference less than or equal to 3 mm.

The authors were encouraged by their initial experience, and felt that the procedure offered reliable stability as assessed by clinical and arthrometric data, excellent postoperative motion, and excellent recovery of quadriceps strength. Their experience provides further documentation that extraarticular augmentation is unnecessary and adds little to intraarticular reconstruction.

Hamstring Tendon

For the sake of space, and because of the significantly reduced morbidity and incidence of patellofemoral pain of arthroscopy-assisted reconstructions versus reconstructions done through an arthrotomy, we review only the results of the former.

Boden et al reported the early results of 20 patients with an average follow-up time of 26 months (range 18–39 months) who had undergone ACL reconstruction using a combined single-stranded semitendinosus, gracilis graft.[235] An extraarticular tenodesis of the iliotibial band was also performed in all patients. Average age of the patients was 20 years (range 17–30 years).

At follow-up no patient was reported to have a Lachman test greater than +1, and all patients had a negative pivot shift. KT-1000 arthrometer measurements demonstrated an average side-to-side difference with a 20-lb anterior force of 1.0 mm. Muscle testing revealed an average of 91% of the normal side for extension, and 93% for flexion. Eighty percent of the patients were reported to have returned to their preinjury level.

Marder et al in a prospective study of 80 consecutive patients with a chronic ACL-deficient knee operated on from 1986 to 1988, compared the results of arthroscopy-assisted ACL reconstructions performed with a 10-mm central-third patellar tendon autograft (PT) and those of double-looped semitendinosus, gracilis grafts (STGS).[71] The procedures were performed in a strict alternating sequence. Because 8 patients were lost to follow-up, 37 PTS and 35 STGS were evaluated. The mean time at follow-up was 29 months (range 24–42 months). There were no statistical differences with respect to age and sex or preoperative laxity in the groups. The postoperative rehabilitation program was identical in both groups.

Subjective evaluation revealed no statistically significant difference between the two groups with respect to average final knee rating score (PT = 39, STG = 42, maximum possible = 50), anterior knee pain with activity, giving-way symptoms, or return to activity.

Objective evaluation revealed that 5 of 37 (14%) PT patients and 4 of 35 (11%) STG patients had +2 or greater patellofemoral crepitus and were symptomatic with activity (not statistically significant). Four PT patients (11%) had patellar tendinitis, versus no STG patients. Final range of motion was similar in both groups except for one PT patient who experienced a 15° loss of extension. No statistical differences were reported between the two groups for the postoperative manual Lachman test or pivot-shift test.

Instrumented laxity tested with a KT-1000 arthrometer at 20 lb revealed average values of 1.6 ± 1.4 mm for the PT patients and 1.9 ± 1.3 mm for the STG group (not statistically significant). A side-to-side difference of 2 mm or less was obtained in 32 of 37 (86%) PT patients and 26 of 35 (74%) STG patients (not statistically significant). Five percent of the PT group (2/37) and 9% of the STG group (3/35) were noted to have a greater than 3-mm side-to-side difference.

Strength testing revealed average peak extension torques at 60°/s of $88 \pm 17\%$ for PT patients and $91 \pm 19\%$ for STG patients (not statistically significant). The average peak flexion torque at 60°/s was $91 \pm 18\%$ for

Table 14-4 Clinical ratings by group

Group	Excellent/Good	Fair	Reoperated
Acute*	23(92%)	2(8%)	–
Chronic*	16(64%)	9(36%)	–
IA	16(67%)	6(25%)	2(8%)
IA/EA"	23(82%)	5(18%)	

*n = 25
n = 24
"n = 28

Reprinted with permission from Grana WA, and Hines R: Arthroscopic-assisted semitendinosus reconstruction of the anterior cruciate ligament. Am J Knee Surg 5:19, 1992.

the PT group and $83 \pm 16\%$ for STG patients (statistically significant).

The authors concluded that at an average follow-up of 29 months, the results of arthroscopy-assisted ACL reconstruction performed using patellar tendon and double-looped semitendinosus, gracilis grafts were comparable.

Grana and Hines reported on their first 50 ACL reconstructions performed between July 1984 and March 1986 using an arthroscopy-assisted technique with a double-looped semitendinosus autograft.[236] The average age of the patients was 24 years (range 14–58). The average follow-up was 3.4 years (range 3–4.9). In 28 of the patients, an iliotibial band tenodesis was performed along with the intraarticular reconstruction. Twenty-five of the reconstructions were performed acutely (within 4 weeks of initial injury), and 25 were chronic.

Follow-up evaluation consisted of a Lysholm subjective clinical rating, Tegner activity scale, manual examination (Lachman and pivot-shift tests), instrumented laxity testing with a Stryker laxity tester using a 13.5-kg force, and a Cybex strength evaluation at 180°/s. The clinical ratings by group are listed in Table 14-4.

Manual examination revealed that 84% of the patients had less than a +1 Lachman test, 85% had a negative pivot-shift test, and 15% had a positive pivot-shift test. Seventy-one per cent of the patients were reported to have returned to their preinjury level of activity.

Instrumented laxity testing with a Stryker laxity testing device with a 13.5-kg force revealed that 75% of the patients had less than a 3-mm side-to-side difference, 15% had a 3- to 5-mm side-to-side difference, and 10% had a greater than 5-mm side-to-side difference.

Hamstring strength testing using a Cybex dynamometer at 180°/s revealed that 44% of the patients had hamstring strength equal to or greater than that of the normal side, 19% of the patients had less than a 10% deficit, and 25% were reported to have greater than a 10% deficit. Quadriceps strength measurements at 180°/s revealed that 44% of the patients had quadriceps strength equal to or greater than that of the

normal side, 21% had less than a 10% deficit, and 23% had greater than a 10% deficit.

Only 6 patients (12%) complained of patellofemoral pain. Nine of fifty-two cases (17%) were considered failures because of repeat surgery or pathologic laxity (>5-mm side-to-side difference, or positive pivot shift, or Lachman test score greater than +1).

Although noting their 17% failure rate, the authors felt that because of the lower incidence of postoperative patellofemoral pain and loss of motion compared with previous reports of patellar tendon reconstructions, this procedure was useful.

Karlson et al reported the results of 64 patients operated on over a 30-month period beginning in 1985 who underwent ACL reconstruction with a combined single-limb semitendinosus, gracilis graft.[204] Thirty-two of the patients had grafts placed in an over-the-top position and 32 through a femoral drill hole. The average time at follow-up was 2.9 years (range 2–4.9 years). The two groups of patients were reported to be similar with respect to age, gender, chronicity of injury, number of meniscectomies, and preoperative activity level.

No statistical differences between the two graft placements were seen with respect to overall knee rating, range of motion, KT-1000 arthrometer measurements, isokinetic strength measurements, and one-leg hop test. The combined average knee ratings were 92 ± 7 for the Lysholm score, 89 ± 7 for the Hospital for Special Surgery score, 92 ± 7 for the Noyes score, and 7 excellent, 41 good, and 0 poor for the International Knee Documentation Committee score.

Instrumented laxity testing with a KT-1000 using a 20-lb force revealed a mean side-to-side difference of 2.1 mm. Nine of the sixty-four (14%) patients were reported to have a greater than 3.5-mm side-to-side difference.

Cybex peak torque measurements at 60°/s revealed average values of 95% for extension and 106% for flexion. At 180°/s the average values were 96% for extension and 100% for flexion. Sixty-nine percent had greater than 90% quadriceps strength, whereas 10% were noted to have less than 80% quadriceps strength. Similar figures were obtained for hamstring strength. The average hop index was 95, with 73% of the patients having a hop index greater than 90, 22% a hop index between 80 and 90, and 5% a hop index less than 80.

Nine of the sixty-four patients (14%) were considered failures because of a greater than 3.5-mm side-to-side difference and the presence of a positive pivot shift. Six of the eight failures were in patients with chronic ACL-deficient knees. Because of the 14% failure rate in this series the authors no longer recommend the use of single-limbed grafts, particularly in chronic ACL-deficient knees.

Aglietti et al, in a prospective study performed in

1989, reported on the results of 60 patients with chronic ACL-deficient knees.[80] The patients were randomly assigned to be reconstructed with either a central-third patellar tendon autograft (PT) in 30 patients or a double-looped semitendinosus, gracilis graft (STG) in 30 patients. There were no significant differences between the two groups as far as age, sex, interval to surgery, or preoperative activity level.

The central-third patellar tendon grafts were fixed with a press fit technique and No. 2 nonabsorbable sutures tied around a screw and washer on the femoral side. The tibial end of the graft was fixed with an interference screw and sutures on the tibial side. The doubled semitendinosus, gracilis grafts were looped around a screw and soft tissue washer on the femoral side and fixed on the tibial side by tying sutures placed in the free ends of the graft around a screw and washer. In 80% of the cases sufficient length was obtained to add a barbed staple on the tibial side. An identical postoperative rehabilitation program was used in both groups and consisted of early passive motion of 0° to 90°. The patients were full weight bearing by 8 weeks.

The average follow-up was 25 months (range 21–39 months). Return to the same sport was reported in 66% of the PT patients and 50% of the STG patients (not statistically significant). A positive grade I pivot shift was noted in 23% of the PT group and 27% of the STG group (not statistically significant). Patellofemoral crepitus was noted in 16% of the PT patients versus 3% of the STG patients ($P = .01$). Two PT knees experienced difficulty regaining full extension.

Instrumented laxity testing with a KT-1000 using a 20-lb force revealed side-to-side differences of less than 3 mm in 53% of the PT and 40% of the patients, between 3.5 and 5 mm in 37% of the PT and 47% of the STG patients, and greater than 5 mm in 10% of the PT and 13% of the STG patients. None of these differences were noted to be statistically significant. The authors noted that in the 24 patients in whom the tendons were of sufficient length to be stapled to the tibia, the average side-to-side difference was 3.7 mm versus 5.4 mm for the group with suture fixation only. This difference was said not to be statistically significant.

Isokinetic extension and flexion peak torque measurements revealed no significant differences between the two groups at 60°, 120°, and 180° per second.

The authors concluded that the only statistically significant differences between the two graft sources was a higher incidence of patellofemoral crepitus in the PT patients; however, there was a trend for hamstring tendon grafts to have less objective stability, particularly if insufficient length prevented rigid fixation on both ends. There was also a trend toward more donor site problems and motion problems in the PT patients.

Sgaglione et al in a retrospective study reviewed 50 patients who had undergone ACL reconstruction with semitendinosus and gracilis tendon grafts between May 1984 and December 1986.[101] Twenty-two of the patients had an acute reconstruction (within 3 weeks of injury), and 29 were treated for chronic ACL deficiency. In the chronic group a doubled semitendinosus graft was used in 75% of patients and a single-stranded combined semitendinosus and gracilis graft was used in 25% (because of inadequate length). In 86% of the acute group a doubled semitendinosus graft was used and in 14%, single-stranded combined semitendinosus and gracilis grafts.

Mean follow-up was 40 months for the acute group and 34 months for the chronic group. Subjective evaluation revealed no statistically significant difference between the two groups, with 77% good to excellent results in the acute group and 75% good to excellent results in the chronic group. Patellofemoral pain was reported in 23% of the acute patients and was rated as mild in 14% and significant in 9%. In the chronic group 14% complained of patellofemoral pain, mild in 10% and significant in 4%. The authors reported that the incidence of significant patellofemoral pain between the two groups (acute = 9%, chronic = 4%) was not statistically significant. Measurable loss of motion was noted in 50% of the acute cases versus 21% of the chronic group (statistically significant).

Manual laxity testing revealed that 95% of the acute reconstructions had a normal or +1 Lachman test versus 82% of the chronic reconstructions. The pivot-shift test was noted to be absent in 95% of the acute reconstructions compared with 82% of the chronic reconstructions. These difference was reported to be statistically significant.

Instrumented laxity testing with a KT-1000 using a 20-lb force revealed that 88% of the acute reconstructions had a side-to-side difference of 3 mm or less as compared with only 61% of the chronic group. One acute patient (5%) had a side-to-side difference greater than 5 mm as compared with five chronic patients (18%). It should, however, be noted that single-stranded grafts were used in 25% of the chronic cases versus only 14% of the acute cases.

The authors concluded that the hamstring tendons provided a good clinical outcome when used to reconstruct acute ACL injuries; however, because of the greater incidence of pathologic motion as evaluated by the Lachman test, pivot-shift test, and instrumented laxity testing, they felt that hamstring tendon grafts lead to a less optimal outcome in chronic patients.

Complications

Recent articles by Graf and Uhr,[90] Roberts et al,[186] Sachs et al,[84] and Brown and Indelicato[87] have discussed the complications of ACL surgery. For a thorough discussion of this topic, the reader is referred to these references. In this section we discuss donor site complications unique to the use of a particular autograft.

Andrews et al have said that donor site problems are the most common complication following ACL reconstruction with a patellar tendon autograft.[69] Potential donor site complications include the following:

1. Patellar tendon rupture
2. Patellar fracture
3. Patellar tendinitis
4. Patellofemoral pain
5. Quadriceps weakness
6. Donor site pain

As discussed in earlier sections, many of these complications may be related to surgical technique and postoperative rehabilitation, and thus may be preventable. Patellar tendon rupture following reconstruction of the ACL with a patellar tendon autograft is certainly a devastating complication. Fortunately the incidence of patellar tendon rupture appears to be quite low, as only sporadic case reports have appeared in the orthopedic literature.

Bonamo et al reported two cases of patellar tendon rupture following reconstruction of the ACL with a quadriceps tendon patellar retinaculum-ligament intraarticular substitute.[85] In both cases the grafts consisted of the central third of the patellar tendon, a 10-mm width, with more than half of the quadriceps aponeurosis overlying the patella in continuity with a 10-mm-wide segment of the central portion of the rectus femoris tendon.

The first case occurred 8 months postoperatively after a sudden jump. At surgical exploration the patellar tendon together with a small fragment of bone was avulsed from the inferior pole of the patella. The second case occurred 4 months postoperatively during a fall. As in the first case the patellar tendon was found to be avulsed from the inferior pole of the patella. After repair of the patellar tendon both patients achieved a near-normal range of motion, but both had persistent quadriceps weakness as evaluated by isokinetic testing. Both patients were said to be able to resume recreational sports.

Langan and Fontanetta also reported a rupture of the patellar tendon following harvest of the central third for ACL reconstruction.[94] This patient's postoperative course was complicated by limited motion; at 6 months the range of motion was reported to be 10° to 90°, with no significant improvement with intense physical therapy by 10 months postoperatively. The patient was also noted to have a persistent extensor lag. A lateral radiograph revealed patella alta, and this finding eventually led to surgical exploration. At surgery the patellar tendon was noted to be avulsed off the inferior pole of the patella without a bony fragment. The medial and lateral portions of the tendon were noted to have slipped off to the side of the patella such that they did not apply a central vector force to allow full extension. Surgical repair was performed, and at 7 months postoperatively the patient had a range of motion from 0° to 105°. Functionally the patient was reported to have had some limitation with stairs.

Daniel et al reported 4 ruptures in 148 patients (2.7% incidence) who underwent ACL reconstruction with a quadriceps tendon patellar retinaculum-ligament graft augmented with a Kennedy ligament-augmentation device.[237] MacKinlay et al have also reported one late quadriceps tendon rupture in a group of 100 patients who underwent reconstruction of the ACL with a quadriceps tendon patellar retinaculum-ligament autograft.[95]

It is interesting to note that 7 of the 11 reported cases of extensor mechanism rupture have involved the quadriceps tendon patellar retinaculum-ligament graft. One possible explanation for this trend is that perhaps the extra dissection of the quadriceps and patellar retinaculum may impair the blood supply to the remaining patellar tendon. Additionally, removing a portion of the rectus femoris tendon from the quadriceps could further weaken the extensor mechanism, predisposing it to rupture. If this hypothesis is true, then it may be wise when harvesting the patellar bone block to minimize surgical dissection of the patellar aponeurosis.

DeLee and Craviotto reported a rupture of the quadriceps tendon after harvest of a central-third patellar-ligament graft for ACL reconstruction.[89] At the time of graft harvest the patellar bone block measured 10 mm in width, 30 mm in length and 5 mm in depth. A 20-mm cortical rim of bone was left intact around the superior pole of the patella, and the defect in the patella was bone grafted at the time of surgery. Six weeks postoperatively, while wearing a brace, the patient slipped and fell and sustained a hyperflexion valgus injury to the operated knee, resulting in an avulsion of the quadriceps tendon from the superior pole of the patella. Following surgical repair the range of motion was reported to be 0° to 140°.

Hardin and Bach recently reported a case of a distal rupture of the patellar tendon following use of the central third of the patellar tendon for ACL reconstruction.[91] The patient was a 42-year-old police officer who was 1 month postoperative and slipped on ice while using crutches. He sustained a hyperflexion injury to the knee. Clinical examination revealed that the patient was unable to actively extend his knee; radiographs were noted to be normal. An MRI demonstrated a large effusion, intact cruciate reconstruction, and a high signal uptake at the distal insertion of the patellar tendon consistent with a complete rupture.

At surgery a ½-in. transverse defect with retraction of the distal patellar tendon was noted. The remainder of the patellar tendon was hypertrophied. Primary repair of the patellar tendon and augmentation with the

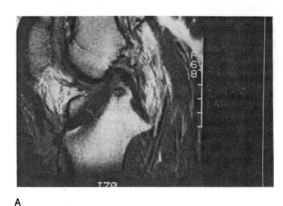

A

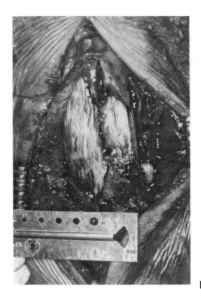

B

Figure 14–68. A. MRI showing distal rupture of the patellar tendon. **B.** Intraoperative photograph. (Reprinted with permission from Hardin and Bach.[91])

gracilis and semitendinosus tendons were performed. The repair was protected with a figure-eight tension-band wire. At follow-up examination, the patient was reported to have a range of motion of 3° to 126°, to be pain free, to be able to perform a normal straight-leg raise, and to have a stable knee (Fig. 14–68).

Zero patellar tendon ruptures have been reported by various authors in large series of patients who have undergone ACL reconstruction with patellar-ligament autografts.[227] Sachs et al reported no patellar tendon ruptures in 360 cases done at the Kaiser Medical Center in San Diego.[84]

In summary, although the complication of patellar tendon rupture following harvest of the central third of the patellar tendon is a major concern, few cases have been reported. The risk of patellar tendon rupture seems to be highest after use of the quadriceps tendon patellar retinaculum-ligament graft, possibly related to the extra surgical dissection required during harvest.

Intraoperative patellar fracture may also occur during the harvest of the patellar bone block. Christen and Jakob reported that between 1980 and 1990 at their institution, 490 ACL and PCL reconstructions were performed in which a central-third patellar tendon graft was harvested.[88] They reported 6 cases of incomplete patellar fracture (fissures) and 3 complete fractures (1.8% incidence). Graf and Uhr pointed out that patellar fracture may not necessarily result in compromise of the clinical result if stable fixation of the fracture is performed so that early motion can be started.[90] This complication can largely be prevented by proper surgical technique such as using a sagittal saw during graft harvesting and avoiding forceful use of osteotomes.

Bonatus and Alexander reported a patellar fracture and avulsion of the patellar tendon following harvest of a central-third patellar-ligament graft.[86] Seven days postoperatively, the patient slipped and fell down a flight of stairs while ambulating with crutches. Radiographs demonstrated a displaced longitudinal fracture through the patella bone block site. At surgery a comminuted patellar fracture (three fragments) was found, as was avulsion of the lateral third of the patellar tendon. The patellar fracture was repaired with lag screws and a tension-band wire. The patellar tendon was repaired with a Bunnell suture and was splinted with an 18-gauge wire. Postoperatively, the patient's course was complicated by a loss of motion requiring arthroscopic debridement and manipulation at 5 months. At 11 months the patient was reported to have returned to full military duty with a normal range of motion and a stable asymptomatic knee. Late patellar fracture has also been reported by McCarroll[96] and Lambert and Cunningham.[93]

Patellar tendinitis has also been reported as a complication following reconstruction of the ACL with a patellar-ligament autograft. Graf and Uhr reported that 6% of their patients mentioned this as a complaint in postoperative follow-up. They noted an association with the initiation of aggressive progressive resistance exercises.[90] The symptoms were reported usually to resolve with rest, anti-inflammatory agents, and an eccentric quadriceps program. Marder et al reported that

11% of their patients who underwent reconstruction with a patellar tendon graft experienced tenderness at the inferior pole of the patella with activities versus 0% with hamstring grafts.[71] Rubinstein et al reported an incidence of activity-related patellar tendinitis of 21% in patients undergoing ACL reconstruction using the central third of the patellar tendon.[97] In another study in which they investigated the isolated donor site morbidity by harvesting a central-third patellar tendon graft from the opposite knee, they reported a 55% incidence of activity-related patellar tendinitis. They felt that the tendinitis was rarely a problem after the first year.

Perhaps the most common donor site complication following ACL reconstruction is patellofemoral pain. It is difficult to know the exact incidence of patellofemoral pain following ACL surgery as this symptom is often not reported in follow-up studies. Also, there is no universally accepted method of evaluating or grading the patellofemoral joint in patients who have undergone knee ligament surgery. Based on reports in the orthopedic literature the incidence of patellofemoral pain appears to be highest in patients who undergo ACL surgery done through an arthrotomy.

Johnson et al reviewed 87 patients who underwent ACL reconstruction using a modification of the Brostrom procedure.[227] The knee joint was entered by division of the medial patellar retinaculum and lateral dislocation of the patella. They reported subpatellar crepitus in 57 of the 87 patients. The subpatellar crepitus was rated mild in 43 of 87 patients (49%) and severe in 14 of 87 patients (16%). The authors noted that mild subpatellar crepitus did not necessarily compromise the clinical result, but that marked crepitus in many cases was the cause of a poor result. In 11 cases (13%) subpatellar crepitus was the cause of an unsatisfactory postoperative result, in the face of a stable knee.

Arendt et al reviewed 37 patients who underwent ACL reconstruction using a medial-third vascularized patellar-ligament graft done through a medial arthrotomy.[232] At the beginning of the study the patients were immobilized in a cast at 45° of flexion for 8 weeks. This was later changed to 2 weeks of immobilization, followed by a controlled motion program. They reported that 55% of the patients complained of anterior knee pain and 69% had crepitation when the patellofemoral joint was examined. They felt that the unacceptably high incidence of patellofemoral problems was due to postoperative immobilization and early institution of a progressive resistance program with an isokinetic machine. The incidence of anterior knee pain was substantially reduced when they modified their postoperative protocol by delaying the start of isokinetic exercises until 16 weeks postoperatively and allowing only high-speed isokinetic exercises through a limited arc of motion.

Sachs et al evaluated 126 patients who underwent ACL reconstruction with either patellar-ligament or hamstring tendon autografts.[83,84] They reported that 24 of the 126 patients (19%) had patellar irritability on examination 1 year after surgery. A significant positive correlation between patellar irritability and loss of extension and a positive correlation between quadriceps weakness and patellar irritability were also noted.

Aglietti et al in a very detailed paper reported on patellofemoral pain in 226 patients who had undergone ACL surgery.[81] The patients were divided into four groups: Group A (43 knees) had an acute Marshall-type repair of the ACL with arthrotomy and semitendinous augmentation. Group B (38 knees) had an acute arthroscopy-assisted reconstruction of the ACL using the semitendinous and gracilis tendons. Group C (76 knees) comprised chronic ACL-deficient knees treated by arthrotomy and reconstruction of the ACL with a central-third patellar-ligament graft. Group D (69 knees) were chronic ACL-deficient knees treated with arthroscopy-assisted ACL reconstruction using the central third of the patellar ligament. The average follow-up was 3 years (range 1–9 years). Cast immobilization was reported to have been used in 53% of group A patients and 72% of group C patients (the open groups). Early motion was reported to have been used in the remainder of the patients in these groups and in all patients in groups B and D (arthroscopic groups).

They classified patellofemoral pain as absent, mild, moderate, and severe. Mild patellofemoral pain was defined as minimal crepitation not volunteered by the patients, moderate patellofemoral pain as asymptomatic patellofemoral crepitus, and severe pain as pain or swelling brought on by flexion activities. The incidences of moderate and severe patellofemoral pain were reported to be 40% (group A), 21% (group B), 24% (group C), and 21% (group D). The difference in patellofemoral pain between the acute open group (group A) and the other groups was highly significant ($P = 0.02$). Arthroscopy-assisted surgery and early motion in acute cases reduced the incidence of moderate and severe patellofemoral pain to that seen in the chronic groups. Severe patellofemoral pain was also found to correlate with a decreased postoperative activity level, but mild or moderate patellofemoral pain was not found to affect the postoperative activity level. Thigh atrophy of 2 cm or greater was found in 75% of the patients with severe patellofemoral pain. An abnormal hop test was reported in 19% of patients with absent or mild patellofemoral pain, in 43% with moderate pain, and in 75% with severe pain. The authors also evaluated postoperative patellar height and reported an overall incidence of 17% patella baja. Arthroscopy-assisted ACL surgery had a significantly lower incidence of patellar baja (12%) versus open ACL surgery (21%). In chronic cases the authors also noted a highly statistically significant correlation between preoperative patellofemoral crepitus and the development of severe and moderate postoperative patellofemoral pain. In patients with preoperative patellofemoral crepitus the postoperative incidence of moderate and severe patellofemoral pain was 47%, versus 19% in those patients with a normal preoperative patellofemoral joint. In the chronic group they found a positive correlation between loss of extension and patellofemoral pain as previously reported by Sachs et al.[83,84] The authors concluded that patellofemoral pain is one of the most common complications following ACL surgery and is related to many factors, including preexisting patellofemoral articular cartilage degeneration, patellofemoral congruence, arthrotomy, nonisometric ligament placement, graft impingement, and inadequate rehabilitation.

O'Brien et al reported a 37% incidence of patellofemoral pain in 80 knees with chronic ACL deficiency that had undergone ACL reconstruction with a central-third patellar-ligament autograft.[26] The procedure was performed through a medial arthrotomy, and postoperatively all patients were treated with 6 weeks of cast immobilization at 30° of flexion. The authors also reported on postoperative changes in the patellar tendon height. In 51 knees preoperative and postoperative lateral radiographs were available to measure changes in the postoperative Insall–Silvati patellar tendon/patellar ratio, a measure of patellar tendon length. They reported that 55% of the knees had on average 20% shortening of the patellar tendon, 25% had no change, and 20% had a relative lengthening. Although they could not demonstrate any statistically significant correlation between patellar pain and the Insall–Salvati ratio, there was a trend for the incidence of patellar pain to increase the more the patellar tendon was shortened or lengthened. The authors felt that the high incidence of patellar pain in their patients may have been related to the 6 weeks of postoperative immobilization. They speculated that the patellar tendon graft source may also have played a role.

Buss et al reported a 26% incidence of patellofemoral pain in 70 patients who underwent arthroscopy-assisted ACL reconstruction using an autogenous patellar tendon graft. Postoperatively no immobilization was used, and all patients were treated with an early motion program.[99]

Sgaglione et al reported incidences of significant patellofemoral pain of 9% in acute knees and 3.6% in chronic knees following arthroscopy-assisted ACL reconstruction using double-stranded hamstring grafts.[101]

On the basis of the preceding reports patellofemoral pain is a very frequent complication following ACL surgery. In most series where this symptom is evaluated as part of the postoperative follow-up, it is perhaps the most common complication. Although the source of postoperative patellofemoral pain is multifactorial there is still controversy regarding the relationship of patellofemoral pain to autograft source.

Marder et al reported a prospective study of 80 patients who were treated in an alternating sequence with arthroscopy-assisted ACL reconstruction using a central-third patellar-ligament autograft or semitendinosus and gracilis autograft.[71] Both patient groups were similar with respect to age, sex, level of activity, and degree of laxity. Both groups underwent a standardized postoperative rehabilitation program. Of patients who underwent reconstruction of the ACL with a patellar-ligament autograft, 8 of 40 (20%) patients had slight patellofemoral pain with activity, and 3 of 40 (8%) had moderate patellofemoral pain with activity. Of patients who underwent ACL reconstruction with the semitendinosus and gracilis tendons, 5 of 40 (13%) had slight patellofemoral pain with activity and 1 of 40 (3%) had moderate pain with activity. Marder et al concluded that there was no statistical significant difference in patellofemoral pain between the two autografts.

Aglietti et al in a retrospective study reported no difference in patellofemoral pain between patients who underwent acute arthroscopy-assisted ACL reconstruction using semitendinosus and gracilis autografts (21%) and those who underwent chronic reconstructions with a central-third patellar-ligament autograft (21%).[81]

Aglietti et al reported a prospective randomized study of 60 patients with chronic ACL-deficient knees.[80] Thirty patients underwent ACL reconstruction with a central-third patellar-ligament graft and 30 with looped semitendinosus, gracilis tendons. The postoperative rehabilitation program was the same for both groups, and included early full extension and flexion, and early partial weight bearing. The authors reported that 16% of the patellar-ligament patients had patellofemoral crepitus versus 3% of the hamstring tendon patients. This difference was found to be statistically significant ($P = 0.01$).

In a further attempt to determine the relationship of patellofemoral pain to graft source, Re et al performed a prospective study of anterior knee pain evaluating 187 patients.[82] Fifty patients with ACL tears were treated nonoperatively, 50 were treated with a semitendinosus and gracilis reconstruction, 50 were treated with patellar tendon reconstruction, and 50 were treated with allograft reconstruction of the ACL. The incidence of anterior knee pain in the nonoperatively treated group was 22%, similar to the figure reported by Buss et al.[238] Preoperatively, 17% of patients undergoing ACL reconstruction using hamstring tendons were noted to complain of anterior knee pain, compared with 14% postoperatively (not statistically significant). For the allograft group, the incidences of anterior knee pain were 22% preoperatively and 26% postoperatively (not statistically significant). The patients undergoing patellar tendon reconstruction were noted to have a 26% incidence of anterior knee pain preoperatively, compared with 47% postoperatively (highly significant, $P = .058$). The authors also reported a statistically significant increase in anterior knee pain between the patellar tendon and hamstring reconstruction groups ($P = .002$). The authors attributed the difference in anterior knee pain between the hamstring tendon reconstructions and the patellar tendon reconstructions to the morbidity associated with the donor site.

Patellofemoral pain and crepitus are common complications following ACL reconstruction. Although many patients are asymptomatic or the symptoms are mild, in some cases the symptoms can be severe. In some clinical series, patellofemoral pain was the most common cause of an unacceptable result in the face of a stable knee.[227,232] Although the exact cause of postoperative patellofemoral pain is not known, it is clear that many factors may increase a patient's risk for the development of patellar pain. Some of the risk factors identified are listed here:

1. Preoperative patellofemoral pain
2. Surgery performed through an arthrotomy
3. Postoperative immobilization
4. Extension loss greater than 5°
5. Flexion loss greater than 10°
6. Graft source (patellar tendon > hamstring, patellar tendon > allograft)

Improvements in surgical technique and postoperative rehabilitation have resulted in a dramatic decrease in patellar pain and crepitus. Based on recent reports,[71,80-82,98-100] the incidence of patellar pain and crepitus following arthroscopy-assisted ACL reconstruction with a central-third patellar tendon autograft is approximately 16 to 47%, versus 3 to 21% for hamstring grafts.[71,80-82,101]

Quadriceps weakness, defined[41,192] as a quadriceps index less than 80, has also been another frequently reported complication following ACL reconstruction using patellar tendon autografts.[83,84,229] It has been reported that 111 of 180 patients (62%) who underwent ACL reconstruction with patellar tendon or hamstring tendon autografts had a quadriceps index less than 80 when their extension torque was evaluated at 60°/s. An additional test, the one-leg hop test, was also used to evaluate quadriceps function. In a previous study Daniel et al described a one-leg hop test performed with the injured and noninjured legs as a measure of lower limb function.[230] On the basis of this study, they felt that a hop index of at least 90 was the goal following reconstruction of the ACL. Sachs et al reported that 116 of their 180 patients (64%) had a hop index less than 90.[83,84] When the data were analyzed by autograft

type, 81 of 116 patients (70%) with patellar tendon reconstructions had a hop index less than 90, versus 35 of 64 patients (55%) with hamstring tendons, a statistically significant difference.

Sachs et al,[83,84] Aglietti et al,[81] and O'Brien et al[26] also noted a statistically significant correlation of quadriceps weakness to patellofemoral pain. Sachs et al reported no difference in hamstring strength after 1 year between ACL reconstructions performed with the hamstring tendon and patellar tendon reconstructions[83,84]; however, they reported a statistically significant difference in quadriceps strength between hamstring and patellar tendon reconstructions. At 1 year, in a group of patients without flexion contractures or patellar irritability, the mean quadriceps index was 72% for patellar tendon grafts versus 83% for hamstring tendon grafts. The authors concluded that graft source alone did influence quadriceps strength at 1 year.

Shelbourne et al, on the other hand, reported a mean quadriceps index of 90 in a large series of patients who had undergone acute open ACL reconstruction using an autogenous patellar-ligament graft followed by an accelerated postoperative rehabilitation program.[145,235] It thus appears that the postoperative rehabilitation program could also play a large role in determining quadriceps strength. Shelbourne and co-workers demonstrated that a postoperative rehabilitation program with early emphasis on full extension and closed-kinetic-chain exercises could minimize patellofemoral pain (which has a negative correlation with quadriceps strength) and maximize early return of quadriceps strength. It is their feeling (personal communication, 1991) that much of the postoperative morbidity reported following ACL reconstruction with a patellar-ligament autograft is directly related to the rehabilitation program used.

Marder et al in a prospective study found mean quadriceps indices of 88 for patellar-ligament autografts and 91 for hamstring tendon grafts and concluded that there was no statistically significant difference in quadriceps function between the two graft sources.[71] Lephart et al have also reported no significant difference in quadriceps strength as measured by a Cybex isokinetic machine at 60°/s and 240°/s among 10 patients who underwent ACL reconstruction with a patellar-ligament autograft and 10 patients who underwent allograft replacement of the ACL.[108] These two studies suggest that harvest of a patellar tendon autograft may not necessarily compromise the extensor mechanism as much as previously thought.

Aglietti et al reported a prospective randomized study comparing the results of patellar tendon autografts with those of looped semitendinosus and gracilis autografts.[80] Peak extension torque was evaluated with a Cybex II dynamometer at 60°, 120°, and 180° per second. The results were as follows:

Speed	Patellar Tendon	Hamstring Tendons
60°/s		
Quadriceps	91%	89%
Hamstrings	98%	94%
120°/s		
Quadriceps	93%	94%
Hamstrings	94%	96%
180°/s		
Quadriceps	94%	95%
Hamstrings	98%	93%

The authors concluded that there was no significant difference between the two graft sources as far as quadriceps and hamstring strength was concerned.

The relationship of graft source to quadriceps weakness is still open to debate. The work by Shelbourne et al suggests that some of the quadriceps weakness previously reported following ACL reconstruction with a patellar tendon graft may be related more to the postoperative rehabilitation program than to graft source.[150,235] Prospective randomized studies by Marder et al[71] and recently Aglietti et al[80] have failed to show a significant difference in quadriceps strength between patellar tendon and hamstring autografts. (See note added in proofs.)

In conclusion, graft site complications are perhaps the most common complication following ACL reconstruction. The incidence of graft site complications appears to be highest following use of a patellar tendon autograft. Fortunately, many of these complications can be prevented or minimized by attention to proper surgical technique, by aggressive postoperative rehabilitation, and by early and aggressive treatment when complications do occur.

Summary

The optimal replacement for a torn anterior cruciate ligament remains controversial. Although one can find proponents for the use of allografts and synthetic ligaments, at present autograft tissues remain the most commonly used substitute. Of the autograft tissues available the central-third patellar tendon graft and hamstring tendon grafts (semitendinosus and gracilis tendons) have been the most extensively studied, and are most frequently used. Although many surgeons consider the central-third patellar tendon graft to be the "gold standard" for ACL reconstruction, this current bias flies in the face of recent studies that have shown no significant difference in stability or functional outcome between central-third patellar tendon and hamstring tendon grafts.[71,80]

Animal and recent human studies indicate that following transplantation, autografts irrespective of the tissue type undergo "ligamentization," a complex biologic process that results in a substitute that grossly and histologically resembles a normal ACL. Although the ACL replacement graft appearance under light microscopy is similar to that of the normal ACL, recent ultrastructural studies using electron microscopy have shown that the ACL replacement graft is collagenized by primarily small-diameter collagen fibrils (<100 nm). The absence of the large-diameter collagen fibril population (>100 nm), which is found in the donor patellar tendon and hamstring tendons and in the normal human ACL, is thought to be one of the causes of decreased tensile strength following transplantation.[59] Although the final biomechanical properties of transplanted autograft tissues are unknown, extrapolation of animal data would suggest that at best, the final tensile strength of the graft is approximately 80% of its initial strength.[52]

Reconstruction of the ACL has evolved from an open procedure involving large capsular incisions, patellar dislocation, and cast immobilization to an arthroscopy-assisted technique with early motion and minimal postoperative immobilization. At present, arthroscopy-assisted ACL reconstruction can be performed using a two-incision technique or the newer single-incision "endoscopic" technique. Although it is our early clinical impression that the endoscopic technique appears to result in less postoperative pain and may allow earlier hospital discharge, it also has a steep learning curve, and the complication rate has been reported to be higher.[173] In our experience the end results of the two-incision and the single-incision techniques are the same. This finding has also been reported by others.[174,175] For the occasional or beginning ACL surgeon the two-incision technique has a lot to recommend, as placement of the femoral tunnel and graft fixation are technically easier. Although the single-incision technique is cosmetically superior and results in less pain in the early postoperative period, it is technically challenging and is probably best reserved for the experienced ACL surgeon.

Based on our fixation studies[73] we feel that the two-incision technique is the preferred method for hamstring tendon grafts, as rigid graft fixation on both ends of the graft can be achieved. Although it is possible to rigidly fix the femoral end of hamstring tendon grafts endoscopically using an endobutton, present methods of fixing the free ends of the tendon graft on the tibia may provide inadequate strength and stiffness if the surgeon wishes to use an accelerated rehabilitation program. This situation is sure to change as stronger, stiffer, and lower-profile methods of soft tissue-to-bone fixation evolve.

Improvements in surgical technique and postoperative rehabilitation have dramatically improved the results of ACL surgery. Recent reports by Aglietti et al,[80,98] Buss et al,[99] Shelbourne et al,[153,235] Marder et al[71], and Bach et al.[234] suggest that using current arthroscopy-assisted surgical techniques, surgeons can achieve approximately a 90% success rate as determined by subjective and objective evaluation for both patellar tendon and hamstring tendon grafts. Postoperative patellofemoral pain, muscle weakness, loss of knee motion, and residual postoperative laxity still remain problems, however. Recent "accelerated" rehabilitation programs following ACL reconstruction with a patellar tendon graft that emphasize early full extension and closed-kinetic-chain exercises have been shown to decrease the incidence of many of these complications without compromising stability.

At present there are no clinical studies documenting the safety of an "accelerated" rehabilitation program following ACL reconstruction with hamstring tendon grafts. For approximately the past 18 months we have been using an "accelerated" rehabilitation program following ACL reconstruction with the double-stranded hamstring technique described in this chapter. Using our described method of hamstring graft fixation we have experienced no cases of graft loosening or loss of stability in the early postoperative period prior to biologic incorporation of the graft. With approximately a 12-month follow-up, it is our clinical impression that the postoperative stability following ACL reconstruction with double-stranded semitendinosus and gracilis grafts is the same as that for patellar tendon grafts. We hope to report a 2-year follow-up of this technique in the future.

Although at present there may be no true "gold standard" for ACL reconstruction, because of their availability, favorable biomechanical properties, early revascularization, and extensive clinical experience, patellar tendon and hamstring tendon autografts will remain commonly used ACL substitutes.

Notes Added in Proofs

Initial Graft Strength

We have recently investigated the effects on the mechanical properties of doubling gracilis and semitendinosus tendons in a paired human cadaver model (unpublished data). The specimens were tested in such a manner so as to create equal tension in both limbs of the doubled tendons. The average age of the specimens (n = 12) was 81 years. The mean failure load of a single strand gracilis tendon was 837 ± 138 N, and 1550 ± 428 N for a doubled stranded gracilis tendon. The mean stiffness of a single stranded gracilis tendon was 160 N/mm, and 340 N/mm for a double stranded tendon. Doubling the gracilis tendon increased the mean ultimate failure load by 85%, and the mean stiffness by 113%. For a single stranded semitendinosus tendon the mean ultimate failure load was 1060 ± 227 N, and 2328 ± 452 N for a double stranded tendon. The stiffness of a single stranded semitendinosus tendon was 213 ± 44 N/mm,

and 469 ± 185 N/mm for a double stranded tendon. Doubling the semitendinosus increased the ultimate failure load and stiffness values by 120%. We feel that this preliminary data does support the hypothesis that doubling a soft tissue graft doubles the failure load and stiffness. As far as we are aware this is the first biomechanical data that proves this point.

Based on our preliminary data, and assuming that the failure load of the composite graft is the sum of the failure load of each doubled graft, a double stranded gracilis, semitendinosus graft (in old specimens) would be expected to have a mean ultimate failure load of 3879 N (this number is higher than that of a 10 mm patellar tendon graft in young specimens as reported by Copper et al[70]).

At the present time we are in the process of performing similar biomechanical studies using tendons from younger specimens. Based on our preliminary biomechanical studies, we feel that the initial mechanical properties of double stranded gracilis, semitendinosus grafts are more than adequate to serve as a replacement for the human ACL. We hope that our further biomechanical studies will finally put to rest the question of whether hamstring tendon grafts are strong enough to serve as biological replacements for the human ACL.

Complications

Harvest of the hamstring tendons appears to cause few donor site complications. Lipscomb et al reviewed 51 who were an average of 26.2 months postoperative following harvest of the hamstring tendons for ACL reconstruction.[239] In the group in which the semitendinosus and gracilis tendons were used, they reported an average hamstring strength of 98% at 60°/sec, and 100% at 240°/sec. When the semitendinosus alone was used the average hamstring strength was 104% at 60°/sec, and 101% at 240°/sec. Quadriceps strength averaged 95% at 60°/sec, and 98% at 240°/sec in both groups. The authors concluded that there was no significant loss of hamstring strength following harvest of the semitendinosus and gracilis tendons for ACL reconstruction. Similar findings have been reported by Aglietti et al, and Karlson et al.[80,204]

Acknowledgments. This project was supported by a grant from the Harvard Community Health Plan Foundation. The authors also thank Mrs. Linda Stafford and Mrs. Vikki Ingrassia for their technical assistance in the preparation of this manuscript.

References

1. Miyasaka KC, Daniel DM, Stone ML, Hirshman P. The incidence of knee ligament injuries in the general population. *Am J Knee Surg.* 1991;4:3–8.

2. Feagin JA. The syndrome of the torn anterior cruciate ligament. *Orthop Clin North Am.* 1979;10:81–90.
3. Fetto JF, Marshall JL. The natural history and diagnosis of anterior cruciate ligament insufficiency. *Clin Orthop.* 1980;147:29–38.
4. Noyes FR, Bassett RW, Grood ES, Butler DL. Arthroscopy in acute traumatic hemarthrosis of the knee. Incidence of anterior cruciate tears and other injuries. *J Bone Joint Surg Am.* 1980;62:687–695.
5. Noyes FR, Mooar PA, Matthews DS, Butler DL. The symptomatic anterior cruciate deficient knee. Part I: The long term function disability in athletically active individuals. *J Bone Joint Surg Am.* 1983;65:154–162.
6. Noyes FR, McGinniss GH, Mooars LA. Functional disability in the anterior cruciate insufficient knee syndrome. Review of knee rating systems and projected risk factors in determining treatment. *Sports Med.* 1984;1:278–302.
7. Paulos LE, Noyes FR, Malek M. A practical guide to the initial evaluation and treatment of knee ligament injuries. *J Trauma.* 1980;20:498–506.
8. Ray JM. A proposed natural history of the symptomatic anterior cruciate ligament. Injuries of the knee. *Clin Sports Med.* 1988;7:697–713.
9. Butler DL, Noyes FR, Grood ES. Ligamentous restraints to anterior–posterior drawer in the human knee. A biomechanical study. *J Bone Joint Surg Am.* 1980;62:259–270.
10. Daniel DM, Malcom LL, Losse G, Stone ML, Sachs R, Burks R. Instrumented measurement of anterior laxity of the knee. *J. Bone Joint Surg Am.* 1985;67:720–726.
11. Daniel DM, Stone ML, Sachs R, Malcom L. Instrumented measurement of anterior knee laxity in patients with acute anterior cruciate ligament disruption. *Am J Sports Med.* 1985;13:401–407.
12. Daniel DM, Stone ML. Instrumented measurement of knee motion. In: Daniel DM, Akeson WH, O'Connor JJ, eds. *Knee Ligaments: Structure, Function, Injury, and Repair.* New York: Raven Press; 1990:421–426.
13. Grood ES, Noyes FR. Diagnosis of knee ligament injuries: Biomechanical precepts. In: Feagin JA, ed. *The Crucial Ligaments.* New York: Churchill Livingstone; 1988:245–260.
14. Noyes FR, Grood ES. Diagnosis of knee ligament injuries: Clinical concepts. In: Feagin JA, ed. *The Crucial Ligaments.* New York: Churchill Livingstone; 1988:261–285.
15. Daniel DM, Stone ML. KT-1000 anterior–posterior displacement measurements. In: Daniel DM, Akeson WH, O'Connor JJ, eds. *Knee Ligaments: Structure, Function, Injury, and Repair.* New York: Raven Press; 1990:427–447.
16. Strobel M, Stedtfeld HW. Evaluation of the ligaments. In: *Diagnostic Evaluations of the Knee.* New York: Springer-Verlag; 1990:118.
17. Torg JS, Conrad W, Kalen V. Clinical diagnosis of anterior cruciate ligament instability in the athlete. *Am J Sports Med.* 1976;4:84–93.
18. Donaldson WF, Warren RF, Wickiewicz T. A comparison of acute anterior cruciate ligament examinations. Initial versus examination under anesthesia. *Am J Sports Med.* 1985;13:5–10.
19. Katz JW, Fingeroth RJ. The diagnostic accuracy of ruptures of the anterior cruciate ligament comparing the Lachman test, the anterior drawer sign, and the pivot shift test in acute and chronic knee injuries. *Am J Sports Med.* 1986;14:88–91.
20. Lee JK, Yao L, Phelps CT, Wirth CR, Czajka Jr, Loz-

man J. Anterior cruciate ligament tears: MRI imaging compared with arthroscopy and clinical tests. *Radiology.* 1988;166:861–864.
21. Müller W. *The Knee: Form, Function, and Ligament Reconstruction.* New York: Springer-Verlag; 1983.
22. Noyes FR, Matthews DS, Mooar PA, Grood ES. The symptomatic anterior cruciate deficient knee. Part II: The results of rehabilitation, activity, modification, and counseling on functional disability. *J Bone Joint Surg Am.* 1983;65:163–174.
23. Noyes FR, McGinniss GH. Controversy about treatment of the knee with anterior cruciate laxity. *Clin Orthop.* 1985;198:61–76.
24. Grood ES, Noyes FR, Butler DL, Suntay WJ. Ligamentous and capsular restraints preventing straight medial and lateral laxity in intact human cadaver knees. *J Bone Joint Surg Am.* 1981;63:1257–1269.
25. Gersoff WK, Clancy WG. Diagnosis of acute and chronic anterior cruciate ligament tears. *Clin Sports Med.* 1988;7:727–738.
26. O'Brien SJ, Warren RF, Wickiewicz TL, et al. Reconstruction of the chronically insufficient anterior cruciate ligament using the central-third of the patellar ligament. *J Bone Joint Surg Am.* 1991;73:278–285.
27. Gollehan DL, Torzilli PA, Warren RF. The role of the posterolateral and cruciate ligaments in the stability of the human knee. *J Bone Joint Surg Am.* 1987;69:233–242.
28. Grood ES, Stowers SF, Noyes FR. Limits of movement in the human knee. *J Bone Joint Surg Am.* 1988;70:88–97.
29. Jakob RP, Hassler H, Staeubli HU. Part II. The reverse pivot shift sign. A new diagnostic aid for posterolateral rotatory instability of the knee (the pathomechanism and distinction from the true pivot shift sign). *Acta Orthop Scand Suppl.* 1981;191:18–32.
30. Malcom LL, Daniel DM, Stone ML, Sachs R. The measurement of anterior knee laxity after ACL reconstructive surgery. *Clin Orthop.* 1985;186:35–41.
31. Dietz GW, Wilcox DM, Montgomery JB. Segond tibial condyle fracture: Lateral capsular ligament avulsion. *Radiology.* 1986;159:467–469.
32. Scuderi GR. The Segond fracture. *Am J Knee Surg.* 1991;4:32–34.
33. Woods GW, Stanley RF, Tellos HS. Lateral capsular sign, x-ray clue to a significant knee instability. *Am J Sports Med.* 1979;7:27–33.
34. Fischer SP, Fox JM, Del Pizzo W, Friedman MJ, Snyder SL, Ferkel RD. Accuracy of diagnosis from magnetic resonance imaging of the knee. *J Bone and Joint Surg Am.* 1991;73:2–10.
35. Barrack RL, Bruckner JD, Inman WS, Alexander AH. The outcomes of nonoperatively treated complete tears of the anterior cruciate ligament in active young adults. *Clin Orthop.* 1990;259:192–198.
36. Daniel DM, Stone ML, Riehl BE, Fithian DC, Rossman DC. Fate of the ACL-injured patient. A prospective outcome study. Presented at the Combined Meeting of the Orthopaedic Association of the English Speaking World; Toronto, Canada; 1992.
37. Hawkins RJ, Misamore GW, Merritt TR. Follow-up of the acute nonoperated isolated anterior cruciate ligament tear. *Am J Sports Med.* 1986;14:205–210.
38. Feagin JA, Blake WP. Postoperative evaluation and result recording in the anterior cruciate ligament reconstructed knee. *Clin Orthop.* 1983;172A:142–147.
39. Minkoff J, Sherman OH. Considerations pursuant to the rehabilitation of the anterior cruciate injures knee. In:

Pandolf KB, ed. *Exercise and Sports Medicine Reviews.* New York: MacMillan; 1987:297–349.

40. Nichols CE, Johnson RJ. Cruciate ligament injuries: Nonoperative treatment. In: Scott N, ed. *Ligament and Extensor Mechanism Injuries of the Knee: Diagnosis and Treatment.* St. Louis: Mosby Year Book; 1991:227–238.
41. Johnson RJ, Beynnon BD, Nichols CE, Restrom PAFH. Current concepts reviewed: The treatment of injuries of the anterior cruciate ligament. *J Bone Joint Surg Am.* 1992;74:140–151.
42. Shelbourne KD, Nitz PA. Anterior cruciate ligament injuries. In: *Sports Medicine. The School Age Athlete.* Philadelphia: WB Saunders; 1991:284–316.
43. Andrews JR, Carson WG. The role of extra-articular anterior cruciate ligament stabilization. In: Jackson DW, Drez D, eds. *The Anterior Cruciate Deficient Knee.* St. Louis: CV Mosby; 1987:168–192.
44. Carson WG. The role of anterolateral extra-articular procedures for anterolateral rotatory instability. *Clin Sports Med.* 1988;7:751–772.
45. Muller W. Kinematics of the cruciate ligaments. In Feagin JA, Jr, ed. *The Crucial Ligaments,* New York, Churchill Livingstone; 1988:217–233.
46. Dye SF, Cannon WD. Anatomy and biomechanics of the anterior cruciate ligament. *Clin Sports Med.* 1988; 17:715–725.
47. Alm A, Stromberg B. Transposed medial third of patellar ligament in reconstruction of the anterior cruciate ligament: A surgical and morphologic study in dogs. *Acta Chir Scand Suppl.* 1974;445:37–49.
48. Amiel D, Kleiner JB, Akeson WH. The natural history of the anterior cruciate ligament autograft of patellar tendon origin. *Am J Sports Med.* 1986;14:449–462.
49. Amiel D, Kuipel S. Experimental studies on anterior cruciate ligament grafts: Histology and biochemistry. In: Daniel DM, Akeson WH, O'Connor JJ, eds. *Knee Ligaments: Structure, Function, Injury, and Repair.* New York: Raven Press; 1990:379–388.
50. Arnoczky SP, Tarvin GB, Marshall JL. Anterior cruciate ligament replacement using patellar tendon: An evaluation of graft revascularization in the dog. *J Bone Joint Surg.* 1982;64:217–224.
51. Arnoczky SP. The vascularity of the anterior cruciate ligament and associated structures. In: Jackson DW, Drez D, eds. *The Anterior Cruciate Deficient Knee.* St. Louis: CV Mosby; 1987:27–54.
52. Clancy WG, Narechania RG, Rosenberg TD, et al. Anterior and posterior cruciate ligament reconstruction in Rhesus monkeys. *J Bone Joint Surg Am.* 1981; 63:1270–1289.
53. Schaefer RS, Gillogly SD, Rak KM. Evaluation of patellar tendon autograft revascularization in anterior cruciate ligament reconstruction using gadolinium–DPTA enhanced magnetic resonance imaging. In: *58th Annual ASSO Meeting Final Program, Anaheim.* 1991.
54. Rougraff B, Shelbourne KD, Gerth PK, Warner J. Arthroscopic and histologic analysis of human patellar tendon autografts used for anterior cruciate ligament reconstruction. *Am J Sports Med.* 1993;21:277–284.
55. Alm A, and Gillquist J. Reconstruction of the anterior cruciate ligament by using the medial third of the patellar ligament. Treatment and results. *Acta Chir Scand.* 1974;140:289–296.
56. Shino K, Inove M, Horibe S, Nagano J, Ono K. Maturation of allograft tendons transplanted into the knee: An arthroscopic and histological study. *J Bone Joint Surg Br.* 1998;70:556–560.
57. Kurosaka M, Abe S, Iguchi T, Fujita N, Yoshiya S,

Hironata K. Light and electron microscopic study of remodeling and maturation of the autogenous graft for anterior cruciate ligament reconstruction. In: *Fourth Congress of ESKA Abstract Book, Stockholm.* 1990:42–43.
58. Abe S, Hirohata K, Iguchi T, Kurosaka M, Yoshiya S. Light and electron microscopic study of remodeling and maturation in autogenous graft for anterior cruciate ligament reconstruction: Second look arthroscopic and histologic study. *Arthroscopy.* 1993;9:394–405.
59. Oakes BW, Frank C, Woo S, et al. Normal ligament: Structure, function, and composition. In: Woo SL-Y, Buckwalter JA, eds. *Injury and Repair of the Musculoskeletal Soft Tissues.* Park Ridge, IL: AAOS, 1988: 45–101.
60. Butler DL. Anterior cruciate ligament: Its normal response and placement. *J Orthop Res.* 1989;7:910–921.
61. Newton PO, Horibe S, Woo SLY. Experimental studies on anterior cruciate ligament autografts and allografts. Mechanical studies. In: Daniel DM, Akeson WH, O'Connor JJ, eds. *Knee Ligaments: Structure, Function, Injury, and Repair.* New York: Raven Press; 1990:389–399.
62a. Noyes FR, Butler DL, Paulos LE, Grood ES. Intraarticular cruciate reconstruction. I. Perspectives on graft strength, vascularization and immediate motion and replacement. *Clin Orthop.* 1983;172:71–77.
62b. Jackson DW, Grood ES, Goldstein JD, et al. A comparison of patellar tendon autograft and allograft used for anterior cruciate ligament reconstruction in the goat model. *Am J Sports Med.* 1993;21:176–185.
63. Clancy WG Anterior cruciate ligament functional instability. A static intra-articular and dynamic extra-articular procedure. *Clin Orthop.* 1983;172:102–106.
64. Lambert KL. Vascularized patellar tendon graft with rigid internal fixation for anterior cruciate ligament insufficiency. *Clin Orthop.* 1983;172:85–89.
65. McLean, I, Deacon O, Oakes B. The final morphology of anterior cruciate ligament grafts. In: *5th Congress of ESKA Abstract Book, Mallorca.* 1992:132–133.
66. Jackson DW, Grood ES, Cohn BT, Arnoczky SP, Simon TM, Cumming JF. The effect of in situ freezing on the anterior cruciate ligament. *J Bone Joint Surg Am.* 1991;73:201–213.
67. Noyes FR, Butler DL, Grood ES, et al. Biomechanical analysis of human ligament grafts used in knee ligament repairs and reconstructions. *J Bone Joint Surg Am.* 1984;66:344–352.
68. Woo SLY, Hollis JM, Adams DJ, et al. Tensile properties of the human femur anterior cruciate ligament-tibia complex. The effects of specimen age and orientation. *Am J Sports Med.* 1991;19:217–225.
69. Andrews JR, Indelicato PA, Noyes FR, Price SP. Surgical controversies: Autografts or allografts for ACL reconstruction. Strategies for rehabilitative orthopaedics. *Biodex Prof Serv.* 1989;1:2–5.
70. Cooper DE, Deng X, Burstein A, et al. The strength of the central third patellar tendon graft: A biomechanical study. *Am J Sports Med.* 1993; 21:818–824.
71. Marder RA, Raskind JR, Carroll M. Prospective evaluation of arthroscopically assisted anterior cruciate ligament reconstruction. *Am J Sports Med.* 1991;19: 478–484.
72. Larson RV. Arthroscopic anterior cruciate ligament reconstruction utilizing double loop semitendinosus and gracilis tendons. In: *11th Annual ANAA Meeting, Book of Abstracts, Instructional Courses and Symposia, Boston.* 1992:124–128.

73. Steiner ME, Hecker A, Brown CH, Hayes WC. ACL graft fixation: Comparison of hamstring tendons versus patellar tendon. In: *18th Annual AOSSM Meeting, Abstracts and Outlines, San Diego*; 1992: *Am J Sports Med.*, in press.

74. Howell SM, Berns GS, Farley TE. Unimpinged and impinged anterior cruciate ligament grafts: MR signal intensity measurements. *Radiology.* 1991;179:639–643.

75. Howell SM, Clark JA, Farley TE. A rationale for predicting anterior cruciate graft impingement by the intercondylar roof: An MRI study. *Am J Sports Med.* 1991;19:276–281.

76. Howell SM, Clark JA, Farley TE. Serial magnetic resonance study assessing the effects of impingement on the MR image of the patellar tendon graft. *Arthroscopy.* 1992;8:350–358.

77. Howell SM. Case report. Arthroscopic roofplasty: A method for correcting an extension deficit caused by roof impingement of an anterior cruciate ligament graft. *Arthroscopy.* 1992;8:375–379.

78. Howell SM, Clark JA. Tibial tunnel placement in anterior cruciate ligament reconstructions and graft impingement. *Clin Orthop.* 1992;283:187–195.

79. Howell SM. Arthroscopically assisted technique for preventing roof impingement of an anterior cruciate ligament graft illustrated by the use of an autogenous double-looped semitendinosus and gracilis graft. *Operative Technique Sports Med.* 1993;1:58–65.

80. Aglietti P, Buzzi R, Zaccherotti G. Patellar tendon versus semitendinosus and gracilis in ACL reconstruction. In: *18th Annual AOSSM Meeting, Abstracts and Outlines, San Diego*: 1992: 29–30.

81. Aglietti P, Buzzi R, D'Andria S, Zaccherott G. Patellofemoral problems after intra-articular anterior cruciate ligament reconstruction. *Clin Orthop.* 1993;288:195–203.

82. Re LP, Weiss RA, Rintz KG, et al. Incidence of anterior knee pain after treatment for anterior cruciate ligament rupture. In: *AOSSM Specialty Day Meeting Book of Abstracts and Outlines, San Francisco.* 1993:21.

83. Sachs RA, Daniel DM, Stone ML, Garfein RF. Patellofemoral problems after anterior cruciate ligament reconstruction. *Am J Sports Med.* 1989;17:760–765.

84. Sachs RA, Reznik A, Daniel DM, et al. Complications of knee ligament surgery. In: Daniel DM, Akeson W, O'Connor J, eds. *Knee Ligaments Structure, Function, Injury, and Repair.* New York: Raven Press; 1990:511–520.

85. Bonamo J, Krinick RM, Sporn AA. Rupture of the patellar ligament after use of its central third for anterior cruciate reconstruction. *J Bone Joint Surg Am.* 1984; 66:1294–1297.

86. Bonatus TJ, Alexander AH. Patellar fracture and avulsion of the patellar ligament complicating arthroscopic anterior cruciate ligament reconstruction. *Orthopedics.* 1991;20:770–774.

87. Brown HR, Indelicato PA. Complications of anterior cruciate ligament reconstruction. *Operative Technique Orthop.* 1992;2:125–135.

88. Christen B, Jakob RP. Fractures associated with patellar ligament grafts in cruciate ligament surgery. *J Bone Joint Surg Br.* 1992;74:617–619.

89. DeLee JC, Craviotto DF. Rupture of the quadriceps tendon after a central third patellar tendon anterior cruciate ligament reconstruction. *Am J Sports Med.* 1991;19:415–416.

90. Graf B, Uhr F. Complications of intra-articular cruciate reconstruction. *Clin Sports Med.* 1988;7:835–848.

91. Hardin GT, Bach BR. Distal rupture of the infrapatellar tendon after use of its central third for anterior cruciate ligament reconstruction: Case report. *Am J Knee Surg.* 1992;5:140–143.

92. Huegal M, Indelicato PA. Trends in rehabilitation following anterior cruciate ligament reconstruction. *Clin Sports Med.* 1988;7:801–811.

93. Lambert KL, Cunningham RR. Anatomic substitution of the ruptured ACL using a vascularized patellar tendon graft with interference fixation. In: Feagin JA, ed. *The Crucial Ligaments.* New York: Churchill Livingstone; 1988:401–408.

94. Langan P, Fontanetta AD. Rupture of the patellar tendon after use of its central third. *Orthop Rev.* 1987; 16:61–65.

95. MacKinlay D, Fowler PJ, Roth JN. Long term review of intra-articular ACL reconstruction augmented with braided polypropylene (Kennedy LAD). In: *Abstracts Book of the 6th Congress of the International Society of the Knee, Rome,* 1989.

96. McCarroll JR. Fracture of the patella during a golf swing following reconstruction of the anterior cruciate ligament—A case report. *Am J Sports Med.* 1983;11:26–27.

97. Rubinstein RA, Shelbourne KD. Preventing complications and minimizing morbidity after autogenous bone–patellar tendon–bone anterior cruciate ligament reconstruction. *Operative Technique Sports Med.* 1993; 1:72–78.

98. Aglietti P, Buzzi R, D'Andria S, Zaccherotti G. Arthroscopic anterior cruciate ligament reconstruction with patellar tendon. *Arthroscopy.* 1992;8:510–516.

99. Buss DD, Warren RF, Wickiewicz, TL, ed al. Arthroscopically assisted reconstruction of the anterior cruciate ligament with use of autogenous patellar-ligament grafts. *J Bone Joint Surg Am.* 1993;75:1346–1355.

100. Schoen JL. Open versus arthroscopically-assisted ACL reconstruction using the central part of the patellar tendon. In: *4th Congress of ESKA Abstract Book, Stockholm.* 1990:141.

101. Sgaglione NA, Del Pizzo W, Fox JM, et al. Arthroscopic-assisted anterior cruciate ligament reconstruction with the pes anserine tendons: Comparison of results in acute and chronic ligament deficiency. *Am J Sports Med.* 1993;21:249–256.

102. Jackson DW, Kurzweil PR. Allografts in knee ligament surgery. In: Scott WN, ed. *Ligament and Extensor Mechanism Injuries of the Knee. Diagnosis and Treatment.* St. Louis: Mosby Year Book; 1991:349–360.

103. Jackson DW, Rosen M, Simon TM. Soft tissue allograft reconstruction: The knee. In: Czitrom AA, Gross AE, eds. *Allografts in Orthopaedic Practice.* Baltimore: Williams and Wilkins: 1992:197–216.

104. Noyes FR, Barber SD, Mangine RE. Bone–patellar ligament–bone and fascia lata allografts for reconstruction of the anterior cruciate ligament. *J Bone Joint Surg Am.* 1990;72:1125–1136.

105. Noyes FR, Barber SD. The effect of an extra-articular procedure on allograft reconstructions for chronic ruptures of the anterior cruciate ligament. *J Bone Joint Surg Am.* 1991;73:882–892.

106. Noyes FR, Barber SD. The effect of a ligament-augmentation device on allograft reconstruction for chronic rupture of the anterior cruciate ligament. *J Bone Joint Surg Am.* 1992;74:960–973.

107. Strum GM, Friedman MJ, Fox JM, et al. Acute anterior cruciate ligament reconstructions. Analysis of complications. *Clin Orthop.* 1990;253:184–189.

108. Lephart SM, Kocher MS, Harner CD, Fu F. Quadriceps strength and functional capacity after anterior cruciate ligament reconstruction. Patellar tendon autograft versus allograft. *Am J Sports Med.* 1993;21:738–743.
109. Noyes FR, Wojtys EM, Marshall MT. The early diagnosis and treatment of developmental patella infera syndrome. *Clin Orthop.* 1991;265:241–252.
110. Fuss FK. Anatomy of the cruciate ligaments and their function in extension and flexion of the human knee. *Am J Anat.* 1989;184:165–176.
111. Fuss FR. Optimal replacement of the cruciate ligaments from the functional–anatomical point of view. *Acta Anat.* 1991;140:260–268.
112. Girgis FG, Marshall JL, Al Monajem ARS. The cruciate ligaments of the knee joint: Anatomical function and experimental analysis. *Clin Orthop.* 1975;106:216–231.
113. Graf B. Isometric placement of substitutes for the anterior cruciate ligament. In: Jackson DW, Drez D, eds. *The Anterior Cruciate Deficient Knee.* St. Louis: CV Mosby; 1987:102–113.
114. O'Brien WJ. Isometric placement of anterior cruciate ligament substitutes. *Operative Technique Orthop.* 1992;2:49–54.
115. Odensten M, Gillquist J. Functional anatomy of the anterior cruciate ligament and a rationale for reconstruction. *J Bone Joint Surg Am.* 1985;67:257–261.
116. Acker JH, Drez D. Analysis of isometric placement of grafts in ACL reconstruction procedures. *Am J Knee Surg.* 1989;2:65–70.
117. Arms SW, Pope MH, Johnson RJ, et al. The biomechanics of anterior cruciate ligament rehabilitation and reconstruction. *Am J Sports Med.* 1984;12:8–18.
118. Howe JG, Wertheimer C, Johnson RJ, et al. Arthroscopic strain gauge measurement of the normal anterior cruciate ligament. *Arthroscopy.* 1990;6:198–204.
119. Sapega AA, Moyer RA, Schneck C, Komalaniranya N. Testing for isometry during reconstruction of the anterior cruciate ligament. *J Bone Joint Surg Am.* 1990; 72:259–267.
120. Brand MG, Daniel DM. Considerations in the placement of an intra-articular anterior cruciate ligament graft. *Operative Techique Orthop.* 1992;2:55–62.
121. Grood ES, Hefzy MS, Noyes FR. Factors affecting the region of the most isometric femoral attachment. Part II: The anterior cruciate ligament. *Am J Sports Med.* 1989;17:208–215.
122. Siddles JA, Larson RV, Garbini JL, Downey DL, Matsen FA. Ligament length relationship in the moving knee. *J Orthop. Res.* 1988;6:593–610.
123. Clancy WG, Nelson DA, Reider B, Narechania RG. Anterior cruciate ligament reconstruction using one-third of the patellar ligament augmented by extra-articular tendon transfers. *J Bone Joint Surg Am.* 1982;64:352–359.
124. Sapega AA. Arthroscopically assisted reconstruction of the anterior cruciate ligament. In: Torg JS, Welsh PR, Shepard RJ, eds. *Current Therapy in Sports Medicine—2.* Philadelphia: BC Decker; 1990:292–297.
125. Penner DA, Daniel DM, Wood P, Mishra D. An in vitro study of anterior cruciate ligament graft placement and isometry. *Am J Sports Med.* 1988;16:238–243.
126. Bylski-Austrow DI, ES Grood, JP Holden, MS Hefzy, DL Butler. Anterior cruciate ligament replacements: A mechanical study of femoral attachment location, flexion angle at tensioning, and initial tension. *J Orthop. Res.* 1990;8:522–531.
127. Melhorn JE, Henning CE. The relationship of the femoral attachment site to the isometric tracking of the anterior cruciate ligament graft. *Am J Sports Med.* 1987;15:539–542.
128. Yoshiya S, Andrish JT, Manley MT, Bauer TW. Graft tension in anterior cruciate ligament reconstruction: An in vitro study in dogs. *Am J Sports Med.* 1987;15:464–470.
129. Burks RT, Leland R. Determination of graft tension before fixation in anterior cruciate ligament reconstruction. *Arthroscopy.* 1988;4:260–266.
130. Schabus R, Fuchs M, Kwasny O. The effect of ACL graft preload on the static pressure distribution in the knee joint. In: *Transactions of the 35th Annual ORS Meeting, Las Vegas.* 1989;14:517.
131. Friedrich NF, O'Brien WR, Muller W, Henning CE. The effects of stress relaxation on initial graft loads during ACL reconstruction. In *AOSSM Specialty Day Book of Abstracts and Outlines, Anaheim.* 1991:11.
132. Holden JP, Grood ES, Butler DL, et al. Biomechanics of fascia lata ligament replacement: Early postoperative changes in the goat. *J Orthop. Res.* 1988;6:639–647.
133. Kurosaka M, Yoshiya S, Andrish JT. A biomechanical comparison of different surgical techniques of graft fixation in anterior cruciate ligament reconstruction. *Am J Sports Med.* 1987;15:225–229.
134. Robertson DB, Daniel DM, Biden E. Soft tissue fixation to bone. *Am J Sports Med.* 1986;14:398–403.
135. Fithian DC, Daniel DM, Casanave A. Fixation in knee ligament repair and reconstruction. *Operative Technique Orthop.* 1992;2:63–70.
136. Matthews LS, Lawrence SJ, Yahiro MA, Sinclair MR. Fixation strengths of patellar tendon–bone grafts. *Arthroscopy.* 1993;9:76–81.
137. Pyne J, Gottlieb DJ, Beynnon BD, et al. Semitendinosus and gracilis tendon graft fixation in ACL reconstructions. In: *Transations of the 38th Annual ORS Meeting, Washington, DC.* 1992;17:245.
138. Paulos LE, Payne FC, Rosenberg TD. Rehabilitation after anterior cruciate ligament surgery. In: Jackson DW, Drez D, eds. *The Anterior Cruciate Deficient Knee.* St. Louis: CV Mosby; 1987:291–314.
139. Van Rens TJG, van den Berg AF, Huiskes R, et al. Substitution of the anterior cruciate ligament: A long-term histologic and biomechanical study with autogenous pedicled grafts of the iliotibial band in dogs. *Arthroscopy.* 1986;2:139–154.
140. Schiavone Panni A, Fabbriciani C, Delcogliano A, Franzese S. Bone–ligament interaction in patellar tendon reconstruction of the ACL. *Knee Surg Sports Traumatol Arthrosc.* 1993;1:4–8.
141. Rodeo SA, Arnoczky SP, Torzilli PA, et al. Tendon healing in a bone tunnel: A biomechanical and histological study in the dog. In: *Transactions of the 39th Annual ORS Meeting, San Francisco*; 1993;18:29. *J Bone Joint Surg.*, in press.
142. Harner CD, Irrgang JJ, Paul JJ, et al. Loss of motion after anterior cruciate ligament reconstruction. *Am J Sports Med.* 1992;20:499–506.
143. Mohtadi NGH, Webster-Bogaert S, Fowler PJ. Limitation of motion following anterior cruciate ligament reconstruction: A case-control study. *Am J Sports Med.* 1991;19:620–625.
144. Shelbourne KD, Wilchens J, Mollabashy A, DeCarlo M. Arthrofibrosis in the acute ACL reconstruction. The effect of timing of reconstruction and rehabilitation protocol. *Am J Sports Med.* 1991;19:332–336.
145. Shelbourne KD, Basle JR. Treatment of combined

anterior cruciate and medial collateral ligament injuries. *Am J Knee Surg.* 1988;1:56–58.

146. Aglietti P, Buzzi R, Zaccherotti G, Andria S. Operative treatment of acute complete lesions of the anterior cruciate and medial collateral ligaments: A 4 to 7 year follow-up study. *Am J Knee Surg.* 1991;4:186–193.

147. Flynn W, Warren RF, Marchand R, et al. Results of early reconstruction of combined injuries to the anterior cruciate ligament and the posterolateral corner of the knee. In: *18th Annual AOSSM Meeting, Abstracts and Outlines, San Diego.* 1992:66.

148. Rubinstein RA, Shelbourne DK. Management of combined instabilities: Anterior cruciate ligament/medial collateral and anterior cruciate ligament/lateral side. *Operative Technique Sports Med.* 1993;1:66–71.

149. Shelbourne KD, Porter DA. Anterior cruciate ligament–medial collateral ligament injury: Nonoperative management of medial collateral ligament tears with anterior cruciate ligament reconstruction. A preliminary report. *Am J Sports Med.* 1992;20:283–286.

150. Shelbourne KD, Nitz P. Accelerated rehabilitation after anterior cruciate ligament reconstruction. *Am J Sports Med.* 1990;18:292–299.

151. Shelbourne KD, Wilchens J. Current concepts in anterior cruciate ligament rehabilitation. *Orthop Rev.* 1990; 19:957–964.

152. Klootwyk TE, Shelbourne KD, DeCarlo MS. Perioperative rehabilitation considerations. *Operative Technique Sports Med.* 1993;1:22–25.

153. Bach BR Arthroscopy-assisted patellar tendon substitution for anterior cruciate ligament insufficiency: Surgical technique. *Am J Knee Surg.* 1989;2:3–20.

154. Jackson DW, Reimen PR. Principles of arthroscopic anterior cruciate reconstruction. In: Jackson DW, Drez D, eds. *Anterior Cruciate Deficient Knee.* St. Louis: CV Mosby; 1987:273–285.

155. Jackson DW, Jennings LD. Arthroscopically assisted reconstruction of the anterior cruciate ligament using a patellar tendon bone autograft. *Clin Sports Med.* 1988;7:785–800.

156. Mott HW. Semitendinosus anatomic reconstruction for cruciate ligament insufficiency. *Clin Orthop.* 1983;172: 90–92.

157. Gomes JL, Marczyk LR. Anterior cruciate ligament reconstruction with a loop or double thickness of semitendinosus tendon. *Am J Sports Med.* 1984;12:199–203.

158. Moyer RA, Betz RJ, Marchetto PA, et al. Arthroscopic anterior cruciate reconstruction using the semitendinosus and gracilis tendons: Preliminary report. *Contemp Orthop.* 1986;12:17–23.

159. Friedman MJ. Arthroscopic semitendinosus (gracilis) reconstruction for anterior cruciate ligament deficiency. *Techniques Orthop.* 1988;2:74–80.

160. Mitchell N, Shepard N. The deleterious effect of drying on articular cartilage. *J Bone Joint Surg Am.* 1989; 71:89–95.

161. Speer KP, Tucker JA, Seaber AV, Callaghan JJ. The effects of air exposure on articular cartilage: A histochemical and ultrastructure evaluation. In: *Transactions of the 36th Annual ORS Meeting, New Orleans.* 1990;15:349.

162. Noyes FR, Mangine RE, Barber S. Early knee motion after open and arthroscopic anterior cruciate ligament reconstruction. *Am J Sports Med.* 1987;15:149–160.

163. Brown HR. Patellofemoral morbidity following intra-articular anterior cruciate reconstruction—A comparison of three surgical techniques and graft source. In: *18th Annual AOSSM Meeting, First Annual Fellow's Research Program, San Diego.* 1992:19.

164. Gillquist J, Odensten M. Arthroscopic reconstruction of the anterior cruciate ligament. *Arthroscopy.* 1988;4:5–9.

165. Shelbourne KD, Klootwyk TE: The miniarthrotomy technique for anterior cruciate ligament reconstruction. *Oper Tech Sports Med.* 1993;1:26–39.

166. Paulos LE, Cherf J, Rosenberg TD. Anterior cruciate ligament reconstruction with autografts. *Clin Sports Med.* 1991;10:469–485.

167. Olson EJ, DiGioia AM, Harner CD, Fu F. Total quadriceps sparing arthroscopic anterior cruciate ligament reconstruction. *Pitts Orthop J.* 1990;1:16–19.

168. Hardin GT, Bach BR, Bush-Joseph CA, Farr J. Endoscopic single-incision anterior cruciate ligament reconstruction using patellar tendon autograft: Surgical technique. *Am J Knee Surg.* 1992;5:144–155.

169. Beck CL, Paulos LE, Rosenberg TD. Anterior cruciate ligament reconstruction with the endoscopic technique. *Operative Technique Orthop.* 1992;2:86–98.

170. Fu F, Olson EJ. Anterior cruciate ligament reconstruction using fresh frozen patellar tendon allografts. In: Parisien JS, ed. *Techniques in Therapeutic Arthroscopy.* New York: Raven Press; 1993:81–89.

171. Yates CK. Endoscopic technique versus two incision technique. In: *10th Annual AANA Meeting, Book of Abstracts and Outlines, Palm Desert.* 1991:38–39.

172. Graf B, Vanderby R, Rothenberg M. The effects of preload, tunnel orientation and chamfering on fatigue failure of patellar tendon grafts at the femoral tunnel. In: *18th Annual AOSSM Meeting, Abstracts and Outlines, San Diego.* 1992:57.

173. Meade TD, Dickson TB. Technical pitfalls of single incision arthroscopy-assisted ACL ligament reconstruction. *Am J Arthrosc.* 1992;2:15–19.

174. Garfinkel MJ, Miller LS, Antich TJ: Endoscopic versus two-incision technique of anterior cruciate ligament reconstruction using patellar tendon autograft. In 19th Annual Meeting American Orthopaedic Society for Sports Medicine, Book of Abstracts and Outlines, Sun Valley, Idaho, 1993:85.

175. Sgaglione NA, Schwartz RE. Comparison of endoscopic and arthroscopically assisted anterior cruciate ligament reconstruction. In 19th Annual Meeting American Orthopaedic Society for Sports Medicine Book of Abstracts and Outlines, Sun Valley, Idaho, 1993:57.

176. Graf B, Rosenberg TD. Endoscopic technique for ACL reconstruction with Pro-Trac tibial guide: Endobutton fixation. Technique paper, Acufex Microsurgical Inc., Mansfield, MA, 1993.

177. Rosenberg TD, Paulos LE, Parker RD, et al. The well-leg support. *Arthroscopy.* 1988;4:41–44.

178. Marzo JM, Warren RF, Arnoczky SP, et al. Arthroscopic meniscal repair: Review of the outside-in technique. *Am J Knee Surg.* 1992;4:164–172.

179. Morgan CD, Casscells SW. Arthroscopic meniscus repair: A safe approach to the posterior horns. *Arthroscopy.* 1986;2:3–12.

180. Cannon WD. Arthroscopic meniscus repair. In: McGinty JB, Caspari RB, Jackson RW, Poehling GG, eds. *Operative Arthroscopy.* New York: Raven Press; 1991:237–251.

181. Scott GA, Jolly BL, Henning CE. Combined posterior incision and arthroscopic intra-articular repair of the meniscus. *J Bone Joint Surg Am.* 1986;68:847–861.

182. Warren LF, Marshall JL. The supporting structures and layers on the medial side of the knee. *J Bone Joint Surg Am.* 1979;61:56–62.
183. Bach BR, Bush-Joseph C. Technical note: The surgical approach to lateral meniscus repair. *Arthroscopy.* 1992; 8:269–273.
184. Seebacher JR, Inglis AE, Marshall JL, Warren RF. The structure of the posterolateral aspect of the knee. *J Bone Joint Surg Am.* 1982;64:536–541.
185. Daluga D, Johnson C, Bach BR. Primary bone grafting following graft procurement for anterior cruciate ligament insufficiency. *Arthroscopy.* 1990;6:205–208.
186. Roberts TS, Drez D, Banta CJ. Complications of anterior cruciate ligament reconstruction. In: Sprague NF III, ed. *Complications in Arthroscopy.* New York: Raven Press; 1989:169–177.
187. Roberts TS, Drez D, Parker W. Prevention of late patellar fracture in ACL deficient knees reconstructed with bone patellar tendon–bone autografts. *Am J Knee Surg.* 1989;2:83–86.
188. Ferrari JD, Ferrari DA. The semitendinosus: Anatomic considerations in tendon harvesting. *Orthop Rev.* 1991; 20:1085–1088.
189. Ivey M, Prud'homme J. Anatomic variations of the pes anserinus: A cadaver study. *Orthopedics.* 1993;16:601–606.
190. Pagnani MJ, Warner JJ, O'Brien SJ, Warren RF. Anatomic considerations in harvesting the semitendinosus and gracilis tendons and a technique of harvest. *Am J Sports Med.* 1993;21:565–571.
191. Warner JP, Warren RR, Cooper DE. Management of acute anterior cruciate ligament injury. In: Tullos HS, ed. *Instructional Course Lectures.* Park Ridge, IL: AAOS; 1991;40:219–232.
192. Cross MJ, Roger G, Kujawa P, et al. Regeneration of the semitendinosus and gracilis tendons following their transection for repair of the anterior cruciate ligament. *Am J Sports Med.* 1992;20:221–223.
193. Doerr AL, Cohn BT, Ruoff MJ, et al. A complication of interference screw fixation in anterior cruciate ligament reconstruction. *Orthop Rev.* 1990;19:997–1000.
194. Anderson AF, Lipscomb AB, Liudahl KJ, Addlestone RB. Analysis of the intercondylar notch by computed tomography. *Am J Sports Med.* 1987;15:547–552.
195. Kieffer DA, Curnow RJ, Southwell RB, et al. Anterior cruciate ligament arthroplasty. *Am J Sports Med.* 1984;12:301–312.
196. Tanzer M, Lenczner E. The relationship of intercondylar notch size and content to notchplasty requirement in anterior cruciate ligament surgery. *Arthroscopy.* 1990; 6:89–93.
197. Odensten M, Gillquist J. A modified technique for anterior cruciate ligament (ACL) surgery using a new drill guide for isometric positioning of the ACL. *Clin Orthop.* 1986;213:154–158.
198. Hewson GF. Drill guides for improving accuracy in anterior cruciate ligament repair and reconstruction. *Clin Orthop.* 1983;172:119–124.
199. Jackson DW, Schaefer RK. Cyclops syndrome: Loss of extension following intra-articular cruciate ligament reconstruction. *Arthroscopy.* 1990;6:171–178.
200. Marzo JM, Bowen MK, Warren RF, et al. Intraarticular fibrous nodule as a cause of loss of extension following anterior cruciate ligament reconstruction. *Arthroscopy.* 1992;8:10–18.
201. Reznik AM, David JL, Daniel DM. Optimizing interference fixation for cruciate ligament reconstruction. In: *Transactions of the 36th Annual ORS Meeting, New Orleans.* 1990;15:519.
202. Brown CH, Hecker AT, Hipp JA, et al. The biomechanics of interference screw fixation of patellar tendon anterior cruciate ligament grafts. *Am J Sports Med.* 1993;21:880–886.
203. Burger RS, Larson RL. Acute ligamentous injury. In: Larson RL, Grana WA, eds. *The Knee: Form, Function, Pathology, and Treatment.* Philadelphia: WB Saunders; 1993:546–552.
204. Karlson JA, Steiner ME, Brown CH. ACL reconstruction using gracilis and semitendinosus tendons: Comparison of through the condyle versus over the top graft placement. In: *18th Annual AOSSM Meeting, Meeting Abstracts and Outlines, San Diego.* 1992:31.
205. Paulos LE, Noyes FR, Grood ES, Butler DL. Knee rehabilitation after anterior cruciate ligament reconstruction and repair. *Am J Sports Med.* 1981;9:140–149.
205. Paulos LE, Wnorowski DC, Beck CL. Rehabilitation following knee surgery. *Sports Med.* 1991;11:257–275.
206. DeMaio M, Noyes FR. Mangine RE. Sports medicine rehabilitation series: Principles for aggressive rehabilitation after reconstruction of the anterior cruciate ligament. *Orthopedics,* 1992;15:385–392.
207. Noyes FR, Mangine RE, Barber SD. The early treatment of motion complications after reconstruction of the anterior cruciate ligament. *Clin Orthop.* 1992;227:217–228.
208. Silfverskiold JP, Steadman JR, Higgins RW, et al. Rehabilitation of the anterior cruciate ligament in the athlete. *Sports Med.* 1988;6:308–319.
209. Seto JL, Brewster CE, Lombardo SL, Tibare JE. Rehabilitation of the knee after anterior cruciate ligament reconstruction. *J Orthop Sports Phys Ther.* 1989;10: 8–18.
210. Steadman JR, Forster RS, Silfverskiold JP. Rehabilitation of the knee. *Clin Sports Med.* 1987;8:605–627.
211. DeMaio M, Mangine RC, Noyes FR, Barber SD. Sports medicine rehabilitation series: Advanced muscle training after ACL reconstruction weeks 6 to 52. *Orthopedics.* 1992;15:757–767.
212. Mangine RE, Noyes FR, DeMaio M. Sports medicine rehabilitation series, Minimal protection program: Advanced weight bearing and range of motion after ACL reconstruction weeks 1 to 5. *Orthopedics.* 1992;15: 504–515.
213. Drez D, Paine RM, Neuschwander D, D'Ambrosia R. Three phase study measuring anterior tibial translation in the ACL deficient knee. In: *Advances on the Knee and Shoulder Course Syllabus, Cincinnati Sports Medicine Meeting.* 1989.
214. Renstrom P, Arms SW, Stanwyck TS, Johnson RJ, Pope MH. Strain within the anterior cruciate ligament during hamstring and quadriceps activity. *Am J Sports Med.* 1986;14:83–87.
215. Noyes FR, Wojtys EM. The early recognition, diagnosis, and treatment of the patella infera syndrome. In: Tullos HS, ed. *Instructional Course Lectures.* Park Ridge, IL: AAOS; 1991:233–247.
216. Paulos LE, Rosenberg TD, Drawbert J, et al. Infrapatellar contracture syndrome. *Am J Sports Med.* 1987;15:331–340.
217. Grood ES, Suntay WJ, Noyes FR, Butler DL. Biomechanics of the knee extension exercise. Effect of cutting the anterior cruciate ligament. *J Bone Joint Surg*

Am. 1984;66:725–734.

218. Palmitier RA, Kai-Nan A, Scott SG, et al. Kinetic chain exercise in knee rehabilitation. *Sports Med.* 1991;11: 404–413.

219. Lutz GE, Palmitier RA, An KN, Chao YS. Comparison of tibiofemoral joint forces during open-kinetic-chain and closed-kinetic-chain exercises. *J Bone Joint Surg Am.* 1993;75:732–739.

220. Ericson MO, Nisell R. Tibiofemoral joint forces during ergometer cycling. *Am J Sports Med.* 1986;14:285–290.

221. Ericson MO, Nisell R, Arborelius UP, et al. Muscular activity during ergometer cycling. *Scand J Rehab Med.* 1985;17:53–61.

221. Richmond JC, Al Assal M. Arthroscopic management of arthrofibrosis of the knee including infrapatellar contracture syndrome. *Arthroscopy.* 1991;7:144–147.

222. Del Pizzo W, Fox JM, Friedman M, et al. Operative arthroscopy for the treatment of arthrofibrosis of the knee. *Contemp Orthop.* 1985;10:67–73.

223. Parisien JS. The role of arthroscopy in treatment of postoperative fibroarthrosis of the knee joint. *Clin Orthop.* 1988;229:185–192.

225. Sprague NF, O'Connor RL, Fox JM. Arthroscopic treatment of postoperative knee fibroarthrosis. *Clin Orthop.* 1982;166:165–172.

226. Richmond JC, Al Assal M. Arthroscopic management of arthrofibrosis of the knee including infrapatellar contracture syndrome. *Arthroscopy.* 1991;7:144–147.

227. Johnson RJ, Eriksson E, Haggmark T, et al. Five to ten year follow-up evaluation of the anterior cruciate ligament. *Clin Orthop.* 1984;183:122–140.

228. Wilk KE, Keirns MA, Andrews JR, et al. Anterior cruciate ligament reconstruction rehabilitation: A six-month follow up of isokinetic testing in recreational athletes. *Isokinet Exercise Sci.* 1991;1:36–43.

229. Daniel DM, Malcom L, Perth H, et al. Quantification of knee stability and function. *Contemp Orthop.* 1982;5: 83–91.

230. Daniel DM, Stone ML, Riehl B, et al. The one leg hop for distance. *Am J Knee Surg.* 1988;1:212–213.

231. Tegner Y, Lysholm J. Rating systems in the evaluation of knee ligament injuries. *Clin Orthop.* 1985;198:43–49.

232. Arendt EA, Hunter RE, Schneider WT. Vascularized patellar tendon anterior cruciate ligament reconstruction. *Clin Orthop.* 1989;44:222–232.

233. Feagin JA, Wills RP, Van Meter CD, et al. Intraarticular anterior cruciate ligament reconstruction without extraarticular augmentation. Two to ten year follow-up. In: *57th Annual AAOS Meeting Final Program, New Orleans.* 1990:85.

234. Reider B. Arthroscopic anterior cruciate ligament reconstruction using patellar tendon. In: Scott WN, ed. *Ligament and Extensor Mechanism Injuries of the Knee.* St. Louis: Mosby Year Book; 1991:239–252.

234. Bach BR, Jones GT, Sweet FA, Hager CA. Arthroscopy assisted anterior cruciate ligament reconstruction using patellar tendon substitution: Two to four year follow up results. Am J Sports Med., in press.

235. Boden B, Moyer RM, Betz R, et al. Arthroscopically assisted anterior cruciate ligament reconstruction: A follow-up study. *Contemp Orthop.* 1990;20:187 194.

235. Shelbourne KD, Whitaker J, McCarroll JR, Rettig AC, Hirshman LD. Anterior cruciate ligament injury: Evaluation of intra-articular reconstruction of acute tears without repair. *Am J Sports Med.* 1990;18:484–489.

236. Grana WA, Hines R. Arthroscopic-assisted semitendinosus reconstruction of the anterior cruciate ligament. *Am J Knee Surg.* 1992;5:16–22.

237. Daniel DM, Woodward EP, Losse GM, et al. The Marshall/MacIntosh anterior cruciate ligament reconstruction with the Kennedy ligament augmentation device. Report of the United States clinical trials. In: Friedman MJ, Ferkel RD, eds. *Prosthetic Ligament Reconstruction of the Knee.* Philadelphia: WB Saunders; 1988:71–78.

238. Buss DD, Skyhar MJ, Galinat BJ, Warren RF, Wickiewicz TL. Conservatively treated anterior cruciate ligament injuries. In: *57th Annual AAOS Meeting, Final Program, New Orleans.* 1990:83.

239. Lipscomb AB, Johnson RK, Synder RB, et al. Evaluation of hamstring strength following use of semitendinosus and gracilis tendons to reconstruct the anterior cruciate ligament. *Am J Sports Med.* 1983; 10:340–342.

15

Posterior Cruciate Ligament Injuries

Timothy E. Foster and Bertram Zarins

Introduction

The diagnosis and treatment of injuries to the posterior cruciate ligament (PCL) and posterolateral structures of the knee have received increased attention over the past decade; however, our knowledge concerning the natural history of PCL tears is small compared with our current understanding of anterior cruciate ligament (ACL) injuries. The PCL has been described as the primary stabilizer of the knee by some authors,[1-3] but despite its apparent anatomic importance there are contradictory reports in the literature concerning the fate of knees that have isolated tears of the PCL.[4-20] A tear of the PCL can result in disability varying from no functional compromise to a severe impairment. The majority of patients who have isolated PCL tears can function with minimal disability; however, if the PCL is torn in combination with injury to the posterolateral structures, significant knee disability can result.

The pertinent anatomy and biomechanics of the knee with reference to the PCL are reviewed. An understanding of the anatomy and function of the PCL and related structures will allow the surgeon to accurately diagnose and treat these injuries.

Mechanisms of Injury

Approximately half of PCL injuries are isolated tears that injure no other knee ligament. An isolated tear of the PCL can occur from a dashboard injury or a fall on a flexed knee. A vehicular accident is the most common mechanism of isolated PCL injury. In a collision, the knee can strike the dashboard of the automobile, driving the tibia posteriorly and tearing the PCL (Fig. 15–1). Many isolated PCL injuries have gone undetected and only recently have received adequate attention;

therefore, PCL injuries have been underreported. The dashboard-type injury to the proximal tibia usually tears the PCL at the tibial attachment site or, less commonly, avulses a fragment of bone with the PCL from the posterior tibia.[11] The dashboard model of injury was demonstrated by Kennedy in the laboratory; the tibia displaced posteriorly an average of 45 mm before the PCL ruptured.[15]

A fall on the flexed knee with the foot in plantar flexion is the second most common mechanism of injury to the PCL (Fig. 15–2). When someone falls in this manner the tibial tubercle hits the ground, forcing the tibia posteriorly and tearing the PCL.[21]

Another mechanism of injury to the PCL that has been described is hyperextension of the knee. The force typically is delivered by an opponent striking the front of the extended knee, or by the players own body weight being shifted to create a posteriorly directed force[14]; however, a hyperextension injury rarely injures the PCL alone, and the ACL is often torn prior to the PCL in such an injury.[22] A rotational mechanism associated with a varus or valgus stress may injure the PCL and collateral ligaments. A varus force to the proximal tibia of a hyperextended knee can result in posterolateral instability.[23]

Incidence

The recognition of injuries to the PCL is increasing. In 1950, O'Donoghue reported that only 9% of knee ligament injuries involved the PCL.[24] Kennedy and Grainger reported a 10% incidence in 1967.[15] Clendenin et al reported a 20% incidence in 1980,[5] and Bianchi said the incidence of PCL tears in patients with knee ligament injuries was 23% in a report in 1983.[25] The largest study to date, describing 500 patients who had knee

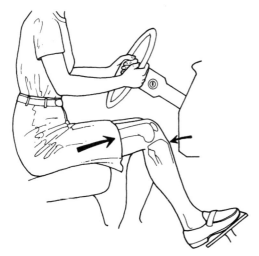

Figure 15-1. Dashboard injury to the knee can result in an isolated tear of the posterior cruciate ligament. The force hitting the area of the tibial tuberosity can drive the tibia posteriorly, rupturing the posterior cruciate ligament. The force hitting the patella can result in patellar fractures or traumatic chondromalacia patella. The force can also be directed posteriorly to injure the hip joint, possibly resulting in posterior dislocation of the hip.

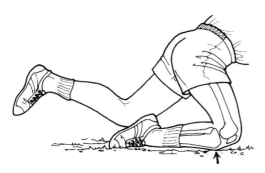

Figure 15-2. A fall on a flexed knee can drive the tibia posteriorly, tearing only the posterior cruciate ligament.

ligament injuries, reported that 7% involved the PCL.[4,26] Clancy et al[4] reported a 10% incidence of PCL injuries in a series of acute and chronic knee ligament injuries.

An isolated injury to the PCL can result in no functional impairment, and therefore, the prevalence of isolated PCL injuries may be higher than reported. A National Football League predraft physical evaluation of 450 college football players revealed a 2% incidence of isolated PCL injuries, many of which were previously unrecognized.[27]

Anatomy

Posterior Cruciate Ligament

The PCL is an intraarticular but extrasynovial structure. The PCL is attached to the tibia posterior to the attachment of the ACL, and, thus, derives its name.[22]

Femoral Attachment

The PCL attaches to the lateral surface of the medial femoral condyle in the posterior region of the intercondylar notch (see Chapter 1B). The femoral attachment is half-moon-shape, with the longitudinal axis directed in the anteroposterior plane of the femur. The femoral attachment of the PCL is only 3 to 5 mm from the articular border of the medial femoral condyle in the intercondylar notch.[22]

Tibial Attachment

The PCL attaches to the tibia 1 cm posterior to the posterior articular surface in a depression between the tibial condyles. There is a broad attachment to the posterior aspect of the tibia, with the bulk of the PCL fibers attaching to a region 13 mm wide (see Chapter 1B).

Midsubstance of Posterior Cruciate Ligament

The PCL is longer and broader than the ACL. Its average length is 38 mm and average width is 13 mm. Anatomic dissections by Girgis et al demonstrated an anterolateral band and a posteromedial band.[22] The anterolateral band of the ligament derives its name from the attachment site of the femur; it forms the bulk of the ligament. The posteromedial band is shorter and runs posteriorly and inferiorly to attach on the medial aspect of the posterior tibial sulcus. The two bands within the PCL function in a similar fashion to the two bands in the ACL. The anterolateral band becomes increasingly tighter as the knee is brought into full flexion. The posteromedial band is taut when the knee is extended. Although it is conceptually attractive to envision the PCL as consisting of two separate bands, the bands are actually inseparable. Cadaveric dissections of 14 knees by Satku and co-workers in 1984 refute the work of Girgis et al; Satku and colleagues state that the ligament is composed of only one band.[19]

Meniscofemoral Ligaments

The anterior meniscofemoral ligament (ligament of Humphrey) attaches to the posterior horn of the lateral meniscus and courses anterior to the PCL. The size of the anterior meniscofemoral ligament can be one third the diameter of the PCL.

The posterior meniscofemoral ligament (ligament of Wrisberg) attaches to the posterior horn of the lateral meniscus and, on occasion, arises from the posterior capsule. It travels posterior to the PCL and attaches to the medial condyle of the femur.

The meniscofemoral ligaments are not constant anatomic features of the human knee. Girgis et al reported that both meniscofemoral ligaments were not observed to be present in any knee, and that in 30% of anatomic specimens both ligaments were absent.[22] Kaplan, however, has identified at least one meniscofemoral ligament in all cadaver knees he dissected.[28] The variable attachments of the posterior meniscofemoral ligaments on the lateral meniscus and capsule may account for this apparent discrepancy.[22]

Blood Supply and Innervation

The PCL receives its blood supply from branches of the middle geniculate artery and branches of the medial and lateral inferior geniculate arteries. The synovium, which encompasses the PCL, has a rich blood supply derived from the middle geniculate artery; the medial and lateral inferior geniculate arteries have minimal contributions as well. The vessels travel in the longitudinal axis of the ligament in the synovium and periligamentous structure.

The PCL is innervated via the posterior articular branch of the tibial nerve. The nerve fibers course parallel to the PCL in the synovium and periligamentous tissue. Mechanoreceptors have been identified within the ligament and these nerve fibers probably contribute a sense of proprioception.[29-31]

Posterolateral Anatomy

The posterolateral aspect of the knee can be divided into three distinct layers. The superficial layer (layer I) is continuous with the deep fascia of the thigh. The deep fascia is confluent with the iliotibial band, which is the aponeurotic tendon of the tensor fascia lata and gluteus maximus. The iliotibial band inserts on the anterolateral aspect of the proximal tibia known as Gerdy's tubercle. The posterior aspect of the superficial layer contains the biceps muscle and aponeurosis.[32]

The middle layer (layer II) consists of the joint capsule and related ligamentous structures. The fibular collateral ligament is attached proximally to the lateral femoral epicondyle and courses distally to the fibular head. The fibular collateral ligament is a rounded structured that is discrete from the lateral joint capsule.

The deep layer (layer III) is composed of the synovium of the knee joint. The popliteus tendon passes deep to the fibular collateral ligament and is separated from the ligament by a small bursa. A synovial membrane of the joint (subpopliteal recess) separates the popliteus tendon from the lateral meniscus.

A detailed anatomic study of the posterolateral region of the knee was published by Seebacher et al in 1982.[33] They divided each tissue layer into sublayers, adding to the complexity of this region.

Functional Anatomy

The PCL is broader and stronger than the ACL and has a tensile strength of approximately 2000 N.[34] The PCL is the primary static stabilizer of the knee and restrains posterior tibial translation.[35,36] Isolated sectioning of the PCL results in posterior translation of the tibia at all degrees of flexion; however, translation is maximal between 75° and 90° and minimal from 0° to 30° of flexion.

The fibular collateral ligament is the primary static stabilizer of the knee that restrains varus rotation at all angles of flexion. The fibular collateral ligament does not have a role in restraining posterior translation of the tibia. The fibular collateral ligament is also a primary restraint to external rotation at all angles of knee flexion; however, at 60° of flexion this role is minimal.[37]

The capsule, including the arcuate ligament, and the popliteus tendon have minimal roles in restraining varus rotation. They play a substantial role in restraining external rotation of the tibia.[37]

An injury to the fibular collateral ligament and the lateral capsule will result in an increase of varus laxity at all angles of flexion and a large increase in external rotational laxity that will be maximum at 30° of flexion. Posterior translation of the tibia increases when both the fibular collateral ligament and the posterolateral capsule are cut.[37]

Combined injury to the PCL, fibular collateral ligament, and lateral capsule results in a large increase in posterior tibial translation, varus laxity, and external tibial rotation at all angles of knee flexion.[37] Isolated injury of the fibular collateral ligament or the posterolateral capsule may be difficult to recognize; however, a combined injury to these structures is usually not difficult to detect.

Associated Injuries

If a patient sustains a dashboard-type injury to the knee or falls on a flexed knee, an isolated tear of the PCL can result. In other mechanisms of injury, isolated tears of the PCL are uncommon; the force required to rupture the PCL is usually dissipated in the soft tissues surrounding the knee, disrupting other ligamentous and cartilaginous restraints as well. In the San Diego Kaiser study "isolated" ACL tears represented 48% of total knee ligamentous injuries as compared with "isolated" PCL injuries which accounted for only 4% of knee injuries.[26]

In 29 patients who had PCL tears reported by Hughston et al in 1980, all had injuries to additional knee structures.[38] Twenty-two had associated ACL tears, 26 had associated MCL tears, 2 had fibular collateral ligament injuries, and one patient had medial and lateral collateral ligament injuries. Hughston also reported that 24 of the 29 patients (83%) sustained medial meniscal tears. Hughston stated that PCL injury is always associated with other knee ligament injury.[39]

Loos et al reported on 102 patients who had PCL injuries, 59 of whom were treated acutely with operative intervention.[40] Twenty-six patients had coexistent ACL tears, 27 had medial collateral ligament tears, 18 had lateral ligaments tears, and 17 patients had medial meniscal tears.[40]

Diagnosis

The cornerstone of the management of ligamentous injuries to the knee is early diagnosis and treatment. There have been several reports in the literature of patients who had undiagnosed PCL tears who presented with late disability.[41] Loos and co-workers reported that in 43 of 102 patients the PCL injuries were unrecognized.[40]

There are several reports concerning the late recognition of PCL injuries; however, awareness of this injury has increased since 1980.[5,16,42,43] A patient who has been involved in a motor vehicle accident should be evaluated for knee ligament injuries. A patient who has a femoral fracture should be suspected of having knee ligament injuries until proven otherwise.

The degree of symptoms in an acute knee injury often correlates with the mechanism of injury. A high-velocity motor vehicle accident that results in a dashboard-type injury can injure the PCL alone or in combination with other supporting structures of the knee. After high-velocity injury the knee is typically painful, swollen, and ecchymotic and has obvious laxity. The absence of a hemarthrosis in a severely injured knee suggests capsular tearing with fluid extravasation into the soft tissue surrounding the knee.[1] An isolated

injury to the PCL, such as from a fall on a flexed knee, may present at the opposite end of the spectrum. Such a patient can have minimal symptoms. Patients who have isolated PCL injuries frequently deny pain and have a mild or no hemarthrosis.[4]

Patients who have chronic tears of the PCL have symptoms that are quite different from those of acute injuries. Patients who have symptomatic chronic PCL tears often describe knee disability; however, they do not have the same sense of instability as do patients who have ACL injuries.[4,44] The patients who have PCL injuries often notice the symptoms during the pushoff phase of the running cycle or while descending stairs. An injury to the ACL typically results in the inability of an athlete to change direction quickly; however, athletes who have isolated PCL tears usually return to sports.

Physical Examination

In the acute injury the knee and leg should be inspected for signs of direct impact. A complete neurovascular examination of the lower extremities is imperative, especially in patients who have sustained high-velocity injuries and in patients who are suspected of having had a knee dislocation that has spontaneously reduced. Injuries to the peroneal nerve are frequently associated with posterolateral capsular disruption.[45,46]

Posterior Drawer Test

The posterior drawer test assesses the posterior translation of the tibia with respect to the femur (Fig. 15–3). The test is graded on a similar scale as the anterior drawer.[47] The quality of the endpoint of the translation is also evaluated as being "firm" or "soft."

The posterior drawer test should be performed with the knee between 70° and 90° of flexion; in this position the PCL is the major static stabilizer. At 90° of flexion

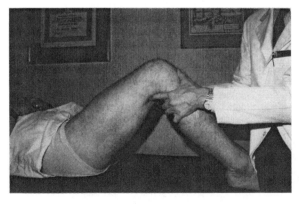

Figure 15–3. Method of examining a knee to detect the posterior drawer sign: Both knees are flexed at 90° and the examiner sits on the feet. The examiner grasps the proximal tibia with both hands. The tips of the thumbs are used to palpate the distal ends of the femoral condyle while the bases of the thumbs are used to palpate the proximal tibia. The index fingers are kept extended to ensure that the hamstring muscles remain relaxed during the procedure. The other fingers are used to move the tibia in an anteroposterior direction.

the contribution of collateral and capsule structures to stability is eliminated.[35-37] In the posterior drawer test, the knee is flexed to 90° and positioned in neutral rotation. The examiner stabilizes rotation and position of the foot by sitting on it. The examiner places his or her thumbs over the anterior aspect of the flexed knee, with the tips of the thumbs on the femoral condyles and the thenar eminences resting on the proximal tibia. The index fingers are extended to palpate the tension in the patient's hamstring tendons during the examination to ensure relaxation of these muscles. The remaining fingers gently grasp the posterior aspect of the tibia. The thumbs are used to feel the relative position of the contour of the femoral condyles in relation to the tibial plateau. Anterior and posterior forces are applied to the tibia and the degree of translation is assessed. The contralateral knee is always examined for comparison.

It is often difficult to determine if a drawer sign is anterior or posterior. In a patient who has a torn PCL the examiner may feel an increase in anterior translation and confuse this with a positive anterior drawer

sign. This "false-positive" sign results from starting the test with the tibia in a posteriorly subluxated position. If a knee has an apparent positive anterior drawer sign at 90° of flexion and negative Lachman and pivot shift signs, the examiner should be alert to a torn PCL. Some authors have suggested that a positive anterior drawer test performed with the tibia in internal rotation is indicative of an injury to the ACL and PCL.[1,48]

The posterior drawer sign is often negative in an acutely injured knee in which multiple ligaments, including the PCL, are torn.[1] A positive posterior drawer sign will become evident later in a chronic state.

Posterior Sag Sign

In 1903, Robson recognized that a tear of the PCL resulted in a posterior "rollback" of the tibia in relation to the femur; he coined the term *posterior sag sign*.[49] This test is similar to the posterior drawer test. The lateral contours of the knee are evaluated with both knees flexed 90° (Fig. 15–4A).

A
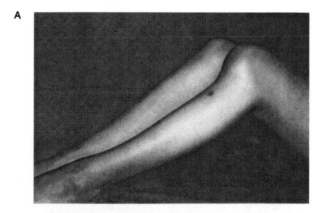

B
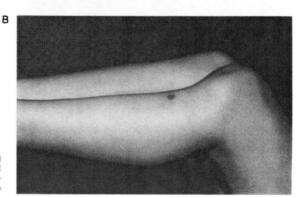

Figure 15–4. A. Right knee marked posterior sag caused by rupture of the posterior cruciate ligament and chronic posterior tibial subluxation. **B.** An alternate method of eliciting the posterior sag with the hips and knees flexed to a 90° position.

A similar method of looking for a posterior sag was described by Godfrey (Fig. 15–4B).[50] The hip and knee of both extremities are flexed 90° while the heels are held by the examiner. The contour of the knees is evaluated from the side.

Genu Recurvatum

If a knee hyperextends beyond 10° or 15° it is usually indicative of tears of both cruciate ligaments (Fig. 15–5). If a knee hyperextends only 5° or 10°, this motion is usually accompanied by slight external rotation of the tibia. This test is called the external rotation recurvatum test; it indicates that the PCL is probably intact but that the ACL and internal structures are lax.

The external rotation recurvatum test was described by Hughston et al in 1976.[1,23] The test was designed to evaluate the competency of the posterolateral structures including the fibular collateral ligament, popliteus tendon, arcuate ligament, and ACL. The test is performed by lifting the extended leg from the examining table by the big toe. A test is positive if the knee externally rotates as it hyperextends. Biomechanical studies performed by Girgis et al indicate that a hyperextension injury must first tear the ACL before the PCL is injured.[22] A positive external rotation recurvatum test,

therefore, implies an injury to the ACL, posterolateral structures, and usually an intact PCL.[22,51] If the knee goes into straight hyperextension, it usually means that the PCL is also torn.

Reverse Pivot Shift

The reverse pivot shift is performed with the knee in flexion and the tibia externally rotated. A valgus stress is applied to the leg and the knee is gradually extended. In a positive test, the tibia starts in a posteriorly subluxated position when the knee is flexed, and as the knee is extended the tibia reduces at 30° of flexion (Fig. 15–6).[52]

A reverse pivot shift test is not specific for injury to posterolateral structures because a positive test can be elicited in normal knees.[12,52] A positive reverse pivot shift is significant only if it differs from that for the uninjured knee and if the patient has a history of knee trauma consistent with injury to the posterolateral structures.

Quadriceps Active Test

The quadriceps active test was described by Daniel as an "active test" compared with the previously described tests that are passive.[53] A muscular contraction is used to move the tibia.

The vector force of the quadriceps muscle as it acts through the patella tendon in a normal knee at 90° of flexion is directed posteriorly. If the PCL is torn and the tibia is in a posteriorly subluxated position (posterior sag), the force is directed anteriorly. The active quadriceps test is performed with the knee at 90° of flexion and with the patient's foot resting on the examination table (Fig. 15–7). The examiner sits on the patient's foot to prevent the foot from moving. The patient is asked to contract the quadriceps muscle by sliding the leg down the examination table against resistance, that is, to extend the knee. The contraction of the quadriceps muscle should result in little or no movement of the tibia in a normal knee. If the PCL is torn, the contraction of the quadriceps muscle results in 4 to 6 mm of anterior translation of the tibia from its original "posterior sag" position.[53] The test can also be performed by firmly grasping the ankle of the patient in a sitting position and asking her or him to forcefully extend the knee but allowing no extension.

Varus–Valgus Stress Test

Excess laxity to varus and valgus stress tests may indicate injury to the PCL. Hughston et al maintain that the most reliable test for laxity as a result of PCL injury is the varus–valgus stress test with the knee in full extension.[1] Gollehon's work based on a biomechanical study suggests that varus instability in full extension can

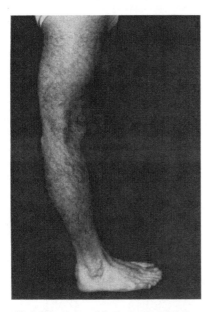

Figure 15–5. Lateral view of the patient in a standing position demonstrating excessive straight recurvatum of the right knee as a result of rupture of both the cruciate ligaments and posterior capsule.

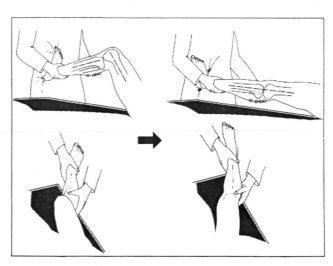

Figure 15–6. Reverse pivot shift sign: To examine the right knee the examiner rests the foot on the right side of the pelvis. The left hand is supported on the lateral side of the leg. The knee is flexed 70° to 80° resulting in external rotation of the tibia as a result of posterior subluxation of the lateral tibial plateau. As the knee is extended and an axial load and valgus force are applied, the lateral tibial plateau suddenly reduces at 20° flexion. The reduction comes from a posterior subluxation in external rotation to a final position of reduction and neutral rotation. (Reprinted with permission from Jakob et al.[52(p19)])

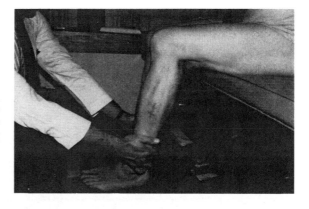

Figure 15–7. Quadriceps active test: With the patient in the seated position, the examiner firmly grasps the patient's ankle. The patient actively tries to extend and flex the knee while the examiner holds the knee fixed at a 90° angle. A positive test is anterior tibial translation while the patient is actively extending the knee. This occurs when the quadriceps muscle force pulls the tibia forward from a posteriorly subluxated position if the patient has a torn posterior cruciate ligament.

result from an injury to the fibular collateral ligament and posterolateral structures with an uninjured PCL.[37] Excess laxity to varus stress in full extension indicates injury to the fibular collateral ligament, the posterolateral structures, and possibly the PCL and ACL.

Instrumented Knee Testing

Several instruments are available that give a quantitative measure of tibial translation. These include the KT1000, Genucom, and Acuflex Knee Signature System. The arthrometer measurements are useful to permit the comparison of knee laxity before and after surgical treatment. Except for the quadriceps active test, instrumented testing of posterior knee laxity is not reliable because of the difficulty in establishing the normal anteroposterior position of the tibia at 90° of flexion.

Radiographic Evaluation

Routine radiographic evaluation of the knee consists of four views: anteroposterior, lateral, tunnel, and tangential taken at 30° of flexion. If a PCL tear is suspected, a lateral view can be taken with the knee flexed 90° (Fig. 15–8) and posterior stress applied; a comparison view of the opposite knee should also be obtained. The lateral radiograph should be specifically evaluated for the presence of avulsion of a fragment of bone at the tibial attachment of the PCL (Fig. 15– 9).

The advent of magnetic resonance imaging (MRI) has significantly increased diagnostic accuracy of knee liga-

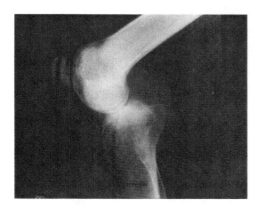

Figure 15-8. Lateral radiograph of a knee showing chronic posterior tibial subluxation caused by a complete tear of the posterior cruciate ligament.

ment injuries. The T1 image provides the best anatomic detail, and the T2 image yields additional information with reference to hemorrhage, edema, and joint effusion.

The PCL is best visualized in a sagittal plane and has very low signal intensity (black) on the T1 image (Fig. 15-10). The intact PCL will often show small areas of "artifact" on routine MRI evaluation and these should not be confused with a PCL tear. A knee surface coil can be used to improve imaging resolution. If the liga-

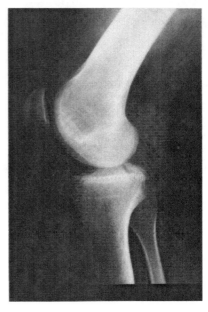

Figure 15-9. Lateral radiograph of a knee showing avulsion fracture of the tibial attachment of the posterior cruciate ligament.

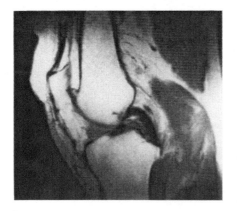

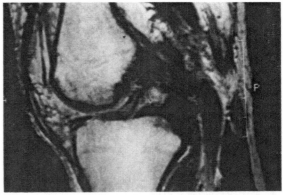

A   B

Figure 15-10. A. Magnetic resonance imaging of the knee sagittal section showing a normal posterior cruciate ligament. **B.** Magentic resonance image of the knee showing a complete tear of the posterior cruciate ligament. The popliteal artery was injured at the time of knee injury and the artery was repaired.

A

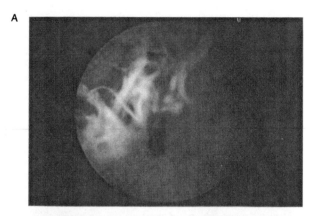

B

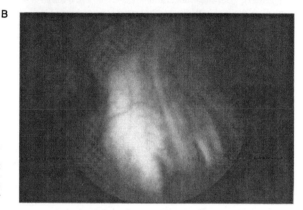

Figure 15–11. A. Arthroscopic visualization of an acute isolated tear of the posterior cruciate ligament. **B.** The anterior cruciate ligament in this patient appears lax because the tibia is subluxated posteriorly. This lax appearance of the ligament should not be misinterpreted as stretching of the anterior cruciate ligament.

ment is adequately visualized on scanning with a surface coil the accuracy rate for diagnosis of injury approaches 100%.[54]

Arthroscopy

Arthroscopy is not usually a good method to diagnose a torn PCL; however, a torn PCL can sometimes be clearly seen (Fig. 15–11A). If the PCL is torn, the ACL will appear to be lax secondary to posterior subluxation of the tibia (Fig. 15–11B).

Natural History of PCL Tears

The treatment of an isolated PCL tear is controversial because our knowledge of the long-term natural history of this condition is lacking and because the surgical treatments currently available have variable results. Clancy et al have described patellofemoral joint and

medial compartment degenerative changes in patients who have chronic PCL tears; they studied 33 patients who underwent operative reconstruction of the PCL at least 1 month after injury.[4] The average patient had sustained the injury 3 years prior to surgery. Clancy et al noted at the time of arthrotomy that 64% of the patients had degenerative changes in the medial compartment; only 31% of these changes were evident on radiographs.[4] They also noted that articular cartilage degeneration was far more common in patients who had sustained PCL injuries 2 years or longer prior to reconstruction, leading Clancy et al to conclude that progressive deterioration of articular cartilage occurred over time following rupture of the PCL.

The conclusions of Clancy et al agree with earlier work done by Kennedy in 1967. Kennedy and Grainger described 57 patients who had PCL injuries who were treated nonoperatively; 44% of the patients developed significant degenerative changes.[15] Degenerative changes were also described by Cross and co-workers in 62 patients who had PCL injuries treated nonoperatively; 42% of these patients eventually developed symptoms that required operative intervention.[44] The authors concluded that PCL tears will eventually lead to degenerative arthritis of the knee.

Torg et al described radiographic evidence of degenerative changes in knees that have a PCL injury; however, these changes were more common in knees that had combined ligament injuries than in knees that had isolated PCL tears.[20] Torg et al stated that the "functional outcome could be predicted on the basis of the instability type." They concluded that patients who had isolated tears of the PCL did not require operative intervention; however, patients who sustained a PCL tear plus other ligament tears had a significantly higher incidence of poor functional outcomes.[20] This work is in agreement with that of Satku et al who reported on 48 patients who had torn PCLs.[19] They concluded that the most important factor in determining the functional outcome of patients with PCLs who were treated without surgery was the presence of additional ligament injuries.

Parolie and Bergfeld reported on the long-term results of 25 athletes who had isolated PCL tears treated nonoperatively.[18] Sixty-eight percent returned to their previous level of athletic function. The authors emphasized the need for a quadriceps muscle rehabilitation program. Fifty-two percent of the patients reported occasional knee pain. Radiographic evidence of degenerative changes were identified in 36%.[18]

The San Diego Kaiser PCL Follow-up Study evaluated 17 patients who had isolated PCL tears 11 to 45 months after injury.[26] Three patients had meniscal tears subsequent to the initial injury. Mild pain was present in 71% of the patients and swelling was noted in 18%. No patient in this study described instability.[26]

It is our observation that patients who have isolated PCL tears can usually return to athletics after a rehabilitation program. The natural history of PCL injury differs from that of an ACL tear in that there are very few episodes of instability in a knee that has a torn PCL, and the menisci are at an only slightly increased risk for a secondary tear compared with a knee that has a torn ACL. Patients who have isolated PCL injuries may have occasional effusions that are self-limiting and are activity related. The major complaint is a vague discomfort, which usually does not limit the patient's activities.

Patients who have PCL tears as well as other ligament injuries are likely to develop knee instability, meniscus tears, and degenerative articular cartilage changes. Patients who have complex instability are in a different functional category than patients who have isolated PCL tears. Our treatment protocol attempts to differentiate between these two groups.

Treatment of Acute Isolated PCL Tears

The majority of patients who have isolated PCL tears should be treated nonoperatively. Most will achieve good functional results with rehabilitation and possibly bracing of the injured knee. Current surgical techniques do not have predictably good results and surgery has not been shown to decrease the risk of developing degenerative changes in the joint. Therefore, patients who have isolated PCL tears are counseled concerning the injury, degree of expected dysfunction, and possible long-term effects.

An MRI scan can be obtained to document ligament injury and to assess subchondral bone damage. The knee is placed in a splint with the knee extended for 1 week to allow soft tissue swelling to subside. The patient begins isometric quadriceps exercises within days of the injury. Rehabilitation is begun after the acute swelling subsides. The patient is instructed on a quadriceps muscle strengthening program 1 to 2 weeks after the initial injury. The knee immobilizer is removed 1 week postinjury for daily range-of-motion exercises. We prefer that the patient regains full quadriceps muscle strength before returning to competitive athletics. The patient is followed at yearly intervals.

Surgical Treatment of PCL Tears

Reconstructive procedures for PCL tears include primary repair of the ligament or replacement of the ligament with an autogenous tissue graft, allograft, or prosthetic ligament. Operative procedures have been described including primary ligament repair[25,38,55,56]; substitution using semitendinosus tendon graft,[25,55–57] fascia lata,[58–60] or meniscus[61,62]; and transfer of the medial head of the gastrocnemius.[5,17,38,41,56,63]

We currently prefer to use autogenous or allograft tissue to reconstruct the PCL. We prefer to use the middle one third of the patellar tendon if using autograft or the Achilles tendon if using allograft.

Isometric Points for PCL Reconstruction

Although there is controversy on whether or not isometric points truly exist, studies have been done to find the best attachment points to the femur and tibia for PCL grafts.[64,65]

A study by Bomberg et al found that changing the location of the femoral hole had a marked effect on the length of a PCL graft during knee motion.[65] Sites located anterior to the most isometric point resulted in greater tension with knee flexion, whereas sites posterior to the isometric point resulted in greater tension with extension (Fig. 15–12). Moving the femoral hole superiorly into the intercondylar roof or inferiorly on the lateral aspect of the medial femoral condyle did not

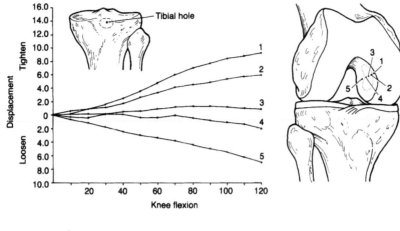

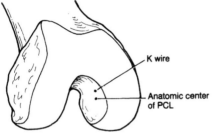

Figure 15–12. Results of an experimental cadaver study showing elongation of a simulated PCL graft if the tibial hole is located at the center of the attachment of the PCL to the tibia and the femoral hole is varied (F1 through F5) at several knee flexion angles. The K-wire should be located several millimeters anterior to the anatomic center of the PCL to compensate for eccentric placement of the graft following overdrilling of the K-wire using a larger drill. (Adapted with permission from Bomberg et al.[65])

affect the change in length of the graft. Change in location of the tibial hole had little effect on the length of the graft, whereas moving the femoral hole caused significant changes in length.

We believe that the tibia guide pin should be positioned at or slightly distal to the center of the tibial attachment of the PCL. The femoral guide pin should be placed at the edge of the intercondylar fossa, at the corner created by the roof of the intercondylar fossa and its medial wall. If the guide pin will be overdrilled using a 10-mm cannulated drill, the pin should be placed 5 mm posterior to the edge of the articular cartilage.

PCL Reconstruction Using Achilles Tendon Allograft

An Achilles tendon allograft has several potential advantages as a PCL replacement. It is large and has a high tensile strength. The great density of organized collagen in the tendon contributes to its strength. The potential disadvantages include possibility of transmission of disease and rejection and weakness of fixation of the tendon end of the graft.

The graft can be inserted with the aid of arthroscopic visualization. A 30° fore oblique arthroscope is introduced via an anteromedial portal. An anteromedial portal is used for introduction of instruments that are used to debride the PCL stump. A 70° fore oblique arthroscope is introduced via a posteromedial portal and the posterior tibial condyle is cleared of soft tissues. An arthroscopic PCL drill guide (Acuflex Microsurgical, Inc, 575 University Avenue, Norwood, MA 02062, or Arthrex Inc, 3050 North Horseshoe Drive, Naples, FL 33942) is introduced through the anteromedial portal and its tip is placed in the posterior suclus 1 cm below the joint line.

A guidewire is drilled through the proximal tibia from anterior to posterior. The tibial drill guide is placed at the anterior tibia approximately 5 cm distal to the joint line and 1 cm medial to the tibial tubercle (Fig. 15–13). The hole should avoid injuring the pes anserinus tendons and tibial collateral ligament. The tibial tunnel should be angled approximately 45° to the long axis of the tibia (see Fig. 15–17A). A more horizontal tunnel may create difficulty later in the procedure when passing the graft and a more vertical tunnel may be too long. Extreme caution must be exercised when drilling. The knee is flexed to 90° to relax the posterior neurovascular structures. The K-wire is advanced to the posterior tibial cortex and a fluoroscopic or radio-

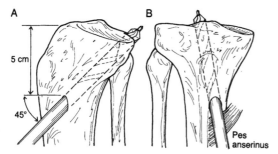

Figure 15–13. Lateral view of the tibia showing a guidewire overdrilled with a cannulated drill. The entry point for the hole is approximately 5 cm distal to the joint line. The angle is approximately 45° in relation to the long axis of the tibia. The exit point of the hole in the back of the tibia is several millimeters below the superior surface of the tibia centrally.

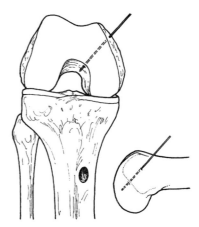

Figure 15–14. The guidewires have been drilled from the area of the medial epicondyle to enter the joint in the intercondylar area 5 mm from the edge of the articular cartilage. The drill point is several millimeters anterior to the center of the PCL attachment to the femur.

graphic image is obtained to evaluate the position and obliquity of the K-wire. The K-wire is then drilled through the posterior cortex under fluoroscopic control and with direct arthroscopic visualization via the posteromedial portal. A stop should be placed on the wire to prevent drilling it in too deeply.

A small skin incision is made in the anteromedial leg at the entry site of the K-wire and the soft tissues are cleared. A 10- to 11-mm cannulated drill is passed over the K-wire and used to drill the tibia. Extreme caution is used when drilling to prevent pushing the K-wire ahead of the drill and to prevent the drill point from catching on neurovascular tissues as it exits the posterior tibia. The tip of the rotating drill can catch soft tissues and pull them from a distance. Direct fluoroscopic and arthroscopic visualization is maintained.

The tip of the guide for drilling the medial femoral condyle is placed through the anteromedial arthroscopy portal. The tip of the guide is placed very close to the articular surface of the medial femoral condyle, 5 mm medial to the top of the intercondylar notch[12,14] (Fig. 15–14). A K-wire is drilled through the medial femoral condyle while viewing with an arthroscope in the anterolateral portal. A small skin incision is made over the K-wire near the medial epicondyle and the guidewire is overdrilled using a 9- to 10-mm cannulated drill.

The Achilles tendon allograft is prepared on a separate table by a surgical assistant. A whip stitch is placed in the proximal end of the tendon using No. 5 Ethibond suture. The calcaneal end of the graft is fashioned into a 25-mm-long by 10-mm-wide bone block. Three holes are drilled through the bone in two different planes. Heavy sutures (No. 5 Ethibond) are passed through the holes.

An 18-gauge wire or heavy suture is advanced through the tibial tunnel to the posterior tibia, then anteriorly into the intercondylar notch and out through the medial femoral tunnel. The allograft is passed from the tibial tunnel into the femoral tunnel using the 18-gauge wire or suture as a leader. The proximal end of the graft is advanced first; therefore, the soft tissue portion of the graft lies within the femoral tunnel and the bone block is within the tibial tunnel (Fig. 15–15).

The bone block within the tibial tunnel is secured using an interference fit screw. The knee is extended to 0° and manual tension is applied to the graft. The posterior tibial subluxation reduces when the knee is extended. The sutures attached to the proximal end of the allograft are tied to a screw placed in the femur adjacent to the tunnel.

Midthird Patellar Tendon Graft

A graft commonly used to replace the PCL is a midthird patellar tendon autograft or allograft.[21] Bone from the inferior pole of the patella and tibial tuberosity is left attached to the graft (Fig. 15–16). The procedure is performed as described earlier; however, a posteromedial incision is made to expose the posterior tibia. The posteromedial incision allows direct retraction of the peroneal artery and tibial nerve, thus decreasing the possibility of neurovascular injury. The tip of the K-wire that is passed through the proximal tibia can be visualized and palpated as it enters the posterior tibial cortex; therefore, fluoroscopic control is not necessary. The bone blocks in the tibial and femoral tunnels are both secured with interference screws with the knee in an extended position (Fig. 15–17).

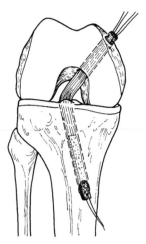

Figure 15–15. An Achilles tendon allograft has been passed through the tibial hole in retrograde manner, leaving the bone plug in the tibial tunnel. The tendinous portion of the graft has been pulled forward in the joint and out through the femoral hole. An interference screw will be placed in the tibial tunnel. The sutures attached to the proximal end of the tendon allograft will be tied around a screw placed in the distal femur.

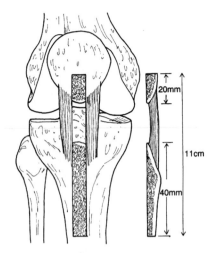

Figure 15–16. Midthird patellar tendon autograft. When used to replace a PCL the patellar portion of the graft is approximately 20 mm long. A short graft is easier to pass through the tibial and femoral tunnels. The tibial portion of the graft is 40 mm long. Leaving this section of bone long will allow it to extend most of the length of the tibial tunnel and make it easier to engage the interference fit screw.

Postoperative Care

The knee is placed in a splint in extension. The patient may bear weight fully on the leg in the brace using crutches for support starting on the first postoperative day. The brace is locked in full extension; however, care must be taken to avoid hyperextension of the knee to prevent stretching the graft. Isometric quadriceps setting exercises are started on postoperative day 2 and continue throughout the course of rehabilitation. The patient may begin a closed-chain quadriceps muscle stregthening program during the second week as well as stationary cycling with minimal resistance. We do not allow athletes to return to competition for 9 to 12 months after surgery.

Treatment of Acute PCL Avulsion Fractures

The surgical fixation of acute avulsion fractures of the PCL from the tibia has been recommended by many authors.[6,10,11,66,67] The results are reported to be quite good in restoring knee stability. The operative procedure to reattach the avulsion fragment is technically easier than a ligament reconstruction. The objective results are superior to those of nonoperative treatment.

The surgical procedure is performed with the patient in a prone position. A direct posterior approach is used.

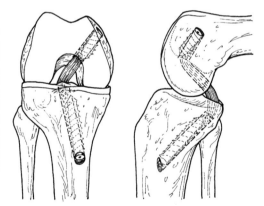

Figure 15–17. Location of midthird patellar tendon graft in the tibia and femoral tunnels and the location of the interference fit screws.

The avulsion fracture is reattached to the tibia using a single half-thread cancellous screw (Fig. 15–18). The patient is placed in a hinged brace with the knee flexed to 30° to release tension on the ligament. The patient is immobilized for 10 days before a range-of-motion program is instituted.

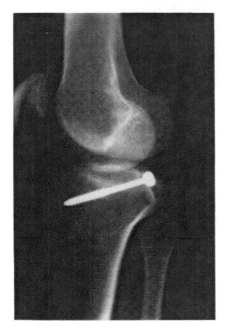

Figure 15–18. Lateral radiograph of a knee showing a screw that has been used to fix an avulsion fracture of the posterior tibia with the attached PCL (same patient as in Fig. 15–9).

Treatment of PCL Tears With Posterolateral Instability

A tear of the PCL with additional injury to the posterolateral structures can produce significant disability; therefore, we recommend acute surgical repair of the lateral capsule and ligaments and primary reconstruction of the PCL using a midthird patellar tendon autograft or Achilles tendon allograft. Postoperatively the knee is placed in a hinged brace for 1 week, locked in extension. The hinges are unlocked at 1 week and the patient begins to work on range-of-motion exercises.

Treatment of Acute Posterolateral Instability

A patient who has an acute tear of the PCL and posterolateral structures is treated with early surgery. We have not been completely satisfied with secondary reconstructive procedures for posterolateral instability; therefore, we recommend early repair of the injured structures. There have been several reports of satisfactory results with early repair of the posterolateral structures. Surgery is delayed for 7 to 14 days to allow soft

tissue swelling to subside; then a primary repair of the torn posterolateral tissues is performed. The arcuate ligament complex and popliteus tendon are repaired primarily and the capsule is repaired where torn. If the PCL is torn, the ligament is replaced using a graft as previously described.

Postoperatively, the knee is placed in a hinged brace locked at 30° of flexion for 2 weeks after surgery. The patient performs isometric quadriceps muscle exercises during this time. The patient is maintained on touchdown weight bearing for 2 to 3 weeks postoperatively. The rehabilitation progresses gradually with range-of-motion and quadriceps strengthening exercises.

Surgical Treatment of Chronic PCL Tears and Chronic Posterolateral Instability

The reconstruction of a chronic PCL tear combined with posterolateral laxity is difficult, and the results have been variable. Reconstructive procedures should correct laxity caused by the PCL tear and the posterolateral structures to be effective.

Patients who have chronic posterolateral laxity, a significant varus alignment to the lower extremity, and a lateral thrust in the stance phase of gait are candidates for a high tibial valgus osteotomy.

A transfer of the biceps femoris tendon is recommended for reconstruction of chronic posterolateral laxity. We have had variable success using this procedure; however, Clancy reports consistently good results using this technique.[21]

Conclusion

Patients who have isolated tears of the PCL may do quite well functionally but appear to be somewhat predisposed to develop early degenerative joint changes. A combined tear of the PCL and posterolateral structures often heralds the beginning of chronic instability with progressive joint degeneration; therefore, early surgical repair is advisable.

The management of injuries to the PCL and associated structures is complex. There are very few prospective studies with long-term results to guide our treatment of these injuries.

References

1. Hughston JC, Andrews JR, Cross MJ, Moschi A. Classification of knee ligament instabilities. Part 1. The medial compartment and cruciate ligaments. *J Bone Joint Surg Am.* 1976;58:159–172.
2. McCluskey G, Blackburn T. Classification of knee ligament instabilities. *Phys Ther.* 1980;60:1575–1577.
3. Cain TE, Schwab GH. Performance of an athlete with straight posterior knee instability. *Am J Sports Med.* 1981;9:203–208

4. Clancy WG, Shelbourne KD, Zoellner GB, Keene JS, Reider B, Rosenberg TD. Treatment of knee joint instability secondary to rupture of the posterior cruciate ligament. Report of a new procedure. *J Bone Joint Surg Am.* 1983;65:310–322.
5. Clendenin MB, DeLee JC, Heckman JD. Interstitial tears of the posterior cruciate ligament of the knee. *Orthopedics.* 1980;3:764–772.
6. McMaster WC. Isolated posterior cruciate ligament injury: Literature review and case reports. *J Trauma.* 1975;15:1025–1029.
7. Ogata K. Posterior cruciate reconstruction using iliotibial band. Preliminary report of a new procedure. *Arch Orthop Trauma Surg.* 1983;101:107–110.
8. Strand T, Molster AO, Engesaetter LB, Raugstad TS, Alho A. Primary repair in posterior cruciate ligament injuries. *Acta Orthop Scand.* 1984;55:545–547.
9. Tillberg B. The late repair of torn cruciate ligaments using menisci. *J Bone Joint Surg Br.* 1977;59:15–19.
10. Trickey EL. Rupture of the posterior cruciate ligament of the knee. *J Bone Joint Surg Br.* 1968;50:334–341.
11. Trickey EL. Injuries to the posterior cruciate ligament: Diagnosis and treatment of early injuries and reconstruction of late instability. *Clin Orthop.* 1980;147:76–81.
12. Cooper DE, Warren RF, Warren JJ. The posterior cruciate ligament and posterolateral structures of the knee: Anatomy, function, and patterns of injury. In: Tullos HS, ed. *Instructional Course Lectures.* Chicago: American Academy of Orthopaedic Surgeons; pp. 1991;40:249–270.
13. Dandy DJ, Pusey RJ. The long-term results of unrepaired tears of the posterior cruciate ligament. *J Bone Joint Surg Br.* 1982;64:92–94.
14. Fowler PJ, Messieh SS. Isolated posterior cruciate ligament injuries in athletes. *Am J Sports Med.* 1987;15:553–557.
15. Kennedy JC, Grainger RW. The posterior cruciate ligament. *J Trauma.* 1967;7:367–377.
16. Kennedy JC, Roth JH, Walker DM. Posterior cruciate ligament injuries. *Orthop Digest.* 1979;Aug/Sept:19–31.
17. Kennedy JC, Galpin RD. The use of the medial head of the gastrocnemius muscle in the posterior cruciate deficient knee. Indications, technique, results. *Am J Sports Med.* 1982;10:63–74.
18. Parolie JM, Bergfeld JA. Long-term results of nonoperative treatment of isolated posterior cruciate ligament injuries in the athlete. *Am J Sports Med.* 1986;14:35–38.
19. Satku K, Chew C.N. and Seow H. Posterior cruciate ligament injuries. *Acta Orthop Scand.* 1984;55:26–29.
20. Torg JS, Barton TM, Pavlov H, Stine R. Natural history of the posterior cruciate ligament-deficient knee. *Clin Orthop.* 1989;246:208–216.
21. Clancy WG. *Posterior Cruciate and Posterolateral Instability.* Instructional Course lecture. Chicago: American Academy of Orthopaedic Surgeons; 1991.
22. Girgis FG, Marshall JL, Monajem ARS. The cruciate ligaments of the knee joint. *Clin Orthop.* 1975;106:216–231.
23. Hughston JC, Norwood LA. The posterolateral drawer test and external rotational recurvatum test for posterolateral rotatory instability of the knee. *Clin Orthop.* 1980;147:82–87.
24. O'Donoghue DM. Surgical treatment of fresh injuries to the major ligaments of the knee. *J Bone Joint Surg Am.* 1950;32:721.
25. Bianchi M. Acute tears of the posterior cruciate ligament: Clinical study and results of operative treatment in 27 cases. *Am J Sports Med.* 1983;11:308–314.
26. Daniel DM, Akeson WH, O'Connor JJ. *Knee Ligaments: Structure, Function, Injury and Repair.* New York: Raven Press; 1990:481–503.
27. Bergfeld JA. Posterior cruciate and posterolateral instability. In: Tullos HS, ed. *Instructional Course Lectures.* Chicago: American Academy of Orthopaedic Surgeons; 1991;40.
28. Kaplan EB. Some aspects of functional anatomy of the human knee joint. *Clin Orthop.* 1962;23:18–29.
29. Kennedy JC, Weinberg HW, Wilson AS. The anatomy and function of the anterior cruciate ligament as determined by clinical and morphological studies. *J Bone Joint Surg Am.* 1974;56:223–235.
30. Marshall JL, Arnoczky SP, Rubin RM, Wickiewicz TL. Microvasculature of the cruciate ligament. *Phys Sports Med.* 1979;7:87–91.
31. Wladmirow B. Arterial sources of blood supply of the knee joint in man. *Acta Med.* 1968;47:1–10.
32. Hoppenfeld S, deBower P. *Surgical Exposures in Orthopaedics.* Philadelphia: JB Lippincott; 1984:423–426.
33. Seebacher JR, Inglis AE, Marshall JL, Warren RF. The structure of the posterolateral aspect of the knee. *J Bone Joint Surg Am.* 1982;64:536–541.
34. Kennedy JC, Hawkins RJ, Willis RB, Danylchuk KD. Tension studies of human knee ligaments. *J Bone Joint Surg Am.* 1976;58:350–355.
35. Grood ES, Stowers SF, Noyes FR. Limits of movement in the human knee. Effect of sectioning the posterior cruciate ligament and posterolateral structures. *J Bone Joint Surg Am.* 1988;70:88–97.
36. Butler DL, Noyes FR, Grood ES. Ligamentous restraints to anterior–posterior drawer in the human knee. *J Bone Joint Surg Am.* 1980;62:259–270.
37. Gollehon DL, Torzilli PA, Warren RF. The role of the posterolateral and cruciate ligaments in the stability of the human knee. *J Bone Joint Surg Am.* 1987;69:233–242.
38. Hughston JC, Bowden JA, Andrews JR, Norwood LA. Acute tears of the posterior cruciate ligament: Results of operative treatment. *J Bone Joint Surg Am.* 1980;62:438–450.
39. Hughston JC. The posterior cruciate ligament in knee joint stability. *J Bone Joint Surg Am.* 1969;51:1045–1046.
40. Loos WC, Fox JM, Blazina ME, DelPizzo W, Friedman MJ. Acute posterior cruciate ligament injuries. *Am J Sports Med.* 1981;9:86–92.
41. Insall JN, Hood RW. Bone-block transfer of the medial head of the gastrocnemius for posterior cruciate insufficiency. *J Bone Joint Surg Am.* 1982;64:691–699.
42. Liljedahl SO, Nordstrand A. Injuries of the ligaments of the knee. Diagnoses and results of operation. *Injury.* 1969;1:17–24.
43. Lysholm J, Gillquist J, Liljedahl S. Arthroscopy in the early diagnosis of injuries to the knee joint. *Acta Orthop Scand.* 1981;52:111–118.
44. Cross MJ, Fracs MB, Powell JF. Long-term follow-up of posterior cruciate ligament rupture: A study of 116 cases. *Am J Sports Med.* 1984;12:292–297.
45. Baker CL, Norwood LA, Hughston JC. Acute posterolateral rotatory instability of the knee. *J Bone Joint Surg Am.* 1983;65:614–618.
46. DeLee JC, Riley MB, Rockwood CA. Acute straight lateral instability of the knee. *Am J Sports Med.* 1983;11:404–411.
47. Zarins B, Adams M. Knee injuries in sports. *N Engl J Med.* 1988;318:950–961.
48. Hughston JC, Andrews JR, Cross MJ, Moschi A. Classification of knee ligament instabilities. Part II. The later-

al compartment. *J Bone Joint Surg Am.* 1976;58:173–179.

49. Robson AWM. Ruptured crucial ligaments and their repair by operation. *Ann Surg.* 1903;37:716–718.

50. Godfrey JD. Ligamentous injuries of the knee. In: Ashtron JP Sr, ed. *Current Practice in Orthopaedic Surgery.* St. Louis: CV Mosby; 1973;5.

51. Marshall JL, Warren RF, Fleiss DJ. Ligamentous injuries of the knee in skiing. *Clin Orthop.* 1975;108:196.

52. Jakob RP, Hassler H, Staeubli HU. Observations on rotatory instability of the lateral compartment of the knee: Experimental studies on the functional anatomy and the pathomechanism of the true and the reverse pivot shift sign. *Acta Orthop Scand.* 1981;52(suppl 191):1–32.

53. Daniel DM, Stone ML, Barnett P, et al. Use of quadriceps active test to diagnose posterior cruciate ligament disruption and measure posterior laxity of the knee. *J Bone Joint Surg Am.* 1988;70:386–391.

54. Polly DW, Callaghan JJ, Sikes RA, et al. The accuracy of selective magnetic resonance imaging as compared with arthroscopy of the knee. *J Bone Joint Surg Am.* 1988; 70:192–198.

55. Barrett GW, Savoie FH. Operative management of acute PCL injuries with associated pathology. Long-term results. *Orthopedics.* 1991;14:687–692.

56. Fleming RE, Blatz DJ, McCarroll JR. Posterior problems in the knee: Posterior cruciate insufficiency and posterolateral rotatory insufficiency. *Am J Sports Med.* 1981; 9:107–113.

57. Lipscomb AB, Johnston RK, Snyder RB. The technique of cruciate ligament reconstruction. *Am J Sports Med.* 1981;9:77–81.

58. Bosworth DM, Bosworth BM. Use of fascia lata to stabilize the knee in cases of ruptured crucial ligaments. *J Bone Joint Surg.* 1936;18:178–179.

59. Cubbins WR, Conley AH, Callahan JJ, Scuderi CS. A new method of operating for the repair of ruptured cruciate ligaments of the knee joint. *Surg Gynecol Obstet.* 1932;54:299–306.

60. Cubbins WR, Callahan JJ, Scuderi CS. Cruciate ligaments. A resume of operative attacks and results obtained. *Am J Surg.* 1939;18:481–485.

61. Coleman HM. Cruciate ligament repair using meniscus. *J Bone Joint Surg Br.* 1956;38:778.

62. Lindstrom N. Cruciate ligament plastics with meniscus. *Acta Orthop Scand.* 1959;29:150–151.

63. Roth JH, Bray RC, Best TM, Cunning LA, Jacobson RP. Posterior cruciate ligament reconstruction by transfer of the medial gastrocnemius tendon. *Am J Sports Med.* 1988;16:21–28.

64. Schmidt TA, Hughston JC, Jacobson KE. Acute posterolateral rotatory instability of the knee. AAOS Presentation, 1992, Washington.

65. Bomberg BC, Acker JH, Boyle J, Zarins B. The effect of posterior cruciate ligament loss and reconstruction on the knee. *Am J Knee Surg.* 1990;3:85–96.

66. Meyers MH. Isolated avulsion of the tibial attachment of the posterior cruciate ligament of the knee. *J Bone Joint Surg Am.* 1975;57:669–672.

67. Torisu T. Avulsion fracture of the tibial attachment of the posterior cruciate ligament. *Clin Orthop.* 1979;143:107–114.

16

Collateral Ligament Injuries

Mark S. McMahon and Arthur L. Boland

Recently, there has been an increased anatomic, biomechanical, and clinical understanding of both the intact and injured collateral ligaments of the knee. This greater understanding has resulted in an evolution of our approach toward surgical treatment and rehabilitation of the traumatized medial and lateral collateral ligaments.

Anatomy

Medial Collateral Ligament

The medial collateral ligament (MCL) takes its origin from the medial epicondyle of the femur, inserting on the tibia approximately 4 cm distal to the joint line (Fig. 16–1). Warren and Marshall described a three-layered organization of the medial aspect of the knee.[1] Layer 1 includes the crural fascia and is external to the superficial MCL. The crural fascia is defined by the fascial insertion of the sartorius muscle. The gracilis and semitendinosus tendons lie posteromedially between layers 1 and 2.

Layer 2 consists of the superficial MCL, the primary static stabilizer to valgus stress. The origin of the superficial MCL is reinforced by the vastus medialis obliquus. The superficial MCL has been shown to consist of both vertical and oblique portions which function differently with knee joint motion.[2] The vertical fibers remain taut throughout the range of motion of the knee, with the oblique portion becoming lax with flexion. These oblique fibers are considered by Hughston and Eilers to represent a discrete structure commonly termed the *posterior oblique ligament*.[3]

Layer 3 consists of the joint capsule and the deep MCL. The medial meniscus is firmly attached to this layer. The coronary, or meniscotibial, portion of the deep MCL remains a discrete structure, whereas the meniscofemoral portion of the deep MCL may fuse with the overlying superficial MCL. The superficial and deep portions of the MCL fuse posteromedially, blending into the tendon sheath of the semimembranosus.

Lateral Collateral Ligament

The lateral collateral ligament (LCL) originates on the lateral epicondyle of the femur and inserts into the head of the fibula (Fig. 16–2). The lateral aspect of the knee can be considered to consist of three layers.[4] Layer 1 includes the iliotibial tract[5] and the superficial portion of the biceps femoris. The iliotibial tract inserts into Gerdy's tubercle; the biceps femoris inserts into the fibular head.

Layer 2 includes the extracapsular lateral collateral ligament, and is represented anteriorly by the quadriceps retinaculum and posteriorly by the two patellofemoral ligaments and the patellomeniscal ligaments. Layer 3 consists of the joint capsule, including the arcuate and fabellofibular ligaments.

The lateral aspect of the knee can also be divided into anterior, middle, and posterior thirds.[3] The anterior third consists of the joint capsule, which extends posteriorly from the lateral border of the patella and patellar tendon. The middle third includes the iliotibial band and the capsular ligaments deep to it, as well as the LCL, posteriorly. The posterior third is termed the *arcuate complex* and consists of the LCL anteriorly, the arcuate ligament, and the popliteus. The arcuate ligament arches from the posterolateral corner of the tibia to the femur. The popliteus muscle originates posteriorly on the proximal tibia, running laterally and superiorly to insert on the femur just anterior to the LCL. The posterior third of the lateral ligamentous complex is dynamically reinforced by the biceps femoris, popliteus,

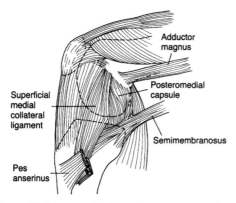

Figure 16–1. The medial ligamentous support consists of the superficial medial collateral ligament, which extends distally under the pes tendons and the deeper capsular ligaments, attaching from the femoral condyle to the meniscus and then to the tibia. The posterior medial capsule, the posterior oblique ligament, is an expansion from the semimembranes. (Reprinted with permission from Hughston JC, Eilers AF. The role of the posterior oblique ligament in repairs of acute medial (collateral) ligament tears of the knee. J Bone Joint Surg Am. 1973;55:923–940.)

and lateral head of the gastrocnemius. The lateral head of the gastrocnemius originates just posterior to the LCL on the femur.

The quadruple complex has been described by Kaplan as providing functional stability to varus stress.[6] The complex includes the iliotibial band, biceps femoris, LCL, and popliteus.

Histology

Ligaments consist of dense, regularly oriented, parallel bundles of collagen which also contain regularly arranged fibroblasts as well as proteoglycans. Following injury to an extraarticular ligament, there is exudation of blood and associated blood products from disrupted vessels, organization of a fibrin clot, vascularization of the fibrin scaffold, proliferation of cells and synthesis of an extracellular matrix, and, finally, remodeling of the repair tissue.[7,8]

Laws and Walton emphasized that MCL lesions heal via a cellular response mediated by fibroblasts, and that an MCL 1 week after a grade II injury possessed only 13% of the tensile strength of a normal MCL.[9] Frank et al showed that the injured MCL healed by bridging scar formation rather than true ligament regeneration, with some residual valgus laxity.[10] Clayton and Weir demonstrated that surgically repaired MCLs had a more normal histologic appearance than nonsurgically treated MCLs.[11] Woo et al demonstrated increased osteoclastic activity, resorption of bone, and disruption of the nor-

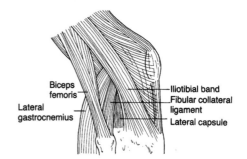

Figure 16–2. The lateral supports consist of the iliotibial band attaching distally at Gerdy's tubercle, the lateral collateral ligament, and the lateral capsule. The popliteus and arcuate ligament support the posterior lateral corner and are deep to the lateral gastrocnemius.

mal attachment of bone to ligament at the femoral and tibial insertion sites of immobilized MCLs.[12] Gomez et al showed that in MCLs that were allowed to heal under tension, cellularity was reduced and collagen alignment was more longitudinally directed compared with MCLs that were allowed to heal without increased tension.[13,14]

Biomechanics

Medial Collateral Ligament

Numerous studies have been performed to assess the mechanical properties of the medial collateral ligament. The MCL normally acts to resist external torque valgus moment and anterior tibial force (when the tibia is externally rotated).[15] Kennedy and Fowler used clinical stress machines to prove that testing for medial laxity should be performed in partial flexion rather than in full extension and that medial capsular ligament injuries need not be present with anterior cruciate ligament (ACL) rupture.[16] Warren et al used similar techniques to identify the superficial MCL as the primary stabilizer of the medial side of the knee against valgus and rotatory stress, and emphasized the importance of the anterior fibers of the superficial MCL.[17] Contraction of the sartorius and vastus medialis muscles has been shown to increase valgus stability substantially; however, the muscles act too slowly to augment the stiffness of the knee so as to prevent injury.[18] Hughston et al emphasized that with an isolated medial compartment tear, the abduction stress test was negative at 0° and positive at 30° of flexion.[19] In addition, the abduction stress test at 0° of flexion was shown to be the most specific test for an acute tear of the posterior cruciate ligament (PCL) with an associated MCL tear.

Grood et al performed selective ligament cutting studies in cadaveric knees and then recorded restraining function as the percentage contribution of each structure in resisting the force applied by the examiner.[20] The MCL provided the primary restraint to valgus stress at both 5° and 25° of flexion from full hyperextension. At 5° the posterior part of the capsule and the cruciate ligaments were important secondary restraints. As flexion increased, the posterior part of the capsule became slack, causing a marked decrease in its restraining action. The deep MCL did not play a major role in valgus stability. Furthermore, with normal knee joint motion, the functional deficit of the MCL in valgus stress is compensated for primarily by the ACL; that is, the ACL appears to play a vital role in resisting valgus laxity.[21] Thus the pathologic increase in valgus laxity in isolated MCL injuries is much smaller than was believed previously, and the initial healing process of the injured MCL can take place without much mechanical disturbance because of the existence of an intact ACL. An intact MCL, on the other hand, effectively helps to protect the anterior cruciate ligament in positions of knee flexion.[15,22,23] With the tibia in an externally rotated position, the force generated in the anterior cruciate ligament increased after a resection of the medial collateral ligament.[15]

Several studies have examined the healing properties of traumatized MCLs. Tipton et al[24] and Vailas et al[25] have shown that strength of a healing MCL is improved with increased physical activity. Hart and Dahners demonstrated that active motion of MCL injuries in rats with intact secondary restraints had a statistically significant beneficial effect on the strength of the healing MCL.[26] Goldstein and Barmada showed that at 6 weeks, mobilized MCLs had higher loads to failure than MCLs immobilized for 3 weeks followed by 3 weeks of remobilization.[27] Similarly, Woo et al showed significant reductions in the ultimate load and energy-absorbing capabilities of the bone–ligament MCL complex after immobilization, with increasing failure by tibial avulsion.[12] Furthermore, Woo et al demonstrated that early mobilization of transected canine MCLs in the setting of an intact ACL was superior to surgically repaired and immobilized MCLs in terms of restoration of mechanical properties.[28,29] This was believed to occur as a result of the valgus stability provided by the ACL. Finally, it has been shown by Gomez et al that at 6 weeks, canine knees with a transected and mobilized MCL were twice as lax as control MCLs[13]; however, joints placed under increased tension after transection had valgus laxity 1.5 times that of control MCLs. At 12 weeks, joints with increased stress were not statistically different from controls.

Lateral Collateral Ligament

Selective ligament cutting studies of the LCL have also been performed. Grood et al showed that the LCL was the primary ligament restraint limiting lateral opening of the joint.[20] It provided 54.8% of the total restraint at 5° and 69.2% at 25° of flexion. The cruciate ligaments, primarily the ACL, were found to be important secondary restraints to lateral opening of the knee joint, especially at 5° of flexion. The middle third of the lateral capsule provides little restraining force. The iliotibial tract and the popliteus musculotendinous unit provided little passive restraint; however, a force applied to either the iliotibial band or the biceps tendon, to simulate muscle tension, produced an additional restraint that in vivo presumably would protect the lateral ligaments and capsule.

The lateral capsuloligamentous complex has been shown to play an important role in the rotational stability of the knee. In 1976, Hughston et al published a classification consisting of six types of lateral instability, including anterolateral and posterolateral rotatory instabilities.[30] Anterolateral knee instability, manifested by the pivot shift test,[31,32] is produced by selective cutting of the ACL and lateral capsule.[33] Lipkey et al performed a selective cutting study to determine that deficiency of the ACL must be present for anterolateral rotational instability to occur, and that anterolateral rotational instability is enhanced by sectioning the posterolateral complex in the LCL.[34]

Posterolateral rotatory instability is characterized by posterior subluxation and external rotation of the lateral tibial plateau about the axis of an intact posterior cruciate ligament, and is usually caused by injury to the LCL and arcuate ligament complex.[35] The mechanism of injury is commonly an anteromedial and varus force to the proximal tibia, often with resultant hyperextension.[36] Correct diagnosis of the entity depends on either a positive external rotation–recurvatum test, a positive posterolateral drawer test, or both.[36] When hyperextension is present, there is usually an associated tear of the anterior cruciate ligament. The posterior cruciate ligament is frequently torn in combination with lateral collateral and arcuate ligament injuries.

Evaluation

History

Collateral ligament injuries about the knee are the result of either direct or rotational forces. Isolated disruption of the MCL usually occurs as a result of a direct blow to the lateral aspect of the knee with the leg fixed.[37,38] As a result of the valgus stress, the patient typically experiences a tearing sensation medially and does not recall hearing a "pop." A careful history is of utmost importance in assessing the mechanism of injury. The magnitude of the valgus injury sequentially causes disruption of the primary medial stabilizer (MCL) and possibly the secondary stabilizer, the ACL.[39] Approximately 10% of isolated MCL injuries are believed to occur as a result of noncontact injuries.[37,38]

A concomitant rotational and valgus injury often results in a combined ACL/MCL injury.[1] Combination injuries involving the MCL and ACL may occur in noncontact-type injuries, particularly in an athlete who is making an abrupt pivot in which the tibia goes into valgus relative to the femur.[40] The noncontact type of injury results from a decelerating maneuver in which the forces can be rather substantial.[39]

Similarly, isolated disruption of the LCL usually occurs as a result of a direct varus blow to the medial aspect of the knee with the leg fixed. Once again, a careful history is important to assess the mechanism of injury. Isolated LCL injuries most commonly occur in wrestlers after straight varus stress.[40] A more severe varus stress in full extension also disrupts the posterolateral capsule and PCL. Hyperextension forces tear the ACL first. Lateral instability of the knee is less frequent, but more disabling than medial instability of a comparable amount.[30] Injuries of the lateral stabilizing ligaments of the knee very frequently involve a rotational component. Anterolateral instability occurs as the result of an internal rotation and varus stress of the knee.[30] Although patients typically do not experience instability while walking, they may experience instability when running, decelerating suddenly, or "cutting." In a patient with posterolateral instability, the mechanism of injury typically involves an anteromedial and varus force to the proximal tibia with resultant hyperextension.[36] Patients typically report that standing is uncomfortable or painful, and that they have a sensation the knee is bent too far backward and does not become normally stabilized with extension.[30]

Physical Examination

The patient with an isolated MCL or LCL injury does not typically manifest a significant joint effusion, insofar as the collateral ligaments are extraarticular structures. Inspection may, however, reveal a more localized and somewhat more superficial area of swelling corresponding in location to the capsuloligamentous complex in question. Swelling usually occurs within several hours. Gait evaluation is helpful in assessing chronic collateral ligament injuries. A medial thrust indicates medial collateral and posteromedial capsule laxity. A lateral thrust indicates lateral collateral and posterolateral capsule laxity. Likewise, tenderness to palpation is usually quite discrete in location. In the case of an MCL injury, the point of maximal tenderness may occur anywhere from the medial femoral condyle to a point 6 to 7 cm along the tibial shaft, along the distal course of the superficial tibial collateral ligament. Localized tenderness at either the origin or insertion suggests avulsion rather

than an intrasubstance tear. LCL disruption is manifested by tenderness to palpation anywhere from the lateral epicondyle to the fibular head. In addition, the normally taut, discrete nature of the LCL, with the joint placed under a varus stress, is replaced by a softer, more boggy quality on palpation. The anterior, middle, and posterior thirds of both the medial and lateral capsules should be specifically and individually palpated.

Hunter et al found that a high correlation exists between tears of the vastus medialis obliquus (VMO) from its femoral attachment and tears of the medial compartment ligaments from their respective femoral attachments.[41] VMO disruptions should be assessed both by direct palpation of the muscle and by assessment of patellar instability, as this finding will have therapeutic and surgical implications. An associated subluxation of the patella must also be ruled out with these valgus injuries.

Evaluation of an MCL injury must include a valgus stress test, which may reveal medial joint space widening, pain, or both. Pain is more likely in incomplete MCL tears. The examiner places the palm of one hand just proximal to the lateral joint line, with the valgus stress imparted by the palm of the other hand just proximal to the medial malleolus. The findings of Grood et al discussed previously, mandate that the knee be stressed in both 0° and 25° of flexion.[20] Joint laxity to valgus stress at 25° that disappears at 0° is suggestive of an isolated MCL tear. Laxity at both 0° and 25° suggests a combined MCL and cruciate injury, as the cruciates are important secondary stabilizers of the knee at 0° of flexion. A positive valgus stress test at 0° necessitates performance of a Lachmann test and posterior drawer test to assess cruciate integrity. An anterior drawer test with the foot in 15° external rotation (Slocum test) can be used to demonstrate posteromedial capsule disruption.[42] Grood et al stated that 4 to 8 mm of joint opening greater than that found in the contralateral normal knee implies significant injury to the collateral ligament.[20]

An isolated LCL injury is evaluated in a similar, although opposite, manner. To perform the varus stress test, the examiner places the palm of one hand just proximal to the medial joint line and imparts a varus force with the palm of the other hand, which is placed just proximal to the lateral malleolus. Once again, the knee should be stressed in both 0° and 25° of flexion, with laxity at 0° suggesting cruciate injury. Anterolateral instability may be demonstrated by a pivot shift test[31] and, if present, confirms the presence of an ACL tear. If posterolateral instability is suspected, the examiner should perform a posterior drawer test with the tibia in neutral rotation, as well as in external rotation.[35,36] A reverse pivot shift should also be performed[43]; however, an increase in external rotation of the tibia on the femur at 30° of flexion when compared with the normal side is the most sensitive test for posterolateral instability.

Radiologic Workup

Standard radiographs are helpful to rule out tibial plateau fractures or growth plate injuries, both of which may produce varus or valgus laxity. A lateral capsular sign[44] or Segund[45] fracture, that is, capsule avulsion of the edge of the lateral tibial plateau, is suggestive of an ACL tear. Roentgenographic evidence of fractures of the fibular head or Gerdy's tubercle suggests lateral knee ligament injury.[46] After a chronic MCL injury, an x-ray may reveal evidence of calcification at the origin of the MCL, that is, the Pellegrini–Steida phenomenon.

Magnetic resonance imaging is useful in evaluation of collateral ligament injuries. A complete tear of an MCL is seen as a loss in continuity of the normal dark band, with a bright signal intensity in the precise area of disruption on T2-weighted images.[47] Subacute tears may manifest as a thickened, buckled, and homogeneously ill-defined low signal band; chronic tears may appear as a thickened ligament with increased signal intensity.[47] On both T1- and T2-weighted images a tear of the lateral collateral ligament is recognized by its complete absence on imaging, by disruption of the straight, homogeneous dark band, or by an area of increased signal intensity within the band.[47]

Classification

Sprains of the ligaments of the knee are graded according to the American Medical Association's recommendation.[48]

First-degree sprain, or grade I tear, is tear of a minimum number of fibers (microtears, or less than one third) of the ligament, with localized tenderness and no instability or laxity.

Second-degree sprain, or grade II tear, is tear of more ligamentous fibers (one to two thirds), with more loss of function and more swelling, mild laxity, and noticeable instability.

Third-degree sprain, or grade III tear, involves more disruption of fibers (greater than two thirds) and demonstrable laxity.[49] Sprains are further subdivided according to the amount of joint space widening[49]:

1 + laxity: <0.5-cm opening of joint surfaces
2 + laxity: 0.5- to 1-cm opening of joint surfaces
3 + laxity: >1-cm opening of joint surfaces

Rotatory instabilities have also been classified[19,30,50] and include anteromedial, posteromedial, anterolateral, posterolateral, and combined. The most common combined instabilities are anterolateral–anteromedial, anterolateral–posterolateral, and anteromedial–posterolateral.[49] When grading these instabilities, 0 is normal, 1+ is a translation of 0.5 cm, 2+ is 0.5 to 1 cm, and 3+ is 1 to 1.5 cm.

Principles of Treatment

Nonoperative Treatment

The current trend is toward nonoperative treatment of collateral ligament injuries. Traditionally, grade I and II injuries were treated nonoperatively, with more and more authors now advocating conservative treatment of grade III tears. The trend toward conservative treatment of grade III tears has its origin in the numerous biomechanical studies described previously. The key to success in treating a complete tear of the MCL[38,51] or LCL is to determine that there is no associated structural damage to the cruciates or menisci. This can be accomplished with a careful history and physical examination, with a magnetic resonance imaging scan ordered if necessary. Ellsasser et al, in 1974, described successful nonoperative treatment of MCL tears.[52] Similarly, Fetto and Marshall reported no difference in outcome between surgically and nonsurgically treated MCL injuries.[53] Hastings,[54] Derscheid and Garrick,[55] and Holden et al[56] all reported excellent results with nonoperative treatment of grade I and II MCL injuries. In 1983, Indelicato performed a prospective study that showed that operatively and nonoperatively treated isolated grade III tears of the MCL had similar long-term results, with nonoperatively treated patients returning to sports 3 weeks earlier.[38] Additional studies have confirmed the efficacy of nonoperative treatment of isolated grade III MCL injuries.[51,57,58] Kannus, however, has advised operative repair of isolated grade III injuries to prevent long-term complications such as medial instability, muscle weakness, and osteoarthritis.[59]

Rehabilitation of grade I MCL injury consists of ice and compressive dressing in the acute stage.[60] Limited pain-free range of motion should begin after 1 to 2 days of rest. The patient can then begin quadriceps and hamstring strengthening, as well as resisted knee flexion and extension. If the patient's strength and range of motion are pain free, and comparable to those of the contralateral side, return to sports is allowed.[60]

According to Sweitzer et al, rehabilitation after grade II and III sprains is initiated after a brief period (7–10 days) of immobilization and minimal weight-bearing crutch ambulation.[60] After the initial 3 to 4 days, the patient may remove the immobilizer several times per day to perform pain-free, active range-of-motion exercise, and may also begin hamstring and quadriceps isometric strengthening. After the immobilization period, a hinged knee brace is worn as the patient progresses with range-of-motion and progressive resistive exercises. Weight bearing is gradually increased as pain decreases and quadriceps strength returns.[60] At 3 weeks the patient can progress to isokinetic flexion and extension exercises.[61] With continued use of the brace, the patient is finally progressed to running and agility drills when there are no symptoms of discomfort with either direct palpation of the MCL or valgus stress. The rehabilitation program varies in length, depending on degree of tissue damage initially sustained and performance demands of the patient.[62]

Rehabilitation of isolated LCL injuries mirrors that of isolated MCL injuries. When a patient is first seen, the area is iced and compressed, and a knee immobilizer is applied in full extension. The patient is allowed to ambulate with crutches, partial weight bearing as tolerated. The three grades of LCL injury are treated according to the guidelines described earlier for MCL injuries.

Operative Treatment

Acute Isolated Medial Collateral Ligament Injuries. As noted in the preceding section, isolated MCL injuries can be effectively treated nonoperatively. The surgeon must be sure that there is no evidence of cruciate ligament injury, however, before continuing with the conservative management of the MCL disruption. Those MCL injuries that have resulted from a valgus external rotation force and extend into the posterior medial capsule often result in disruption of the posterior oblique fibers.[31] A continuation of this mechanism of injury may extend into a partial or complete ACL tear as well. In these cases, it is important that the Lachman test be performed carefully. The tibia may externally rotate because of lack of support in the posteromedial corner, and the Lachman test may appear subtly positive (a pseudo-Lachman test). Thus, one must be sure to keep the tibia in neutral rotation as the Lachman test is performed. If the ACl is intact, the Lachman test will have a firm endpoint with the tibia in neutral rotation.

In those cases in which there is any question about the integrity of the ACL, it is advisable either to obtain a magnetic resonance image or to examine the knee under anesthesia with diagnostic arthroscopy. In those athletes who put great demands on their ligamentous supports while involved in cutting, pivoting, and twisting activities, the surgeon should consider surgical repair of the completely disrupted MCL which has extended into the posterior oblique fibers. The author recommends exploring these knees through a median parapatellar incision that extends toward the adductor tubercle. One must be diligent in locating the exact site of injury. Most frequently it is the deep MCL that is torn near its attachment on the femoral condyle. The medial capsular ligament can be torn at the meniscal

tibial attachments below the meniscus, and the superficial fibers can be disrupted deep to the pes anserinus tendons 8 to 10 cm distal to the knee joint. The MCL can be reattached with sutures through drill holes in the femur and the tibia or by using staples or the recently developed suture anchors (Fig. 16–3).

It is important to address the posterior oblique fibers in the posterior medial corner of the knee, reattaching these to the medial epicondylar area and the posterior edge of the MCL as described by Hughston and Eilers.[3] Following repair of the medial collateral and the posterior oblique fibers, the knee should be taken through gentle range of motion to be sure that the repair is not excessively tight. The knee should also be tested for valgus stability both in extension and in 20° to 30° of flexion. If the MCL fibers are of poor quality, the repair may be reinforced with autogenous tissue harvested from the semimembranosus tendon or the adductor tendon. The adductor fibers are turned down from proximal to distal over the medial collateral repair; the semimembranosus can be brought proximally from the tibia up over the collateral to the medial epicondylar region. Postoperatively the knee should be protected in a hinged brace or an immobilizer in 20° to 30° of flexion. Once the swelling and postoperative pain have begun to subside, gentle range of motion can be initiated, either passively or with active assisted exercises. A touchdown weight-bearing gait is acceptable with gradual progression of weight bearing as quadriceps strength and control improve. The authors recommend 6 weeks of protected weight bearing followed by progressive rehabilitation of the quadriceps and hamstring muscles. Full range of motion, no swelling, and functional strength must be obtained before return to strenuous activities is allowed.

Acute Isolated Lateral Collateral Ligament Injuries. Acute isolated LCL injuries rarely require surgical repair. The treating physician, however, must be aware of the patient's overall knee alignment. Those individuals with a varus knee configuration may require more careful protection and follow-up. The authors have not operated on an LCL that was not associated with some other major ligamentous damage.

Chronic Isolated Medial Collateral Ligament Injuries. As most isolated MCL injuries heal satisfactorily when treated appropriately nonoperatively, the chronic MCL injury that requires reconstruction is usually the result of a combined injury that was not recognized or was not successfully treated initially. Patients who have had previous anterior or posterior cruciate ligament reconstructions that have stretched out or failed may have associated MCL damage that did not heal satisfactorily following the reconstruction of the cruciate ligament. Some of these individuals, therefore, have residual

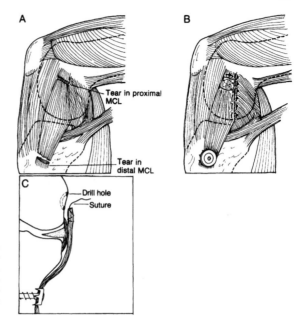

Figure 16–3. A. Disruption of collateral ligament proximally at the femoral attachment and distally near the pes tendons. **B, C.** Medial and frontal views of the repair of the proximal fibers using nonabsorbable sutures placed through drill holes in the bone and the distal fibers reattached with a soft tissue screw. MCL, medial collateral ligament.

anterior/posterior laxity as well as chronic medial instability. If the anterior or posterior laxity is mild, then the MCL reconstruction may be the procedure needed to stabilize the knee more effectively. It is important, however, to emphasize that the late MCL reconstruction will, indeed, stretch out if the anterior and/or posterior cruciate laxity is extensive. The surgeon must therefore be convinced that there is no further need for cruciate reconstruction before attempting an isolated MCL reconstruction.

The authors have used autogenous tissue to perform chronic MCL reconstructions. The semitendinosus tendon, bone/patellar tendon complexes, and adductor or semimembranosus tendons have all been used. When the old medial collateral ligament is detached from the medial epicondyle and advanced superiorly, it is not isometric and has typically stretched out. One may choose to remove the attachment from the medial femoral condyle and then recess it more deeply into the bone at the anatomic site of the femoral condyle; however, the substance of the MCL in chronic instabilities may be inadequate to maintain good stability.

The semitendinosus tendon can be harvested with a tendon stripper, and then, by use of a large needle, the tendon can be threaded through the MCL and the posterior capsule using a baseball stitch configuration and attached to the medial epicondyle (Fig. 16–4). A bony bed in the subchondral bone should be prepared, and the semitendinosus either stapled or secured with a screw-and-washer technique. Any additional length of

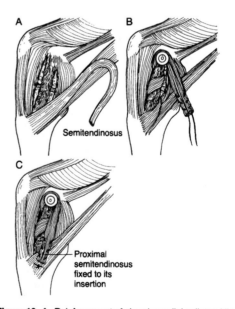

Figure 16–4. Reinforcement of chronic medial collateral ligament laxity with semitendinosus tendon. **A.** Semitendinosus harvested and detached proximally. **B.** Semitendinosus passed through the medial capsule, attached proximally with soft tissue screw. **C.** Remaining tendon brought distally to reinforce repair. The posterior oblique ligament may be advanced anteriorly to the semitendinosus.

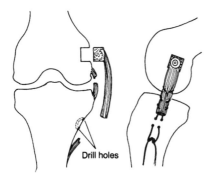

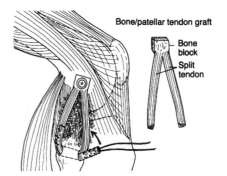

Figure 16–5. Reconstruction of medial collateral ligament with bone/patellar tendon complex. The bone fragment is secured into the femoral condyle with a cancellous screw. The patellar tendon is fixed to the tibia with nonabsorbable sutures into drill holes.

Figure 16–6. Reconstruction of the lateral collateral ligament using a bone/patellar tendon complex. The bone fragment is secured into a trough at the lateral condyle with a cancellous screw. The patellar tendon is split. One arm is passed from anterior to posterior, and the other from posterior to anterior, through a drill hole in the fibula. The ends are sutured with nonabsorbable sutures.

tendon can be folded back distally to reinforce the repair down onto the tibia. The authors have also used a bone/patellar tendon complex, from either the same or the contralateral leg. The bone fragment is secured into the medial femoral condyle with a screw and then the patellar tendon is extended distally and attached into the tibia below the joint (Fig. 16–5). It is also acceptable to use allografts (either bone/patellar tendon or Achilles tendon, with a portion of os calcis) to perform a similar reconstruction. When additional tissue is needed for further reinforcement, the procedure described above, using either the semimembranosus tendon or the adductor tendon, can be employed.

When the repair is completed, the knee should be examined to be sure there is satisfactory range of motion. Stability should be tested gently in extension and in 30° of flexion. Postoperatively the knee should be protected in a hinged brace or splint. Gentle range of motion for flexion and extension is started as soon as the soft tissue swelling allows.

Chronic Isolated Lateral Collateral Ligament Injuries. As was pointed out earlier, isolated LCL injuries heal satisfactorily without surgery. As in the case of chronic MCL injuries, there are usually combined injuries that have either been overlooked or inadequately treated. One must be diligent to exclude the combined posterior cruciate and posterolateral injuries. These are frequently overlooked. The authors have performed isolated LCL injury reconstructions in a few patients in whom the accompanying anterior or posterior cruciate ligament had already been reconstructed. In those cases in which the ipsilateral patellar tendon has already been used, the contralateral patellar tendon may be harvested to reconstruct the LCL. The iliotibial band and biceps tendons are also sources of material for reconstruction

of the LCL. In reconstructing the LCL, the patellar tendon is used with bone only on one end. The bone fragment is countersunk into a defect created on the lateral femoral condyle at the normal attachment of the LCL (Fig. 16–6). A drill hole is then made in the fibular head from anterior to posterior, and the patella tendon is split longitudinally. Half of the patellar tendon is passed from anterior to posterior through the fibular head, and the other tail is brought from posterior to anterior. The ends are sutured to each other with nonabsorbable sutures.

A strip of autogenous iliotibial band can also be used to reconstruct the LCL. Fixation at the lateral epicondyle can be achieved with a staple, though the author recommends a screw and washer. The iliotibial band is fed through the fibula from anteriorly to posteriorly, and then back up to the adductor tubercle as described earlier. Another satisfactory graft for the lateral collateral ligament is the biceps tendon. One can take a portion of the biceps tendon, detach it proximally, leaving it attached to the fibular head, and then direct the proximal end up to the lateral epicondyle, securing it with a staple or screw and washer.

Postoperatively patients with LCL injury reconstructions should be protected from varus forces. Either a hinged brace or cast is used initially to immobilize the knee for approximately 6 weeks. Gentle range of motion can be initiated as soon as the soft tissues allow. A hinged knee brace should be used to protect the knee, however, during the early weight-bearing period.

Acute Combined Tears of the Medial Collateral and Anterior Cruciate Ligaments. Treatment of acute MCL injuries in combination with a torn ACL has changed significantly over the past few years. Because of the reported complication of arthrofibrosis following acute repairs of the ACL with associated MCL disruption, many surgeons favor splinting these knees temporarily to protect the MCL before proceeding to repair or reconstruct the anterior cruciate ligament. The knee is allowed to move in flexion/extension as soon as possible to regain strength in the quadriceps muscle. Once the patient has recovered functional extension and flexion, the ACL is reconstructed using bone/patellar tendon/bone or a similarly acceptable graft, such as the semitendinosus gracilis. Following completion of the ACL reconstruction, the knee is then examined for valgus laxity at both 0° and 30° of flexion. Most frequently, reconstructing the ACL gives good control of the medial instability. If, however, there is still residual laxity in the medial and posteromedial capsule, it is recommended that these structures be addressed surgically. An incision can be made over the medial epicondyle and along the collateral ligament to the posterior medial corner. A preoperative magnetic resonance image often shows the site of damage of the MCL structure. The medial collateral ligament can then be repaired as described previously under Acute Isolated Medial Collateral Ligament Injuries. It is important in these cases that the posterior oblique ligament be repaired as well. Following the completion of the anterior cruciate and medial compartment repairs, the knee should be carried through a range of motion, and the knee stressed gently at 0° and 30° of flexion to be sure that there is no residual instability. Postoperative care is similar to that for an isolated ACL reconstruction. The knee should be splinted in extension. Active flexion and passive extension exercises can also be used in the immediate postoperative period, as recommended for isolated ACL reconstructions. It is important that the medial collateral and posterior oblique repairs be done in such a way that they do not limit full extension passively.

Acute Combined Tears of the Collateral and Posterior Cruciate Ligaments

Knees that have PCL injuries as well as collateral ligament disruption are usually the result of very severe trauma. They are difficult to treat and an exact diagnosis must be made before proceeding. Often these knees have been significantly subluxed, dislocated, or both. Once the soft tissue swelling and acute bleeding have subsided, and once one is confident there is no neurovascular compromise in the popliteal area, it is recommended that the knee be examined under anesthesia and the ligaments stabilized. The PCL injury may, at times, be reparable, as it frequently is pulled away from its femoral or tibial attachment. Sutures can be placed in the stump of the posterior cruciate and then reattached through drill holes into the anatomic attach-

ments on the tibia or the femur. These primary repairs can be augmented with an autogenous semitendinosus graft or with allograft material, if the surgeon feels it is necessary. In those cases in which the substance of the PCL is not sufficient for repair, a formal reconstruction can be performed using the patient's autogenous bone/patellar tendon/bone or an allograft patellar tendon or the Achilles tendon. In these injuries with multiple ligamentous damage, using allografts is quite helpful, as it reduces the amount of soft tissue dissection needed to complete the procedure.

Once the PCL is reconstructed, it is essential again to test the stability of the collateral ligament. If the MCL and posterior oblique are still unstable, then repair of the collateral ligament should be performed as described in the previous section. At the completion of the procedure, the knee should be tested for range of motion and stability. If one is satisfied with the quality of the tissues repaired, then a continuous passive motion machine may be used between 0° and 30°. Further flexion in a PCL reconstruction can be potentially harmful if the tibia subluxes posteriorly in flexion. It is safer to place the knee in full extension to maintain good position of the tibia relative to the femur. Touchdown weight-bearing gait is allowed, with the knee being protected in a splint or brace for at least 6 weeks. It is important to avoid active or resisted hamstring exercises during the first 4 to 6 weeks following a PCL repair, as this may produce posterior translation of the tibia on the femur, stretching out the PCL reconstruction.

Acute combined LCL ligament injuries are often seen in association with posterior and posterolateral ligament injuries. Those cases involving the PCL and the posterolateral corner are very disabling and must be addressed surgically. Magnetic resonance imaging is very helpful in more specifically locating the site of injury. The acute PCL injury is repaired or reconstructed, as described previously in this section. The entire lateral complex must be explored surgically. Often, the LCL is avulsed from the fibula, sometimes with a fragment of bone. The popliteus tendon can also be disrupted from its femoral attachment or more distally at the posterolateral corner of the tibia. These need to be repaired surgically, along with the posterior cruciate reconstruction. The avulsed fibular collateral ligament with a bone fragment should be sutured back down into the proximal fibula (Fig. 16-7). The bone fragment itself is generally too small to allow screw fixation. Heavy, nonabsorbable sutures can be placed in the ligament and then brought out through drill holes in the fibula. When the lateral collateral ligament is disrupted within its substance, or adjacent to the femoral attachment, sutures can be used to secure it into the lateral epicondyle.

Postoperatively these knees must be protected from varus force. A splint, cast, or hinged brace may be

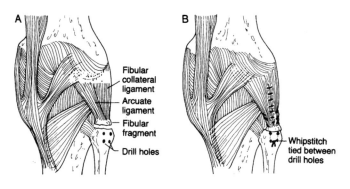

Fibular collateral ligament
Arcuate ligament
Fibular fragment
Drill holes

Whipstitch tied between drill holes

Figure 16–7. Repair of an acute avulsion of the fibular collateral ligament. The fibular collateral ligament is secured using nonabsorbable sutures passed through drill holes in the fibula.

used, depending on the preference of the surgeon. As was noted in the previous section, it is important to prevent posterior translation of the tibia by placing these knees in extension. Gentle range of motion from 0° to 30° may be tolerated, depending on the quality of the repair.

Chronic Combined Collateral Ligament Injuries

As most chronic medial collateral or lateral collateral ligament injuries are associated with either an anterior or a posterior cruciate ligament disruption, it is essential that these central ligaments be reconstructed first. Once the anterior and/or posterior cruciate ligament is reconstructed, the collateral ligaments must be addressed again. As in the case of acute combined disruptions, once the anterior and/or posterior cruciate reconstruction is performed, very often the medial or lateral collateral laxity is much improved. There are, however, cases in which it is essential to go on to reconstruct the medial and/or lateral ligament complexes. When this is necessary, the authors recommend the procedures described earlier for chronic medial and/or lateral collateral ligament reconstructions. Autogenous tissues such as the semitendinosus tendon, bone/patellar tendon/bone

complex, or adductor or semimembranosus tendons can be used to reinforce the MCL. In chronic instability, however, it may be preferable to use allografts such as bone/patella tendon or Achilles tendon for delayed reconstruction of the MCL.

The chronic combined LCL injury most frequently is seen in association with posterior cruciate and posterolateral instability. Following reconstruction of the PCL with autogenous bone/patellar tendon/bone or allograft, the lateral collateral ligament and posterolateral corner (arcuate ligament) must be addressed. We have used the procedure described by Clancy transferring the biceps tendon up to the lateral epicondyle (Fig. 16–8). This effectively reconstructs the LCL and also helps to stabilize the arcuate ligament posterolaterally. It is also possible to reconstruct the LCL and reinforce the posterolateral corner with the iliotibial band. This tendon is harvested and passed through the tibia from anterior to posterior up to the lateral epicondyle and then back to the fibular head (Fig. 16–9). There are a variety of procedures for posterolateral instability; however, no long-term follow-up studies have clearly proven the efficacy of these techniques. The authors have used a variety of procedures but, most recently, have favored the Clancy biceps reconstruction for the lateral collateral and pos-

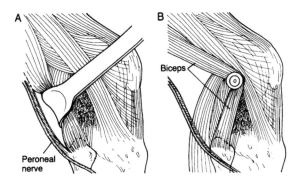

Biceps

Peroneal nerve

Figure 16–8. Reconstruction for chronic posterior lateral instability. The peroneal nerve must be identified and protected. The biceps femoris tendon is mobilized and fixed into a bone trough at the lateral femoral condyle with a cancellous screw.

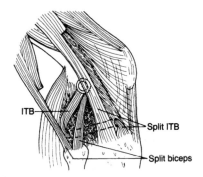

ITB

Split ITB

Split biceps

Figure 16–9. Reconstruction for chronic posterior lateral instability. The iliotibial band (ITB) is harvested and passed through a drill hole in the tibia up to the lateral condyle. A portion of biceps tendon may also be detached proximally and secured to iliotibial band with a soft tissue screw on the lateral condyle.

terolateral corner in combination with bone/patellar tendon/bone reconstruction of the posterior cruciate ligament.

These knees are placed in full extension to protect the knee from posterior subluxation and to allow the posterolateral reconstruction to become secure. Gentle range of motion from 0°–30° may be undertaken if the patient and therapist are careful not to allow any posterior translation of the tibia on the femur.

Results

Conservatively treated patients with isolated collateral ligament injuries do quite well. In general, the delay of return to athletic endeavors correlates well with the grade of injury. Patients with mild grade I injuries may occasionally return to the preinjury activities after 7 to 14 days, whereas those with severe grade III injuries may require as long as 12 weeks. Derscheid and Garrick found that patients with grade I sprains returned to full, unprotected participation after an average of 10.6 days of time lost, whereas those with grade II sprains returned after 19.5 days; neither group showed an appreciably increased likelihood of reinjury.[55] Holden et al reported that conservatively treated athletes with grade I and II tears of the MCL were able to return to full competition at an average of 21 days.[56] Indelicato et al found that the average time from injury to return to full contact drills in patients with grade III MCL tears was 9.2 weeks.[51] In addition, only 8 of 21 players with grade III MCL injuries examined at an average of 46 months postinjury had no detectable clinical valgus laxity when compared with the other knee, although residual laxity did not appear to have any influence on their ability to return to competitive athletics. Jones et

al reported that athletes with grade III MCL injuries who were treated conservatively were able to return to competitive sports at a mean time of 34 days.[57]

Although conservative therapy is the treatment of choice for isolated collateral ligament injuries, Kannus has reported residual medial laxity after grade II tears, as well as a high frequency of medial instability and posttraumatic osteoarthritis in conservatively treated knees with grade III MCL tears[59]; however, many of these patients were found to develop severe anteromedial and anterolateral instability, leading to speculation that many of the original injuries were not isolated to the medial collateral ligament.

Complications and Pitfalls

The preceding discussion draws attention to an overriding pitfall in treating injuries to the collateral ligaments, that is, opting for surgical treatment (with its attendant risks of neurovascular injury, infection, and postoperative stiffness, as well as cosmetic considerations) when nonoperative treatment would suffice. Of course the decision to treat conservatively should be made only after associated injuries, such as cruciate and meniscal injuries, are ruled out. An early magnetic resonance image is helpful in this regard. Meniscal injuries are relatively rare, although they may have an occurrence rate as high as 13%.[59] Associated cruciate ligament injuries must be carefully ruled out before initiating conservative therapy.

Similarly, acute, straight lateral instability of the knee, as described by DeLee et al,[46] in which an LCL injury is combined with PCL injury, may be ruled out by a stable varus stress test at 0° of flexion.

References

1. Warren LF, Marshall JL. The supporting structures and layers on the medial side of the knee: An anatomical analysis. *J Bone Joint Surg Am.* 1979;61:56–62.
2. Brantigan OC, Voshell AF. The tibial collateral ligament: Its function, its bursae, and its relation to the medial meniscus. *J Bone Joint Surg Am.* 1943;25:121–131.
3. Hughston JC, Eilers AF. The role of the posterior oblique ligament in repairs of acute medial (collateral) ligament tears of the knee. *J Bone Joint Surg Am.* 1973; 55:923–940.
4. Seebacher JR, Inglis AE, Marshall JL, Warren RF. The structure of the posterolateral aspect of the knee. *J Bone Joint Surg Am.* 1982;64:536–541.
5. Terry GC, Hughston JC, Norwood LA. The antomy of the iliopatellar band and iliotibial tract. *Am J Sports Med.* 1986;14:39–45.
6. Kaplan EB. Some aspects of functional anatomy of the human knee joint. *Clin Orthop.* 1962;23:18–29.
7. Arnoczky SP. Physiologic principles of ligament injuries and healing. In: Scott WN, ed *Ligament and Extensor Mechanism Injuries of the Knee: Diagnosis and Treatment.* St. Louis: Mosby Year Book; 1991.

8. Jack EA. Experimental rupture of the medial collateral ligament of the knee. *J Bone Joint Surg Br.* 1950;32:396–402.

9. Laws G, Walton M. Fibroblastic healing of grade II ligament injuries. *J Bone Joint Surg Br.* 1988;70:390–396.

10. Frank CB, Schachar N, Dittrick D. Natural history of healing in the repaired medial collateral ligament. *J Orthop Res.* 1983;1:179–188.

11. Clayton ML, Weir GJ Jr. Experimental investigations of ligamentous healing. *Am J Surg.* 1959;98:373–378.

12. Woo SLY, Gomez MA, Sites TJ, Newton PO, Orlando CA, Akeson WH. The biomechanical and morphological changes in the medial collateral ligament of the rabbit after immobilization and remobilization. *J Bone Joint Surg Am.* 1987;69:1200–1211.

13. Gomez MA, Woo SLY, Amiel D, Harwood F, Kitabayashi L, Matyas JR. The effects of increased tension on healing medial collateral ligaments. *Am J Sports Med.* 1991;19:347–354.

14. Gomez MA, Woo SLY, Inoue M, Amiel D, Harwood FL, Kitabayashi L. Medial collateral ligament healing subsequent to different treating regimens. *J Appl Phys.* 1989;66:245–252.

15. Shapiro MS, Markolf KL, Finerman GAM, Mitchell PW. The effect of section of the medial collateral ligament on force generated in the anterior cruciate ligament. *J Bone Joint Surg Am.* 1991;73:248–256.

16. Kennedy JC, Fowler PJ. Medial and anterior instability of the knee: An anatomical and clinical study using stress machines. *J Bone Joint Surg Am.* 1971;53:1257–1260.

17. Warren LF, Marshall JL, Girgis F. The prime static stabilizer of the medial side of the knee. *J Bone Joint Surg Am.* 1974;56:665–674.

18. Pope MH, Johnson RJ, Brown DW, Tighe C. The role of the musculature in injuries to the medial collateral ligament. *J Bone Joint Surg Am.* 1979;61:398–402.

19. Hughston JC, Andrews JR, Cross MJ, Moschi A. Classification of knee ligament injuries. I. The medial compartment and cruciate ligaments. *J Bone Joint Surg Am.* 1976;58:159–172.

20. Grood ES, Noyes FR, Butler DL, Suntay WJ. Ligamentous and capsular restraints preventing straight medial and lateral laxity in intact human cadaver knee. *J Bone Joint Surg Am.* 1981;63:1257–1269.

21. Inoue M, McGurk-Berleson E, Hollis JM, and Woo SLY. Treatment of medial collateral ligament injury. I. The importance of anterior cruciate ligament on the varus-valgus knee laxity. *Am J Sports Med.* 1987;15:15–21.

22. Ahmed AM, Hyder A, Burke DL, Chan KH. In vitro ligament tension pattern in the flexed knee in passive loading. *J Orthop Res.* 1987;5:217–230.

23. Shoemaker SC, Markolf KL. Effects of joint load on the stiffness and laxity of ligament-deficient knees. An in-vitro study of the anterior cruciate and medial collateral ligaments. *J Bone Joint Surg Am.* 1985;67:136–146.

24. Tipton CM, James SL, Mergner KW, Tcheng TK. Influence of exercise on strength of medial collateral ligaments of dogs. *Am J Physiol.* 1970;218:894–902.

25. Vailas AC, Tipton CM, Matthes RD, Gart M. Physical activity and its influence on the repair process of medial collateral ligaments. *Connect Tissue Res.* 1981;9:25–31.

26. Hart DP, Dahners LE. Healing of medial collateral ligaments in rats. *J Bone Joint Surg Am.* 1987;69:1194–1199.

27. Goldstein WM, Barmada A. Early mobilization of rabbit medial collateral ligament repairs: Biomechanic and histopathologic study. *Arch Phys Med Rehabil.* 1984;65:239–242.

28. Woo SLY, Inoue M, McGurk-Burleson E, Gomez MA. Treatment of the medial collateral ligament injury. II. Structure and function of canine knees in response to differing treatment regimens. *Am J Sport Med.* 1987;15:22–29.

29. Woo SLY, Gomez MA, Inoue M, Akeson WH. New experimental procedures to evaluate the biomechanical properties of healing canine medial collateral ligaments. *J Orthop Res* 1987;5:425–432.

30. Hughston JC, Andrews JR, Cross MJ, Moschi A. Classification of knee ligament instabilities. II. The lateral compartment. *J Bone Joint Surg Am.* 1976;58:173–179.

31. Galway RD. The pivot shift syndrome. In: Proceedings of the New Zealand Orthopaedic Association. *J. Bone Joint Surg Br.* 1972;54:558.

32. Galway RD, Beaupre A, MacIntosh DL. Pivot shift: A clinical sign of symptomatic anterior cruciate insufficiency. In: Proceedings of the Canadian Orthopaedic Association. *J Bone Joint Surg Br.* 1972;54:763–764.

33. Johnson LL. Lateral capsular ligament complex: Anatomical and surgical considerations. *Am J Sports Med.* 1979;7:156–160.

34. Lipke JM, Janecke CJ, Nelson CL, et al. The role of incompetence of the anterior cruciate and lateral ligaments in anterolateral and anteromedial. *J Bone Joint Surg Am.* 1981;63:954–959.

35. Hughston JC, Jacobson KE. Chronic posterolateral rotatory instability of the knee. *J Bone Joint Surg Am.* 1985;67:351–359.

36. Hughston JC, Norwood LA. The posterolateral drawer test and external rotation recurvatum test for posterolateral rotatory instability of the knee. *Clin Orthop.* 1980;147:82–87.

37. Hughston JC, Barrett GR. Acute anteromedial rotatory instability: Long-term results of surgical repair. *J Bone Joint Surg Am.* 1983;65:145–153.

38. Indelicato PA. Non-operative treatment of complete tears of the medial collateral ligament of the knee. *J Bone Joint Surg Am.* 1983;65:323–329.

39. Scott WN, Insall JN. Injuries of the knee. In Rockwood CA Jr, Green DP, Bucholz RW, eds. *Rockwood and Green's Fractures in Adults.* Philadelphia: JB Lippinott; 1991.

40. Rettig A. Medial and lateral ligament injuries. In: Scott WN, ed. *Ligament and Extensor Mechanism Injuries of the Knee: Diagnosis and Treatment.* St. Louis: Mosby Year Book; 1991.

41. Hunter SC, Marascalco R, Hughston JC. Disruption of the vastus medialis obliques with medial knee ligament injuries. *Am J Sports Med.* 1983;11:427–431.

42. Slocum DB, Larson RL. Rotatory instability of the knee: Its pathogenesis and clincial test to demonstrate its presence. *J Bone Joint Surg Am.* 1968;50:211–225.

43. Jakob RP, Hassler H, Staeubli HU. Observations on rotatory instability of the lateral compartment of the knee: Experimental studies on the functional anatomy and pathomechanisms of the true and reversed pivot shift sign. *Acta Orthop Scand.* 1981;52(suppl 191):1–32.

44. Woods GW, Stanley RF, Tullos HS. Lateral capsular sign: X-ray clue to a significant knee instability. *Am J Sports Med.* 1979;7:27–33.

45. Segond P. Recherches cliniques et experimentales sur les epanchements sanguines du genou par entorse. *Pro. Med.* 1879;1:279.

46. DeLee JC, Riley MB, Rockwood CA. Acute straight lateral instability of the knee. *Am J Sports Med.* 1983;11:404–411.

47. Glashow JL, Friedman MJ. Diagnosis of knee ligament injuries: Magnetic resonance imaging. In: Scott WN, ed. *Ligament and Extensor Mechanism Injuries of the Knee: Diagnosis and Treatment.* St. Louis: Mosby Year Book; 1991.

48. American Medical Association, Committee on the Medical Aspects of Sports. *Standard Nomenclature of Athletic Injuries.* Chicago: The Association; 1968:99–101.

49. Mont MA, Scott WN. Classification of ligament injuries. In: Scott WN, ed. *Ligament and Extensor Mechanism Injuries of the Knee: Diagnosis and Treatment.* St. Louis: Mosby Year Book; 1991.

50. American Orthopaedic Society for Sports Medicine Research and Education Committee, 1976.

51. Indelicato PA, Hermansdorfer J, Hyegel PT. Non-operative management of complete tears of the medial collateral ligament of the knee in intercollegiate football players. *Clin Orthop.* 1990;256:174–177.

52. Ellsasser JC, Reynolds FC, Omohundro JR. The non-operative treatment of collateral ligament injuries of the knee in professional football players. *J Bone Joint Surg Am.* 1974;56:1185–1190.

53. Fetto JF, Marshall JL. Medial collateral ligament injuries of the knee: A rationale for treatment. *Clin Orthop.* 1978;132:206.

54. Hastings DE. The non-operative management of collateral ligament injuries of the knee joint. *Clin Orthop.* 1980;147:22–28.

55. Derscheid GL, Garrick JG. Medial collateral ligament injuries in football. Non-operative management of grade I and grade II sprains. *Am J Sport Med.* 1981;9:365–368.

56. Holden DL, Eggert AW, Butler JE. The non-operative treatment of grade I and II medial collateral ligament injuries to the knee. *Am J Sports Med.* 1983;11:340–344.

57. Jones RE, Henley MB, Francis P. Nonoperative management of isolated grade III collateral ligament injury in high school football players. *Clin Orthop.* 1986;213:137–140.

58. Sandberg R, Balkfors B, Nilsson B, Westlin N. Operative versus non-operative treatment of recent injuries to the ligaments of the knee—A prospective randomized study. *J Bone Joint Surg Am.* 1987;69;1120.

59. Kannus P. Long-term results of conservatively treated medial collateral ligament injuries of the knee joint. *Clin Orthop.* 1988;226:103–112.

60. Sweitzer RW, Sweitzer DA, Saraniti AJ. Rehabilitation for ligament and extensor mechanism injuries. In: Scott WN, ed. *Ligament and Extensor Mechanism Injuries of the Knee: Diagnosis and Treatment.* St. Louis: Mosby Year Book; 1991.

61. Steadman JR. Rehabilitation of first- and second-degree sprains of the medial collateral ligament. *Am Sports Med.* 1979;1:300–302.

62. Ritter AM, McCarroll J, Wilson FD, Carlson SR. Ambulatory care of medial collateral ligament tears. *Phys Sports Med.* 1983;11:47.

17

Dislocation of the Knee

Kevin D. Plancher and John M. Siliski

Introduction

Traumatic knee dislocations are uncommon but devastating injuries. They include a disparate group of knees that have a variable pattern of ligament disruption, but may also include open wounds, nerve injury, vascular injury, compartment syndrome, intraarticular fracture, and meniscal tears. Limb salvage and restoration of function require thorough evaluation and complex treatment. This chapter reviews the management of dislocations, including the associated vascular and neurologic injuries.

History

The severity and rarity of this injury were discussed by Sir Astley Cooper as early as 1824.[1] In his treatise on dislocations and fractures of the joint he stated, "Of this I have only seen one instance and I conclude it, therefore, to be a rare occurrence and there are scarcely any accidents to which the body is liable which more imperiously demand immediate amputation than these." Birkett in 1850 was one of the first to attempt closed reduction under general anesthesia.[2] Unfortunately, this irreducible dislocation was ultimately amputated. With the advent of roentgenograms in 1895, accurate diagnosis and descriptions of knee dislocations became possible.

There has been a long controversy concerning the treatment of acute ligamentous injury in knee dislocations. In 1937, Conwell and Alldredge in reviewing seven cases stated that closed reduction under general anesthesia with prolonged immobilization yielded gratifying results. In the same article, however, they did admit that some of their cases had considerable instability in the knee after 5 months.[3] In 1963, Kennedy advo-

cated early ligament repair when severe damage is present.[4] Meyers and Harvey in 1971 agreed with this plan and recommended repair of all structures involved in a knee dislocation.[5,6] In 1972, Taylor et al reported that nonoperative treatment of knee dislocations was the method of choice.[7] Sisto and Warren in 1985 and Roman et al in 1987 reported better stability but poorer motion in operatively versus nonoperatively treated cases.[8,9] As late as 1986, Downs and MacDonald advocated external fixation with a plastic cylinder cast for 6 to 8 weeks as the treatment of choice for traumatic knee dislocations with popliteal injuries.[10] Siliski and Plancher in 1989 noted better stability, motion, and knee scores in patients who had undergone operative treatment.[11]

Today, with available techniques of ligament repair and reconstruction, it appears that more favorable results occur in patients treated with early ligament repair.[8,9,12–15]

Anatomy

Knee dislocations are usually accompanied by disruption of many of the soft tissues, including ligaments and menisci. The reader is referred to Chapter 1 regarding general knee anatomy and to Chapters 14, 15, 16, and 18 regarding isolated ligament and meniscal injuries. The basic principles of isolated injuries must be brought together in the management of the complex patterns seen in knee dislocations.

Arterial and neurologic damage is often associated with dislocation of the knee because of the regional anatomy. The popliteal artery (Fig. 17–1) is tethered proximally by the adductor hiatus and distally by the fibrous arch of the soleus. During a complete knee dislocation, there may be insufficient excursion of

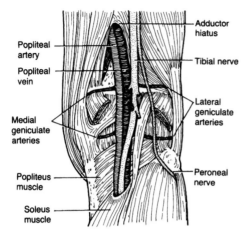

Figure 17-1. Anatomy of the popliteal artery and peroneal nerve.

this artery, causing a traction tear and/or thrombosis. Although there is a collateral vascular anastomosis around the knee joint, these vessels do not provide adequate circulation to the lower leg when injury to the popliteal artery has occurred.[16]

The tibial nerve, which also crosses the popliteal fossa, is not tethered by structures as is the artery and, therefore, has less chance of injury. The peroneal nerve, however, is tethered distally as it passes around the fibular neck. Peroneal nerve palsy is a common occurrence in a knee dislocation, especially with a medial dislocation.

Epidemiology

Epidemiologic data on knee dislocations are limited. As this injury is uncommon, it is essential to combine several studies to arrive at meaningful data. In previous reports of knee dislocations it appears that the male:female ratio is 4:1, with a peak incidence during the third decade of life. Two thirds of dislocations are results of motor vehicle accidents, with sports-related and industrial injuries making up the other largest segments.[3,4,8,9,11,18-20]

Classification

Complete dislocations of the knee have been designated as anterior, posterior, lateral, medial, and rotatory (anteromedial, anterolateral, posteromedial, posterolateral) with respect to the displacement of the tibia in relation to the femur[4] (Fig. 17-2).

In reviewing the literature, Green and Allen, in 1977, found incidences of 30% anterior, 22% posteri-

or, 15% lateral, 4% medial, 4.5% rotatory, and 24.5% unspecified.[21] Other studies have found similar percentages.[22,23] At the Massachusetts General Hospital, in a review of 48 patients, we found 7% anterior, 30% posterior, 11% medial, 2% lateral, 29.5% rotatory, and 2.5% indeterminate.[15] It is clear from most studies that approximately one half of knee dislocations are anterior or posterior, and it is these types that carry the highest risk of vascular injury.

Anterior dislocations are thought to be produced by hyperextension of the knee joint.[4] As the knee hyperextends, the posterior capsule and the cruciate ligaments tear. If hyperextension is severe enough, the popliteal artery is injured. Posterior dislocations often result from a direct blow to the tibia with the knee flexed, as often seen in a dashboard-type injury. A tremendous amount of force is required to produce a posterior dislocation, and this accounts for the frequent arterial injury. Our finding of a large percentage of posterior dislocations in the Massachusetts General Hospital study can best be explained by the high frequency of motor vehicle accidents as the mechanism of injury.[15]

The direction of dislocation, although a simple scheme of classification, does not identify the specific structures injured. Examination under anesthesia is the best method, short of surgical exploration, to identify which ligaments are torn. In most knee dislocations both cruciate ligaments and one collateral ligament complex will be disrupted; however, both collateral ligament complexes may be injured. There are isolated cases in which only one cruciate ligament has been disrupted. The authors have seen one case of a posterior knee dislocation in which only the posterior cruciate ligament was avulsed from the femur (Fig. 17-3). A wide array of ligamentous injuries can therefore be seen in knee dislocations.

Knee dislocations can also be classified by criteria such as open versus closed, fracture dislocations, and high versus low energy. Often the dislocation resulting from a high-energy injury has associated open wounds and intraarticular fracture (Fig. 17-4). When the ligamentous injury is combined with other aspects such as meniscal tears, open wounds, associated intraarticular fractures, and neurovascular injuries, each case takes on an almost unique character.

One other "type" of dislocation requires mention: the spontaneously reduced or "transiently" dislocated knee. This injury is at risk for underdiagnosis and undertreatment. A delay in diagnosis may occur with potentially limb-threatening consequences.[24-37]

Diagnosis and Physical Findings

The critical first step is to make the diagnosis of a knee dislocation. Complete knee dislocation may be defined as a grossly unstable knee as determined by roentgeno-

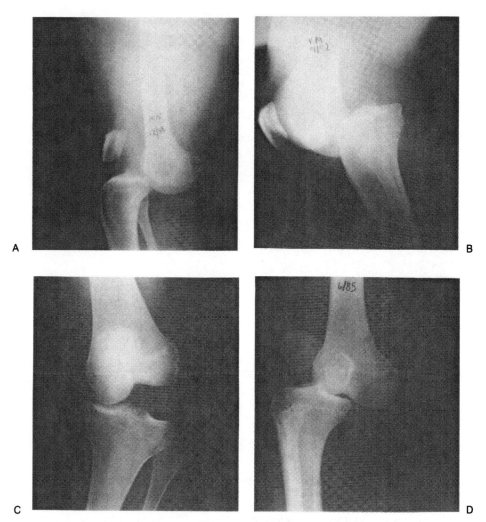

Figure 17-2. Dislocation of the knee. **A.** Anterior. **B.** Posterior. **C.** Medial. **D.** Lateral.

gram or by clinical examination. We include in our definition of knee dislocation those knees that at the time of presentation are reduced but in which both cruciate ligaments and at least one collateral ligament is disrupted. The diagnosis of a dislocated knee is simple when it arrives in the emergency room grossly deformed. An x-ray may be needed to define the exact source of the deformity, which may be the result of a knee dislocation, fracture dislocation, or periarticular fracture. Longitudinal manual traction should be applied to the deformed knee, a splint should be applied, and an x-ray obtained. A knee dislocation may have

been reduced at the scene of an accident or during splinting and transport to a hospital. Such a knee on first inspection may appear relatively benign, because bleeding may diffuse through the torn capsule into the calf and thigh rather than collect in the knee joint. It is essential that stress testing of the ligaments be performed to ensure that the appropriate diagnosis is made. Even without anesthesia, the knee can be gently evaluated for hyperextension and for anteroposterior and varus–valgus instability at 20° of flexion. This occult presentation of a knee dislocation is at risk for underdiagnosis and undertreatment, particularly in the

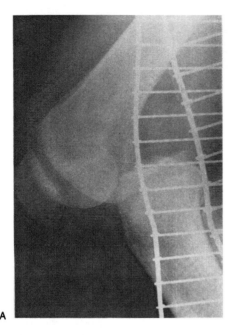

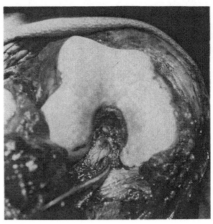

Figure 17-3. **A**. Posterior dislocation of the knee. **B**. Operative findings of an isolated posterior cruciate ligament avulsion. The posterior cruciate ligament was reattached to the femur with excellent motion, stability, and function at 4-year follow-up.

A

multiple-trauma patient. If an occult popliteal artery injury is present, a potentially limb-threatening situation will exist.

Radiographic Evaluation

Plain x-rays of the knee after a dislocation may reveal no abnormality other than soft tissue swelling. If the knee is reduced at the time of x-ray, an unremarkable set of films may be obtained. Subtle subluxation of the knee may be present, however, providing a clue that some significant ligament injury has occurred.

Bone fragments in the intercondylar notch typically represent avulsion fragments on the ends of the anterior or posterior cruciate ligaments, where they have been pulled off the femur or tibia (Fig. 17-5). Unless the fragments are large and in close proximity to their origin, it may not be possible by x-ray to determine to which ligament the fragments are attached; however, the presence of such fragments suggests that at least one cruciate ligament has sustained injury and that if a surgical repair is attempted, reattachment of the ligament may be possible.

Avulsion fragments may also occur related to the collateral ligaments (Fig. 17-6). These may occur at the level of the femur or below the joint at the level of the fibular head and medial tibia. The presence of such fragments suggests that at the time of surgical repair

direct reattachment of a ligament to its bony avulsion site may be possible.

Magnetic resonance imaging (MRI) studies may provide additional information regarding ligament and bony injury prior to surgery (Fig. 17-7). MRI may be able to distinguish ligament avulsion from midsubstance tear, as well as to identify meniscal tears and contusion of the articular surfaces.

Associated Injuries

Complications associated with complete knee dislocations are common and threaten limb preservation and function.

Vascular Injury

Vascular injury with ischemia is a limb-threatening complication of knee dislocations.[23] The reported incidence of popliteal artery injury in the setting of knee dislocation varies from one report to another, most likely reflecting referral patterns and mechanism and energy of injury. Most reports note an incidence of popliteal artery injury of 5 to 30%.[8,9,16,21,25,27,30,33,35-46]

Certainly the management of traumatic arterial injuries in the lower extremity has been a challenge. Hoover in 1961 reported that 67% of patients with knee dislocation and arterial injury required an amputa-

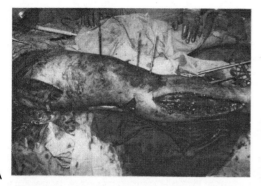

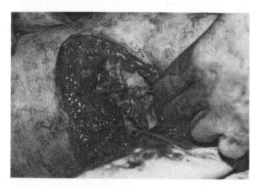

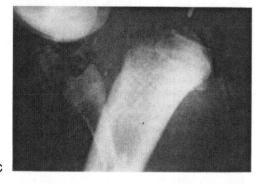

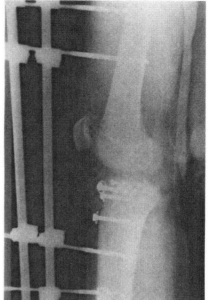

Figure 17-4. A. High-energy lower extremity injury with femoral fracture, tibia fracture, compartment syndrome, and knee dislocation. **B.** Open wound over popliteal fossa with exposed tibia and posterior cruciate ligament. The popliteal artery was patent by arteriogram. **C.** Lateral x-ray showing associated fracture of the tibial plateau. Through a small anterior incision the fractures were fixed and the cruciate ligaments and patellar tendon reattached. **D.** External fixator stabilizing the knee and permitting wound management of the knee and calf.

tion.[30] Kennedy reported on a similar series, with an amputation rate of 71%.[4] Untreated injuries of the popliteal artery resulted in a high incidence in amputations in a military population as was reported by DeBakey and Simeone.[47] These authors reported an amputation rate of 72.5% secondary to ischemia in patients with major lower extremity arterial injuries during World War II. During the Korean War, as a result of improved vascular surgical techniques, the amputa-

tion rate in a similar set of patients was lowered to 32%.[48] The amputation rate, however, remained 32% during the Vietnam War.[23] In 1949, Miller and Welch using frogs and an experimental model had shown that arterial repair must be performed within 8 hours of injury. After 8 hours, damage to the muscles in the calf is irreversible and, if extensive, often leads to amputation.[22] In 1977, Green and Allen reported an amputation rate of 86% if vascular repair or reconstruc-

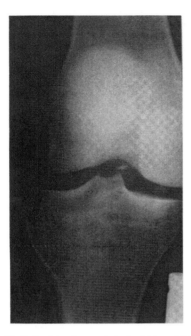

Figure 17–5. Avulsion fragments in the intercondylar notch, originating from the tibial eminence and attached to the anterior cruciate ligament.

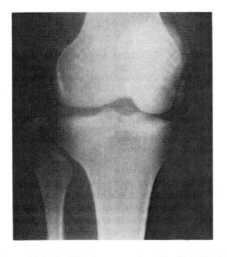

Figure 17–6. Avulsion fragments from the tip of the fibula and medial femoral condyles are radiographic evidence of avulsions of the lateral and medial collateral ligaments.

tion was not done within 8 hours of injury.[41] Wolma showed that vascular injury in a knee dislocation often leads to a poor prognosis. He found that if ischemic time was less than 6 hours, there was an 8.3% amputation rate, whereas ischemic time greater than 6 hours led to a 50% amputation rate.[49] O'Donnell and coworkers at the Massachusetts General Hospital recommended arteriography in every case of knee dislocation because of the serious consequences of arterial injury and the sometimes benign initial appearance of the limb.[36]

The vascular status of a dislocated or grossly unstable knee must be evaluated immediately. Palpation of the posterior tibial and dorsalis pedis arteries should be performed by tactile exam. Treatment of the dislocated knee with manual traction to reduce the joint may relieve pressure on a compressed popliteal artery to restore previously absent pulses. If the pulses are not present and the knee joint has been reduced, evaluation by Doppler studies is in order. If there is any diminution of pulse pressure compared with the other limb, arteriogram or surgical exploration is mandatory (Fig. 17–8). If time constraints are an issue and taking the patient to vascular radiology may jeopardize limb salvage, the arteriogram should be done in the operating room as the patient is prepared for surgery. A single injection arteriogram with a single x-ray usually will provide sufficient information to guide the vascular surgeon.

If pulses in the foot are present and Doppler studies are normal, arteriography may not be mandatory. We have noted in our review of knee dislocations seen at the Massachusetts General Hospital during the past two decades that 20 cases did not have arteriograms performed.[15] None of these resulted in subsequent clinical vascular problems. There is, however, a risk that if an arteriogram is not performed, an unidentified intimal tear may be missed. The tear may progress to arterial thrombosis if the patient is not anticoagulated, resulting in a vascular emergency.

Peripheral nerves are affected by decreased blood flow. Changes in motor strength and/or sensory exam may be a clue to a popliteal artery thrombosis. Distinguishing between a true nerve injury, ischemic neuropathy, and a limb too painful to move voluntarily may be difficult to do clinically. When treating a patient with a knee dislocation, as Lefrak in 1976 noted, this scenario mandates an arteriogram.[32]

When vascular repair is needed, the contralateral saphenous vein is usually used to maintain the integrity of the ipsilateral venous superficial system. Reversed saphenous vein grafting is the standard technique for repair of a lacerated or thrombosed popliteal artery.

When popliteal artery injury occurs, limb salvage is the primary concern. There is often a race to achieve revascularization within 8 hours of injury. The ischemia time typically results in a compartment syndrome that

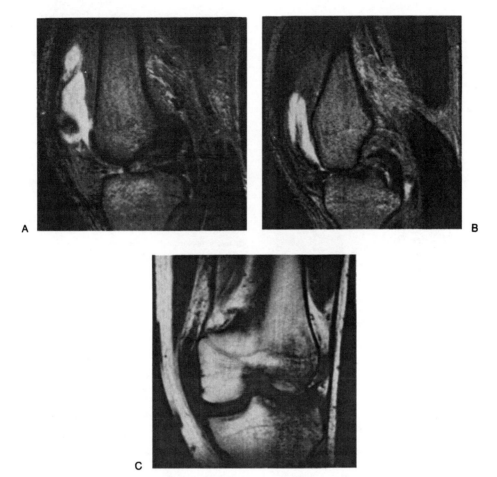

Figure 17-7. Magnetic resonance image of a knee dislocation. **A.** Anterior cruciate ligament avulsed from tibia. **B.** Posterior cruciate ligament avulsed from femur. **C.** Edema at proximal end of medial collateral ligament, suggesting avulsion from femur. Bone contusion of lateral femur and tibia also present.

requires fasciotomies of the calf. There are some who would advocate doing ligament repair and reconstruction at the time of the revascularization and fasciotomy. It is our belief that these surgeries should be staged. After revascularization and fasciotomies, the reduced knee can be stabilized with splints or an external fixator. Anticoagulation is instituted, and the extremity is followed for maintenance of adequate blood flow to the foot. If all proceeds satisfactorily regarding revascularization and fasciotomies, the patient can be returned to the operating room at approximately 7 to 10 days,

and repair of ligaments, menisci, and fractures performed. This second surgery can be done as an "elective" procedure with optimal planning and support for a complicated orthopedic procedure.

In the setting of an intimal injury, identified by initial arteriogram, we recommend that the patient be anticoagulated with the knee splinted in 15° of flexion. Anticoagulation is maintained for a week, at which time it may be safely discontinued if no clinical vascular problems have developed. The orthopedic injuries may then be repaired in an elective and controlled setting.

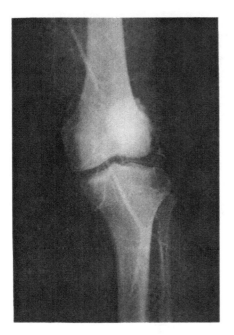

Figure 17–8. Arteriogram of dislocated knee with popliteal artery thrombosis. Saphenous vein grafting of the artery resulted in limb salvage.

Neurologic Injuries

Neurologic injuries, usually peroneal palsy, are unfortunately common and usually permanent when associated with dislocation of the knee. The incidence of peroneal nerve injury ranged from 14% in Kennedy's series to 40% in the study reported by Sisto and Warren.[4,9] In our own series, 44% of patients had a peroneal nerve palsy, with 78% of these being permanent.[15] Tibial nerve injury is uncommon and may be difficult to distinguish from the effects of compartment syndrome and ischemia.

As early as 1971, Meyers et al stated that the prognosis for return of function after peroneal nerve damage is extremely poor.[5,6] At the time of surgery, the usual findings are that the nerve is in continuity, but edematous and hemorrhagic. Severe traction injuries may result in a nerve that is damaged over 10 cm or more. If exposed at the time of early ligament repair, the nerve may be tagged with nonabsorbable sutures to help guide nerve grafting done at a later date. Even if the nerve does not recover acutely, prediction of a permanent nerve palsy can often be done by 2 months postinjury.[15] As 50% or more of these palsies are permanent, an aggressive approach with sural nerve

cable graftings may be warranted. This area is under investigation presently, but insufficient data are currently available to recommend for or against its use. Permanent peroneal nerve palsies may be treated with braces (ankle–foot orthoses), tendon transfers, and hindfoot fusions.[50]

Treatment

The closed dislocation without vascular injury can typically be reduced and splinted in the emergency room, and admitted for subsequent surgery to be done at an optimal time during the first few days after injury. Knee dislocations, because of the extensive ligamentous, capsular, meniscal, and associated fracture disruptions, cannot be treated with early motion as can isolated ligament injuries. The choice for the surgeon is either nonoperative treatment with 8 weeks of immobilization or early repair of the orthopedic structures followed by early motion and rehabilitation.

Nonoperative Treatment

In the absence of significant soft tissue problems, a dislocated knee may be treated with closed reduction with gentle longitudinal traction, followed by casting in approximately 15° of flexion for 8 weeks, as advocated by Taylor et al.[7] A reduction may be maintained by adding a large Steinman pin across the knee, passing from the tibia into the femur in the intercondylar region (Fig. 17–9). The pin may break because of the high forces transmitted across the tibiofemoral joint, and casting must be used while the pin is in place. If used, the pin should be removed at 8 weeks. Most reports of closed treatment have begun knee motion and rehabilitation after 6 to 8 weeks of immobilization

"Olecranonization" of the patella is another option available when acute surgical treatment of ligamentous injuries is not considered appropriate. This technique is performed by placing a large Steinman pin vertically through the patella and into the tibial eminence (Fig. 17–10). A complication that may be seen with this technique is infection at the insertion site over the patella. As this pin is not crossing the tibiofemoral joint, the pin may be less likely to break than a pin connecting the tibia and femur. The knee can even be moved with active assisted range-of-motion exercises in a hinged brace. Insufficient information exists to advocate the routine use of this technique.

When a knee dislocation with a major soft tissue problem exists, several options can be pursued. One method of treatment is closed reduction and casting, with a window or bivalving the cast to manage the soft tissues.[51] Another option is the use of an external fixator across the knee joint, which can provide immobilization and, at the same time, wide access to the

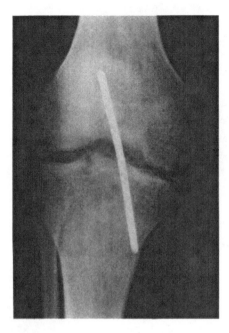

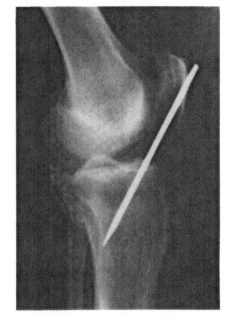

Figure 17-9. Tibial femoral transfixion pin for augmentation of cast immobilization.

Figure 17-10. Olecranonization of the patella.

soft tissues. External fixation may be used as definitive immobilization for 8 weeks or may be used briefly to manage soft tissues. A leg that has undergone vascular repair and compartment releases can be immobilized for 7 to 10 days with an external fixator until ligament repair can be done safely.

Examination Under Anesthesia

Prior to surgical repair, a thorough examination under anesthesia should be performed for instability. In particular, one should look for hyperextension, anterior and posterior laxity at 20° and 90°, varus and valgus instability, and rotatory instability (Fig. 17-11). If disrupted, the lateral collateral ligament will be absent as a discrete structure at the posterolateral corner. Swelling over the medial and lateral ligament complexes usually correlates with instability and the subsequent findings at surgery.

Examination is important to confirm the diagnosis of multiple ligament instability and to help guide the choice of incisions. If the posterolateral structures remain intact, then a second incision will not be required. Even with both cruciate and the medial collateral ligaments disrupted, the knee will be stable to varus stress at 20° if the posterolateral structures remain intact.

There is a small role, if any, for arthroscopy in most cases of knee dislocations. If examination under anesthesia reveals multiple ligament instabilities, as is typical, the surgical repair is an open one. As well, the damaged capsule no longer provides a closed space, and arthroscopy fluid may track up and down the leg creating a problem with soft tissue swelling and even a compartment syndrome. A "dry" arthroscopy may be performed, but is not considered by the authors to be an essential workup in addition to the examination under anesthesia. In the very rare cases where there has been a knee dislocation but the examination under anesthesia does not suggest multiple ligament instability, an arthroscopy may be considered to clarify what structures need to be repaired.

Surgical Techniques

Most commonly, a tourniquet can be used and repair of all orthopedic structures completed within 2 hours. If there has been a vascular injury, use of a tourniquet should be discussed with the vascular surgeon participating in the case.

An anteromedial vertical skin incision is used to approach the cruciate ligaments and medial structures (Fig. 17-12). A medial parapatellar arthrotomy is per-

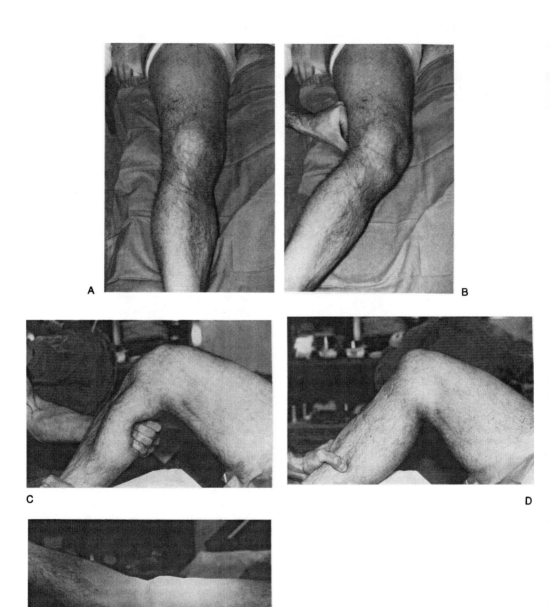

Figure 17–11. Examination under anesthesia after a right knee dislocation sustained in a skiing injury. **A.** Reduced without lateral laxity. **B.** Marked medial laxity on valgus stress. **C.** Anterior drawer. **D.** Posterior drawer. **E.** Hyperextension.

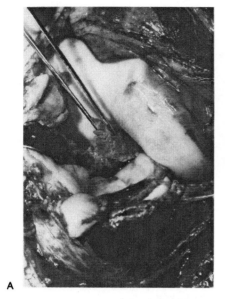

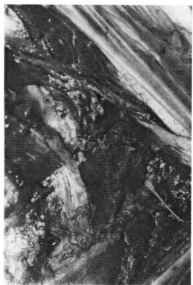

A

C

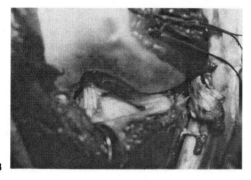

B

Figure 17-12. Intraoperative photographs of same case shown in Figure 17-11. **A.** Anteromedial exposure showing posterior cruciate ligament avulsion from the femur, with peripheral detachment of the medial meniscus. The anterior cruciate ligament has a midsubstance tear, and the medial collateral ligament and medial capsule are completely disrupted. **B.** Reattached posterior cruciate ligament, reconstructed anterior cruciate ligament performed with patellar tendon autograft, and reattached medium meniscus. **C.** Reattached medial capsule, with final steps to reattach medial collateral ligament to the tibia with screw and ligament washer.

formed, and the patella is retracted laterally to gain exposure of the intercondylar region. The lateral compartment can be inspected sufficiently to determine whether there is injury to the lateral meniscus. Typically, when there is a lateral meniscal tear, it is associated with disruption of the posterolateral corner, and the lateral meniscus is repaired subsequently at the time of lateral exposure. The cruciate ligaments are identified and their injuries determined to be either midsubstance or avulsions. Injury to the medial meniscus is sought for, and treatment planned. The medial skin flap can be pulled posteromedially, and the entire capsule and medial collateral ligament inspected. The ends of avulsed structures and the edges of torn structures are tagged for subsequent repair.

After initial inspection of the joint, and identification of the structures that need repair, the surgeon should return to the cruciate ligaments. With an anteromedial arthrotomy, both cruciate ligaments can be reattached or reconstructed using open techniques. On the basis of patient and surgeon preference, midsubstance cruciate ligament tears may be reconstructed with either autograft or allograft. In this setting, a disadvantage of autografting is that two cruciate ligaments may need reconstruction. The harvesting of autografts takes more surgical time, and adds further morbidity to an already extensive procedure. Allografts have the advantage in this situation of shortening operating time and being available in unlimited quantity. If patellar tendon allografts are to be used, they can be prepared by an assis-

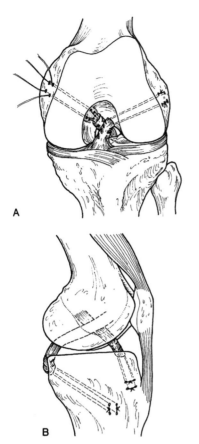

Figure 17–13. Reattachment of the cruciate ligaments, using techniques described by Marshall et al.[52] **A.** Reattachment to the femur. **B.** Reattachment to the tibia.

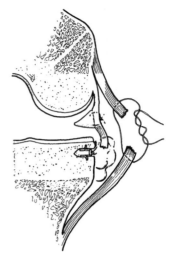

Figure 17–14. Examples of repair techniques of the medial structures. Peripheral detachment of the meniscus is sutured to the capsule (coronary ligament). Capsular avulsions are reattached to the tibia. Midsubstance ligament tears are sutured together.

tant on a side table, while guidewires and drill holes are placed in the femur and tibia for the anterior and/or posterior cruciate ligaments. The patellar tendon grafts can then be placed across the joint, but left unsecured until the additional repairs are completed in the medial compartment.

If cruciate ligaments are avulsed from any attachment site and are thought to have a good blood supply, the surgeon may elect to reattach these rather than use a graft. Reattachment can be performed as described by Marshall et al[52] (Fig. 17–13). Because of the instability of the joint, even the attachment of the posterior cruciate ligament to the tibia can be performed easily under direct vision, as the tibia can be brought quite far forward in the presence of tears of both cruciate ligaments. We have used No. 5 nonabsorbable sutures placed as whipstitches in the ends of the cruciate ligaments. Two

sutures are used, leaving four ends at the periphery of the avulsed ligament. Guidewires, with holes in the tips, can be drilled using a ligament guide system so that the four sutures can be passed through bone to be tied over a bone bridge on the femur and tibia. The base for the ligament reattachment should be curetted or burred to a bleeding surface to promote healing. Although there are controversies regarding the success of reattachment of cruciate ligaments, our experience has been quite satisfactory with this technique in the setting of a knee dislocation.[15] As (1) ligament avulsion is very common in knee dislocations, (2) the reattachment is a very quick and simple procedure, (3) the clinical results are very good, and (4) the occasional isolated cruciate ligament reconstruction for a failed reattachment is relatively simple, at the current time it seems reasonable to reattach cruciate ligament avulsions in knee dislocations.

Repair of the medial compartment structures progresses from posterior to anterior and from deep to superficial. The exact nature of the repair will depend on structures injured and the level of injury (Fig. 17–14). The medial meniscus is commonly detached from the coronary ligament and capsule. Appropriate suturing should be done to reattach the medial meniscus. Rarely, the medial meniscus must be excised because of complex tearing through the avascular portion. The posteromedial capsule should be repaired, either by direct suturing or by reattachment to the tibia if avulsed. This can be done either by passing sutures

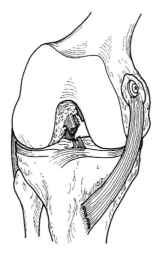

Figure 17–15. Examples of reattachment of the superficial medial collateral ligament. Staples, or cancellous screws with ligament washers, may be used at either reattachment site.

through holes in the tibia placed from front to back or by using anchor sutures. The capsular repair then proceeds anteriorly. The medial collateral ligament is sometimes avulsed with a piece of bone from the medial femoral condyle (Fig. 17–15). If this is the case, reattachment may be relatively easy with a cancellous screw with tendon washer or staples. Likewise, the ligament may be avulsed from the medial face of the tibia, where attachment of the avulsion is quick and simple. If torn midsubstance, the medial collateral ligament is sutured directly to itself.

Repair through the anteromedial exposure is done most easily if grafts and sutures are placed, but not tied, until everything is ready to be secured. The increased mobility of the lax knee makes exposure for all aspects of the repair easier and safer. In general, we prefer to reduce the knee and tension both cruciate ligaments while they are secured in place, either tying sutures or inserting interference screws for reconstructions. We then proceed with tying down the medial structures, working from posterior to anterior and deep to superficial. The medial arthrotomy can then be closed over drains. If the lateral side of the knee also requires repair, that can be done before or after securing in place all of the cruciate and medial repairs.

Surgical exposure of the posterolateral corner is best done with a vertical incision approximately 10 cm long just anterior to the fibular head. The peroneal nerve should be protected posteriorly behind the knee and inferiorly as it passes around the fibular neck. Usually what is encountered is disruption of most of the structures on the posterolateral and lateral side of the knee

(Fig. 17–16). The initial step is to identify all damaged structures, tagging midsubstance tears and avulsed ends of reparable structures. The general process is similar to that on the medial side of the knee. One should work from posterior to anterior and from deep to superficial. The popliteal vessels and tibial nerve may be seen in the deep recesses of this exposure. They, like the peroneal nerve, should be protected. The posterolateral and lateral capsule is typically torn midsubstance or avulsed from the tibia, similar to the medial side of the joint. The capsule is repaired, often simultaneously with reattachment of a peripheral tear of the lateral meniscus. The popliteus tendon may be avulsed from the femur, and if so it can be reattached. Sometimes, it is avulsed from the femur along with the lateral collateral ligament. More often, the popliteus muscle is disrupted at the junction with its tendon. In such cases it may not be reparable. It is unclear how significant loss of the popliteus may be in an injury as extensive as a knee dislocation. The biceps femoris may be avulsed from the fibula along with the insertion of the lateral collateral ligament. In such cases, the two may be simultaneously reattached to the fibula with sutures passed through bone at the tip of the fibula. The biceps femoris muscle may be torn at the junction with the tendon, in which case repair may be difficult. Midsubstance tendinous tears can be sutured together. The lateral collateral ligament may be avulsed from either the femur or the fibula or may be torn midsubstance. It is either reattached to its avulsion site or brought together using whipstitches at the ends of the midsubstance tear. The iliotibial band is commonly avulsed from the tibia and it can often be reattached using a cancellous screw with ligament washer. The peroneal nerve should be inspected gently. This usually requires no further dissection than what has been done for soft tissue repair. If a nerve palsy existed prior to surgery and if a portion of the nerve is noted to be severely damaged, it may be tagged with nonabsorbable sutures at the ends of the damaged section to help guide potential future nerve grafting.

After completion of repairs through the anteromedial and lateral exposures, the wounds are closed over suction drains. The knee is placed in a hinged brace and early motion begun with a continuous passive motion machine.

Open Wounds

Dislocations with open wounds should be taken to the operating room emergently for standard irrigation and debridement. There are certain open knee dislocations in which much of the repair can be done without significant further exposure and trauma to the soft tissues. Closure of the deep structures to repair the joint capsule will in part accomplish some of the repairs, particu-

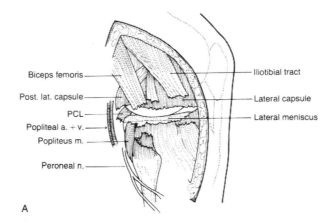

Biceps femoris
Post. lat. capsule
PCL
Popliteal a. + v.
Popliteus m.
Peroneal n.

Iliotibial tract
Lateral capsule
Lateral meniscus

A

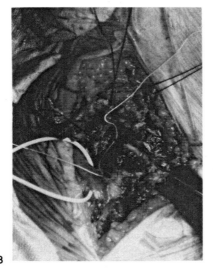

B

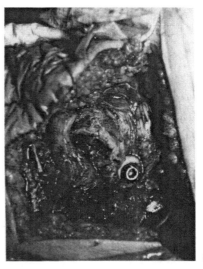

C

Figure 17-16. Structures on the posterolateral corner that are visualized through a vertical incision. Torn or avulsed structures are identified and tagged. Repair procedure from posterior and deep to anterior and superficial. **A**. Diagram of injured structures. **B**. Operative exposure with tagging of damaged structures. The peroneal nerve is identified and protected with a spaghettio. **C**. Completed lateral repair, with screw and ligament washer reattaching iliotibial band. The peroneal nerve is seen at the superficial posterior edge of the incision.

larly to the medial and lateral structures. The knee joint should be reestablished as a closed space if possible, with drains left within the joint. Skin should be left open for subsequent repeat irrigation and debridement and appropriate closure or coverage as needed. If further wound management is expected to be simple, bracing or splinting may be chosen. If wound management is expected to be complicated and prolonged, an external fixator may be used spanning the knee joint. If the soft tissues permit repair or grafting of the ligamentous injuries, this may be done as a staged but early proce-

dure. If soft tissue wounds and concerns about infection are still present a few weeks after injury, then it may be better to complete nonoperative management of the residual orthopedic injuries and apply reconstructive procedures at a more distant date in the future.

Irreducible Dislocations

Irreducible dislocations are uncommon although they have been described.[42,53-56] What has been noted at surgical exploration of these cases is soft tissue interposed between the femur and tibia. Emergency treatment is required to reduce the knee with an open exposure. It is reasonable in this condition to proceed immediately with complete repair of the ligaments, menisci, and associated fractures.

Rehabilitation

Because each case of knee dislocation has some special aspects to the injury, a standardized therapy protocol is not as useful as for isolated ligament injuries; however, some basic principles do exist for this group of injuries.

The basic goal of nonoperative treatment is to allow healing of the capsule and collateral ligaments so at least varus and valgus stability is reasonably restored in the setting of a reduced joint. Most authors recommended initial mobilization for 6 to 8 weeks, followed by weight bearing, passive and active range of motion, and muscle strengthening.

Operative treatment in some series has been reported to result in a poorer range of motion than nonoperative treatment.[8,9] Immobilization after surgical treatment seems to increase stiffness. The goal of operative treatment should therefore be to restore anatomy with sufficient strength of the repair so that early passive motion can begin immediately postoperatively. Because of the multiple capsular and ligamentous repairs required for a dislocation, it is not possible to protect the knee in ways that can be done for isolated ligament injury and repair. Because, in general, significant ligament instability is not a problem after secure ligamentous repair, and because stiffness has been a major issue after surgical repair, we recommend passive and active assisted range of motion of the knee during the first month after surgery, with a goal of achieving nearly full extension, and flexion greater than 90° within the first month. We believe that minor clinical laxity is a lesser evil than a knee that is dysfunctional because of stiffness. Minor laxity of the posterior cruciate ligament appears to be well tolerated. The occasional patient who has had an ACL reattachment that fails can be treated with a relatively simple reconstruction.

Although many patients achieve good and excellent results after knee dislocation, the injury still represents a devastating injury to the knee. Most patients do lose some motion and do not recover entirely normal ligament stability.[15]

References

1. Cooper AP. *A Treatise on Dislocations and Fractures of the Joints*. 2nd ed. Boston: Lilly, Wait, Carter and Hendee; 1832:132.
2. Birkett J. Compound dislocation of the knee. *Lancet*. 1850;2:703.
3. Conwell HE, Alldredge RH. Complete dislocations of the knee joint. *Surg Gynecol Obstet*. 1937;64:94–101.
4. Kennedy JC. Complete dislocation of the knee joint. *J Bone Joint Surg Am*. 1963;45:889–904.
5. Meyers M, Harvey JP Jr. Traumatic dislocation of the knee joint. *J Bone Joint Surg Am*. 1971;53(1):16–29.
6. Meyers M, Moore T, Harvey JP Jr. Follow-up notes on articles previously published in the journal. Traumatic dislocation of the knee joint. *J Bone Joint Surg Am*. 1975;57(3):430–433.
7. Taylor AR, Arden GP, Rainey HA. Traumatic dislocation of the knee. A report of forty-three cases with special reference to conservative treatment. *J Bone and Joint Surg. Br*. 1972;54:96–102.
8. Roman PD, Hopson CN, Zenni EJ Jr. Traumatic dislocation of the knee: A report of 30 cases and literature review. *Orthop Rev*. 1987;16:917–924.
9. Sisto DJ, Warren RF. Complete knee dislocation: A follow-up study of operative treatment. *Clin Orthop*. 1985;198:94–101.
10. Downs AR, MacDonald P. Popliteal artery injuries: Civilian experience with sixty-three patients during a twenty-four year period (1960 through 1984). 4(1):55–62, 1986.
11. Siliski JM, Plancher K. Dislocation of the knee. AAOS Meeting, 1989.
12. Flandry FC, Schwarts MG, Hughston JC. Long term followup of operatively treated knee dislocation. Paper 394, AAOS Annual Meeting, 1991.
13. Frassica FJ, Sim FH, Staeheli JW, Pairolero PC. Dislocation of the knee. *Clin Orthop*. 1992;263:200–205.
14. Montgomery TJ, Hughes JL, Roberts TS, Saboie FH, White JH. Orthopaedic management of dislocations of the knee: Comparison of surgical reconstruction and immobilization. Paper 49, AAOS Annual Meeting, 1992.
15. Plancher KD, Siliski JM. Dislocations of the knee. In press.
16. Doporto JM, Refique M. Vascular insufficiency complicating trauma to the lower limb. *J Bone Joint Surg Br*. 1969;51:680–685.
17. Montgomery JB. Dislocation of the knee. *Orthop Clin North Am*. 1987;18:149–156.
18. Anderson RL, Goldner JL. Dislocation of the knee. *Arch Surg*. 1943;46:598–603.
19. Gross M. Dislocation of the knee. *Orthop Grand Rounds*. 1988;5(1):2–6.
20. Kremchek TE, Welling RE, Kremchek EJ. Traumatic dislocation of the Knee. *Orthop Rev*. 1989;18(10):1051–1057.
21. Green NE, Allen BL. Vascular injuries associated with dislocation of the knee. *J Bone Joint Surg Am*. 1977;59:236–239.
22. Miller HH, Welch CS. Quantitative studies on the time factor in arterial injuries. *Ann Surg*. 1949;130:428.
23. Savage R. Popliteal artery injury associated with knee dislocation improved outlook? *Am Surg*. 1980;46(11):627–632.
24. Aho AJ, Inberg MV, Wegelius U. Dislocation of the knee with total reputare of the popliteal artery. *Acta Chir Scand*. 1971;137:387–389.
25. Alberty RE, Goodfried G, Boyden AM. Popliteal artery injury with fractural dislocation of the knee. *Am J Surg*. 1981;142(1)36–40.
26. Applebaum RR, Yellin AE, Weaver FA, Obergi J, Pentecost M. Role of routine arteriography in blunt lower extremity trauma. *Am J Surg*. 1990;160(2):221–225.
27. Bell WW, Jacocks MA, Carmichael DH. Popliteal artery injury associated with knee dislocation. *J Okla State Med Assoc*. 1984;77:418–421.

28. Chervu A, Quinones-Baldrich WJ. Vascular complications in orthopaedic surgery. *Clin Orthop.* 1988;235:275–288.
29. Hill JA, Rana NA. Complications of posterolateral dislocation of the knee· Case report and literature review. *Clin Orthop.* 1981;154:212–215.
30. Hoover NW. Injuries of the popliteal artery associated with fractures and dislocation. *Surg Clin North Am.* 1961;41:1099–1112.
31. Janes JM, Ghormley RK. Sequelae of vascular injuries. *Am J Surg.* 1950;80:799–804.
32. Lefrak EA. Knee dislocation. An illusive cause of critical arterial occlusion. *Arch Surg.* 1976;111(9):1021–1024.
33. Liedenberg F, Cloete GNP, Dommisse GF, Wyk FA. Injuries of the popliteal artery associated with dislocation of the knee. *Afr Med J.* 1970;44(4):81–86.
34. MacGowan W. Acute ischemia complication limb trauma. *J Bone Joint Surg Br.* 1968;50(3):472–481.
35. McCoy GF, Hannon DG, Barr RJ, Templeton J. Vascular injury associated with low-velocity dislocations of the knee. *J Bone Joint Surg Br.* 1987;69:285–287.
36. O'Donnell TF, Brewster DC, Darling BC, Veen H, Waltham AA. Arterial injuries associated with fractures and/or dislocations of the knee. *J Trauma.* 1977;17:775–784.
37. Settembrini PG, Spreafico G, Zannini P. Popliteal artery injuries associated with knee dislocation. *Cardiovasc Surg.* 1981;22(2):135–140.
38. Cone JB. Vascular injury associated with fracture-dislocations of the lower extremity. *Clin Orthop.* 1989;43:30–35.
39. Dart CH Jr, Braitman HE. Popliteal artery injury following fracture of dislocation of the knee. Diagnosis and management. *Arch Surg.* 1977;112(8):969–973.
40. Eger M, Huler J, Hirsch M. Popliteal artery occlusion assciated with dislocation of the knee joint. *Br J Surg.* 1970;57(4):315–317.
41. Frykberg ER, Crump JM, Vines FS, et al. A reassessment of the role of arteriography in penetrating proximity extremity trauma: A prospective study. *J Trauma.* 1989;29(8):1041–1051.
42. Goldman H. Complete dislocation of the knee with rupture of the popliteal vessels. *J Int Coll Surg.* 1953;19(2):237–242.
43. Jones RE, Smith EC, Bone GE. Vascular and orthopaedic complications of knee dislocations. *Surg Gynecol Obstet.* 1979;149:554–558.
44. Shields L, Mital M, Cave EF. Complete dislocation of the knee: Experience at the Massachusetts General Hospital. *J Trauma.* 1969;9:192–215.
45. Varnell RM, Coldwell DM, Sangeorzan RJ, Johansen KH. Arterial injury complicating knee disruption, third place winner: Conrad Jobst Award. *Am Surg.* 1989;55(12):699–704.
46. Welling RE, Kakkasseril J, Cranley JJ. Complete dislocation of the knee with popliteal vascular injury. *J Trauma.* 1981;21:450–453.
47. DeBakey ME, Simeone FA. Battle injuries in World War II. *Ann Surg.* 1946;123:534.
48. Ziperman HH. Acute arterial injuries in the Korean War: A statistical study. *Ann Surg.* 1954;139:1–8.
49. Wolma FJ. Arterial injuries of the legs associated with fractures and dislocations. *Am J Surg.* 1980;140:806.
50. Siliski JM, Voss F. Lower extremity nerve palsies. In: Gelberman RH, ed. *Operative Nerve Repair and Reconstruction.* Philadelphia: JB Lippincott; 1991.
51. Connolly JF, Yao J. Fracture dislocation of the knee managed by closed reduction. *Nebr Med J.* 1983;69(8):275–277.
52. Marshall JL, Warren RF, Wickiewicz TL, Reider TL, Reider B. The anterior cruciate ligament: A technique of repair and reconstruction. *Clin Orthop.* 1979;143:97.
53. Brennan JJ, Krause ME, MacDonald WF. Irreducible posterolateral dislocation of the knee joint with grossly intact cruciate ligaments. *Am J Surg.* 1962;104:117–119.
54. Clarke HG. Dislocation of the knee with capsular interpositions. *Proc R Soc Med.* 1942;35:759.
55. Quinlan AG. Irreducible, posterolateral dislocation of the knee with button-holing of the medial femoral condyle. *J Bone Joint Surg Am.* 1966;48:1619–1621.
56. Quinlan AG, Sharrard WW. Posterolateral dislocation of the knee with capsular interposition. *J Bone Joint Surg Br.* 1958;40(4):660–663.

Bibliography

Chapman JA. Popliteal artery damage in closed injuries of the knee. *J Bone Joint Surg.* 1985;67(3):420–403.
Collins HJA, Jacobs JK. Acute arterial injuries due to blunt trauma. *J Bone Joint Surg Am.* 1961;43:193–197.
Dhillon KS, Teng TK. Traumatic dislocation of the knee. *Med J Malaysia.* 1987;42(3):173–176.
Esser WR. Anterior dislocation of the knee joint: Report of a case. *J Am Osteopath Assoc.* 1975;12:1159–1197.
Ford GL, Goodner JL. Dislocation of the knee joint. *North Carolina Med J.* 1959;20:463–468.
Griswold AS. Irreducible dislocations of the knee joint. *J Bone Joint Surg Am.* 1951;33(3):787–791.
Gustilo RB, Anderson JT. Prevention of infection in the treatment of one thousand and twenty-five open fractures of long bones. *J Bone Joint Surg Am.* 1976;58:453.
Gustilo RB, Mendoza RM, Williams DN. Problems in the management of type III (severe) open fractures. A new classification of type III open fractures. *J Trauma.* 1984;24:742.
Helferich H. *On Fractures and Dislocations.* London: The New Syndenham Society; 1899:137–138.
Hughston JC. Acute tears of the posterior cruciate ligament. *J Bone Joint Surg Am.* 1980;62:438.
Insall JN, Ranawat C, Aglietil P, Shine J. A comparison of four models of total knee-replacement prostheses. *J Bone Joint Surg Am.* 1976;58:754.
Kobayashi S, takei T, Tagi R, Mamiya N. Reconstruction of the four major ligaments in an unstable knee joint after dislocation by solvent-preserved human fascia lata transplantation. A case report. *Arch Orthop Trauma Surg.* 1989;108(4):246–249.
Levitsky KA, Berger A, Nicholas GG, Vernick CG, Wilber JH, Scagliotti CJ. Bilateral open dislocation of the knee joint. A case report. *J Bone Joint Surg Am.* 1988;70:1407–1409.
Marin EL, Bifulco SS, Fast A. Obesity, a risk factor for knee dislocation. *Am J Phys Med Rehab.* 1990;69(3):132–134.
McCutchan JD, Gillham NR. Injury to the popliteal artery associated with dislocation of the knee: Palpable distal pulses do not negate the requirement for arteriography. *Injury.* 1989;20(5):307–310.
Mitchell JL. Dislocation of the knee. *J Bone Joint Surg.* 1930;12:640.
Moore JM. Fracture—Dislocation of the knee. *Clin Orthop.* 1981;156:128–140.

Mubarak SJ, Owen CA. Double-incision fasciotomy of the leg for decompression in compartment syndromes. *J Bone Joint Surg Am.* 1977;59:184.

Myles JW. Seven cases of traumatic dislocation of the knee. *Proc R Soc Med.* 1967:60:279–281.

Nystrom M, Samini S, Ha'Eri GB. Two cases of irreducible knee dislocation occurring simultaneously in two patients and a review of the literature. *Clin Orthop.* 1992;277: 197–200.

O'Donoghue DH. An analysis of end results of surgical treatment of major injuries to the ligaments of the knee. *J Bone Joint Surg.* 1955;37:1–13.

Pearsall AW, Schuller D. Anterior knee, dislocation: Case report and discussion. *Orthopedics.* 1990;13(2):231–233.

Reckling FW, Peltier LF. Acute knee dislocations and their complications. *J Trauma.* 1969;9:181–190.

Rich NM, Hughes CW. Vietnam vascular registry: A preliminary report. *Surgery.* 1969;65(1)218–226.

Sherry E. Complete dislocation of the knee. *Med J Aust.* 1985;142(10):577.

Shelbourne KD, Porter DA, Clingman JA, McCarroll JR,

Rettig AC. Low velocity knee dislocations. *Orthop Rev.* 1991;20:995–1004.

Siliski JM. Traumatic dislocation of the knee. In: Scott WN, ed. *Ligament and Extensor Mechanism Injuries of the Knee. Diagnosis and Treatment.* St. Louis: Mosby Yearbook; 1991.

Smillie IS. *Injuries of the Knee Joint.* 3rd ed. Edinburgh/London: E & S Livingston Ltd: 1962:213.

Spencer AD. The reliability of signs of peripheral vascular injury. *Surg Gynecol Obstet.* 1962;115:490–494.

Stain SC, Yellin AE, Weaver FA, Pentecost MJ. Selective management of nonocclusive arterial injuries. *Arch Surg.* 1989;24:1136–1141.

Thompsen PB, Rud B, Jensen UH. Joint stability and motion after traumatic dislocation of the knee. *Acta Orthop Scand.* 1984;55(3):278–283.

Walls RM, Rosen P. Traumatic dislocation of the knee. *J Emerg Med.* 1984;(6):527–531.

Weimann S, San-Nicolo M, Sandbichler P, Hafele G, Flora G. Civilian popliteal artery trauma. *J Cardiovasc Surg.* 1987;28(2):145–151.

18
Meniscal Repair and Replacement

Steven P. Arnoczky, Julie Dodds, and Daniel E. Cooper

Introduction

The menisci are C-shaped disks of fibrocartilage interposed between the condyles of the femur and tibia. Once described as the functionless remains of leg muscle,[1] the menisci were relegated to an obscure role within the knee and were often removed with impunity. Unfortunately, the importance of the menisci to the well-being of the knee was often appreciated only after they were removed and the attendant degenerative joint changes became evident.[2-5] Subsequent clinical and basic science studies defined the critical role of the menisci in the complex biomechanics of the knee and underscored the importance of preserving these structures whenever possible.[3-21]

Over the last 10 years meniscal repair has taken the place of traditional meniscectomy in the treatment of certain meniscal injuries.[7,22-40] The advent of arthroscopy and arthroscopic surgical techniques has increased the surgeon's ability to diagnose and treat meniscal lesions.[16,22,27,30,33,35,36,38,39] Although partial and even subtotal meniscectomy must still be done on occasion, meniscal repair has become the preferred procedure to preserve both the meniscus and the subsequent well-being of the knee joint.

Recent experimental and clinical investigations into the use of meniscal allografts have provided some intriguing information regarding the possibility of using such techniques to replace the meniscus and thereby eliminate, or at least minimize, the degenerative changes attendant to meniscectomy.[41-54]

This chapter examines the role of the meniscus in knee joint function, the basic science rationale of meniscus repair, and the clinical progress made in the preservation of the meniscus through repair and replacement techniques.

Meniscal Function

The function of the menisci has been clinically inferred by the degenerative changes that accompany its removal. Fairbank described radiographic changes following meniscectomy which included narrowing of the joint space, flattening of the femoral condyle, and the formation of osteophytes (Fig. 18–1).[2] These changes were attributed to the loss of the weight-bearing function of the meniscus. More sophisticated biomechanical studies have demonstrated that at least 50% of the compressive load of the knee joint is transmitted through the meniscus in extension, while approximately 85% of the load is transmitted in 90° of flexion.[6] In the meniscectomized knee the contact area is reduced approximately 50%.[6] This significantly increases the load per unit area and results in articular cartilage damage and degeneration (Fig. 18–2). Partial meniscectomy has also been shown to significantly increase contact pressures.[8,29] In an experimental study resection of as little as 15 to 34% of the meniscus increased contact pressures by over 350%.[17] Thus, even partial meniscectomy does not appear to be a benign procedure.[8-10,31]

Another proposed function of the meniscus is that of shock absorption. By examining the compressive load-deformation response of the normal and meniscectomized knee it has been suggested that the viscoelastic menisci may function to attenuate the intermittent shock waves generated by impulse loading of the knee during gait.[17,20] Studies have shown that the normal knee has a shock-absorbing capacity about 20% higher than knees that have undergone meniscectomy.[20] As the inability of a joint system to absorb shock has been strongly implicated in the development of osteoarthritis,[55] the meniscus would appear to play an important role in maintaining the health of the knee joint.

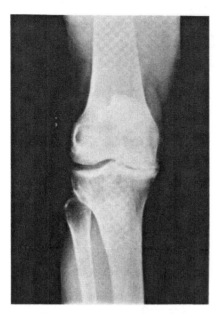

Figure 18–1. Radiograph of a knee illustrating the degenerative changes within the medial compartment joint secondary to medial meniscectomy.

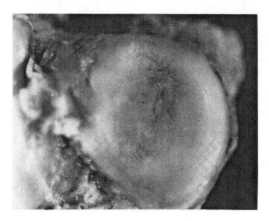

Figure 18–2. Photograph of the lateral tibial plateau of a cadaver knee illustrating the articular cartilage degeneration resulting from an absent lateral meniscus.

In addition to their role in load transmission and shock absorption, the menisci are thought to contribute to knee joint stability. Although meniscectomy alone may not significantly increase joint instability, studies have shown that meniscectomy in association with anterior cruciate ligament insufficiency significantly increases the anterior laxity of the knee.[13]

Because the menisci serve to increase the congruity between the condyles of the femur and tibia they contribute significantly to overall joint conformity (Fig. 18–3). It has been suggested that this function is also synergistic with the lubrication of the articular surfaces of the joint.[56] Although this hypothesis has never been proven it does suggest another important function of the menisci.

Finally, the menisci have been suggested as proprioceptive structures providing a feedback mechanism for joint position sense. This has been inferred from the presence of type I and type II nerve endings observed in the anterior and posterior horns of the menisci.[57,58]

In summary the proposed functions of the menisci include load bearing, shock absorption, joint stability, lubrication, and proprioception. Loss of the meniscus, in part or in total, significantly alters these functions and predisposes the joint to degenerative changes. Because acute, traumatic tears of the meniscus usually occur in young (13- to 40-year-old), active individuals, the need to preserve the meniscus and thus minimize these degenerative changes is of paramount importance.[56] The development of techniques to "save the meniscus" has all but replaced traditional total meniscectomy in the treatment of meniscal lesions. Although partial meniscectomy is still required in many instances, research into new techniques of meniscal repair may one day make even this procedure obsolete.

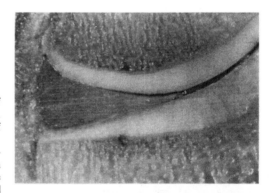

Figure 18–3. Frontal section of the medial compartment of a human knee illustrating the articulation of the meniscus with the condyles of the femur and tibia. (Reprinted with permission from Warren RF, Arnoczky SP, Wickiewicz TL. Anatomy of the knee. In: Nicholas JA, Hershman EB, eds. *The Lower Extremity and Spine in Sports Medicine.* St. Louis: CV Mosby; 1986;657–694.)

Basic Science of Meniscal Repair

Although Thomas Annandale was credited with the first surgical repair of a torn meniscus in 1883,[59] it was not until 1936 when King published his classic experiment on meniscus healing in dogs that the actual biologic limitations of meniscus healing were set forth.[60] King demonstrated that for meniscus lesions to heal they must communicate with the peripheral blood supply.[60] It is apparent, therefore, that a detailed knowledge of the vascular anatomy of the human meniscus must predicate a rationale approach to repair.

Vascular Anatomy of the Meniscus

The vascular supply to the medial and lateral menisci of the knee originates predominantly from both the medial and lateral genicular arteries (both inferior and superior branches).[61] Branches from these vessels give rise to a perimeniscal capillary plexus within the synovial and capsular tissues of the knee joint. This plexus is an arborizing network of vessels that supplies the peripheral border of the meniscus about its attachment to the joint capsule (Fig. 18–4). These perimeniscal vessels are oriented in a predominantly circumferential pattern, with radial branches being directed toward the center of the joint (Fig. 18–5). Anatomic studies have shown that the degree of peripheral vascular penetration is 10 to 30% of the width of the medial meniscus and 10 to 25% of the width of the lateral meniscus. The middle genicular artery, along with a few terminal branches of the medial and lateral genicular vessels, also supplies vessels to the menisci through the vascular synovial covering of the anterior and posterior horn attachments. These synovial vessels penetrate the horn attachments

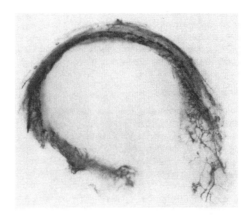

Figure 18–4. Superior aspect of a medial meniscus after vascular perfusion with India ink and tissue clearing with a modified Spaltholz technique. Note the vascularity at the periphery of the meniscus as well as at the anterior and posterior horn attachments. (Reprinted with permission from Arnoczky and Warren.[61])

and give rise to smaller vessels which enter the meniscal horns for a short distance and end in terminal capillary loops.

A small reflection of vascular synovial tissue also is present throughout the peripheral attachment of the medial and lateral menisci on both the femoral and tibial articular surfaces. This "synovial fringe" extends for a short distance over the articular surfaces of the meniscus and contains small, terminally looped vessels.

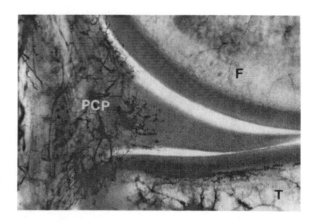

Figure 18–5. Frontal section of the medial compartment of the knee following vascular injection and tissue clearing. Branching radial vessels from the perimeniscal capillary plexus (PCP) penetrate the peripheral border of the medial meniscus. F = femur, T = tibia. (Reprinted with permission from Arnoczky and Warren.[61])

Although this vascular synovial tissue is intimately adherent to the articular surfaces of the menisci, it does not contribute vessels to the meniscus per se. As will be seen later, however, this synovial fringe contributes markedly to the reparative response of the meniscus.

Vascular Response to Injury

As was noted previously, the vascular supply of the meniscus is an essential element in determining its potential for repair. Of equal importance is the ability of this blood supply to support the inflammatory response characteristic of wound repair. Clinical and experimental observations have demonstrated that the peripheral meniscal blood supply is capable of producing a reparative response similar to that observed in other connective tissue.[62,63]

Following injury within the peripheral vascular zone, a fibrin clot forms that is rich in inflammatory cells. Vessels from the perimeniscal capillary plexus proliferate through this fibrin "scaffold," accompanied by the proliferation of undifferentiated mesenchymal cells. Eventually, the lesion is filled with a cellular, fibrovascular scar tissue that "glues" the wound edges together and appears continuous with the adjacent normal meniscal fibrocartilage. Vessels from the perimeniscal capillary plexus, as well as a proliferative vascular pannus from the "synovial fringe," penetrate the fibrous scar to provide a marked inflammatory response (Fig. 18–6).[62]

Experimental studies have shown that radial lesions of the meniscus extending to the synovium are completely healed with fibrovascular scar tissue by 10 weeks (Fig. 18–7).[6] Modulation of this scar into normal-

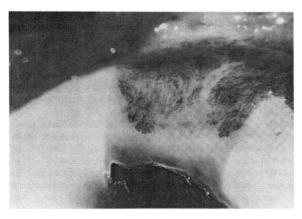

Figure 18–6. Photograph of a healing radial tear in the medial meniscus of a dog 6 weeks following injury. The lesion is healing with fibrovascular scar tissue. Note the proliferative vascular pannus from the synovial fringe over the surface of the repair. (Reprinted with permission from Arnoczky and Warren.[62])

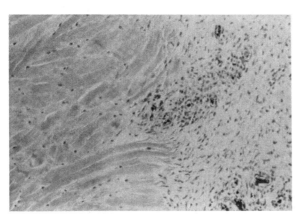

Figure 18–7. Photomicrograph of a healing dog meniscus at the junction of the fibrovascular scar and the normal adjacent meniscal tissue. Hematoxylin and eosin; x100. (Reprinted with permission from Arnoczky and Warren.[62])

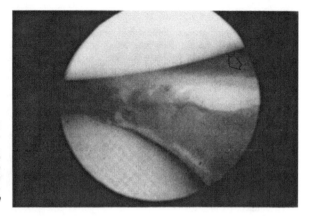

Figure 18-8. Arthroscopic view of a peripheral tear of a human meniscus. Note the vascular granulation tissue present at the margin of the lesion. This would be classified as a red–white tear. Also note the proliferation of the synovial fringe over the femoral surface of the meniscus. (Reprinted with permission from Arnoczky SP, Torzilli PA. Cartilage biology. In: Hunter, Funk, eds. *Rehabilitation of the Injured Athlete.* St. Louis: CV Mosby; 1984.)

appearing fibrocartilage, however, requires several months. It should be stressed that the initial strength of this repair tissue, as compared with the normal meniscus, is thought to be minimal. Further study is required to delineate the biomechanical properties of this repair process.

The ability of meniscal lesions to heal has provided the rationale for the repair of peripheral meniscal injuries, and several reports have demonstrated excellent results following primary repair of peripheral meniscal injuries.[23–26,28,30,34,38] Postoperative examinations of these peripheral repairs have revealed a process of repair similar to that noted in the experimental models.[36]

When examining injured menisci for potential repair, lesions are often classified by the location of the tear relative to the blood supply of the meniscus and the "vascular appearance" of the peripheral and central surfaces of the tear. The so-called red–red tear (peripheral capsular detachment) has a functional blood supply on the capsular and meniscal side of the lesion and obviously has the best prognosis for healing. The red–white tears (meniscus rim tear through the peripheral vascular zone) has an active peripheral blood supply, and the central (inner) surface of the lesion is devoid of functioning vessels (Fig. 18–8). Theoretically, these lesions should have sufficient vascularity to heal by the aforementioned fibrovascular proliferation. The white–white tears (meniscus lesion completely in the avascular zone) are without blood supply and theoretically cannot heal.[64]

Although meniscus repair has generally been limited to the peripheral vascular area of the meniscus (red–red and red–white tears), a significant number of lesions occur in the central, avascular portion of the meniscus (white–white tears). Experimental and clinical observations have shown that these lesions are incapable of healing and have thereby provided the rationale for partial meniscectomy.[60,62,64] In an effort to

"extend" the level of repair into these avascular areas techniques have been developed that provide vascularity to these white–white tears. These techniques include vascular access channels[62] and synovial abrasion.[29]

The concept of vascular access channels stems from the fact that lesions connected to the peripheral vascularity of the meniscus will heal by the aforementioned process. Experimental studies have shown that a lesion in the avascular portion of the meniscus connected to the peripheral blood supply via a vascular access channel can heal through a normal process[60,62,64]; however, because the creation of a large enough vascular access channel may disrupt the normal peripheral architecture of the meniscus other methods of vascular ingrowth have been proposed.[65] These include the creation of vascular tunnels,[65] pedicle grafts of synovium,[65] and synovial abrasion.[29] The latter technique involves the stimulation of the synovial fringe on both the femoral and tibial surfaces of the meniscus. This is intended to produce a vascular pannus that will migrate into the lesion and, it is hoped, support a reparative response. A recent study has demonstrated that an exogenous fibrin clot placed in a stable lesion in the avascular portion of the meniscus can support a reparative response similar to that seen in the vascular area.[66] The clot provides potent chemotactic and mitogenic stimuli as well as a scaffold on which the cellular response is supported.[66] This technique may allow the repair of avascular lesions anywhere in the meniscus or optimize the repair of lesions in areas of marginal vascularity. Clinical studies are currently under way to determine the applicability of this repair technique.

On the basis of these basic science investigations, surgical repair has been widely accepted as the treatment of choice for certain meniscal lesions. This acceptance has also led to the development of a number of surgical techniques with which to accomplish this goal.

Clinical Indications and Techniques

When considering meniscal repair the surgeon must consider the many factors that may affect its result. These include location of the tear, the extent and type of tear, the chronicity of the tear, the age of the patient, and the presence of associated injuries such as cruciate ligament insufficiency. Although a few partial-thickness or short (< 5 mm) stable tears can be treated nonoperatively with expected healing,[67] the majority of clinically evident tears will require surgical intervention. In general, meniscal repair has proved most successful in treating longitudinal, acute, tears in the vascular periphery of the meniscus in young individuals with stable knees. Although other types of meniscal tears (radial, flap, complex tears) have been repaired,[36] the long-term success of these types of repair has yet to be demonstrated.

The question of meniscal repair in an unstable knee has long been a topic of debate among orthopedic surgeons; however, biomechanical studies have documented the role of the meniscus in providing a certain measure of anteroposterior stability in the anterior cruciate deficient knee.[13] Inferred from this data is the fact that the meniscus must experience increased loads in these unstable joints and therefore place meniscal repairs at risk. Follow-up evaluation of meniscal repairs reflects this concern in the high rates of re-tearing that have been reported in anterior cruciate ligament deficient joint.[26,28,29,34-37]

Initial attempts at meniscal repair were limited to peripheral detachments of the meniscus, the so-called red–red tears. These lesions were approached through a longitudinal incision in the area of the meniscal tear. This "open" technique is technically demanding and provides the surgeon only limited access to the central portion of the meniscus.[24-27] Thus, only the most peripheral lesions can be repaired through this approach. Clinical follow-up of these open repairs of red–red tears demonstrated a success rate of 84 to 100% based primarily on the relief of clinical symptoms.[23,26,28,40] Although the results of open repair were better in acute rather than chronic tears, healing was reported in tears repaired up to 7 years after injury.[28]

The advent of arthroscopy permitted better visualization of the menisci. Through the arthroscope the surgeon could gain access to all aspects of the meniscus, and with the development of arthroscopic surgical techniques the repair of the more central red–white as well as the peripheral red–red meniscal tears was possible.

Three types of arthroscopic meniscal repair have been described. Although the specific technique used depends on meniscal tear location and surgeon preference, all have been shown to yield comparable results.

The "inside-out" meniscal suturing technique was proposed by Henning and co-workers[36] and modified by Cannon,[68] Rosenberg et al,[34] Clancy and Graf.[69] In this technique, the tear is first defined arthroscopically and the edges of the meniscal lesion are debrided. A posterolateral or posteromedial exposure is then made to allow the retrieval of sutures. The posteromedial incision is made just anterior to the sartorius tendon with the knee flexed and taken down to the posterior joint capsule just anterior to the semimembranosus. Care is taken to protect the sartorial branch of the saphenous nerve. The posterolateral incision dissects between the anterior border of the biceps femoris and the iliotibial band at the level of the joint line. The lateral head of the gastrocnemius muscle is elevated from the posterolateral capsule to allow suture retrieval. With the knee flexed, the peroneal nerve lies posterior to the surgical dissection. After capsular exposure is gained, a single- or double-cannula system is used to pass sutures through the meniscus, across the tear, into the peripheral rim of the meniscus, and out the posterior capsule (Fig. 18–9). A popliteal retractor is used to avoid piercing the popliteal neurovascular structures with needle passage. Approximately every 4 to 5 mm sutures are placed alternately on the upper and lower surfaces of the menisci. If anterior cruciate ligament (ACL) reconstruction is performed concurrently, sutures may be tied prior to or following reconstruction (see Graf, BK, personal communication, 1992).

The "outside-in" technique as described by Warren[39] and Morgan and Casscells[33] was developed as an attempt to avoid the neurovascular complications originally encountered with the "inside-out" technique. As in the previously described technique the meniscal tear is identified and prepared arthroscopically and the posterior medial or posterolateral capsule exposed. An 18-gauge spinal needle is then passed from the posterior capsule through the rim, across the tear, and into the meniscus under arthroscopic visualization (Fig. 18–10). A suture is then passed through the needle into the joint and brought out through an anterior portal. A large knot is tied in the end of the suture and the knot pulled back into the meniscal body by pulling the "tail" of the suture (Fig. 18–11). This process is repeated every 4 to 5 mm, alternating the knot on the upper and lower meniscal surfaces as needed to stabilize the tear. The "tail" ends of the suture are then tied over the posterior capsule.

The most recent development in meniscal suturing is the all-inside method.[70] This method is applicable to posterior horn tears only and is a good adjunct to the other methods to allow safe access to the most central tears of the medial or lateral meniscus. A posterolateral or posteromedial portal with an arthroscopic cannula is used for placement and tying of a suture that passes

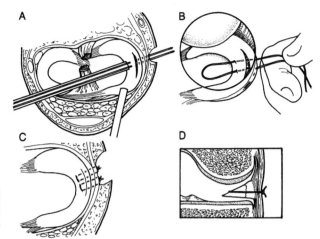

Figure 18–9. Drawing of the "inside-out" technique of meniscal repair showing (**A**) placement of needles through the lesion, (**B**) the horizontal mattress suture in place, (**C**) the sutures tied subcutaneously, and (**D**) the orientation of the sutures through the meniscal tear.

through the meniscal rim and body. Specialized suturing and knot tying instruments are necessary for this type of repair.

As previously noted, several procedures have been proposed to enhance tear vascularity to improve healing rates. Fibrin clot injection[29,66] is performed by obtaining 50 to 75 mL of blood via venipuncture and precipitating a fibrin clot by stirring the whole blood in a glass vessel. The clot is rinsed with saline to remove excess red blood cells and injected into the tear site prior to

tensioning of the repair sutures. Henning has reported an improvement in healing rate from 59 to 92% with this procedure.[71] Vascular access channels, created through the peripheral meniscal rim using multiple needle sticks or trephines, have also resulted in improved healing rates.[36,62,65] When vascular access channels are used, care must be taken to avoid complete disruption of the rim architecture as this is the key to maintaining the "hoop stresses" within the meniscus, which, in turn, maintain the normal load-bearing status of the

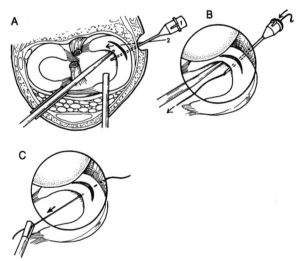

Figure 18–10. Drawing of the "outside-in" technique of meniscal repair showing (**A**) placement of an 18-gauge spinal needle across the meniscal lesion, (**B**) passage of the suture material through the needle, and (**C**) grasping of the suture to pull it out of an anterior portal.

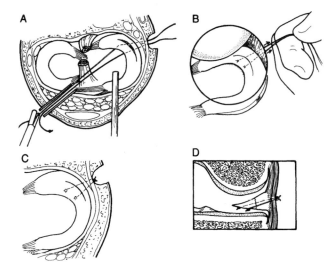

Figure 18–11. Drawing of the "outside-in" technique of meniscal repair showing **(A)** two sutures placed across the meniscal injury and exiting an anterior portal, **(B)** the sutures being pulled flush with the meniscal surface after knots have been tied in the end of the sutures, **(C)** the free ends of the sutures being tied together subcutaneously, and **(D)** the orientation of the sutures through the meniscal tear.

meniscus.[8,18] Synovial abrasion is a relatively simple technique that has been shown to enhance healing in clinical cases.[36]

Postoperative Care

Postoperative rehabilitation following meniscal repair has varied widely among surgeons. It is probably best individualized by patient age, tear type, tear location, and stability of repair. Fu has shown that knee flexion past 70° creates posterior horn excursions of 5.1 mm medially and 11.2 mm laterally.[72] Even the most stable posterior repairs may not be able to withstand this degree of motion early in the healing phase. Weight bearing is usually limited for the first 6 weeks and agility and contact stresses are avoided during the first 6 months. Jogging, cycling, and swimming are allowed when strength and range of motion are adequate.[26] When a concomitant ACL reconstruction is performed, rehabilitation normally follows the ACL protocol with minimal alteration for the repaired meniscus.

Results

Results of meniscal repair have been documented by clinical symptoms, second-look arthroscopies, arthrograms, and, most recently, magnetic resonance imaging (MRI). Lack of clinical symptoms has been shown to be a good indicator of healed meniscal tears as noted on second-look arthroscopy.[73] MRI does not appear to be able to distinguished healed, partially healed, and unhealed meniscal tears in early studies.[74]

Early results of the healing of open and arthroscopic repairs have been reported as 80% or higher.[28,29,33,34] DeHaven reported an 89% success rate at 5 years.[26] At 10 years, a 79% success rate was noted with normal weight-bearing radiographs in 81% of these patients, suggesting adequate meniscal function.[75] Healing rates have been documented to be higher in tears with rim widths greater than 3 mm[76] or 4 mm.[68] Higher healing rates were also noted in patients who have undergone ACL reconstructions.[26,34,76] This may be due to the fact that the joints are stable as well as having increased bleeding (and resulting fibrin clots) following ACL reconstruction. Morgan documented 74 second-look arthroscopies following meniscal repair.[70] Eighty-four percent of tears were noted to be healed, with all nonhealed tears in ACL-deficient knees. Healing rates as a function of tear length have yielded inconsistent results, with increased healing in shorter tears noted by Cannon[68] but not by Buseck and Noyes.[76]

Complications

All arthroscopic procedures have a reported complication rate of 1.5%; meniscal repairs have a rate of 1.2%.[77] As arthroscopic meniscal repair involves posteromedial or posterolateral incisions, the main complications associated with this procedure are related to these incisions and needle passage out the posterior capsule. Saphenous nerve, peroneal nerve, and popliteal nerve and vessel injuries have been reported.[33,34] Fortunately, as this complication has been recognized its incidence has been decreasing.

Meniscal Replacement

Although preservation of the meniscus is now axiomatic, not all meniscal lesions are reparable and total or subtotal meniscectomy is still required in some cases. Because of the deleterious effects of total meniscectomy on the knee joint, alternatives to total removal are being sought. These alternatives include replacement of the removed meniscus with an allograft or synthetic prosthesis.

Allografts

Allograft tissues such as bone, articular cartilage, and fascia have been used in orthopedic surgery for many years.[78–91] When allograft tissues are used as replacement materials, several factors must be taken into consideration. These include (1) the potential antigenicity of the graft; (2) the method of preservation and/or secondary sterilization; and (3) the ability of the graft to maintain (or reestablish) its viability, normal biology, and normal material and functional properties within the host environment. Although substantial amount of information is available regarding these considerations in bone and articular cartilage, experimental and clinical investigations have only recently begun to explore these parameters with regard to meniscal transplantation.

Antigenicity. Meniscal tissue, like articular cartilage, is thought to be an "immunologically privileged" tissue. This is because the meniscal cells, which harbor the major histocompatibility antigens on their surface, are isolated from the host's immune system by a dense extracellular matrix.[82,87] Clinical and experimental studies using fresh menisci alone and fresh menisci as components of fresh osteochondral allografts have not demonstrated any evidence of a rejection or immunologic response.[46,53,92] In addition, experimental studies evaluating the use of "processed" (cryopreserved, fresh-frozen, freeze-dried) meniscal allografts showed no signs of an immune response at any time during the postoperative period.[43,44,46,48–51,53,54]

Preservation. Although experimental and clinical investigations have suggested that fresh menisci can be successfully used as allografts the logistical considerations involved in performing such fresh transplants are substantial. These include locating and preparing an appropriate recipient and performing the harvest and implantation within a 12- to 18-hour time frame. In addition, the inability to adequately screen donors for transmittable diseases within this period may further limit its applicability. The ability to preserve meniscal allografts for long periods would allow for more complete donor screening and a potentially larger bank of meniscal sizes from which to choose.

The methods of preservation for meniscal tissue are essentially the same as for other connective tissues and include controlled-rate freezing (cryopreservation), deep-freezing, and freeze-drying (lyophilization). Although the use of fresh meniscal tissue has the previously noted limitations, the ability to maintain cell viability at the time of transplantation may be advantageous. This concept is based on the finding in articular cartilage of a change in the material properties of nonviable articular cartilage following transplantation.[93,94] The desire to maintain cell viability yet allow storage for long periods has led to the development of cryopreservation techniques that can ensure cell viability following storage.

Several experimental studies have examined the effects of cryopreservation on meniscal tissue and have documented cell viability ranging from 10 to 50% of normal controls.[41,44,46,51] A recent study has, however, shown that after transplantation of a fresh meniscal allograft, no evidence of donor cells could be found 8 weeks after transplantation (see Jackson, DW, personal communication, 1991). This inability of donor cells to survive in the host environment challenges the rationale of transplanting viable meniscal cells and may reflect a cytotoxic process associated with an occult immunologic response. Obviously, more work is needed to determine the role of cell viability in the ultimate fate of meniscal allografts.

Unlike controlled-rate freezing, the preservation techniques of deep-freezing and freeze-drying effectively kill all the cells within the tissue. Although these preservation techniques allow the meniscus to be stored for longer periods they also permit the use of secondary sterilization techniques on the tissue. The two most common methods of secondary sterilization are ethylene oxide and gamma radiation.

Ethylene oxide has been used to sterilize other connective tissues such as bone, fascia lata, and tendon. It is most commonly used in association with freeze-drying preservation techniques. Freeze-dried, ethylene oxide-sterilized fascial and patellar tendon grafts have been used to reconstruct the anterior cruciate ligament; however, an increased incidence of joint effusions following their use and the findings of ethylene oxide by-products in one of these joints have raised many questions regarding this sterilization technique.[95]

In gamma radiation low dosages of gamma radiation from cobalt-60 are used to sterilize tissues. Although precise procedures and dosages have been established to ensure the bactericidal action of gamma radiation, its reliability in killing the human immunodeficiency virus type 1 (HIV-1) without adversely affecting the material properties of the tissue is still questionable.

Allograft Biology and Biomechanics. The long-term ability of a meniscal allograft to survive and function within the knee joint is essential for its success as a therapeutic modality. Over the last several years numerous experimental studies have examined the biologic and biomechanical fate of meniscal allografts, in animal models.[43,44,46,50–54]

An experimental study using cryopreserved menisci showed that 6 months following transplantation, the meniscal allografts were healed to the peripheral capsular tissues by dense fibrous connective tissue.[44] The periphery of the menisci were revascularized in a pattern similar to that observed in normal control menisci.[44] Biochemical analysis of these allografts at 6 months demonstrated that the proteoglycan component of the extracellular matrix was similar in composition to normal control menisci.[44] In addition, biomechanical analysis of the transplants demonstrated no change in the elastic modulus or tensile strength over control values.[52]

In studies using deep-frozen and freeze-dried menisci,[48] it was found that deep-frozen menisci were repopulated with fibroblasts from the host and were revascularized in a pattern similar to that of normal menisci. In freeze-dried menisci, however, this revascularization process extended throughout the tissue and the allografts appeared completely remodeled by 6 months.[48] This remodeling included an apparent shrinkage in the size of the allograft menisci.[48]

A recent study demonstrated that although deep-frozen menisci were capable of being repopulated with cells from the host, a subtle remodeling phenomenon appears to accompany this repopulation.[43] Microscopic analysis of these repopulated grafts reveal a change in the collagen architecture of the superficial and subsuperficial layers of the meniscus.[43] These changes may result in an alteration of the material properties of the

meniscus in these areas and thus make the meniscus more susceptible to injury.[43] Additional long-term biomaterial studies are required to examine the consequences of this remodeling phenomenon.

Clinical Experience. The initial clinical experience with meniscal allografts was gleaned from the results of massive proximal tibial osteochondral allografts in patients undergoing tumor resection for limb salvage.[86,87] In these cases the menisci were left attached and transplanted as part of the total allograft. Although the contribution of the meniscus to the overall clinical success of these transplants is difficult to assess, this experience suggested that meniscal transplantation was at least feasible.

An indication of the fate of the meniscus when transplanted as part of an osteochondral allograft has been reported.[53] In this study, menisci were transplanted as part of a fresh, small-fragment, osteochondral allograft of the proximal tibial plateau. Arthroscopic "second looks" at these menisci as long as 8.5 years postoperatively found them to be viable on gross and histologic evaluation. This evaluation, albeit limited, provided evidence that a transplanted fresh meniscal allograft was viable several years postoperatively.[53] In addition, the study showed no evidence of a rejection response at the time of evaluation.[53]

The preceding experience has provided some of the clinical basis for the transplantation of isolated meniscal allografts.[42] The first report on isolated meniscal allografts came from Munich and documented the use of deep-frozen and freeze-dried meniscal allografts in 22 patients.[42,48,50] The patients in this study all had ACL reconstruction using a patellar tendon and a meniscal allograft (Fig. 8–12). At a minimum follow-up time of

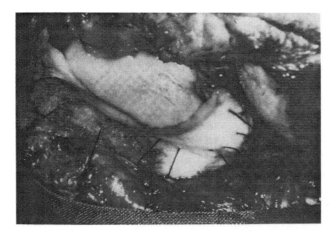

Figure 18–12. Operative photograph showing the exposure of the medial compartment of the human knee and the placement of sutures in the peripheral aspect of a meniscal allograft. (Reprinted with permission from Arnoczky and Milachowski.[42])

24 months (range 24–50 months), the patients with deep-frozen allografts demonstrated good to excellent clinical results using the Lysholm knee score, whereas the freeze-dried meniscal allografts were less successful. Arthroscopic "second looks" in 19 of these patients at various intervals revealed that the menisci appeared to be healed firmly to the peripheral capsular tissues in 18 cases (Fig. 18–13).[42,48,50] There was one case in which the meniscus failed to heal to the peripheral capsule and was removed. The report also noted that although both the deep-frozen and freeze-dried menisci appeared to "shrink" in size following transplantation, the shrinkage associated with the freeze-dried menisci appeared more pronounced (Fig. 18–14). In addition, increased synovial reactions and articular cartilage degeneration were noted in the freeze-dried transplants. These clinical findings coupled with similar findings in animals models suggest that freeze-drying may not be an appropriate processing method for meniscal allografts.[42]

Another clinical study reports on a minimum 2-year follow-up (range 24–44 months) of six fresh meniscal allografts.[45] All patients demonstrated clinical improvement postoperatively and "second-look" arthroscopic examinations of four of the patients revealed normal-appearing menisci. The menisci were firmly healed to the peripheral capsular tissues and showed no evidence of shrinkage.

Although the aforementioned clinical studies provide only limited insight into the efficacy of meniscal allografts the clinical experience with meniscal allografts

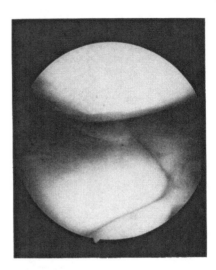

Figure 18–14. Arthroscopic photograph showing the appearance of a freeze-dried meniscal allograft 14 months following transplantation. Although the meniscus is firmly attached to the joint capsule, the meniscus has decreased in size and appears abnormal. (Reprinted with permission from Arnoczky and Milachowski.[42])

continues to increase. Yet, because meniscal transplantation is usually associated with other reconstructive procedures of the knee (ligament reconstruction, osteochondral allograft, osteotomy, etc) the clinical assessment of meniscal allografts is likely to be confounded by several variables. In addition, variations in tissue processing techniques, surgical indications, and the amount of degenerative joint disease present at the time of surgery may further hinder the critical evaluation of meniscal transplantation.

Synthetic Meniscal Replacement

The creation of a synthetic prosthesis that could mimic the normal functional and material properties of a biologic meniscus is a difficult challenge. Not only must the prosthesis be strong enough to withstand tremendous shear, compressive, and tensile forces, it also must be viscoelastic enough to imitate the shock-absorbing function of the normal tissue. In addition, it must be synergistic (both biologically and biomechanically) with the articular cartilage of the femur and tibia. Although these are formidable parameters to duplicate, the creation of such a prosthesis may provide an interesting solution to total meniscectomy. Preliminary work is under way to develop a collagen-based template that will support the regeneration of new meniscus.[96]

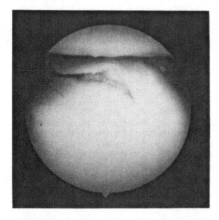

Figure 18–13. Arthroscopic photograph showing the appearance of a deep-frozen meniscal allograft 24 months following transplantation. The meniscus is firmly attached to the joint capsule at its periphery and shows no signs of degeneration. (Reprinted with permission from Arnoczky and Milachowski.[42])

References

1. Sutton JB. *Ligaments: Their Nature and Morphology.* London: MK Lewis & Co; 1897.
2. Fairbank TJ. Knee joint changes after meniscectomy. *J Bone Joint Surg Br.* 1948;30:664–670.
3. Johnson RJ, Kettlekamp DB, Clark W, Leaverton P. Factors affecting late results after meniscectomy. *J Bone Joint Surg Am.* 1974;56:719–729.
4. Krause WR, Clemson MS, Pope MH, Johnson RJ, Wilder DG. Mechanical changes in the knee after meniscectomy. *J Bone Joint Surg Am.* 1976;58:599–604.
5. Tapper EM, Hoover NW. Late results after meniscectomy. *J Bone Joint Surg Am.* 1969; 51:517–526.
6. Ahmed AM, Burke DL. In vivo measurement of static pressure distribution in synovial joints. Part I. Tibial surface of the knee. *J Biomech Eng.* 1983;105:201–209.
7. Arnoczky SP, Cooper DE. Meniscal repair. In: Goldberg VM, ed. *Controversies of Total Knee Arthroplasty.* New York: Raven Press; 1991;291–302.
8. Baratz ME, Fu FH, Mengato R. Meniscal tears: The effect of meniscectomy and of repair on intra-articular contact areas and stresses in the human knee. *Am J Sports Med.* 1986;14:270–275.
9. Cox JS, Cordell LD. The degenerative effects of medial meniscal tears in dog's knees. *Clin Orthop.* 1977;125:236–242.
10. Cox JS, Nye CE, Schaeffer WW, Woodstein IJ. The degenerative effect of partial and total resection of the medial meniscus in dogs. *Clin Orthop.* 1975;109:178–183.
11. Fukubayashi T, Kurosawa H. The contact area and pressure distribution pattern of the knee. A study of normal and osteoarthritic knee joints. *Acta Orthop Scand.* 1980;51:871–880.
12. Kettlekamp DB, Jacobs AW. The tibio-femoral contact area: Determinations and implications. *J Bone Joint Surg Am.* 1972;54:349–356.
13. Levy M, Torzilli PA, Warren RF. The effect of medial meniscectomy on anterior–posterior motion of the knee. *J Bone Joint Surg Am.* 1982;64:883–888.
14. McGinty JB, Geuss LF, Marvin RA. Partial or total meniscectomy? *J Bone Joint Surg Am.* 1977;59:763–766.
15. Mow VC, Arnoczky SP, Jackson DW. *Knee Meniscus: Basic Science and Clinical Foundations.* New York: Raven Press; 1992.
16. Radin EL, Burr DB. Meniscal function and the importance of meniscal regeneration in preventing late medial compartment osteoarthritis. *Clin Orthop Relat Res.* 1982; 171:121–126.
17. Seedholm BB, Hargreaves DJ. Transmission of the load in the knee joint with special reference to the role of the menisci, Part II. *Eng Med.* 1979;8:220–228.
18. Shrive NG, O'Connor JJ, Goodfellow JW. Loadbearing in the knee joint. *Clin Orthop Relat Res.* 1978;131:279–287.
19. Veth RPH, Den Heeten GJ, Jansen HWB, Nielsen HKL. Repair of the meniscus. An experimental investigation in rabbits. *Clin Orthop.* 1983;175:258–262.
20. Voloshin AS, Wosk J. Shock absorption of meniscectomized and painful knees. A comparative in vivo study. *J Biomed Eng.* 1983;5:157–161.
21. Walker PS, Erkman MJ. The role of the menisci in force transmission across the knee. *Clin Orthop Relat Res.* 1975;109:184–192.
22. Barber FA, Stone RG. Meniscal repair. An arthroscopic technique. *J Bone Joint Surg Br.* 1985;67:39–41.
23. Cassidy RE, Shaffer AJ. Repair of peripheral meniscal tears: A preliminary report. *Am J Sports Med.* 1981; 9:209.
24. DeHaven KE. Peripheral meniscal repair: An alternative to meniscectomy. *J Bone Joint Surg Br.* 1981;63:463.
25. DeHaven KE. Meniscus repair: Open vs. arthroscopic. *Arthroscopy.* 1985;1:173–174.
26. DeHaven, KE. Meniscus repair in the athlete. *Clin Orthop.* 1985;198:31–35.
27. DeHaven KE. Meniscectomy versus repair: Clinical experience. In: Mow VC, Arnoczky SP, Jackson DW, eds. *Knee Meniscus: Basic and Clinical Foundations.* New York: Raven Press; 1992;131–139.
28. Hamberg P, Gillquist J, Lysholm, J. Suture of new and old peripheral meniscal tears. *J Bone Joint Surg Am.* 1983;65:193.
29. Henning CE, Lynch MA, Clark JR. Vascularity for healing of meniscus repairs. *Arthroscopy.* 1987;3:13–18.
30. Jacob RP, Staubli HU, Zuber K, Esser M. The arthroscopic meniscal repair: Technique and experience. *Am J Sports Med.* 1988;16:137–142.
31. Lynch MA, Henning, and Glick KR Jr. Knee joint surface changes: Long-term follow-up meniscus tear treatment in stable ACL reconstructions. *Clin Orthop* 1983;172:148–153.
32. Marshall SC. Combined arthroscopic/open repair of meniscal injuries. *Contemp Orthop.* 1987;14:15–24.
33. Morgan CD, Casscells SW. Arthroscopic meniscus repair: A safe approach to the posterior horn. *Arthroscopy.* 1986; 2:3–12.
34. Rosenberg TD, Scott SM, Coward DB, et al. Arthroscopic meniscal repair evaluated with repeat arthroscopy. *Arthroscopy.* 1986;2:14–20.
35. Ryu RK, Dunbar WH. Arthroscopic meniscal repair with two year follow-up: A clinical review. *Arthroscopy.* 1988; 4:168–173.
36. Scott GA, Jolly BL, Henning CE. Combined posterior incision and arthroscopic intra-articular repair of the meniscus. An examination of factors affecting healing. *J Bone Joint Surg Am.* 1986;68:847–861.
37. Sommerlath K. Prognosis of repaired and intact menisci in unstable knees: A comparative study. *Arthroscopy.* 1988;4:93–95.
38. Stone RG, Van Winkle GN. Arthroscopic review of meniscal repair: Assessment of healing parameters. *Arthroscopy.* 1986;2:77–81.
39. Warren RF. Arthroscopic meniscal repair. *Arthroscopy.* 1985;1:170–172.
40. Wirth C. Meniscus repair. *Clin Orthop.* 1981;157:153.
41. Arnoczky SP, McDevitt CA, Schmidt MB, Mow VC, Warren RF. The effect of cryopreservation on canine menisci. *J Orthop Res.* 1988;6:1–12.
42. Arnoczky SP, Milachowski KA. Meniscal allografts: Where do we stand? In: Ewing JW, ed. *Articular Cartilage and Knee Joint Function: Basic Science and Arthroscopy.* New York: Raven Press; 1990;129–136.
43. Arnoczky SP, O'Brien SJ, DiCarlo E, Warren RF. Cellular repopulation of deep-frozen meniscal autografts—An experimental study in the dog. *Arthroscopy.* 1992;8:428–436.
44. Arnoczky SP, Warren RF, McDevitt CA. Meniscal replacement using a cryopreserved allograft—An experimental study in the dog. *Clin Orthop.* 1990;252:121–128.
45. Garrett JC, Stevenson RN. Meniscal transplantation in the human knee: A preliminary report. *Arthroscopy.* 1991;7:57–62.
46. Jackson DW, McDevitt CA, Astwell EA, Arnoczky SP, and Simon TM. Meniscal transplantation using fresh and

cryopreserved allografts: An experimental study in goats. *Trans Orthop Res.* 1990;15:221.

47. Jackson DW, Simon TM. Biology of meniscal allograft. In: Mow VC, Arnoczky SP, Jackson DW, eds. *Knee Meniscus: Basic and Clinical Foundations.* New York: Raven Press; 1992;141–152.

48. Milachowski KA, Weismeier K, Erhardt W, Remberger K. Transplantation of meniscus—An experimental study in sheep. *Sportverletzung Sportschaden.* 1987;1:20–24.

49. Milachowski KA, Weismeier K, Wirth CJ. Homologous meniscus transplantation. Experimental and clinical results. *Int Orthop.* 1989;13:1–11.

50. Milachowski KA, Weismeier K, Wirth CJ, Kohn D. Meniscus transplantation—Experimental study and first clinical report. *Am J Sports Med.* 1987;15:626.

51. Milton J, Flandry F, Terry G, et al. Transplantation of viable, cryopreserved menisci. *Trans Orthop Res.* 1990; 15:22.

52. Schmidt MB, Arnoczky SP, Mow VC, Warren RF. Biomechanical evaluation of cryopreserved meniscal allografts. *Trans Orthop Res Soc.* 1986;11:458.

53. Zukor DJ, Cameron JC, Brooks PJ, et al. The fate of human meniscal allografts. In: Ewing JW, ed. *Articular Cartilage and Knee Joint Function: Basic Science and Arthroscopy.* New York: Raven Press: 1990;147–152.

54. Zukor DJ, Rubins IM, Daigle MR, et al. Allotransplantation of frozen, irradiated menisci in rabbits. *Trans Orthop Res.* 1990;15:219.

55. Radin EL, Rose RM. Role of subchondral bone in the initiation and progression of cartilage damage. *Clin Orthop.* 1986;213:34–40.

56. Arnoczky SP, Adams ME, DeHaven K, Eyre DR, Mow VC. The meniscus. In Woo SL-Y, Buckwalter J, eds. *NIAMS/AAOS Workshop on the Injury and Repair of the Musculoskeletal Soft Tissues.* Park Ridge, IL: American Academy of Orthopaedic Surgeons; 1988;487–537.

57. O'Connor BL, McConnaughey JS. The structure and innervation of cat knee menisci, and their relation to a "sensory hypothesis" of meniscal function. *Am J Anat.* 1978;153:431–442.

58. Wilson AS, Legg PG, McNeur JC. Studies on the innervation of the medial meniscus in the human knee joint. *Anat Rec.* 1969;165:485–492.

59. Annandale T. An operation for displaced semilunar cartilage. *Br Med J.* 1885;1:779.

60. King D. The healing of the semilunar cartilages. *J Bone Joint Surg.* 1936;18:333–342.

61. Arnoczky SP, Warren RF. Microvasculature of the human meniscus. *Am J Sports Med.* 1982;10:90–95.

62. Arnoczky SP, Warren RF. The microvasculature of the meniscus and its response to injury—An experimental study in the dog. *Am J Sports Med.* 1983;11:131–141.

63. Cabaud HE, Rodkey WG, Fitzwater JE. Medial meniscus repairs: An experimental and morphological study. *Am J Sports Med.* 1981;9:129–134.

64. Arnoczky SP. Gross and vascular anatomy of the meniscus and its role in meniscal healing, regeneration, and remodeling. In: Mow VC, Arnoczky SP, Jackson DW, eds. *Knee Meniscus: Basic and Clinical Foundations.* New York: Raven Press; 1992:1–14.

65. Gershuni DH, Skyhar MJ, Danzig LA, Camp J, Hargens AR, Akeson WH. Experimental models to promote healing of tears in the avascular segment of canine knee menisci. *J Bone Joint Surg Am.* 1989;71:1363–1370.

66. Arnoczky SP, Warren RF, Spivak JM. Meniscal repair using an exogenous fibrin clot. An experimental study in dogs. *J Bone Joint Surg Am.* 1988;70:1209–1217.

67. Weiss CB, Lunberg M, Hanburg D, DeHaven KE, Gillquist J. Non-operative treatment of meniscal tears. *J Bone Joint Surg Am.* 1989;71:811–822.

68. Cannon WD. Arthroscopic meniscal repair. In: McGinty J, ed. *Operative arthroscopy.* New York: Raven Press; 1991;237–251.

69. Clancy WG, Graf BK. Arthroscopic meniscal repair. *Orthopaedics.* 1983;6:1125–1128.

70. Morgan CD. The all-inside meniscus repair. *Arthroscopy.* 1991;7:120–125.

71. Henning CE, Lynch M, Yearout K, Vequist S, Stallbaumer R, Decker K. Arthroscopic meniscal repair using an exogenous fibrin clot. *Clin Orthop.* 1990;252:64–72.

72. Fu F. Meniscal motion. Presented at the Arthroscopy Association of North America Annual meeting, 1990.

73. Morgan CD. Meniscal repair. Presented at the American Orthopaedic Society for Sports Medicine Annual Meeting, 1989.

74. Deutsch AL, Mink JH, Fox JM, et al. Peripheral meniscal tears: MR findings after conservative treatment or arthroscopic repair. *Radiology.* 1990;176:485, 488.

75. DeHaven KE. Meniscal repair. Presented at the American Orthopaedic Society for Sports Medicine Annual Meeting, 1991.

76. Buseck M, Noyes FR. Arthroscopic evaluation of meniscal repairs after anterior cruciate ligament reconstruction and immediate motion. *Am J Sports Med.* 1991;19:489–494.

77. Small NC. Complications in arthroscopic surgery performed by experienced arthroscopists. *Arthroscopy.* 1988; 4:215–221.

78. Arnoczky SP, Ashlock MA, and Warren RF. Replacement of the anterior cruciate ligament using a patellar tendon allograft: An experimental study. *J Bone Joint Surg Am.* 1986;68:376.

79. Aston JE, Bentley G. Repair of articular cartilage surfaces by allografts and articular and growth-plate cartilage. *J Bone Joint Surg Br.* 1986;68:29.

80. Brown KLB, Cruess RL. Bone and cartilage transplantation in orthopaedic surgery: A review. *J Bone Joint Surg Am.* 1982;64:270.

81. Campbell CJ, Ishida H, Takahashi H, Kelly F. The transplantation of articular cartilage. *J Bone Joint Surg Am.* 1963;45:1570.

82. Elves MW. The study of transplantation antigens on chondrocytes from articular cartilage. *J Bone Joint Surg Br.* 1974;56:178–185.

83. Elves MW. Bone and cartilage grafting and organ transplantation. In: Owen R, Goodfellow J, Bullough PM, eds. *Scientific Foundations of Orthopaedics and Traumatology.* London: Heineman; 1980;273.

84. Friedlander GE, Strong DM, Sell KW. Studies on the antigenicity of bone. I. Freeze-dried and deep-frozen allografts in rabbits. *J Bone Joint Surg Am.* 1976;58:854.

85. Langer F, Czitrom A, Pritzker KP, Gross AE. The immunogenicity of fresh and frozen allogeneic bone. *J Bone Joint Surg Am.* 1975;57:216.

86. Lexer E. Joint transplantation and arthroplasty. *Surg Gynecol Obstet.* 1925;41:782–800.

87. Mankin HJ, Doppel SH, Sullivan TR, Tomford WW. Osteoarticular and intercalary allograft transplantation in the management of malignant tumors of bone. *Cancer.* 1982;50:613–630.

88. Minami A, Ishii S, Ogino T, Oikawa T, Kubayashi H. Effect of the immunological antigenicity of the allogeneic tendons on tendon grafting. *Hand.* 1983;14:111.

89. Mnaymneh W, Malinin T. Massive allografts in surgery of

bone tumors. *Orthof Clin North Am.* 1989;20:3:455–467.

90. Shino K, Kawasaki T, Hirose J, Gotoh I, Inoue M, Ono K. Replacement of the anterior cruciate ligament by an allogeneic tendon graft: An experimental study in the dog. *J Bone Joint Surg Br.* 1984;66:672.

91. Tomford WW, Fredericks GR, Mankin HJ. Cryopreservation of intact articular cartilage. *Trans Orthop Res Soc.* 1982;7:176.

92. Keene GCR, Paterson RS, Teague DC. Advances in arthroscopic surgery. *Clin Orthop.* 1987;224:64–70.

93. Black J, Shadle CA, Parsons JR, Brighton CT. Articular cartilage preservation and storage. II. Mechanical indentation of viable, stored articular cartilage. *Arthritis Rheum.* 1979;22:1102–1108.

94. Brighton CT, Shadle CA, Jiminez SA, Irwin JT, Lane JM, Lipton M. Articular cartilage preservation and storage. I. Application of tissue culture techniques to the storage of viable articular cartilage. *Arthritis Rheum.* 1979;22:1093–1101.

95. Jackson DW, Windler GE, Simon TS. Intra-articular reaction associated with the use of freeze-dried, ethylene oxide sterilized, bone–patellar tendon–bone allografts in the reconstruction of the anterior cruciate ligament. *Am J Sports Med.* 1990;18:1–10.

96. Stone KR, Rodkey WG, Webber RJ, McKinney LA, Steadman JR. Development of a prosthetic meniscal replacement. In: Mow VC, Arnoczky SP, Jackson DW, eds. *Knee Meniscus: Basic and Clinical Foundations.* New York: Raven Press; 1992;165–173.

19

Injuries of the Proximal Tibiofibular Joint

Mark G. Franco and Bernard R. Bach, Jr

Introduction

Isolated dislocation of the proximal tibiofibular joint is an uncommon knee injury. It was first described by Nelaton in 1874.[1] Several cases undoubtedly go unrecognized. A review of the literature by Lyle in 1925 collected only 41 total cases in the literature, and a second review of the literature in 1974 by Ogden revealed a total of only 108 reported cases.[2,3] Dislocations of the proximal tibiofibular joint occur most frequently in young males, particularly during sports participation. Some of those sports reported to have resulted in proximal tibiofibular dislocation are parachuting, lacrosse, soccer, dancing, horseback riding, wrestling, rugby, skiing, gymnastics, and judo.[4-10] The majority of these injuries are attributed to indirect trauma, although a direct injury mechanism is possible. During World War II, a change in the landing technique taught at the US Parachute School in which the parachutists were instructed to land with the ankles held firmly together resulted in a decrease in ankle fractures, but an increase in the number of proximal tibiofibular dislocations.[11]

Although proximal tibiofibular dislocations are rarely catastrophic, they can result in significant knee impairment and require recognition and appropriate treatment to prevent long-term disability.

Anatomy

Although the anatomy of the knee, including collateral cruciate ligaments and menisci, is extensively reported, less is known about the proximal tibiofibular joint. It is a diarthrodial articulation between the posterior/inferior aspect of the lateral tibial condyle and the anterior/medial surface of the fibular head (Fig. 19–1). The two opposing articular facets are flat and oval with virtually no inherent stability.[5] The joint is held together by a strong, thick anterior capsular ligament and a weaker posterior capsular ligament.[1,8,12-15] The proximal tibiofibular joint communicates with the knee joint space in approximately 10% of adults.[16] The joint is reinforced posteriorly by the popliteus tendon and superiorly by the biceps insertion and fibular collateral ligament.[3-8,14] The inclination of the proximal tibiofibular joint is variable from 0° to 70° with most reflecting an obliquity between 10° and 30°.[3,15,16] Joint obliquity has a role in stability, with the larger, horizontal articulations being more stable. The horizontal inclination allows greater fibular rotation and, therefore, greater ankle dorsiflexion as shown by Barnett and coworkers.[15,17-19] In addition to dissipating rotational stresses, the proximal tibiofibular joint may have the additional roles of dissipating compressive loads up to one sixth body weight and dissipating tensile forces resulting from lateral bending moments.[3,15,20,21]

The common peroneal nerve crosses from posterior and wraps around the neck of the fibula just distal to the head. It may therefore be susceptible to injury, particularly with posterior dislocations of the fibular head.[12,13,22]

Classification

Two classification systems are applicable to the proximal tibiofibular joint. The first classification relates to the obliquity of the proximal tibiofibular joint and the second classification describes the direction of fibular head dislocation.[3,15]

The original classification of proximal tibiofibular joint articulations was proposed by Barnett, who categorized the joint into three types. Type 1 had a horizontal orientation with inclination from 0° to 30°.

347

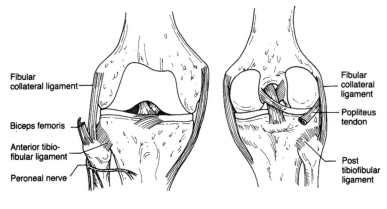

Fibular
collateral ligament

Biceps femoris

Anterior tibio-
fibular ligament

Peroneal nerve

Fibular
collateral
ligament

Popliteus
tendon

Post
tibiofibular
ligament

Figure 19–1. The proximal tibiofibular joint is reinforced anteriorly by a strong capsular ligament and posteriorly by a weaker capsular ligament. Posterior support is provided by the popliteus tendon. The fibular collateral ligament and biceps femoris tendon provide support superiorly.

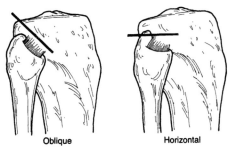

Oblique   Horizontal

Figure 19–2. Oblique proximal tibiofibular joints have an inclination greater than 20° and horizontal joints have an inclination less than 20°. (Adapted with permission from Ogden.[3])

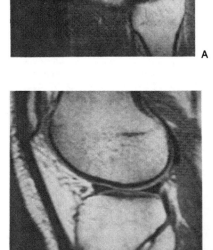

The surface area was greater than 20 mm². A type 2 articulation was a "large" oval surface frequently communicating with the knee. A type 3 articulation was small (less than 15 mm²) and inclined greater than 30°.[18] Ogden simplified this to only two joint types, eliminating type 2 because of ambiguity, and he arbitrarily assigned 20° as the limit between horizontal and oblique articulations (Figs. 19–2 and 19–3).[3,15] The horizontal articulations allow for increased rotational motion at the proximal tibiofibular joint, which results in increased ankle dorsiflexion as described by Barnett and Ogden.[15,19] Horizontal articulations have a larger surface area averaging 26 mm², compared with the average of 17 mm² for the oblique proximal tibiofibular joints.[3,15] Increased obliquity is suggested to result in instability and may predispose to increased risk of proximal tibiofibular dislocation. A review of 84 anatomic

$\longrightarrow$

Figure 19–3. These lateral cuts on magnetic resonance imaging nicely demonstrate horizontal (**A**) and oblique (**B**) angles of joint inclination.

and 117 radiographic specimens revealed that the slight majority (60%) are oblique. The distribution of joint obliquity does not conform to a bimodal, horizontal versus oblique pattern. Instead, the obliquity measurements tend to cluster between 10° and 30°, and represent a normal bell-shaped distribution.[3,15] Increased obliquity may predispose the joint to instability and increased risk of dislocation.

A classification for proximal tibiofibular dislocations was also proposed by Ogden, in which there are four general types (Fig. 19–4). Type 1 is not a true dislocation but rather a subluxation and accounts for nearly

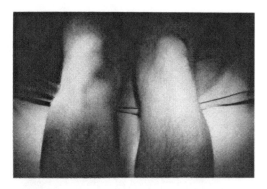

Figure 19–5. An unreduced anterolateral dislocation of the right proximal tibiofibular joint. Note the fullness and deformity. This patient could not be reduced under anesthesia and required an open reduction and internal fixation. (Photograph courtesy of John A. Bergfeld, MD, Director, Sports Medicine Section, The Cleveland Clinic, Cleveland, OH.)

one fourth of cases. Type 2 is an anterolateral dislocation (Fig. 19–5). It is the most common, accounting for 88% of true dislocations. Type 3 dislocations are posteromedial and account for 7%. Type 4, a superior dislocation, is the least common (4%). It is associated with an ankle fracture, interosseous membrane injury, or tibia shaft fracture.[3,10,24,25]

Evaluation

The evaluation of all knee injuries begins with a careful history, examination, and appropriate x-rays. The history of the injury often reflects the mechanism of injury resulting in proximal tibiofibular dislocation. A typical history is a sports injury with a fall in a position of foot plantar flexion and inversion combined with knee flexion, adduction, and internal rotation, with associated external rotation at the hip.[3–6,10,14,22,24] The patient may have tried to regain his or her balance at the time of injury.[26] Often a snap or pop is felt followed by sharp pain along the lateral aspect of the knee, possibly radiating to the lateral ankle. The pain is increased with dorsiflexion of the ankle and decreased with plantar flexion. There may be associated dysesthesia over the dorsal and lateral aspects of the foot. Knee extension is limited and painful. Hemarthrosis and knee joint effusion are not encountered but the fibular head may be quite prominent and tender to palpation, particularly with anterolateral dislocations.

Ligamentous stability of the knee should be documented, particularly with respect to cruciate and collateral ligament function. Usually knee ligament stability is normal in the setting of tibiofibular dislocation.

As with all knee injuries, appropriate radiographs

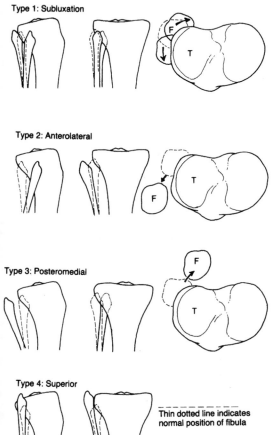

Type 1: Subluxation

Type 2: Anterolateral

Type 3: Posteromedial

Type 4: Superior

Thin dotted line indicates normal position of fibula

Figure 19–4. Type 1 instability is classified as a subluxation. Type 2 is an anterolateral dislocation. Type 3 is a posteromedial dislocation. Type 4 is a superior dislocation of the tibiofibular joint. (Adapted with permission from Ogden.[3])

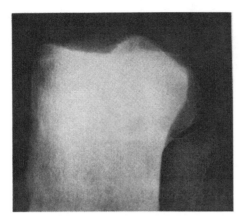

Figure 19-6. An oblique x-ray of the knee in 45° to 60° of internal rotation projects the proximal tibiofibular joint in profile, allowing assessment of width and inclination of the joint. (Reprinted with permission from Resnick et al.[16])

should be obtained, particularly anteroposterior (AP) and lateral projections. An additional view that is beneficial in evaluating the proximal tibiofibular joint is an oblique projection with the knee in 45° to 60° of internal rotation (Fig. 19-6).[14,16] This brings the proximal tibiofibular articulation into profile, so that the width and inclination of the joint space can be assessed.

Resnick reported on the anatomic–pathologic and radiographic correlation of proximal tibiofibular joint injuries.[16] He demonstrated an oblique radiodense line on the lateral projection that was consistent with the subchondral condensation of the tibial facet. When the entire fibular head was projected in front of this sloping line, an anterior lateral dislocation was diagnosed. With posteromedial dislocations, the fibular head projected

entirely posterior to this sloping radiodense line and there was very little overlap between the proximal tibia and the head of the fibula (Fig. 19-7). Evaluation of the proximal tibiofibular joint should be included on all x-rays of acute knee injuries.

Principles of Treatment

The factors that need to be considered when treating subluxations and dislocations of the proximal tibiofibular joint include acute versus chronic injury, type of dislocation, severity of symptoms, and peroneal nerve involvement. Most acute dislocations can be reduced closed but may require general anesthesia.[2-4,7,10,14,22,24]

Anterolateral dislocations are reduced by flexing the knee and, with direct pressure, translating the fibular head posteriorly. A snap or pop is felt at the time of reduction, and after reduction, the joint is usually stable. This is followed by a short period of immobilization (3 weeks) in a long leg cast[3,4,7,13,19,26] with the knee in slight flexion and the ankle dorsiflexed; alternatively, a compressive elastic wrap for 2 to 3 weeks or no protection has been proposed.[7,10,26,27]

Acute posteromedial dislocations also can usually be reduced closed; however, they are more frequently unstable following closed reduction. If instability is noted, temporary percutaneous pin fixation at the caudal aspect of the tibiofibular joint will enhance stability. During pinning the position of the peroneal nerve must be noted and avoided.[4,24]

Open reduction is rarely necessary for anterolateral or posteromedial acute dislocations.[2,4,5,10] Anderson reported two anterolateral dislocations that could not be acutely reduced closed and required open reduction by levering the fibular head over the lateral prominence of the tibia.[4] The taut fibular collateral ligament had locked the fibular head in its dislocated position, thus preventing closed reduction. Ogden recommends open

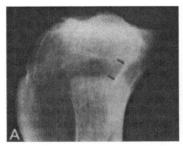
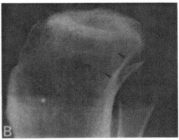

Figure 19-7. A radiodense line shows the position of subchondral bony condensation of the tibial facet. **A.** Lateral radiographs showing the fibula head anterior to this line reflect type 2 dislocations. **B.** Lateral radiographs in which the entire fibular head is posterior to this radiodense line indicate type 3 dislocations. (Reprinted with permission from Resnick et al.[16])

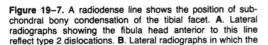

reduction with fibular collateral ligament and capsular repair followed by temporary pin fixation for posteromedial dislocations.[10]

Superior dislocations (type 3) are usually associated with tibia fractures or severe ankle injuries.[28] Following appropriate management of these associated injuries, the superior dislocation is usually reduced and stable.[4,24,25] If they are unstable, temporary pin fixation is advised.

Peroneal nerve injury may be associated with proximal tibiofibular dislocation or instability. Ogden, Lyle, and Levy reported peroneal nerve palsies following posteromedial dislocations.[2,3,29] Shelbourne noted a peroneal nerve injury associated with a superior dislocation.[25] For persistent peroneal nerve symptoms following previous proximal tibiofibular joint dislocation or instability, fibular head resection has been reported to be successful in alleviating these symptoms.[3,4,10,12,19] Arthrodesis of the proximal tibiofibular joint is also beneficial in alleviating peroneal nerve irritation[2,4,10,12,17,19] and persistent instability; however, pain and impaired ankle function make this procedure undesirable.[3,5,10,12,19]

Additional treatment options in mild chronic instability include biceps rehabilitation and a compressive tennis elbow or Chopat strap about the proximal aspect of the fibula. Giachino reported two cases of ligamentous reconstruction for chronic instability following anterior dislocation.[13] A strip of biceps tendon and deep crural fascia were used to reconstruct the capsular ligaments (Fig. 19–8). Giachino reported good results at 7 months and $3\frac{1}{2}$ years following ligamentous stabilization.[13] Ligamentous reconstruction may be considered in the skeletally immature patient and high-caliber athlete, where fibular head resection has relative contraindications.

We have had one experience with a similar procedure using a strip of distally based iliotibial band to stabilize the fibular head (Fig. 19–9). Our patient had functioned well for nearly a decade after a posterior cruciate ligament reconstruction and presented to our office with new symptoms of paresthesias on the dorsum of her foot following a tennis injury. Her physical examination revealed a grade I posterior drawer, increased posterolateral spin and thigh foot angles consistent with posterolateral instability, and posteromedial fibular head subluxation which was tender and reproduced her clinical symptoms. We addressed her posterolateral instability by performing a popliteus bypass procedure using autogenous middle-third patellar tendon, and used a central strip of distally based iliotibial band placed through a drill hole in the fibular head and looped back

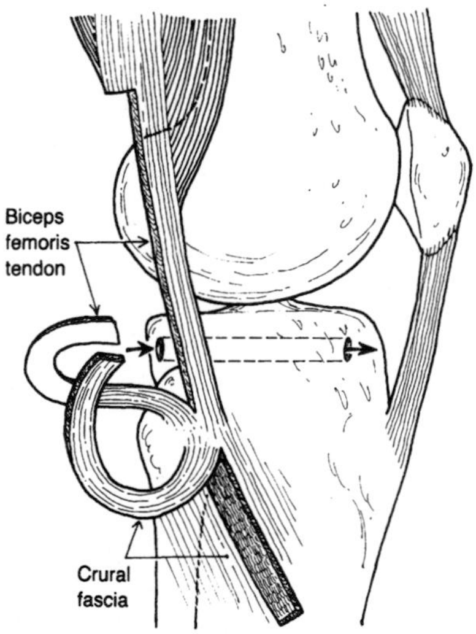

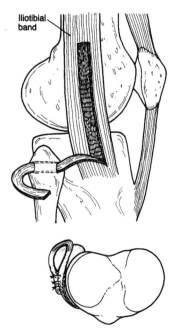

Figure 19–8. Giachino reported two cases of ligamentous reconstruction for chronic instability using a strip of the biceps femoris tendon and a strip of crural fascia secured in a drill hole through the lateral tibial plateau. (Adapted with permission from Giachino.[13])

Figure 19–9. We have used a strip of distally based iliotibial band rerouted through the fibular head and looped anteriorly and secured on itself ot treat chronic symptomatic posteromedial subluxation.

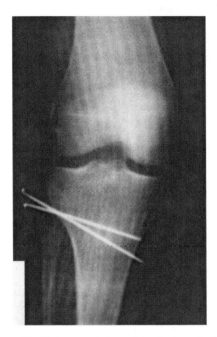

Figure 19–10. Anteroposterior radiograph demonstrating K-wire fixation of the proximal tibiofibular joint.

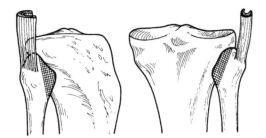

Figure 19–11. An oblique matched partial fibular head resection may allow for decompression and pain relief of the proximal tibiofibular joint without compromising the fibular styloid or lateral collateral ligament.

on itself to stabilize the fibular head. She has done extremely well and returned to recreational athletics 18 months postoperatively.

In summary, the treatment options that have been reported for acute proximal tibiofibular dislocations include closed reduction with immobilization, closed reduction with immobilization, closed reduction and temporary pin fixation (Fig. 19–10), and open reduction with soft tissue and capsule repair combined with temporary K-wire fixation. Fibular head resection, ligamentous stabilization, and arthrodesis are the treatment options for chronic symptomatic dislocations or chronic instability. We do not recommend arthrodesis.

Postoperative Management

There is no uniform agreement among authors regarding postoperative management. After reduction of an acute dislocation, if the reduction is stable, no temporary pin fixation is indicated. A temporary elastic bandage and protected weight bearing for 3 months have been suggested.[3,4,7,8,10,19,26] If pin fixation is used, it should be removed in 4 to 6 weeks and weight bearing postponed until pin removal.[5,7] Type 3 dislocations are more likely to show instability and require pin fixation.

Complications

The long-term complications following proximal tibiofibular injuries include persistent pain, instability, and the development of peroneal nerve symptoms. Although arthrodesis may alleviate these symptoms, associated ankle morbidity makes this inadvisable.[2–4,12,17,19,26] Resection of the fibular head appears to be the treatment of choice.[3,4,12,19] A partial matched fibular head resection with maintenance of the fibular styloid allows for decompression and pain relief without compromising the lateral collateral ligament (Fig. 19–11)[19] (also see Wickiewicz, TL, personal communication). Ligamentous reconstruction may also stabilize the joint thus minimizing peroneal nerve irritation, but there is little reported experience of this technique.[13] We are aware of two painful proximal tibiofibular joints with prolonged persistent symptoms that responded favorably to partial fibular head resection and three with chronic persistent instability that had a satisfactory response following ligamentous reconstruction[13] (also see Wickiewicz, TL, personal communication). One should be cognizant of the posterior relationship of the fibula to the tibia when performing pinning as the senior author (BRB) has seen one patient referred after pinning of the proximal tibiofibular joint in whom the pins were placed errantly and did not make contact with the tibia (Fig. 19–12).

Results

Veth et al reported that eight of ten patients developed radiographic evidence of degenerative joint disease in the proximal tibiofibular joint during a follow-up of 4 to 6 months following dislocation.[30] Seven of the ten patients were asymptomatic. Two experienced persistent pain over the lateral aspect of the knee, particularly when rising from a chair. One of these two demonstrated residual instability, and one patient had complaints of persistent peroneal nerve dysesthesia. Knee

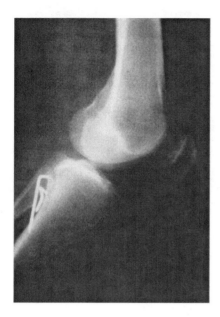

Figure 19–12. This lateral radiograph demonstrates that one must be cognizant of the posterior relationship of the fibular head to the tibia when performing a percutaneous fixation of the joint. The K-wires are not engaging the tibia.

and ankle range of motion and functional stability were reported as normal. Of these ten patients, six had a prior anterolateral dislocation, two posteromedial dislocation, one superior dislocation, and one subluxation. Initial treatment had consisted of closed reduction and symptomatic management in these ten patients.

Anderson reported two anterolateral dislocations that required open reduction and internal fixation with a temporary percutaneous pin.[4] These two had persistent mild symptoms at 7 and 9 months. A posteromedial dislocation, which was treated closed, produced mild to moderate pain and subjective instability at 3 years of follow-up.

Ogden reported that six of fourteen patients with anterolateral dislocations treated by closed reduction were asymptomatic at 9 to 44 months of follow-up.[19] Eight had persistent symptoms following closed reduction. Four of these underwent arthrodesis, which alleviated their knee symptoms but resulted in ankle pain, and the four remaining patients underwent fibular head resection, which alleviated their symptoms.

Summary

Proximal tibiofibular dislocations and subluxations are uncommon injuries but need to be considered in the differential diagnosis of lateral knee pain. Radiographic examination is often helpful; however, radiographic changes are subtle and may be missed. Acute dislocations can usually be reduced closed but may need temporary pin fixation if the proximal tibiofibular joint is unstable following closed reduction. The closed reduction is performed by flexing the knee to 90° and directing manual pressure posteriorly for type 1 dislocations and anteriorly for type 2 dislocations. Anterolateral dislocations are more common, are usually the result of indirect mechanism, and are usually stable following closed reduction. Posteromedial dislocations are frequently the result of direct trauma, are more likely to have associated peroneal nerve symptoms, and are less stable following closed reduction. Although proximal tibiofibular injuries are not commonly diagnosed, they may have long-term impairment requiring surgical management.

References

1. Nelaton A. *Elements de pathologie chirurgicale*. Paris: Balliere; 1874;292.
2. Lyle HM. Traumatic luxation of the head of the fibula. *Ann Surg*. 1925;82:635–639.
3. Ogden JA. Subluxation and dislocation of the proximal tibiofibular joint. *J Bone Joint Surg Am*. 1974;56:145–154.
4. Anderson K. Dislocation of the superior tibiofibular joint. *Injury*. 1985;16:494–498.
5. Crothers OD, Johnson JTH. Isolated acute dislocation of the proximal tibiofibular joint. *J Bone Joint Surg Am*. 1973;55:181–183.
6. Halbrecht JL, Jackson DW. Recurrent dislocations of the proximal tibiofibular joint. *Orthof Rev*. 1991;20:957–960.
7. Harvey GP, Woods GW. Anterolateral dislocation of the proximal tibiofibular joint. Case report and literature review. *Am J Knee Surg*. 1991;4:151–153.
8. Parkes JC II, Zelko RR. Isolated acute dislocation of the proximal tibiofibular joint. *J Bone Joint Surg Am*. 1973;55:177–180.
9. Thomason PA, Linson MA. Isolated dislocation of the proximal tibiofibular joint. *J Trauma*. 1986;26:192–195.
10. Turco VJ, Spinella AJ. Anterolateral dislocation of the head of the fibula in sports. *Am J Sports Med*. 1985; 13:209–216.
11. Lord CD, Coutts JW. A study of the typical parachute injuries occurring in 250,000 jumps at the parachute school. *J Bone Joint Surg*. 1944;26:547–557.
12. Dennis JB, Rutledge BA. Bilateral recurrent dislocations of the superior tibiofibular joint with peroneal nerve palsy. *J Bone Joint Surg Am*. 1958;40:1146–1148.
13. Giachino AA. Recurrent dislocations of the proximal tibiofibular joint. *J Bone Joint Surg Am*. 1986;68:1104–1106.
14. Ogden JA. Dislocation of the proximal fibula. *Diagn Radiol*. 1972;105:547–549.
15. Ogden JA. The anatomy and function of the proximal tibiofibular joint. *Clin Orthof Relat Res* 1974;101:186–191.
16. Resnick D, et al. Proximal tibiofibular joint: Anatomic-pathologic–radiographic correlation. *Am J Roentgenol*. 1978;131:133–138.

17. Baciu C, Tudor AL, Olaru I. Recurrent luxation of the superior tibiofibular joint in the adult. *Acta Orthop Scand*. 1974;45:772–777.
18. Barnett CH, Napier JR. The axis of rotation of the ankle joint in man. Its influence on the form of the talus and mobility of the fibula. *J. Anat*. 1952;86:1–9.
19. Ogden JA. Subluxation of the proximal tibiofibular joint. *Clin Orthof Relat Res*. 1974;101:192–197.
20. Katchis SD, Scott WN. Dislocation of the proximal tibiofibular joint. In: Scott WN, ed. *Ligament and Extensor Mechanism Injuries of the Knee—Diagnosis and Treatment*. St. Louis: CV Mosby; 1991;383–388.
21. Preuschoft H. Die Mechanische Beanspuchung der Fibula bie Primaten. *Gegenbaurs Morph J*. 1971;117:211.
22. Owen R. Recurrent dislocation of the superior tibiofibular joint. *J Bone Joint Surg Br*. 1968;50:342–345.
23. Novich MM. Adduction injury of the knee with rupture of the common peroneal nerve. *J Bone Joint Surg Am*. 1960;42:1372–1376.
24. Falkenberg P, Nygaard H. Isolated anterior dislocation of the proximal tibiofibular joint. *J Bone Joint Surg Br*. 1983;65:310–311.
25. Shelbourne KD, Pierce RO, Ritter MA. Superior subluxation of the fibular head associated with a tibia fracture. *Clin Orthof Relat Res*. 1981;60;172–174.
26. Sijbrandij S. Instability of the proximal tibio-fibular joint. *Acta Orthof Scand*. 1978;49;621–626.
27. Ginnerup P, Sorensen VK. Isolated traumatic luxation of the head of the fibula. *Acta Orthof Scand*. 1978;49:618–620.
28. Herscovici D Jr, Fredrick RW, Behrens F. Superior dislocation of the fibular head associated with a tibial shaft fracture: Case report and review of the literature. *J Orthof Trauma*. 1992;6(1):116–119.
29. Levy M. Peroneal nerve palsy due to superior dislocation of the head of the fibula and shortening of the fibula. *Acta Orthof Scand*. 1975;46:1020.
30. Veth RPH, Clasen HJ, Kingma LM. Traumatic instability of the proximal tibiofibular joint. *Injury*. 1981;13:159–164.

Part 5

Late Reconstructive Problems and Complications

20
Management of the Stiff Knee After Trauma and Ligament Reconstruction

Christopher D. Harner, Mark D. Miller, and James J. Irrgang

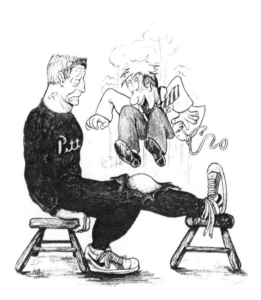

Introduction

The "stiff knee," which has been referred to as "arthrofibrosis," "infrapatellar contracture syndrome," "patella infera," "ankylosis," and various other names, is unfortunately an all too common complication of both fracture management and knee ligament surgery. The etiology of this difficult problem is as diverse as the terms used to describe it. It can be related to inadequate reduction or fixation of intraarticular fractures, prolonged traction or immobilization, infection, and ligament surgery (both intra- and extraarticular) to highlight only a few associated risk factors.

The knee is a unique joint in that patients tolerate loss of flexion more than loss of extension. A 5° to 10° flexion contracture results in quadriceps weakness, patellofemoral pain, and a "bent knee" gait.[1,2] Patients often will tolerate 10° to 20° loss of flexion and still function quite well. The major problem with flexion loss occurs in athletes who are no longer able to sprint.[3]

With this exception, flexion loss is much better tolerated than extension loss, which affects activities of daily living. This is an important concept in decision making for management of the stiff knee.

Much of our previous work has been directed at management of the stiff knee following ligament surgery[4]; however, many of the same problems and treatment principles apply to management of the stiff knee following fracture treatment. Prevention, early recognition, and a well-thought-out treatment plan are critical in the management of the stiff knee. We begin this chapter with a discussion of knee stiffness that results from individual fractures about the knee, and then discuss the recognition and management of the stiff knee following ligament reconstruction.

Fracture Management and the Stiff Knee

Overview

Loss of motion following trauma is multifactorial. Stiffness can follow prolonged immobilization, traction, intraarticular and extraarticular fracture fixation, and other conditions and treatments. Some authors have noted that it is sometimes difficult to determine if loss of motion is secondary to prolonged immobilization in and of itself or is caused by soft tissue injury.[5] Regardless of the etiology, the pathophysiology that leads to stiffness is similar. Initially there is an inflammatory phase followed later by fibrosis and adhesions of the soft tissues. Soft tissues affected include muscles, tendons, capsular structures, and the cruciate ligaments. In addition, bony causes (malreduction, nonunions) can also contribute to loss of motion.

Traction

Traction alone has long been implicated as a cause of knee stiffness. Some authors have noted that knee stiffness is *the most common problem* following traction treatment.[6,7] Winat, in a study of the effect of traction on knee motion, noted that no patient regained full motion, and half of his patients had less than 90° of motion following prolonged traction therapy.[8] Fortunately, prolonged traction has fallen out of vogue for treatment of most injuries, but its detrimental effect on knee motion must be recognized.

Fractures

Distal Femur

Fractures of the femoral shaft and distal femur can lead to contractures secondary to extra- or intraarticular pathology. Extraarticular adhesions that lead to an extension contracture have been attributed to four causes[9]:

1. Fibrosis of the vastus intermedius with tethering of the rectus femoris to the femur
2. Shortening and adhesion of the medial and/or lateral vastus expansions over the distal femur
3. Adhesions of the patella to the femoral condyles
4. Shortening of the rectus femoris itself

Flexion contractures can result from prolonged immobilization in a position of flexion.[10] Associated findings with extraarticular adhesions include an abrupt stop to active and passive motion and an extension lag. Patellar adhesions are best recognized by assessing patellar mobility as compared with the uninvolved knee.[11]

Management

Location of adhesions and timing of treatment are critical in the management of patients with loss of motion following trauma. Adhesions can be located extraarticularly (eg, muscle tendon unit, capsule, collateral ligaments) or can be intraarticular (intercondylar notch scarring, cruciate ligament injury, meniscal pathology). Following any trauma, initial adhesions are hemorrhagic and inflammatory in character and remain theoretically amenable to closed treatment. As the inflammatory process progresses, however, these initial inflammatory adhesions become fibrotic leading to a permanent contracture, which can be treated only by surgical intervention. It has been our experience that if initial adhesions and loss of motion are not addressed by the 6-week postinjury/surgery point, then fibrosis often sets in, leading to permanent contracture. If the loss of motion can be addressed prior to 6 weeks, often aggressive physical therapy combined with possible closed manipulation under anesthesia can lead to a successful outcome with respect to range of motion.

Unfortunately, following fracture treatment the surgeon is limited by his or her ability to aggressively treat loss of motion and still protect fracture fixation. In these difficult cases where range of motion cannot be instituted until adequate fracture healing, one must accept the possibility for developing loss of motion and explain this to the patient at the outset. In these cases, often a second and sometimes a third surgical procedure may be necessary to regain adequate range of motion following fracture healing.

Extraarticular adhesions that have not gone on to develop fibrotic changes are best managed by aggressive physical therapy, which may include hospitalization. The use of an extension dropout cast can be very effective for the elimination of flexion contractures between 10° and 15° (Fig. 20–1). Continuous passive motion (CPM) is often extremely helpful in regaining flexion loss. In the early phases of loss of motion (<6 weeks) closed manipulation under anesthesia should be considered in patients who fail to improve with physical therapy. Manipulation in our hands has, however, been

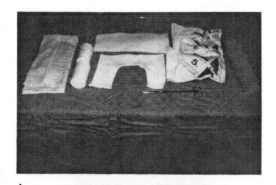

A

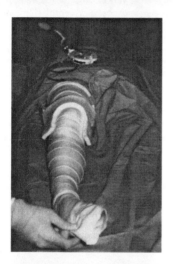

B

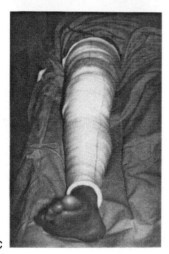

C

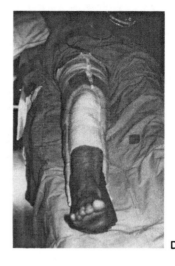

D

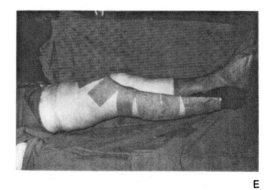

E

Figure 20–1. Extension dropout cast. **A.** Materials used in creation of an extension dropout cast from left to right: Stockinette, cast padding, felt, 5-in. fiberglass casting material, scissors, moleskin protective padding. **B.** Placement of cast padding and felt. *Note:* A rectangular piece of felt is placed on the posterior aspect of the thigh superiorly. The horseshoe-shaped piece of felt is placed on the anterior portion of the thigh just above the patella. **C.** Fiberglass casting material is placed over the well-padded leg, being careful to protect the edges. The area to be cut out is marked with a marking pen. **D.** The anterior portion of the cast up to the area just above the patella is removed and padded with moleskin protective material. The superior aspect of the cast is split longitudinally on the anterior surface; however, the cast padding is not split. This allows for removal and donning of the cast. **E.** Lateral picture demonstrating the completed cast with towels placed under the heel to allow full extension. The cast is used daily as part of the treatment.

more effective for loss of flexion than loss of extension. We usually perform the closed manipulation under epidural anesthesia and continue this anesthesia for several days following the manipulation. This procedure should be used with extreme caution in patients who are osteopenic or have significant chondromalacia of the patella. Forceful manipulation in patients with osteopenia can result in fracture. Aggressive manipulation in patients with underlying chondromalacia may lead to irreversible articular cartilage damage.

In the later stages of loss of motion, surgical intervention may be required. As noted earlier, the adhesions (intraarticular and extraarticular) often become fibrotic, resulting in irreversible loss of motion that cannot be corrected by closed treatment. One of the most common causes of extraarticular adhesions is scarring and shortening of the extensor mechanism. This is most common following comminuted midshaft fractures and distal femur fractures. In this setting, the quadriceps mechanism becomes damaged; because fracture fixation is often tenuous, immediate motion is delayed or limited. The traditional surgical intervention for this problem is a quadricepsplasty[12] (Fig. 20–2). It is important in this procedure that all adhesions be released. The rectus femoris, vastus medialis, and vastus lateralis often adhere down to the bone and must be released in a subperiosteal fashion to reestablish the normal excursion of the quadriceps mechanism. In the chronic situation the quadriceps mechanism will become shortened, thus requiring a lengthening procedure. Our preferred technique is a quadricepsplasty of the scarred and contracted quadriceps tendon using a "pie crusting" technique. A No. 11 blade is used to make small, transverse incisions over the quadriceps mechanism, thus avoiding a Z-plasty incision which we feel weakens the extensor mechanism significantly. When excessive adhesions make the quadriceps nonfunctional, removal of the damaged tissue and insertion of a fresh-frozen allograft (Achilles tendon or patellar tendon) have been successful in our experience.

With respect to loss of extension, in the majority of cases the etiology is secondary to parapatellar adhesions and fat pad scarring. Rarely is the cause secondary to posterior capsular scarring and contracture of the hamstring tendons. Our surgical approach to loss of extension is discussed under to ligament surgery. This is important because we feel the approach to loss of extension is release of scar tissue in the anterior aspect of the knee rather than release and lengthening of the hamstring tendons and posterior capsular structures. Postoperative management following release of extraarticular adhesions should include an extension dropout cast for extension and CPM for flexion. Again, epidural anesthesia is extremely helpful for the first 48 hours following surgery. Finally, postoperatively we start the patient on a 6-day tapering course of oral methylprednisolone.

Other causes of loss of knee motion following distal femoral fractures include malreduction of fractures, misdirected hardware, intraarticular adhesions, and posttraumatic arthritis. If either of the first two problems are identified early, reoperation is indicated. Intraarticular adhesions, which will be the focus of the section on ligament reconstruction that follows, should be approached in an algorithmic fashion. Aggressive physical therapy, manipulation under anesthesia, and arthroscopic or open lysis of adhesions each have a place in the management of these problems. Again, the

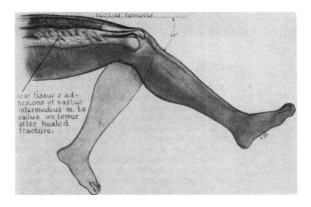
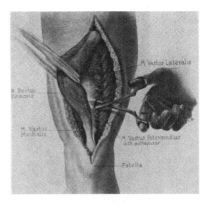

A   B

Figure 20–2. **A.** Adhesions of the vastus intermedius and lysis of adhesions that may occur with femoral fractures. **B.** Lysis of adhesions. (Reprinted with permission from Thompson.[12])

administration of oral steroids following surgical intervention may be beneficial. A recent study on the effects of parenteral steroids following acute fractures in a rabbit model did demonstrate statistically significant decreases in joint stiffness[13]; however, the clinical efficacy has not been proven in controlled clinical trials.

Indications for osteotomy to improve range of motion are limited to those cases in which malunion is present. Careful preoperative planning with long cassette film and computed tomography scan is often extremely helpful in planning out the osteotomy prior to surgical intervention.

Posttraumatic arthritis is best treated with physical therapy and anti-inflammatory agents. Often salvage procedures such as an osteotomy, fusion, and arthroplasty are required in the long term.

Patella Fractures

Fortunately, many of the problems with loss of motion following open reduction and internal fixation of patellar fractures have been overcome with early motion that is possible with newer tension-band wire techniques. Nevertheless, contractures can still occur in this setting. In our experience, loss of flexion is more common than loss of extension following patella fractures. Treatment is similar to the approach outlined earlier and consists of intensive physical therapy, occasionally manipulation, and arthroscopic lysis of adhesions. Complications associated with manipulation include articular cartilage damage, quadriceps rupture (especially following patellectomy), and development of a "boutonniere"-type

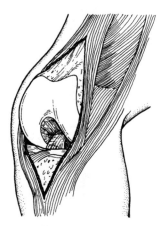

Figure 20-3. Boutonniere-type deformity of the extensor mechanism with herniation of the distal femur through the defect of the central portion of the patellar tendon following patellectomy and manipulation. (Reprinted with permission from Noble and Jajek.[14])

deformity in patients with a longitudinal fracture/retinacular disruption[14] (Fig. 20-3).

Extensor mechanism length disparity is an unusual problem in isolated patellar fractures. Occasionally, quadricepsplasty (as described earlier) may be required in refractory cases of quadriceps contracture. Even more unusual is the case of excessive length of the extensor mechanism. This can present with a "giving way" sensation,[15] and some authors have recommended a Maquet procedure in this setting.[16]

Proximal Tibia

Although knee stiffness is often implicated in *extra*articular fractures of the tibia, many of these cases are likely associated with unrecognized *intra*articular knee injuries.[17,18] In fact, more recent reports have indicated that the incidence of residual knee stiffness in *extra*articular fractures was small, and the amount of stiffness was clinically insignificant.[19] Intraarticular fractures of the proximal tibia should be evaluated using the same approach outlined earlier for intraarticular fractures of the distal femur.

Knee Dislocation

Stiffness is a common sequela of knee dislocation. The literature is inconsistent in reported incidence of loss of motion with operative versus nonoperative treatment. Sisto and Warren reported on results of 16 patients and noted that overall there was minor loss of motion with operative repair and significant loss of motion with cast treatment. They attributed this to the earlier, more aggressive rehabilitation program that could be initiated with early repair.[20] Likewise, Meyers and Harvey reported decreased motion and poorer results with nonoperative management of ligamentous injuries.[21] On the other hand, Roman et al noted that operatively treated patients had better stability but less motion, particularly extension.[22] Scott and Insall conclude their discussion on this subject with this comment: "In view of the problem with stiffness, it seems reasonable to advocate open repair in all situations in which vascular anastomosis has been reestablished or in active patients."[23]

It is our policy to do ligamentous reconstruction as soon as it can be safely done. Once completed, range of motion can be started. We have more difficulty regaining flexion than extension in these cases, primarily because our postoperative protocol involves immobilization in full extension. This helps reduce the joint and provides the least strain on our cruciate ligament reconstruction. When we begin flexion (1 week postop) it is done with a therapist supervising and controlling posterior tibial sag. We avoid CPM in these cases because of posterior gravitational forces on the tibia. Often it will take these patients 6 to 9 months to regain

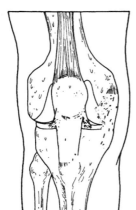

Figure 20-4. Adhesions adjacent to the medial collateral ligament, a common location of adhesions in the knee.

3. Technical errors in graft placement
4. Timing and extent of surgery

We discuss each factor at length in the sections that follow.

Intercondylar Notch Scarring

Intercondylar notch scarring (ICNS) is the result of bleeding into the intracondylar notch area which scarifies and produces a mechanical block to extension. Patients with ICNS usually present with loss of extension only. They usually complain of morning stiffness which improves with activities. Some patients complain of a "catching" sensation with knee extension. Patellar mobility is usually normal, and swelling is minimal.

Prevention of ICNS is based on an adequate notch-

their full flexion. If they are not making progress by the sixth month, then we will consider a manipulation and possible open adhesiolysis. We have not had good success with arthroscopy alone in this setting of complex ligamentous injury and repair. Arthroscopy alone has been helpful following anterior cruciate ligament (ACL) reconstruction with loss of extension only (see next section). Finally, it is the combination of posterior cruciate ligament (PCL)/medial collateral ligament (MCL) that gives the greatest chance of loss of flexion. In these cases, it is important to release adhesions between the MCL and femoral condyle to reestablish the normal cam mechanism of the medial femoral condyle and MCL (Fig. 20-4).

Ligament Surgery

Loss of motion is the most common complication following knee ligament surgery. Significant loss of motion is defined as loss of extension greater than 10° and/or loss of flexion greater than 125°.[4] Of course, as with trauma, loss of knee extension is more devastating to the patient because of the effects on normal gait pattern. In general, ACL reconstruction more often results in loss of extension, whereas PCL reconstruction patients lose flexion. Medial collateral ligament reconstruction/repair has the highest rate of stiffness, with both flexion and extension equally involved. In our experience lateral collateral ligament (LCL)/posterior corner surgery has a low incidence of associated loss of motion. To simplify the approach to the stiff knee we have categorized the etiology into four areas:

1. Intercondylar notch scaring
2. Capsulitis

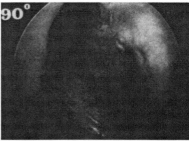

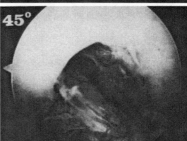

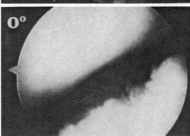

Figure 20-5. View of the anterior cruciate ligament graft at various degrees of knee extension, demonstrating the importance of an adequate notch plasty and clearance of the graft.

plasty. After graft placement, the knee is flexed and extended while the graft is visualized arthroscopically (Fig. 20–5). We do not hesitate to extend our notchplasty if there is any evidence of impingement. ICNS is also minimized if patients are splinted in extension postoperatively and therapy is initiated early.[24] We feel that it is important to reestablish a normal gait as soon as possible following ACL surgery.

Treatment of ICNS is enhanced by early recognition. Physical therapy including the use of an extension dropout cast (see Fig. 20–1) is central to the treatment of ICNS. The extension dropout cast provides a continuous stretch and, with overnight use, allows an increase in and maintenance of extension. Additionally, stretching and strengthening of the quadriceps are emphasized. If extension fails to improve with physical therapy or if ICNS is not recognized until more than 3

months postoperatively, then arthroscopic debridement of the intracondylar notch and, if necessary, revision notchplasty and adhesiolysis may be required (Fig. 20–6). The patient is placed in an extension dropout cast postoperatively, and therapy is initiated immediately. Results of surgery are variable. DeHaven reports good to excellent results in only half of patients treated. Motion was significantly improved, but functional capacity was often limited.[3] In our study, however, approximately 70% of patients who developed loss of motion after ACL reconstruction had a second surgical procedure with subsequent good to excellent results.

Capsulitis

Capsulitis, or as it is sometimes called in its later stages, infrapatellar contracture syndrome, is similar in some ways to adhesive capsulitis of the shoulder, and is a result of periarticular inflammation and swelling. Extracapsular fibrous bands are formed, severely limiting motion[25] (Figs. 20–7 and 20–8).

The etiology of this complex problem is unclear. A hereditary predisposition may be present in some patients (eg, keloid formers). Other possibilities include an autoimmune disorder, persistent bleeding with excessive stimulation of the healing cascade, and growth factor abnormalities.[26] Wahl and Renstrom have suggested that the process is related to an imbalance between collagen synthesis and degradation.[27]

Constant pain, quadriceps weakness, and a flexion contracture are common. Diffuse tenderness, effusion, and loss of motion, including flexion and extension as well as decreased patellar mobility, are seen clinically. Paulos et al defined the natural history of this problem

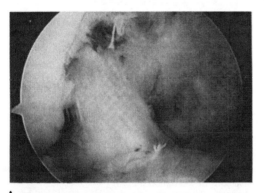

A

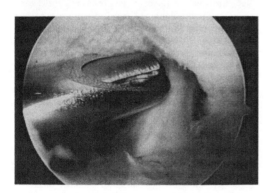

B

Figure 20–6. A. Arthroscopic view of intercondylar notch scarring. **B.** Addressing intercondylar notch scarring with an arthroscopic shaver.

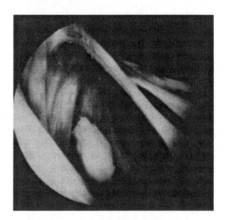

Figure 20–7. Extracapsular fibrous bands seen at our arthroscopy. (Reprinted with permission from Sprague et al.[25])

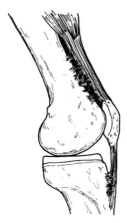

Figure 20–8. Extracapsular fibrous band extending from the proximal pole of the patella to the anterior surface of the femur. (Reprinted with permission from Sprague et al.[25])

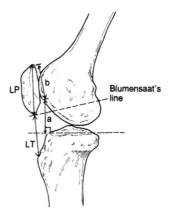

Figure 20–9. Composite illustration demonstrating three popular methods of evaluating patellar height: (1) *Blumensaat's line*: With the knee flexed 30°, the lower pole of the patella should lie on a line extended from the intercondylar notch. If the patella is above this line it is considered patella alta. (2) *Insall–Salvati index*: LT/LP = 1.0 (normal). An index greater than 1.2 is usually considered patella alta. An index less than 0.8 is usually considered patella baja. (3) *Blackburne and Peel index*: a/b = 0.8 (normal). An index greater than 1.0 is considered patella alta. Data have been taken from: (1) Blumensaat C. Die Lageabweichunger und Verrenkungen der Kniescheibe. *Ergeb Chir Orthop.* 1938;31:149–223. (2) Insall J, Salvati E. Patella position in the normal knee joint. *Radiology.* 1971;101:101–104. (3) Blackburne JS, Peel TE. A new method of measuring patellar height. *J Bone Joint Surg (Br.* 1977;59:241–242.)

in three stages.[1] Paulos and co-workers addressed this problem and referred to it as infrapatellar contracture syndrome. We feel, however, that the true pathology is a capsulitis that can secondarily involve the patella and extensor mechanism.[4] Capsulitis can be broken down into three phases:

Stage	Description	Primary Feature
I	Acute inflammatory	Common, usually reversible
II	Fibrotic	Irreversible, usually requires surgery
III	Patella baja	Rare, poor prognosis

Prevention of capsulitis is difficult, but should focus on early recognition. The prodromal stage is very common in the early postoperative period. Fortunately, only a small percentage of patients progress to subsequent stages. Stage III, associated with patella baja (patella infera), is best appreciated on lateral radiographs using measurements previously described[28] (Fig. 20–9).

Treatment of stage I capsulitis consists of the use of nonsteroidal anti-inflammatory agents or a short course of oral steroids and gentle protected range of motion. Aggressive stretching should be avoided. Once a patient progresses to stage II, loss of motion is usually not reversible without surgical intervention. If a patient does not improve by 3 months postoperatively, surgery is considered. We routinely admit patients to the hospital and, under epidural anesthesia, perform arthroscopic adhesiolysis focusing primarily on the intercondylar notch and fat pad. Often an arthrotomy and/or a lateral release is required to restore motion and normal patel-

lar tracking (Fig. 20–10). An extension dropout cast is placed in the operating room and then used at bedtime. Postoperatively, the epidural catheter is left in place for pain management, we prescribe a short course of methylprednisolone and physical therapy is initiated at the bedside. We concentrate on achieving extension first, and some patients may ultimately require a second manipulation to regain flexion at a later date. Progression to stage III is rare but portends a poor prognosis. Treatment of these patients requires an arthrotomy and often salvage procedures such as a proximal tibial tubercle slide, patellectomy, and possibly a total knee arthroplasty.[29]

Figure 20–10. Operative case demonstrating removal of fibrotic tissue. **A.** Medial arthrotomy demonstrating scar tissue underneath the patellar tendon. **B.** Creation of a plane to excise the scar tissue. **C.** Scar tissue after excision. **D.** Note changes on the medial femoral condyle from proliferative scar tissue. Note also lateral release and removal of scar tissue from the lateral incision. **E, F.** Preoperative range of motion prior to scar tissue removal. **G, H.** Postoperative range of motion following scar tissue removal.

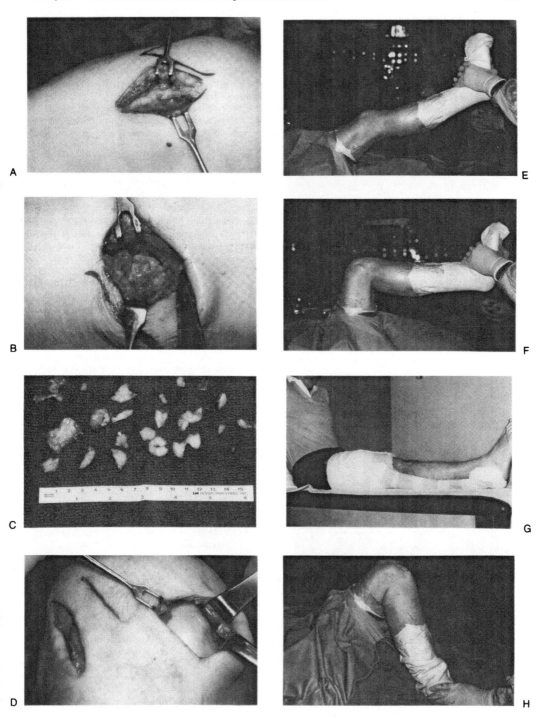

Technical Errors With Surgery

An ACL graft placed too anterior on the tibia can impinge at the intercondylar notch and block extension (Fig. 20–11). Excessive tension on ACL grafts can also prevent full extension. Alternatively, excessive tension on (PCL) grafts blocks flexion. Prevention of knee stiffness secondary to incorrect graft placement simply involves meticulous attention to detail in proper graft positioning. In ACL surgery, we, like other surgeons, have modified our tibial tunnel position to the posterior portion ot the ACL "footprint." Femoral tunnel placement is ideally located at the 10 o'clock position (right knee), with the centroid of the tunnel 5 to 7 mm anterior to the posterior cortex. With proper technique, femoral tunnel positioning can be achieved with either "rear-entry" or "endoscopic" techniques. Regardless of whether a "two-incision" or "endoscopic" technique is used, it is critical to ensure that the edge of the tunnel abuts the posterior femoral cortex.

Failure to adequately debride the joint, and the area adjacent to the tibial tunnel in particular, can lead to the development of what Jackson has termed the *Cyclops syndrome.*[30] In this condition, a nodule of peripheral fibrous tissue located anterolateral to the tibial tunnel can lead to impingement and loss of motion postoperatively. In our experience, this fibrous tissue usually comes from the tibial tunnel drilling breaking off the anterior aspect of the ACL insertion. This bone–ligament stump is then advanced into the notch, with graft passage acting as an impinging process with knee extension. It is important that the base of the graft be viewed in full extension at the completion of the case to eliminate this error.

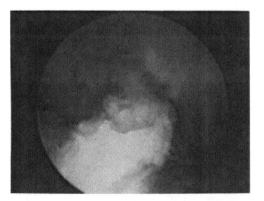

Figure 20–11. Arthroscopic view of anteriorly placed graft demonstrating impingement.

Timing and Extent of Surgery

Although several recent reports have emphasized the high incidence of stiff knee with acute ligament reconstruction,[31,32] this has long been recognized.[33] Although there is no formal consensus regarding the appropriate time period, most surgeons recommend delaying operative reconstruction for 2 to 3 weeks. At this point the pain and swelling will have subsided and range of motion and quadriceps control will have been restored. It is often helpful to initiate physical therapy during this period. Our approach to the acutely injured knee is to try and delay the surgery until the acute inflammatory phase of the injury has subsided and the range of motion has improved. This may vary from patient to patient depending on many factors.

A stiff knee is also common in ligament reconstructions requiring concomitant extraarticular surgery, combined ligament repairs, and meniscal repairs.[4,34] Efforts to prevent this complication in these patients should be emphasized. For extraarticular procedures, surgery should be avoided if nonoperative treatment is acceptable, as in many medial collateral ligament injuries. If surgery is required, anatomic procedures are favored over plications and advancement, and early motion is advocated. Even the extra surgery associated with graft harvesting may lead to an increased incidence of stiff knee. In our recent review, we found that autograft had twice the incidence of loss of motion compared with allograft reconstruction.[4] Reconstruction of combined ligamentous injuries requires aggressive therapy postoperatively. The incidence of stiffness following meniscal repair is reduced by tying sutures with the knee near full extension and, again, stressing early motion.

With regard to PCL injuries, our experience has been that loss of flexion is more common after reconstruction. This most likely occurs because we are reproducing the anterolateral bundle in surgery and this bundle tightens with flexion. Loss of extension is uncommon following PCL reconstruction. In the majority of cases these patients usually regain full range of motion by 6 to 9 months postoperatively, rarely requiring manipulation or surgical adhesiolysis.

Clinical Studies

We have recently completed a retrospective clinical review of loss of motion following ACL reconstruction to evaluate the treatment recommendations we outlined earlier.[24] We compared the results of 244 ACL reconstructions done during 1986–1989 with 231 ACL reconstructions done in 1990–1991. In the earlier group our rehabilitation protocol included initial immobilization in flexion, prolonged limited weight bearing, and delayed quadriceps rehabilitation. In 1990 we revised our postoperative rehabilitation to include immobilization in full extension, early passive range of motion (0–90°), weight bearing as tolerated, and early quadriceps rehabilitation. Additionally, the second group of patients all had delayed reconstruction, allowing range of motion and strength to improve prior to surgery. As a result of these modifications, we reduced our incidence of loss of extension greater than 10° from 7.4 to 1.7%. In both groups, loss of motion was about equally divided between ICNS and capsulitis.

Conclusions

Whether it follows fracture management or ligament surgery, treatment of the stiff knee is a difficult problem. In postfracture care, extraarticular causes may be more common and extensor mechanism adjustment is sometimes necessary. Stiffness following ligament surgery can have a variety of causes; however, the two most common causes are intercondylar notch scarring and capsulitis. In PCL reconstructive surgery, loss of flexion is more common, but usually will correct by 6 to 9 months postoperatively. Treatment is best directed at prevention, but late recognition may require a combination of surgery and aggressive physical therapy. Newer ligament rehabilitation programs that emphasize splinting in extension followed by early motion can markedly decrease the incidence of the stiff knee.

References

1. Paulos LE, Rosenberg TD, Drawbert J, Manning J, Abbott P. Infrapatellar contracture syndrome: An unrecognized cause of knee stiffness with patella entrapment and patella infera. *Am J Sports Med.* 1987;15:331–341.
2. Sachs RA, Daniel DM, Stone ML, et al. Patellofemoral problems after anterior cruciate ligament reconstruction. *Am J Sports Med.* 1989;17:760–765.
3. DeHaven K. Arthrofibrosis of the knee. In: *Proceedings, Sports Medicine Course,* American Academy of Orthopaedic Surgery, Steamboat Springs, CO, March 1992.
4. Harner CD, Irrgang JJ, Paul J, Dearwater S, Fu FH. Loss of motion after anterior cruciate ligament reconstruction. *Am J Sports Med.* 1992;20:499–506.
5. Russell TA, Taylor JC, LaVelle DG. Fractures of the tibia and fibula. In: Rockwood CA Jr, Green DP, Bucholz RW, eds. *Rockwood and Green's Fractures in Adults.* 3rd ed. New York: JB Lippincott; 1991;1915–1982.
6. Carr CR, Wingo CH. Fractures of the femoral diaphysis. A retrospective study of the results and costs of treatment by intramedullary nailing and by traction and a spcia cast. *J Bone Joint Surg Arm.* 1973;55:690–700.
7. Rowntree M, Getty CJM. The knee after midshaft femoral fracture treatment: A comparison of three methods. *Injury.* 1981;13:125–130.
8. Winat EM. The use of skeletal traction in the treatment of fractures of the femur. *J Bone Joint Surg Am.* 1949;31:87–93.
9. Albright JP. Musculotendinous problems about the knee. In: Evarts CM, ed. *Surgery of the Musculoskeletal System.* New York: Churchill Livingstone; 1983;7:195–234.
10. Smillie IS. *Diseases of the Knee Joint.* Edinburgh: Churchill-Livingstone; 1974.
11. Kolowich PA, Paulos LE, Rosenberg TD, Farnsworth S. Lateral release of the patella: Indications and contraindications. *Am J Sports Med.* 1990;18:359–365.
12. Thompson T. Quadricepsplasty to improve knee function. *J Bone Joint Surg Am.* 1944;26:366–379.
13. Grauer JD, Kabo JM, Dorey FJ, Meals RA. The effects of dexamethasone on periarticular swelling and joint stiffness following fracture in a rabbit hind limb model. *Clin Orthop.* 1989;242:277–284.
14. Noble HB, Jajek MR. Boutonniere-type deformity of the knee following patellectomy and manipulations. *J Bone Joint Surg Am.* 1984;66:137–138.
15. Sorensen KH. The late prognosis after fracture of the patella. *Acta Orthop Scand.* 1964;34:198–212.
16. Kaufer H. Mechanical function of the patella. *J Bone Joint Surg Am.* 1971;53:1551–1560.
17. McAndrew MP, Pontarelli W. The long-term follow-up of ipsilateral tibial and femoral diaphyseal fractures. *Clin Orthop.* 1988;232:190–196.
18. Templeman DC, Marder RA. Injuries of the knee associated with fractures of the tibial shaft. Detection by examination under anesthesia. *J Bone Joint Surg Am.* 1989;71:1392–1395.
19. Pun WK, Chow SP, Fang D, et al. A study of function and residual joint stiffness after functional bracing of tibial shaft fractures. *Clin Orthop.* 1991;267:157–163.
20. Sisto DJ, Warren RF. Complete knee dislocation: A follow-up study of operative treatment. *Clin Orthop.* 1985;198:101.
21. Meyers M, Harvey JP. Traumatic dislocation of the knee joint. *J Bone Joint Surg Am.* 1971;53:16.
22. Roman PD, Hopson CN, Zenni EJ. Traumatic dislocation of the knee: A report of 30 cases and literature review. *Orthop Rev.* 1987;16:33.
23. Scott WN, Insall JN. Injuries of the knee. In: Rockwood CA Jr, Green DP, Bucholz RW, eds. *Rockwood and Green's Fractures in Adults.* 3rd ed. Philadelphia: JB Lippincott; 1991.
24. Harner CD, Fu FH, Irrgang JJ, Paul JJ. Recognition and management of the stiff knee following arthroscopic anterior cruciate ligament reconstruction—Recent experience. Scientific Exhibit 1407, American Academy of Orthopaedic Surgery annual meeting, Washington, DC, 1992.
25. Sprague NF, O'Connor RL, Fox JM. Arthroscopic treatment of postoperative knee fibroarthrosis. *Clin Orthop.* 1982;166:165–172.
26. Renstrom AFH. Complications of anterior cruciate ligament surgery. Presented at 5th Annual Panther Sports Medicine Symposium, Pittsburgh, PA, April 1992.
27. Wahl S, Renstrom R. Fibrosis in soft tissue injuries. In: Leadbetter WB, Buckwalter JA, Gordos SL, eds. *Sports Induced Inflammation.* American Academy of Orthopaedic Surgeons; Park Ridge, IL:1990.
28. Noyes FR, Wojtys EM, Marshall MT. The early diagnosis and treatment of developmental patella infera syndrome. *Clin Orthop.* 1991;265:241–252.
29. Canton J, Deschamps G, Chambat P, et al. Les Rotules basses: A propos de 128 observations. *Rev Chir Orthop.* 1982;68:317–325.
30. Jackson DW, Schaefer RK. Cyclops syndrome: Loss of

extension following intraarticular anterior cruciate ligament reconstruction. *Arthroscopy*. 1990;6:171–178.

31. Mohtadi NGH, Webster-Bogaert S, Fowler PJ. Limitation of motion following anterior cruciate ligament reconstruction. A case control study. *Am J Sports Med*. 1991;19:620–625.

32. Shelbourne KD, Wilckens JH, Mollabashy A, DeCarlo M. Arthrofibrosis in acute anterior cruciate ligament re-construction: The effect of timing of reconstruction and rehabilitation. *Am J Sports Med*. 1991;19:332–336.

33. Palmer I. On the injuries to the ligaments of the knee joint: A clinical study. *Acta Chir Scand*. 1938;81 (suppl 53).

34. Graf B, Uhr F. Complications of intra-articular anterior cruciate reconstruction. *Clin Sports Med*. 1988;7:785–800.

21
Nonunions and Malunions About the Knee

Jeffrey Mast

Introduction

The frequency of serious fractures of the lower femur and the upper tibia continues to be considerably large and therefore challenges the fracture surgeon with complex injuries associated with high complication rates.[1-5] As a result, a significant group of patients present with instabilities and deformities in the region of the knee joint that require thorough evaluation of their problems to plan and carry out optimum solutions. Execution of these corrective procedures demands knowledge of methods that may be employed to correct three-dimensional deformity. Internal fixation must be applied to the corrected extremity so that limb function and healing may occur simultaneously.

Because the knee is the central joint of the weight-bearing lower extremity it is extremely sensitive to instability and malalignment. Proper function of the knee joint depends on normal alignment. Alignment of the knee is normal when the mechanical axis of the lower extremity passes through its center. When this condition is present, the joint surfaces of the femur and tibia along with their ligamentous and muscular stabilizers act in such a way as to minimize shear forces and transmit compressive loads evenly and symmetrically across the largest possible area of articular surface (Fig. 21–1).[6,7] On the other hand, abnormal alignment disrupts this balance in the knee and leads to asymmetric overloading of the knee joint which predisposes to degenerative disease (Fig. 21–2).[8,9]

Instability arising from a nonunion of the distal femur or the proximal tibia causes such a profound disability that bracing and external support are required for function of the limb. Malunion of these same bones is associated with an unsightly extremity that is dysfunctional and results in posttraumatic arthrosis which is related to the degree of deformity and period of its existence.[9]

The purpose of this chapter is to discuss the author's approach to the evaluation, planning, and surgical technique used in the management of these cases.[10]

Clinical Evaluation

Patient evaluation begins with the history of the injury which should include the date and details of the original accident. It is important to know if the original fracture was open or closed and whether or not there was associated nerve or vascular injury. Details of the initial treatment and any subsequent treatment should be documented. Of prime importance is to determine if the extremity was at any time infected or if any special procedures were necessary to repair vessels or nerves or provide for soft tissue coverage.

Depending on the nature of the residual problem, nonunion or malunion, the patient may complain of pain and/or instability in the area of the deformity or pain in the region of adjacent joints. These complaints may be magnified by the patient's activity. In the office setting the patient may be freely mobile or may depend on external support for ambulation.

The physical examination must assess the static and dynamic functional alignment in the frontal, sagittal, and horizontal planes. Of the various deformities those of abnormal torsion may be the most difficult to appreciate. These deformities are evaluated by observing the patient standing, viewed from the front and from the side. Where possible, "sighting" down the axis of the extremity is carried out, but unfortunately is limited to the leg and foot. The patient is next asked to walk and the characteristic of the gait is recorded. A search for compensatory mechanisms is carried out.

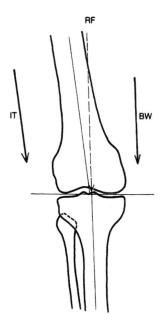

Figure 21-1. Diagram of loading of the knee under normal conditions. BW = the vector of the body weight, IT = the counteracting muscular pull of the iliotibial tract. The reactive force (RP) passes through the center of the knee along the mechanical axis of the lower extremity.

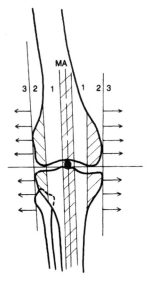

Figure 21-2. Diagram of the relationship of the location of the mechanical axis (MA) to the relative indication for operative correction. When the mechanical axis falls into zone 3, there is an absolute indication for correction. In zone 2, there is a relative to absolute indication for correction. In zone 1, there may be a relative indication for operative correction. (Redrawn with permission from Müller and Müller.[8])

In addition to the general orthopedic examination, specific attention should be paid to leg length measurements, range of motion of the joints, coexisting ligamentous instability, and the neuromuscular status. Peripheral pulses must be sought and evaluated in terms of the normal side or in terms of the examiner's sense of what should be normal, if there is no normal side.

The condition of the soft tissues surrounding and adjacent to the deformity is of paramount importance. The presence of a draining sinus or a thin unyielding adherent soft tissue envelope will certainly limit or redirect the surgical methods to be used.

Radiographic Evaluation

The standard anteroposterior and lateral projections should be taken with the central ray focused on the deformity. These radiographs should be taken at a distance of 1 m so that magnification remains constant in all studies.

Markers are available for use in conjunction with the x-ray study that may allow exact calibration of the magnification to be determined.[3] With deformities adjacent to the knee joint enough of the proximal or distal shaft must be included on the same radiograph to allow precise localization of the anatomic axis of the bone. Control radiographs of the patient's normal side are taken with exactly the same settings and projections as were used for the involved side. These are important studies and will be used for planning the corrections. Additionally, limb alignment radiographs are necessary to coordinate and check the changes planned from the standard views. The author uses 51-in. film exposed at a distance of 2.1 m. Hip, knee, and ankle are all visible on these studies, making the relationships between the anatomic and mechanical axes of the lower extremity easier to visualize.

Recently, computed tomography (CT) scanning with axial superimposition of hip, knee, and ankle has been used to demonstrate the degree of rotational deformity present.[11] In addition, by sighting down the mechanical axis of the extremity through the superimposed CT cuts from the midportions of these respective joints, it is possible to see the marked deviations created by the angular deformities viewed on the plain x-rays.

Although the preceding studies do well to document the static aspects of malunions, nonunions demand further studies to evaluate other aspects of their status. These studies must address both the biologic and the mechanical conditions present. From the standard radiographic views, we may define nonunions as being hypertrophic, normotrophic, and atrophic based on the amount of osteogenic activity present at the nonunion site.[12,13] Adjunctive to these studies is the performance of stress x-rays. This simple procedure can define the planes and quantify the degree of instability.

As has been pointed out by surgeons versed in the Ilizarov technique, it is valuable to characterize nonunions in terms of their mobility.[14] A nonunion may be described as being stiff or, at the other extreme, lax. As one would expect, the degree of mobility usually parallels the degree of biologic activity. Stiff nonunions are usually hypertrophic; lax nonunions, oligotrophic or atrophic. In addition, knowing the direction in which a nonunion becomes stable is also valuable information, as the surgical procedure can be designed to exploit this situation to obtain compression of two bony surfaces and achieve stable fixation.

Another radiographic technique valuable in the evaluation of nonunions is tomography. This time-honored technique can demonstrate the existence of a sequestrum or allow evaluation of the interface between the two fragments to demonstrate an avascular wedge or fragment. When a synovial pseudoarthrosis is suspected, a bone scan showing the characteristic pattern of increased uptake at the terminal aspect of the bone ends with a relatively "cold" cleft between them is confirmatory.[12,13]

Planning

From the history and physical examination, specific problems should raise the possibility of the need for specialty assistance. The patient with a history of a vascular injury or in whom the peripheral pulses are absent or diminished may require a preoperative angiogram to assess vascular status. Likewise the findings of a poor soft tissue sleeve in the region of the deformity, with otherwise satisfactory perfusion to the limb, will necessitate a reconstructive soft tissue procedure to solve this problem before correction and internal fixation can safely be carried out.

Patients with infection complicating their problem require a staged reconstruction. The principle depends on debridement of necrotic tissue including bone and stabilization using an appropriate implant or external fixation.[15] When a significant defect exists the author uses polymethylmethacrylate–antibiotic cement, formed in the shape of the missing segment as a spacer[16]; the technique is similar to the use of a temporary filling by a dentist doing "root canal" surgery. Following successful elimination of the focus of infection and related drainage the "spacer" is removed and autologous cancellous bone graft is inserted into the defect. Cultures of the exudate, pseudomembrane, and bone are taken

at the time of the debridement, and specific antibiotic therapy is continued during the treatment period and empirically for 6 weeks following the cancellous bone grafting.

The Use of Tracings

Preoperative drawings are made from the pertinent x-rays. Tracing of the x-rays with subsequent manipulation of the fragments is essential to understanding the corrective surgery and the steps that will be needed to accomplish it. Malunions are easier to plan than nonunions, because the deformity is static and the surgeon has the opportunity to plan an osteotomy that will best solve the problems of the specific deformity. The goal in the usual case is to correct the deformity completely. If the deformity is unilateral and the patient is prearthrotic, the deformity is corrected to the normal axis and

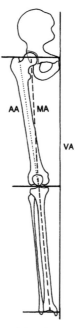

Figure 21-3. Diagram of the axial relationships of the lower extremities in the frontal plane. The vertical axis (VA) is drawn perpendicular to the ground. The mechanical axis (MA) of the ankle, knee, and hip joint can be then defined as being on a line at right angles to the vertical axis at the level of the joint. The mechanical axis of the leg is the same as the anatomic axis (AA) of the tibia, whereas the anatomic axis of the femur joins the mechanical axis of the lower extremity at an angle of 6°. The mechanical axis of the lower extremity is convergent to the vertical axis at an angle of 3°. (Redrawn with permission from Müller and Müller.[8])

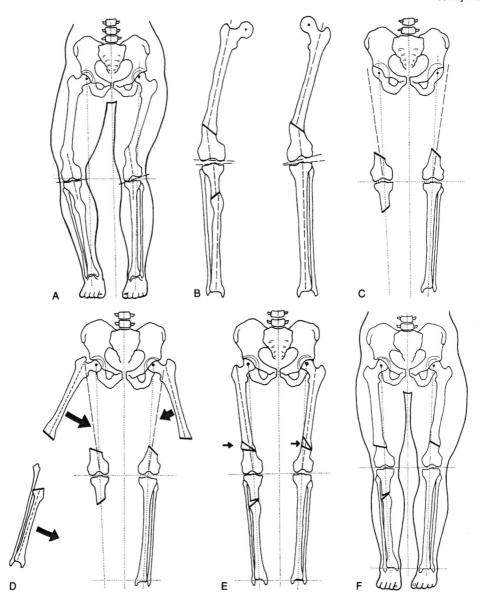

Figure 21-4. A generic frontal plane planning technique using the normal limb axes. Such a case may be planned using long alignment films of the involved extremity(ies). Usually, similar methods are used but with regional axes, to avoid working with such large sheets of paper. This is a hypothetical case of an adult female with posttraumatic "wind-blown" deformities of the lower extremities. She has had bilateral supracondylar femur fractures and a right proximal tibia fracture. All fractures have healed. **A** Tracing of the weight-bearing alignment films. The vertical and mechanical axes of the lower extremity and knee joints have been drawn into their proper positions. **B.** Separate tracings are made of the right and left limbs including their respective anatomic axes. A line is drawn across the bone connecting the contour changes of the medial and lateral cortex of each deformity. This line is usually near the region of the intersection of the anatomic axis. **C.** On a fresh piece of paper are traced the pelvis and the vertical axis along with perpendiculars at the level of the knee and ankle (mechanical axis of the knee joint and ankle joint). The distal femur, proximal tibia, and knee

shape of the normal side; when an arthrosis exists a slight overcorrection to unload the involved side becomes the operative goal.

The plane of reference is selected by reviewing the radiographs. The plane of reference is the plane in which the most significant angulation exists. If the deformity exhibits equal angulations in both the anteroposterior and lateral projections, then the plane of the deformity is inconveniently located halfway between the two standard projections. Although for small angulations this represents no barrier to planning, for larger ones, planning may be better carried out in a different projection. This projection should correspond to an anatomic area for which there is surgical access. Success both in planning, and in the subsequent surgical execution of the plan, depends on knowledge of the normal joint relationships to the anatomic and mechanical axes of the long bones (Fig. 21–3).

Planning of complicated corrections about the knee that are bilateral may be accomplished by the generic methods illustrated in the hypothetical case in Figure 21–4 (Mueller ME, Ganz R, personal communication, 1983).

In the case of nonunions, planning with drawings may be more difficult. Nonunions are variably mobile; as a result, static x-rays may not represent the true relationships of the proximal to the distal fragment. Stress films that force the instability into a fixed relationship may be necessary to obviate this problem. These views also indicate in which direction, if any, the nonunion becomes stable.

The goal in planning for nonunions is to obtain union and to restore the bone as near as possible to its original size and shape. In doing so, the biomechanics of the extremity are optimized. Corrections of malaligned nonunions are planned in the same manner as has been described for malunions, once the appropriate x-rays have been obtained. The axes of the primary distal and proximal fragments are traced into the respective fragments and the fragments with their axes are retraced on separate pieces of tracing paper. They are then manipulated until the requirements of reduction are fulfilled.

With a nonunion, the causative factors must be sought and the nonunion characterized as being hypertrophic, atrophic, or normotrophic. With this in mind the mechanism for obtaining the reduction and fixation

of the nonunion may be developed and included in the plan as part of the kinetics of the operative procedure. The need for a bone graft will depend on the type of nonunion and the manner in which correction will be obtained.

Many instruments and implants are useful in corrective reconstructive surgey in the region of the knee joint. The author relies heavily on the distraction force provided by external fixators or the "distractors" (Fig. 21–5).

On the femoral side of the joint the condylar blade plate (Synthes) is the implant of choice as the fixed-angle relationship between blade and plate lends itself to relatively easy corrective procedures. The device can be placed with planning so the correction is completed when the proximal fragment is reduced to the plate (Figs. 21–6 and 21–7).

Principles

The aim of the surgical procedure is to achieve optimal loading of the knee joint by reestablishment of the proper location of the mechanical axis of the knee joint.

The mechanical axis of the lower extremity is a line that connects the centers of the hip and ankle and passes through the center of the knee. As has been stated by others,[7,8] deviations from the normal location of this axis which exists in malunions in the region of the knee provide a guide for the selection of patients for corrective osteotomy.

As a general rule posttraumatic deformities are most accurately corrected at the site of the original injury. From this standpoint, timing of the surgical procedure becomes important. In the usual circumstances, one should not allow a malreduction to become a malunion. Correcting a poorly executed internal fixation is most easily accomplished in the first few weeks when the un-united fracture can once more be approached, the implants removed, the problem corrected, and stable internal fixation applied. In some cases because of compromised skin, infection, or other coexisting problems, another surgical intervention may be contraindicated. In such cases malalignment may persist to become a malunion or perhaps a malaligned nonunion that must be addressed later after the complicating circumstance has been resolved.

---

joints are retraced at their proper locations at the intersection of the mechanical axis of the lower extremity and the mechanical axis of the knee. **D**. The femurs can now be brought back into the tracing and realigned to the distal femurs already in their corrected position at the knee. This produces the tracing seen in the next figure. **E**. Rotating the femoral shafts at the center of the hip until alignment at the supracondylar level is correct allows one to measure the angular correction needed in the frontal plane to achieve the desired correction. Note that at this time all the anatomic and me-

chanical deficiencies of the hypothetical case have been corrected. **F**. Tracing of the lower extremities with the corrections pictorially completed (the osteotomy wedge was cut from the distal fragment) and the soft tissue outlines redrawn. Fixation of the osteotomies may be carried out with an angled blade plate (condylar plate lateral or 90° plate medially) depending on the requirements of the individual case and the desires of the surgeon. The surgical tactic can then be resolved in terms of steps based on the critical position of the seating chisel in the distal femur.

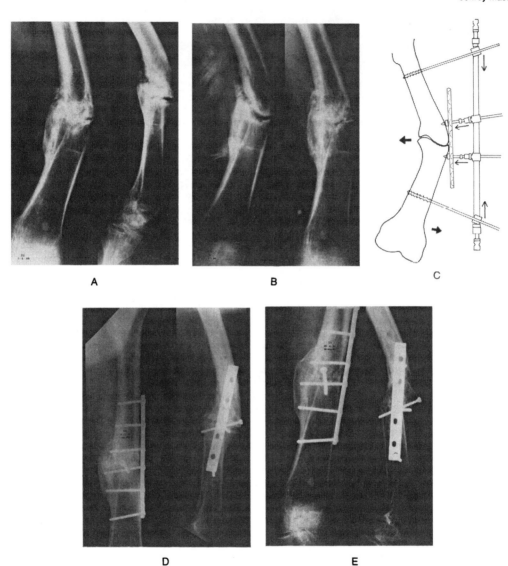

Figure 21–5. A. Anteroposterior and lateral radiographs of a 78-year-old man with a 3-year-old nonunion of the mid-distal third of the left femur. The patient had been treated for the last 2 years with a simple thigh lacer, because he had severe atherosclerotic vascular disease and was status post bypass surgery. The patient had a marked varus deformity and was having knee pain as well as pain in the contralateral hand from the constant use of a cane. This patient was a poor surgical candidate. It was felt that the essentials of the correction should be carried out with as minimal an operative procedure as possible. **B.** Stress films taken in the radiology suite. On the left is shown the stress in varus. Note how the patient's nonunion is unstable in varus, but with the valgus stress, as shown on the right, there is compression of the cartilage in the lateral defect and stabilization of the femur. This finding may be exploited during the operative procedure by pressing laterally. This places the medial callus under tension and the lateral cartilage in the nonunion under compression. High forces will be needed to gain a correction, and therefore an important part of the case is the determination of how this may be accomplished in surgery. **C.** Drawing of the nonunion showing a method that may be used to accomplish the correction in a relatively atraumatic way. In this example an external fixator is used with two large Schantz screws inserted proximally and distally at right angles to the femoral shaft axis. They are then attached by standard adjustable clamps

If old fracture lines are still identifiable, the obvious tactic is to mobilize these fracture surfaces and correct the malreduction at the fracture site. This will sometimes require a limited osteoclasis or partial osteotomy. It is accepted that healed comminution is not disrupted but mobilized "en bloc" in the course of the reconstruction. Such a case is handled similar to a nonunion and may also require a partial osteotomy or limited osteoclasis to achieve proper alignment. When the fracture has completely healed but is malunited, the problem is solved by corrective osteotomy.

In all cases it is essential that stable internal fixation is achieved as part of the surgical procedure. The advantage of planning the osteotomy is that correction of the deformity can be carried out using the implant as a means of correction as well as fixation. Fixed-angle blade plates are particularly well suited to this purpose, and for the author the preferred implant is the condylar blade plate of the ASIF. Using the principles of interfragmentary compression, stable fixation can be achieved that will allow relatively pain-free function in the immediate postoperative period. By treating the patient functionally optimal joint recovery can be achieved (Fig. 21–8).

Distal Femur

The author uses the condylar blade plate for the reasons mentioned earlier to correct malunions and nonunions of the distal femur. This is true regardless of the presence of a varus or valgus deformity. The plate is always applied laterally and opening or closing wedge-type osteotomies are employed depending on the circumstances of the individual case. Figures 21–6 and 21–7 are representative of the planning and execution of surgery of this type of case.

Following successful surgical correction no additional external splintage of any type is employed. The patient is mobilized with crutches or a walker. Weight bearing of 20 to 30 pounds is encouraged on the operated extremity. Union occurs in 6 to 12 weeks. Physical therapy is instituted from the second postoperative day and consists of active assisted range of motion exercises early, followed by assisted resisted range of motion exercises as healing begins to occur. Active resisted exercises with resistance machines round out the rehabilitation program and are monitored with objective functional testing using the uninjured extremity as a control in the final stages.

In most cases the implant is removed at 12 to 18 months following the correction. After plate removal the patient is asked not to participate in contact or other "high-energy" sports for an additional 3 months.

Intraarticular Malunions. Improved training in the management of intraarticular fractures most likely has led to a decline in the number of intraarticular malunions and nonunions. When present, however, their management may be difficult depending on the displacement and the original intraarticular comminution.[17] The solution to the problem may be direct or indirect. An example of a direct solution would be the definition and correction of the articular malunion. An example of an indirect solution would be an osteotomy that redirects weight-bearing loads away from an injured joint surface.

If there exists in the joint a large malunited or displaced and un-united piece of the articular surface, for example, a portion of the medial femoral condyle, the treatment should be directed toward osteotomy and/or mobilization of the fragment, reducing it anatomically and fixing it in its reduced position until healing occurs. The goal is to prevent or delay the onset of posttraumatic osteoarthrosis resulting from significant joint incongruity (Fig. 21–9).[17]

When there has been a crushing or impaction of a significant portion of the weight-bearing articular surface with depression of the surface and secondary instability, then the problem is one of instability and the goal of treatment is to eliminate the depression by elevation of the residual articular surface combined with a buttressing subchondral bone graft, to eliminate the joint instability.

When there was too much intraarticular comminution

(Synthes) to a external fixator tube and open-end compressors are applied at either end. On the lateral aspect or apex of the nonunion, a ten-hole plate is centered over the apex on the proximal and distal fragments, and near the apex, 4.5 Schantz screws have been placed; the tips of which are prevented from penetrating the bone too deeply by 4.5-mm nuts attached to the Schantz screw tips. The Schantz screws are attached to the tubes by standard adjustable clamps. Small open-end compressors from the mini-external fixator set are modified by enlarging their fixation slots so that they can accommodate being attached to 4.5-mm Schantz screws. When they are opened the 4.5mm Schantz screws are pushed against the apex of the nonunion. By this method a hinge is created that can generate enough power to straighten the bone in the frontal plane. A minimal lateral osteoclasis

will be necessary to allow the correction to be fully obtained. No attempt was made to correct the displacement in the sagittal plane because this would require completing the osteotomy resulting in instability. The significant medical problems existing in this patient required a quick operative procedure. **D.** Anteroposterior and lateral projections of the femur at 4 weeks postop. The deformity has been completely corrected in the frontal plane; however, there continues to be slightly increased antecurvatum and the anterior displacement of the proximal fragment persists in the sagittal plane. **E.** At 28 months postop, the patient is healed. He has been free of both external supports and the thigh lacer for 2 years and is extremely pleased with his operative procedure. This case was selected to show how the kinetics of the operation may be developed at the planning stage.

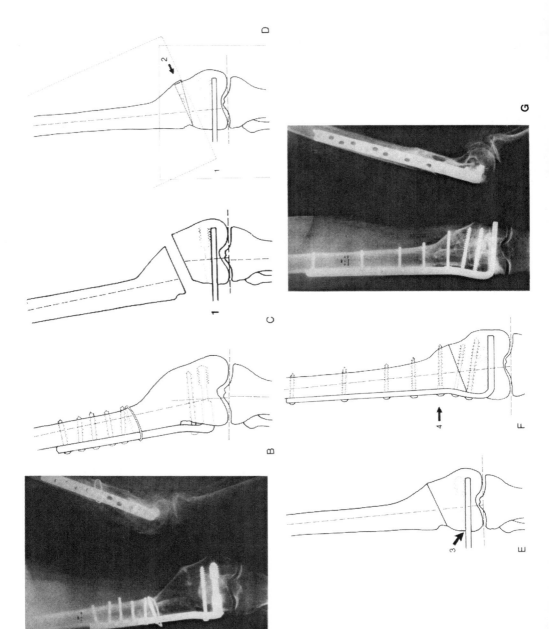

associated with the original injury and early post-traumatic arthrosis exists in a stable joint, a direct correction may be impossible and the best that can be accomplished is an indirect solution to the problem. If, for example, the injury was confined to the medial joint of the tibia, as in a medial plateau fracture, then a valgus osteotomy of the proximal tibia may be indicated (Fig. 21–10). Contrarily, a residual posttraumatic arthrosis of the lateral compartment may require a varus osteotomy to alleviate the patient's symptoms.

Nonunions follow essentially the same principles of treatment, modified by the specific techniques discussed earlier. The postoperative regimen is the same for patients treated by indirect techniques as for patients treated directly for malunion. The postoperative treatment is the same as has been discussed for the distal femur.

Proximal Tibia

The tibia is a straight bone. A straight bone was defined by Milch,[18] as a bone in which the mechanical axis is coaxial with the anatomic axis. Therefore, angular malunions of the tibia are corrected by redirectional osteotomies. These procedures reestablish the proper direction of the mechanical axis of the leg. Posttraumatic deformities of the tibia are frequently associated with displacements as well as angulations. Correction of displacements frequently are important to obtaining an optimum result. Preoperative plans should be formulated for the simultaneous correction of all displacements and angulations (Figs. 21–11 and 21–12).[19]

Postoperatively the foot and leg are placed in a compression dressing made of soft padding material and bias-cut stockinet. The leg is then elevated in a knee CPM machine and continuous passive motion is instituted. On the second postoperative day the patient is ambulated on crutches, 20 to 30 pounds of weight bearing on the operative extremity. The patient remains on crutches with this amount of weight bearing until the bone has healed. Usually this requires 8 to 12 weeks. During the healing period, the patient receives physical therapy tailored individually to encourage the maintenance of a full range of motion of the knee with normal strength.

Complications and Pitfalls

Complications of surgical procedures to correct malunions and nonunions in the region of the knee are not unique to these procedures. They are, however, perhaps more frustrating to the patient and the surgeon, because the patient has already had the unfortunate experience of at least one preceding complication that led to the existing problem. Unfortunately, this does not lessen the fact that the reconstructive attempt is more difficult and, therefore, logically associated with an increased complication rate.

Complications and pitfalls can be divided into those associated with the surgical procedure, those in the immediate postoperative period, and late complications.

All of these cases have in common prior treatment that has failed. When the treatment was a previous open reduction and internal fixation, refixation after correction of the malunion may be difficult. When the initial fixation was with a fixed-angle screw or plate, significant bone loss in the region of the epiphysis may have occurred as a result of motion. Optimum locations

---

Figure 21–6. A, B. Anteroposterior and lateral views of the femur of a 70-year-old woman with osteoporosis. The patient had sustained a femur fracture approximately 12 months prior to being seen in our office. The patient was unable to walk without a walker. She was otherwise in good health although slightly obese. The tracing illustrates the patient's femur in the frontal plane. The patient has a valgus deformity of 10°. **C.** An illustration of the method the author uses for planning such a case. Two fragments are developed based on the deviation from normal on the AP film of the medial and lateral cortical shadows. Each fragment is traced on a separate piece of paper so that it can be manipulated. The most important step is the insertion of the seating chisel to prepare the slot for the 95° condylar plate in the distal fragment. The position of the seating chisel is absolutely critical as it must be parallel to the femur in the frontal plane and in line with the femoral shaft in the sagittal plane. In addition, the direction of the seating chisel must be true as well to the distal femur in the horizontal plane. The technique for insertion of the seating chisel in the distal femur to be treated with a condylar blade plate is well described in other sources. **D.** By manipulating the two tracings on their separate pieces of paper it's possible to correct the deformity in the femur seen in the frontal plane. The overlap medial marked by the arrow in paper 2 determines the angle that must be resected to allow both sides of the osteotomy to be in perfect contact with one another after the correction. Paper 1 again delineates the most important step, which is insertion of the seating chisel parallel to the end of the distal femur. **E.** The tracing is then prepared from the corrected fragments viewed in the last step. In this drawing, attention is turned to the repair of the old hole in the distal epimetaphysis of the distal femur. This hole must be filled with a material able to support the blade of the plate under compressive loads. In this case the plan was to use methylmethacrylate. Its application is depicted by the arrow. **F.** The final tracing showing the desired end result. This tracing should be the documentation of how the final x-ray should appear. This tracing also contains the final steps of the operative procedure including the correct length of plate and the location of the desired fixation. The arrow shows that the first screw in the proximal fragment will be blocked by a nut. This of course will be inserted following the application of tension to the plate. The nut will keep the screw from backing out in the early preoperative stages. This precaution is being taken because of the osteoporosis. **G.** One and one-half years after surgery. The patient has healed and has returned to her normal function.

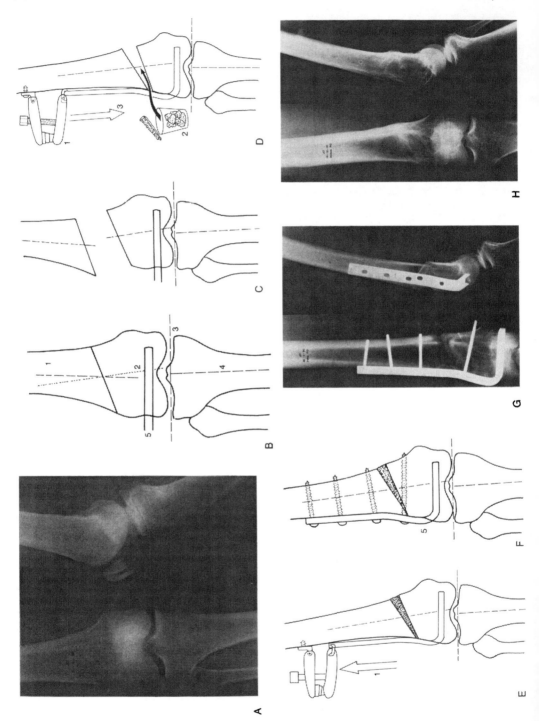

for refixation after correction are compromised. Preoperative planning sometimes must include modification of existing implants or the use of allograft or methylmethacrylate cement (see Fig. 21-6), as attempts to solve these problems. Because of these suboptimal conditions acute loss of fixation with loss of correction is unfortunately too frequently seen.

Because corrective osteotomies demand the use of sharp bone-cutting instruments, and both malunions and nonunions are frequently associated with the proliferation of fibrous tissue as unyielding scar, the chance of an iatrogenic injury to the vessels or nerves is a reality that must be avoided by skilled surgical maneuvers and/or thoughtful planning. In patients whose history, physical examination, or plain x-rays suggest an undue risk for such a complication, an arteriogram with appropriate consultation should help secure the plan of management. Obviously, an occurrence demands the appropriate response to the complication to avoid the permanent disability that can be associated with the event. In high-risk cases a plan that includes arrangements for possibly needed subspecialist help is optimal.

Perhaps the most frustrating type of complication for both surgeon and patient is the failure to obtain complete correction of the deformity. In the author's experience the most common mistake is undercorrection of the deformity. In most cases the error is small and unnoticed by the patient. On a clinical basis the deficit is also usually not readily apparent. Nevertheless, the surgeon in strict postoperative scrutiny is aware of the deficit on the basis of the limb alignment radiographs discussed previously. Rarely is the deficit enough to justify another intervention, but the surgeon is not happy because the case is not perfect and therefore the long-term result may linger in a "guarded" category. Careful perioperative imaging minimizes this complication.

In the immediate postoperative period complications are related to the soft tissues and may consist of hematoma, marginal or full-thickness wound necrosis, compartment syndrome, and deep or superficial infection. To avoid long-term compromise of the results of the reconstructive procedure, prompt diagnosis of these conditions and an effective response are necessary. Because of the general nature of these complications, specific management is not discussed further in this chapter.

Longer follow-up may be associated with the complications of loss of fixation and recurrence of the deformity or the development of a frank nonunion. These complications must be critically studied and the reason for failure identified. The problem must be addressed during the reoperation to finally arrive at a solution with a healed bone and a balanced properly aligned knee.

Summary

Reconstruction of malunions and nonunions in the region of the knee pose stimulating problems for the orthopedic surgeon. The analysis and execution of the surgical solution tax the orthopedist's knowledge of anatomy, biomechanics, fracture healing, and the principles of internal fixation.

This chapter has centered on the approach to the patient through history, physical examination, and evaluation of pertinent radiographic material. Identification of the needs of an individual case has been stressed along with the planning of surgical treatment by means of drawings. Specific examples of representative cases have been presented. Regionally, examples of solutions of cases of both malunions and nonunions of the distal femur, knee joint, and proximal tibia and fibula have been illustrated.

Finally it has been shown that the surgical correction of a case complicated by malalignment or malaligned nonunion is very difficult and, if critically viewed following treatment, usually leaves room for improvement. For this reason, the undertaking of such a case demands the utmost in planning, technical execution, and commitment from the surgical team.

Figure 21-7. Anteroposterior and lateral views of the distal femur and proximal tibia of a 34-year-old male who had a childhood injury to the distal femur. This resulted in a significant varus deformity of the right lower extremity associated with 1 in. of shortening. B. Tracing of the AP x-ray. (1) Existing anatomic axis of the femur. (2) Ideal anatomic axis of the femur. (3) Joint line of the knee. (4) Anatomic axis of the tibia, which is same as the mechanical axis of the lower extremity. (5) Tracing of the seating chisel for the 95° condylar plate traced into the desired location in the frontal plane. C. The distal femur resolved into two fragments, traced on separate pieces of paper. D. Tracing of the distal fragment with the condylar blade plate traced into the distal fragment as well. The proximal fragment is reduced to the plate and an articulating tension device has been drawn in a position of distraction to show how lengthening of 1 in. may be obtained simultaneous with the correction of the varus deformity. In this case cortical cancellous graft and cancellous graft will be added to the opening osteotomy. This can be facilitated by first distracting and increasing the gap until the desired lengthening has been obtained. Following application of bone graft the plate may be tensioned. E. The next stage of the procedure. The bone graft has been added and the plate tensioned. F. Following tensioning of the plate, the screws are inserted. The tracing of the desired end result should approximate the final postoperative x-ray in the frontal plane. G. Two weeks postop. H. Twenty months postop. The metal has been removed. The patient's legs are equal in length. The knee range of motion is unrestricted. The following two cases demonstrate the use of a 95° condylar blade plate to correct both a varus deformity and a valgus deformity in the distal femur. In our hands the technique using this implant is very simple and has been very reliable.

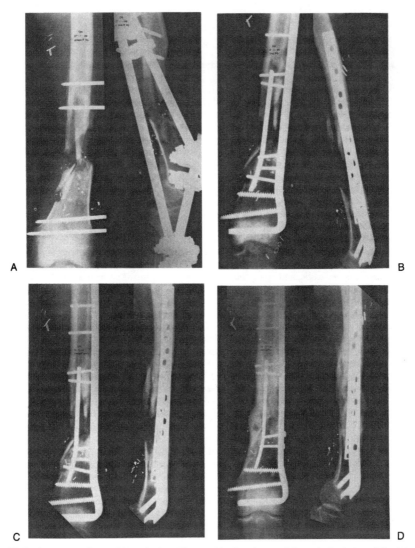

A   B

C   D

Figure 21–8. Anteroposterior and lateral of a 28-year-old man injured 4 months before when hit at close range by a high-velocity bullet. The patient sustained a vascular injury but did not injure any nerve. He was initially admitted to another hospital where vascular repair was carried out after extensive debridement of his wound. The patient was placed in an external fixator and was referred to our office 4 months after his injury. The patient had a segmental defect as can be appreciated and a varus angulation of the distal femur. The limb was short 2½ in. **B.** Anteroposterior and lateral radiographs of the same extremity following the operative intervention. Because of the complex circumstances of the segmental deficiency of bone a special construct was planned. Correction of the deformity was ensured by the use of a 95° condylar blade plate. Note the correct placement of the blade of the plate relative to the distal end of the femur in the frontal plane. The late is 18 holes long and is placed in association with an endosteal narrow 4.5 DC plate that bridges the segmental defect. The endosteal plate has been locked in its intramedullary position by screws that pass through the condy- lar plate and through the holes of the intramedullary plate. The addition of a screw in the montage that blocks the plate medially in the canal ensures that the intramedullary plate is positioned to most effectively provide a temporary medial buttress. This endosteal plate gives additional stability to the construct during the time needed for bone graft added at the same operation to consolidate. **C.** Anteroposterior and lateral x-rays of patient's femur 3 months later and 2 weeks after receiving additional cancellous bone graft. The fixation is stable, the bone density is improving, and consolidation of fractures proximal and distally has occurred. **D.** Sixteen months postop. The patient's femur has healed. There has been full consolidation of the bone graft, with remodeling occurring in the area of the segmental defect. The patient's function is excellent. He has a full range of motion of his knee in both flexion and extension. There is no axial malalignment and the patient's extremity is of equal length of the opposite side. The patient has returned to work. The case is included to show a technique that has been useful in providing a temporary medial buttress during plate fixation.

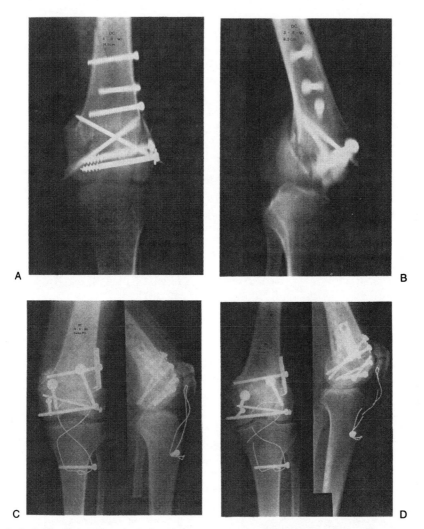

A					B

C					D

Figure 21-9. A, B. Anteroposterior and lateral radiographs of the distal femur of a 19-year-old man. The patient was involved in a Moped versus automobile accident in Mexico. Original radiographs were never available. Apparently, the patient had bilateral femur fractures with bilateral patellar fractures. These radiographs depict the postoperative result of the left femur. A malreduction exists at 8 weeks. Note that both condyles are shortened and the trochlear portion of the distal femur impinges on the anterior tibia. This constitutes an intraarticular malunion. **C.** Anteroposterior and lateral radiographs following reconstruction of the distal femur. The prob-

lem was approached laterally; however, a transpatellar ligament extension was needed medially. The two condyles were osteotomized, reduced, and then distalized as a block. They were fixed by means of lag screws and a posterior lateral buttress plate. **D.** Six-month follow-up AP and lateral radiographs. The articular fragments have healed in the correct position. The patient has recovered function including strength, stability, and range of motion. Note that the wire protecting the repair of the infrapatellar tendon has broken. The patient has returned to work.

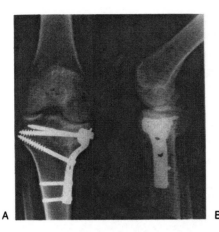

A   B

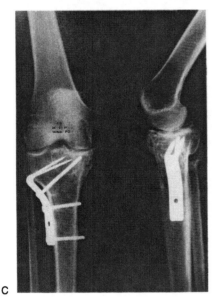

C   D

Figure 21–10. A. Forty-year-old woman with a 2-year-old fracture of the medial tibial plateau. She has a varus deformity and incapacitating medial knee joint pain. There was significant joint depression at the time of the original injury, which was not corrected. **B.** A little over a year after a 16° valgus high tibial osteotomy. The patient has improved but is still not completely pain free. The osteotomy could be criticized as being undercorrected. The goals of such a procedure are to place more load into the healthy lateral side of the joint by redirecting the mechanical axis of the tibia. As a result, symptoms are alleviated and the longevity of the joint can be expected to be improved. This is an example of an indirect solution to the problem of intraarticular malunion.

References

1. Mast J, Jakob R, Ganz R. *Planning and Reduction Techniques in Fracture Surgery.* Berlin: Springer-Verlag; 1989: 1–47.
2. Neer CS II, Granthans SA, Selton ML. Supracondylar-condylar fractures of the adult femur. *J Bone Joint Surg Am.* 1967;49:591–613.
3. Stevens, Peter. M.D. Orthographics.
4. Bucholz RW, Brunbeck RJ. In: Rockwood C, Green W, eds. *Fractures.* 3rd ed. Philadelphia: JB Lippincott; 1991: 1653.
5. Slatis P, Ryoppy S, Huihiuen VM. AOI osteosynthesis of fractures of the distal third of the femur. *Acta Orthop Scand.* 1971;42:162–172.
6. Freeman MAR. *Arthritis of the Knee.* New York: Springer-Verlag; 1980:31–55.
7. Lang J, Wachsmuth W. *Pratische Anatomie.* Bein & Statik; 1972:12–13.
8. Mueller KH, Mueller J. *Indications, Localization and Planning of Post-Traumatic Osteotomies about the Knee.*
9. Pauwels F. Neue Richtlinien Fuer die Operative Behandlung der Coxarthrose. *Vehr Dtsch Orthop Ges.* 1961; 48:332–336.
10. Mast J, Teitge R, Gouda M. Preoperative planning for the treatment of nonunions and the correction of malunions of the long bones. *Orthop Clin North Am.* 1990;21(4).
11. Miller P. *C.T.* Rotational study of the lower extremity. Scientific Exhibit, 78th Scientific Assembly & Annual Meeting of the Radiological Society of North America, Chicago, November 1992.
12. Rosen H. Nonunion and malunion. In: Browner B, Jupiter J, Levine A, Trafton P, eds. *Skeletal trauma.* Philadelphia: WB Saunders; 1992;501–541.
13. Weber BG, Cech O. *Pseudoarthrosis.* Vienna: Hans Huber; 1976;40–44.
14. Schwartsman V, Choi S, Schwartsman R. *Orthop Clin North Am.* 1990;21:639–653.
15. Burri C. *Post-Traumatic Osteomyelitis.* Vienna: Hans Huber; 1975;163–279.
16. Cierny G III, Meder JJ. Approach to adult osteomyelitis. *Orthop Rev.* 1987;16:259–270.
17. Schatzker J. Intra-articular mal- and nonunions. *Orthop Clin North Am.* 1990;21:743–757.
18. Milch H. *Osteotomy of the Long Bones.* Springfield, MA: Thomas; 1947.
19. Paley, Dror, Chaudray M, Pirone AM, Lentz P, Kautz d PA-C. Treatment of malunions and malnonunions of the femur and tibia by detailed preoperative planning and Ilizarov techniques. *Orthop Clin North Am.* 1990;21(4).

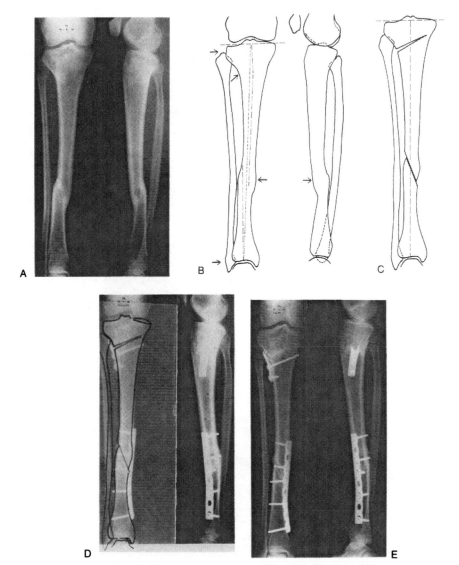

A　　　　　　　　　　　　　B　　　　　　　　　　　　C

D　　　　　　　　　　　　　　　　　　　　　　E

Figure 21–11. A. Anteroposterior and lateral radiographs of
the tibia and fibula of a 20-year-old woman injured 1½ years
previously in a motor vehicle accident. She sustained a pelvic
fracture and a segmental fracture of her right leg. She was
treated nonoperatively for both injuries and developed a valgus deformity associated with a ¾ in. shortening of the right
leg. Note the scars of the previous fractures proximally in the
tibial metaphysis and at the mid-distal third junction of the
tibial diaphysis. Also note that the fibula was not fractured, yet
the tibia underwent shortening. When this occurs one must
look to the ankle or the knee with concern for the distal or
proximal tibia–fibular syndesmosis to explain the consequences of this fracture pattern. **B.** Tracings of the AP and lateral radiographs with arrows drawn at the possible locations
of residual problems. In this case it can be seen that the proximal tibia–fibular joint has been dislocated. The malunion in

valgus of the proximal tibial fracture, although not large at 3°,
is aggravated by the lateralization of the distal fragment of
the tibia. **C.** The preoperative plan derived from the previous
tracing will correct all the deficiencies. Length will be regained by means of an oblique osteotomy of the distal tibia
which will elongate the bone as the lateral shaft displacement
is corrected. Through the intact distal syndesmosis the fibula
will be repositioned. Additionally, an opening lateral based
osteotomy may be used to further regain length and correct
the small angular defomity, restoring the tibia to its physiologic 3° of varus. **D.** Superimposition of the operative plan on
the final surgical result as seen in the postoperative radiographs. The correction is complete. **E.** Anteroposterior and
lateral radiographs 1 month after surgery. Osteotomy lines
are consolidating although at this point the patient is still on
crutches.

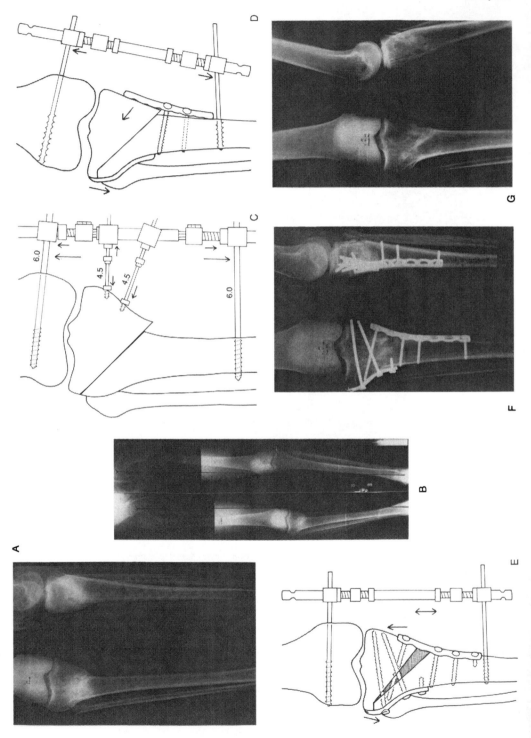

Figure 21–12. A. Anteroposterior and lateral radiographs illustrating the proximal tibia of a 36-year-old man who had suffered this fracture in a motorcycle accident 1 year earlier. Similar to the previous case the fibula has not been broken; rather, the proximal fibula has become dislocated and migrated proximally. **B.** Full-length weight-bearing films demonstrating that the patient's normal side is in varus. As the original fracture involved an intraarticular extension into the lateral tibial plateau, correction of the mechanical axis of the knee beyond the patient's normal side would not be desirable. The lateral displacement of the distal fragment of the tibia will need to be corrected along with the angulation of the malunion. **C.** Anteroposterior tracing of the deformity including the proposed level of osteotomy. The means of carrying out the desired correction with a large external fixator (Synthes) combined with "mini-external fixator" open-end compressors (Synthes) is rendered diagramatically. **D.** Similar AP tracing of the deformity illustrating an alternative means of carrying out the correction using an antiglide plate medially and a hook plate laterally in conjuction with the large external fixator. **E.** Anteroposterior tracing of the desired end result of the surgery. **F.** Final AP and lateral projections of the knee taken 1 week postoperatively. **G.** Final AP and lateral projections of the knee and proximal tibia illustrating the result after metal removal, 27 months after the operation.

22
Arthrodesis of the Knee

Dempsey S. Springfield

History

Symes is credited with doing one of, if not, the earliest knee joint resections sometime around 1835.[1] Symes did his resection for a patient who had tuberculosis involving the knee, but in the early 1800s the conventional treatment of patients with an infected knee (most were due to tuberculosis) was an above-knee amputation. Can you imagine what it must have been like to do a limb salvage operation while your colleagues were doing amputation and having to do the operation without antibiotics or anesthesia? It is said that Symes got the idea of doing a joint resection instead of an amputation from a French surgeon, but the details of how the first knee resection was conceived and done are not available. The operation must have been a success because knee resection soon became a common means of eradicating knee joint infections, and above-knee amputation was reserved only for failure after a resection. There is no information about how these patients functioned, but no doubt the functional results after a knee resection were best in those patients whose knees became the most stable. In all likelihood some of these resection arthroplasties went on to a spontaneous bony union after a period of immobilization, and the patients with a stable arthrodesis of the knee must have functioned better than those with an unstable fibrous union. The idea of intentionally doing an arthrodesis of the knee probably developed slowly during the late 1800s. It was during these same years that elective surgery could more easily be done with the introduction of both anesthesia and aseptic technique. The first arthrodesis is said to have been done in 1878 by Professor Albert.[2] Early attempts at arthrodesis of the knee consisted of little more than excision and prolonged immobilization, but by the early 1900s more aggressive attempts were being made to obtain bony union of the femur and tibia.[3]

In 1911 Goddu stated that metal fixation improved the results of fusion for tuberculous knees.[4] Then in 1913 Osgood said, "The operation of excision of the knee joint is a very old one," and "holding of the nicely approximated bone ends firmly together has definite advantages."[5] And in 1917 Galloway said that knee fusion was not as dangerous as generally believed and that excision of the knee was one of the most useful of operations.[6] He went on to say that success in obtaining a solid fusion was related to how long it took to secure bony union, and he suggested using the patella as a bony bridge and fixing the patella to the femur and tibia with two nails (Fig. 22–1).

This was the beginning of surgeons' publishing their surgical methods to obtain an arthrodesis of the knee. Key in 1932 was probably the first to describe the technique of using external compression with percutaneous wires as a means of stabilizing the bones until the fusion was solid.[7] It was later (1948) that Charnley reintroduced and popularized external compression as a means of immobilizing the bones after total excision of the synovium and articular cartilage to obtain a rapid bony union.[8,9] External fixation became and has continued to be the most popular means of holding the bones rigidly fixed while bony ankylosis is achieved.[10-12] No permanent internal fixation is used with this technique.

Indications

For the first 130 years the indications for a knee arthrodesis remained for the most part unchanged, but since 1970 some of the old indications for arthrodesis are no longer clinical disorders and others are now indications for a total joint replacement. Not only was

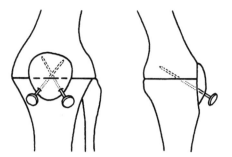

Figure 22–1. By the early 1900s internal fixation was recommended as a means of improving the postoperative stability of the resected joint to increase the chance of obtaining a solid arthrodesis. In one of the earliest methods of fixation suggested, two nails were used to transfix the patella to the tibia and femur.

tuberculosis a common cause of knee infection, but the successful management of joint infection before antibiotics was difficult without total excision of the knee.

Until the early 1950s infection, especially tuberculosis, was the most common indication for knee arthrodesis. Severe degenerative arthritis, usually as a result of trauma, was the second most common indication for an arthrodesis. The other relatively common indication was gross instability of the knee from either muscular paralysis (polio) or a neuropathic joint (Charcot's arthropathy). Pyarthrosis as a result of tuberculosis has become almost a medical curiosity as have polio and Charcot's arthropathy. Since the 1970s degenerative arthritis has been treated with an osteotomy or with a total joint replacement. Thus the discovery of antibiotics for tuberculosis and the development of successful joint replacements have dramatically reduced the need for knee arthrodesis.

The most common current indication for knee arthrodesis is loosening of a total joint endoprosthesis, especially when the loosening is secondary to an infection. It is uncommon for a patient to have a primary knee arthrodesis. Unfortunately, it has become such an uncommon reconstructive operation that it is probably not used as often as it should be. Patients with a history of multiple total knee joint replacement failures and those whose endoprostheses become infected have the most clear indication for an arthrodesis. Knee arthrodesis also is the most appropriate operation for the young active patient with posttraumatic osteoarthritis who needs a strong lower extremity on which to stand and work. Reconstruction after an extraarticular knee joint resection required to manage a bone tumor and the stabilization of a grossly unstable joint caused by a peripheral neuropathy continue to be indications for knee arthrodesis.

Patients with a recurrent failed total knee arthro-

plasty caused by loosening who have sufficient bone may be adequately immobilized with an external compression device, but if they have excessively osteoporotic bone they are probably better served with internal fixation. Those patients having an arthrodesis because of an infected total knee arthroplasty, even when the bone is osteoporotic, are best treated with external fixation initially until their wound is clean. If the external fixation is inadequate after the wound is clean and healed, internal fixation can then be used.[13–18]

The patient with a grossly unstable knee as a result of a neuropathy is probably best treated with an arthrodesis, although a constrained total knee prosthesis may have a place. Soudry and associates did nine total knee replacements in seven patients with classic Charcot or Charcot-like knees with a follow-up of 2 to just over 4 years. Eight of the knees in six patients were functioning well.[19] Whether these knees will continue to do well remains to be seen, but their early results are encouraging. Obtaining an arthrodesis in patients with an unstable knee as a result of a neuropathy has been difficult, and prolonged immobilization has been necessary. This need for prolonged immobilization means that internal fixation, either with a plate or an intramedullary rod, is the fixation of choice.[20]

Reconstruction of a limb after a major resection for a tumor is often best done with an arthrodesis. When only the distal femur or proximal tibia is removed, even when some of the adjacent muscles are resected with the tumor, the knee can be reconstructed and motion maintained. When the entire knee must be removed, however, it is not practical to reconstruct an articulating joint and it is better to do an arthrodesis. An endoprosthetic articulating joint reconstruction done after an extraarticular resection has a weak extensor mechanism, and limited motion and provides limited weight-bearing capacity for the patient. To obtain a stable extremity after an extraarticular resection, the resected joint should be replaced with an intercalary segment. Autogenous bone (nonvascularized and vascularized), allograft bone, and an intercalary endoprosthesis have all been successfully used.[21,22] The choice of intercalary segment used is the surgeon's as there seems to be no difference between the results of reconstruction.

Contraindications

There are few contraindications to arthrodesis of the knee. Charnley reported that he had 11 happy patients with bilateral knee arthrodeses, but it is unlikely that anyone will ever be able to repeat this clinical feat. Bilateral knee arthrosis is a relative, if not absolute, contraindication to knee arthrodesis.[10] For the young patient (less than 50 years of age) with bilateral knee arthritis who needs a strong extremity, there may be a place for an arthrodesis on one side and total knee replacement on the other, although there is little experience with this approach. Usually patients with bilateral disease either are in the age group in which bilateral total knee replacements are acceptable or, if younger, have a systemic disorder that reduces the demands they will put on the knees, making total knee replacement a reasonable option.

The condition of the ipsilateral ankle and foot is the most important potential contraindication. Gait analysis of patients with a knee arthrodesis have shown that stance phase on the arthrodesed side is longer, that ankle motion is reduced, and that there is early heel lift with increased pressure on the metatarsal heads.[23] Although it has not been reported as a contraindication, it is likely that an ipsilateral foot deformity and especially metatarsalgia will adversely affect the functional results of the patient with a knee arthrodesis. This should be considered before advising a patient to have a knee arthrodesis.

For the patient with a knee arthrodesis the most difficult activities are those that require sitting in a limited space or crawling or kneeling.[24-26] Patients who must perform these activities are not good candidates for knee arthrodesis. Usually this does not constitute a contraindication, but it should be discussed with the patient while trying to select the proper reconstruction. The author has seen a patient who had a successful knee arthrodesis converted to an above-knee amputation so he could return to work as a cabinet maker for a yacht-building company.

Position

Numerous suggestions have been made regarding the proper position for the arthrodesed knee, but very few data are available to support the various recommendations. The variables of position include flexion/extension, varus/valgus, and internal/external rotation. Length is an additional variable, although the length of the extremity cannot be adjusted as easily as the other positions, and any shortening can be corrected with a shoe lift.

Flexion is often the only position mentioned by authors, with the amount of flexion recommended varying from 0° to 30°.[13,17,26-29] Most authors suggest between 10° and 15° as the optimal amount of flexion. With the knee in full extension (0° of flexion), which provides the greatest length, the cosmetic appearance is the worst as the knee appears to be hyperextended. When the patient with a fully extended arthrodesis is seated, the extremity is even more difficult to position than when the extremity has a few degrees of flexion. Flexion greater than 15° does not make walking particularly difficult, but the extremity becomes even shorter and again the appearance when the patient is standing is not pleasing. Therefore, 5° to 15° of flexion is best.

The optimal position with respect to varus/valgus is more difficult to select. Most authors have not commented on the varus/valgus position, but those who have, recommend approximately 5° of valgus.[28,29] Probably a better way to select the position of valgus is to select the degree of varus/valgus that positions the hip, knee, and ankle on the weight-bearing axis between the center of body weight and the contact point on the ground[30] (Fig. 22–2). To do this a long weight-bearing radiograph is needed preoperatively to determine the proper degree of valgus.

Rotation of the leg with respect to the thigh is often overlooked as an important variable affecting the stance phase of gait. The rotational position of the foot during gait is determined by the rotational position in which the tibia is fixed to the femur, because the position of

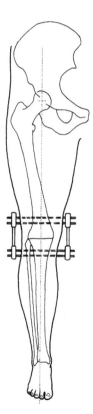

Figure 22–2. The varus/valgus alignment of the arthrodesed knee should position the ankle directly under the hip so that during stance phase, the ground reaction force passes through or near the hip joint. The osteotomes of the tibia and femur should be angled so that they are parallel to the compression pins but still allow the correct amount of valgus (usually 5° to 10°).

the extremity that feels right to the patient is determined by how the femoral head sits in the acetabulum, not how the foot looks on the floor. Therefore, if the tibia is fixed to the femur internally rotated, the patient will walk with the foot internally rotated rather than externally rotating through the hip to position the foot closer to neutral. During normal gait (knee with a full range of motion) the knee begins flexing just as the center of gravity passes over the position of the foot, and the ankle dorsiflexes with knee flexion. Knee flexion and ankle dorsiflexion make it easy for stride length to be maintained. When there is no knee flexion the ankle must maximally dorsiflex during the latter stages of weight bearing to allow the body to move forward. The greater the length of the foot that is out in front of the leg, the more the ankle must dorsiflex to keep the same stride length. When the foot is internally rotated or even neutral, the functional length of the foot is greatest. External rotation of the foot during stance phase has the effect of functionally shortening the foot and helping to keep stride length normal. This external rotation can be obtained if the patient externally rotates the entire extremity during stance phase, but as mentioned, this is not comfortable or easy. It is better to have had the tibia positioned on the femur in 5° to 10° of external rotation at the time of the arthrodesis. If the tibia is internally rotated, the patient cannot externally rotate the limb enough to get the foot out of the way, and the stride length is dramatically shortened. Too much external rotation, although functional, has an unsightly appearance.

The proper length is controversial; some authors recommend that the limb lengths be kept equal, whereas others feel that length is not important.[13,24,29,31] Length can be adjusted with a lift on the shoe. Usually it is more important to get good bone-to-bone contact than to worry about the overall length of the extremity. Only when one is reconstructing a limb after a major osseous resection and is using an intercalary graft, or when the opposite limb is shorter than the operated limb, is it possible to make the limbs the same length. Otherwise, the operated limb is shorter. Up to 3 cm of shortening is easily tolerated; between 1 and 3 cm is probably best. Remember that both flexion and varus/valgus make the limb functionally shorter.

Skin Incision

Any skin incision that provides exposure to the entire knee joint can be used to do an arthrodesis. Usually the patient already has had at least one operation. Whenever possible it is better not to make a new incision, but rather to use a previous one. The exposure should provide complete visualization of the joint so that all of the articular cartilage and intraarticular tissue can be excised. This improves bone-to-bone contact over as broad a surface as possible. The skin should not be dissected from the underlying fascia and muscles, as doing so increases the risk of skin necrosis. When the skin, fascia, and muscle are reflected as a unit, the skin has the best chance of healing. In the multiply operated patient, especially one who has had an infection, the risk of skin edge necrosis is significant. In the unusual case when the arthrodesis is the initial operation the surgeon can use any incision desired, and the author suggests that the surgeon use an incision and exposure that are familiar. The author prefers a straight longitudinal anterior skin incision with a medial parapatellar capsular incision.

Preparation of the Joint

Once the joint is exposed the principal job to be done is debridement of all tissues except healthy viable bone. All cartilage, intraarticular ligaments, necrotic bone, fibrous tissue, and foreign bodies should be removed. As this is being done all efforts should be made to save as much bone as possible. The femoral and tibial condyles can be trimmed to reduce their width if desired, although excessive excision will make the knee look too narrow and the leg unsightly. The surfaces of the bone should be cut so that maximum contact can be achieved with the alignment in flexion, valgus, and rotation as indicated. Resection guides used in knee replacement surgery may be useful in preparing the bone ends. Having broad surfaces of bone with the proper alignment cuts is especially important when external compression is used to immobilize the reconstruction. Adequate fixation with an external fixator requires bony contact sufficient for compression. When the knee has extensive bone loss from prior procedures or after the final debridement, it is better to shorten the leg and achieve good bone contact than to maintain length at the expense of bone contact. Only when an intercalary graft is used can length be adjusted irrespective of the amount of bone removed.

External Fixation Compression

External fixation for compression was introduced by Key in 1932.[6] Key used two turnbuckles on either side of the knee, connecting and compressing two pins, one through the distal femur and the other through the proximal tibia (Fig. 22–3). He was not sure if the compression improved the healing of the bone but he did notice that the reconstruction was more stable, and he was convinced that a stable reconstruction was important. His routine was to use the external compression device with or without a plaster cast for 8 weeks. Then he would remove the pins and put the patient back into a plaster cast for 8 more weeks. The patient was not allowed to bear weight on the extremity until the knee

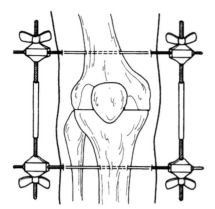

Figure 22-3. The early compression device recommended had only one pin in the tibia and one in the femur. These were connected with a turnbuckle device which could be tightened as necessary. This is not a stable construct, and if the osteotomes were not perfect, it was difficult to hold the tibia and femur in the desired position. Charnley and co-workers used single pins in each bone initially but soon recommended using two in each.[8-10]

was clinically fused, but the first examination for evidence of fusion was not until 16 weeks after surgery.[32] In 1948 Charnley reintroduced and popularized compression with an external device as a means of fusing the knee.[7] Charnley was convinced that the compression improved the rate of healing and the percentage of success. He used one pin in the distal femur and one pin in the proximal tibia in his early reports, but later reported using two pins in each bone.[7-10] He developed a fixation device to compress the bones and said that most of the knees were clinically solid by 8 weeks.

External fixation with compression is currently the most common method used to obtain a solid bony union, even for those patients who have a failed total knee arthroplasty. One advantage of external compression is that it is technically simple and has an excellent rate of union. Recent reports indicate that at least 75% of patients with external fixation compression should successfully fuse.[12,18,28,29,31,33,34] In all reported series patients who had failed total knee arthroplasty accounted for almost all of the failed fusions. Attempts to improve the rate of obtaining a solid bony fusion among patients with a prior failed total knee arthroplasty using newer and more rigid external compression devices have not been successful, and this suggests that the more rigid devices are probably not the answer to a higher incidence of successful arthrodesis.[12]

Pin placement is important and is the most demanding part of the operation. A double frame with two 5-mm titanium pins in the distal femur and two 5-mm titanium pins in the proximal tibia is best. The pins should

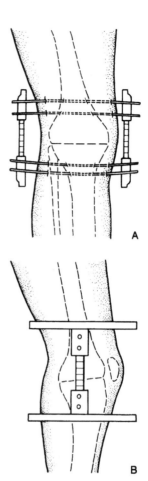

Figure 22-4. Pin placement is important and when done properly, the reconstruction is stable and inadvertent alterations in the position are uncommon. The pins should be parallel to each other and to the osteotomy cuts **(A)** and in the same coronal plane **(B)**. When compressed in this position the joint is extremely stable.

be parallel and in the same plane (Fig. 22-4). This provides the most stable fixation and compression that can be obtained without displacement of the femur on the tibia. Some authors have added an anterior frame with half-pins to the usual double frame to improve the fixation (Fig. 22-5). This makes the placement of transverse pins less critical and may increase the success rate.[30]

It is doubtful that compression actually increases the rate of healing, but the increased rigidity obtained with compression is the important benefit of this method. Cunningham et al have suggested that too much com-

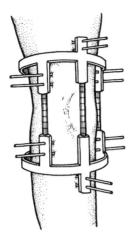

Figure 22–5. More sophisticated devices have been suggested as a means of improving the stability of the reconstruction and may be useful when limited bone is available, but these devices have not improved the incidence of union and are not necessary unless the reconstruction is unstable with the more standard four-pin external compression construction. The anterior half-pins will reduce the risk of the tibia shifting on the femur when there is inadequate bone to obtain sufficient compression and stability.

pression will increase bone loss and that only 200 N is needed.[35] They even showed that excessive compression was quickly lost. Retightening of the compression device is recommended, but more than 200 N is not practical.

There is no standard time to leave the patient in the external compression device. The patient with normal bone and a broad surface for fusion probably will be stable in 8 to 10 weeks, but the patient with minimal bone who had a failed total knee arthroplasty, especially one that had been infected, may take 3 or more months to heal. It is best to leave the compression device on until the radiographs suggest fusion and then examine the patient with the pins in place but the compression device off. If there is no motion, the pins can be removed. The patient's extremity is then placed in a knee cylinder cast for another 8 weeks, during which the patient is encouraged to bear full weight.

Although external compression is the most popular method of immobilizing a knee for fusion, sometimes more permanent fixation is needed. Intramedullary rods and compression plates have been used for these cases. There is little more than anecdotal data regarding these methods of fixation, and they probably should not be used except in special circumstances.

Intramedullary Fixation

A number of surgeons have used intramedullary fixation to immobilize the knee while it fuses.[13,14,16,18,21, 36–38] The two most common indications have been extensive bone loss after debridement of an infected total knee arthroplasty (especially after a failure of fusion with external compression) and reconstruction of a limb from which a tumor has been resected.

When a straight intramedullary rod is used, the position of the knee is 0° of extension and valgus, although the leg can be rotated in any position desired. More commonly a curved rod is used. Long rods with a constant curve, or a curved portion and a straight portion, are available. These rods produce 5° to 10° of flexion but still have no varus or valgus (Fig. 22–6).

A number of surgical techniques to implant the intramedullary rod have been described including the insertion of the rod through a window in the distal tibia or through one in the distal femur.[17] The author prefers to introduce the intramedullary rod in the femur in a retrograde fashion through the distal cut surface of the femur, driving it out the greater trochanter, then driving it back in an antegrade direction into the tibia.[21]

The author usually performs an arthrodesis after a resection of the distal femur or proximal tibia for a tumor. During the past decade he has used an intercalary allograft as the bone graft for the defect created by the tumor resection (usually an extraarticular resection) and a fluted intramedullary rod for fixation. The intramedullary rod has a curve in its proximal portion, but is straight in the distal one third. Once the tumor has been removed and the margins confirmed to be free of tumor, the tibia and femur are reamed to 2 mm greater than the indicated rod diameter (the diameter indicated on the fluted rod is the diameter of the solid part, not the diameter with the flutes). The medullary canal of the allograft is reamed large enough so it can be slipped over the rod (usually 15 or 16 mm for an 11-mm fluted rod). The intramedullary rod is then driven in a retrograde direction proximal through the femur out the greater trochanter until the allograft can be slipped over the exposed rod to leave only 2 cm of the rod exposed. The tibia is positioned on the rod in the desired rotation. The author believes patients function best with 5° to 10° of external rotation. The rod is then driven antegrade into the tibia. The tibia must be held tightly against the intercalary allograft so that contact between the graft and both the femur and tibia is maintained. The rod should be long enough to extend from just below the level of the greater trochanter to well into the metaphysis of the distal tibia (see Fig. 22–6A). The curved portion of the rod provides a minimal amount of flexion, but there is no valgus or varus at the knee. The reamings from the tibia and femur can be

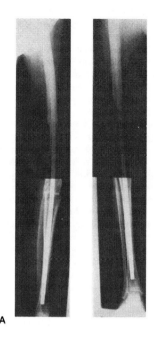

A

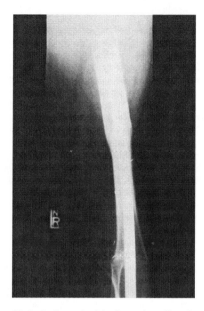

Figure 22-7. Radiograph of the intercalary allograft used to replace the distal femur and knee joint in a patient who had a resection and arthrodesis for an osteosarcoma. The allograft has healed to the patient's femur and tibia and the reconstruction is quite strong.

used as bone graft, as can any bone trimmed from the tibial or femoral condyles. Before the patients are discharged from the hospital they are placed in a long leg brace and allowed to bear weight (up to 40 pounds) immediately. Protected weight bearing is continued until both allograft/host bone junction sites are healed. For those patients not receiving chemotherapy the knee is usually solid in 3 months, but for those patients on chemotherapy the allograft usually does not heal to the host bone until after they have completed their entire course of chemotherapy (Fig. 22-7). The intramedullary rod is not removed.

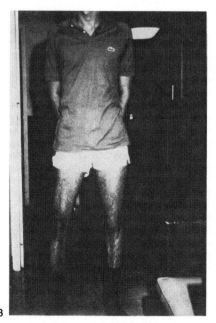

B

⊲————————————————————

Figure 22-6. A. Anteroposterior and lateral radiographs of a patient's lower extremity 7 months after he had an extraarticular resection of an osteosarcoma of the distal femur which had invaded the knee joint. The reconstruction was done with an intercalary fresh-frozen allograft and an intramedullary rod. The rod is straight in the anteroposterior plane but curved in the lateral plane. **B.** When the patient is standing the extremity looks almost normal. The slight anterior bow provided by the curved intramedullary rod improves the appearance of the leg.

Plate Fixation

The use of compression plates is attractive. Only a minimal amount of additional exposure is necessary, and most surgeons are familiar with compression plates. The plates can be bent to position the leg in any amount of flexion, valgus, and rotation desired, and by the use of two or more plates a very strong reconstruction can be achieved. The only disadvantage is that often the distal femur and proximal tibia are osteoporotic and the quality of the fixation compromised. In addition, the distal portion of the medial plate will be subcutaneous. Lucas and Murray recommended using two $\frac{1}{32}$-in.-thick, $\frac{1}{2}$-in.-wide, and 8-in.-long compression plates positioned 90° to each other and bent as needed to achieve 15° of knee flexion.[15] They keep the patients non-weight bearing on two crutches for 12 weeks and then partial weight bearing until the fusion looks solid on the radiograph.

When a resection has been done and an intercalary graft, either allograft or autograft, has been chosen to reconstruct the limb, compression plates can be used for fixation. Using plates reduces the extent of additional exposure, and this may be important if the margin of the resection is later discovered to be inadequate. In addition, the quality of the bone of a patient with a bone tumor is usually normal and plate fixation in this healthy bone is excellent.

Neuropathic Joint

Neuropathic knees are often unstable and painful, and nonoperative management is usually unsatisfactory. Although total knee arthroplasty is not absolutely contraindicated in these patients, there is a higher incidence of complication. The surgeon and patient should be confident that the neurologic condition is stable and that further destruction of the knee is not likely before choosing to do a total joint replacement.[19] When these criteria are not met the treatment should be an arthrodesis. For an unknown reason it is more difficult to obtain an arthrodesis in a neuropathic joint (only about 55% of them are successfully fused) than in a joint with degenerative arthritis (better than 90% fuse). Compression arthrodesis is not as successful in neuropathic joints as in other degenerated joints, and intramedullary fixation is recommended as it has been more successful than other types of fixation.[20]

Complications

The most significant complication, aside from an acute postoperative complication, is nonunion of the arthrodesis. As was indicated earlier, the nonunion rate is between 20 and 25%. Some of these cases can be salvaged with the use of an intramedullary rod, which may allow the fusion to become solid. In some cases even when the bones do not fuse the rod and fibrous tissue can provide sufficient immobilization that the patient functions well. The function of patients with an ununited, unstable arthrodesis is usually poor and most of these patients will have to have an amputation to ambulate without the assistance of two crutches.

The second most important complication is a fracture of the ipsilateral femur or tibia through a pin tract. This usually occurs when a patient is unprotected immediately after the pins are removed. Non-weight bearing or toe-touch weight bearing for 6 to 8 weeks after pin removal is recommended. Fracture has not been a problem for patients with an intramedullary rod.

Pin tract infections are the most common complication when an external fixator is used, but these have been only a minor problem and are easily managed. They usually can be prevented by predrilling the pin holes and carefully releasing the soft tissues, especially the skin, so that there is no tension against the pins.

Injury to the neurovascular structures has been reported to occur when putting in the pins for the external fixator. These should be rare and can be prevented by attention to the local anatomy while drilling in the pins.

Postoperative Care

As soon after the operation as comfort permits (1 or 2 days) the patient is allowed to ambulate on crutches bearing only the weight of the leg on the ground. A knee cylinder cast should probably be used for those patients with a clean wound and external fixation. The patient who has had an infection and needs wound care can be managed without a cast, but often the osteopenic bone has inadequate strength and a cylinder cast should be considered for these patients once the wound is healed. Patients with intramedullary rod fixation should have a long leg brace to improve their rotational stability. (The author does not use a step cut between the allograft and host bone. The step cut is difficult to do and may increase the risk of fracture.) Those patients with plate fixation do not require a cylinder cast unless their bone is osteoporotic.

The most important early rehabilitative activity required is maintaining ipsilateral ankle motion, especially ankle dorsiflexion. Increased ankle dorsiflexion improves the gait pattern by allowing a more normal stride length. There is a tendency for the patient with a knee arthrodesis toward loose ankle motion, and aggressive therapy to maintain and improve ankle dorsiflexion is recommended. No other special activities are needed.

Functional Results

There are few long-term follow-up reports of function for patients with a successful arthrodesis. The author agrees with published reports that patients with an arthrodesis complain most about the difficulties of using public transportation, sitting in a theater or sports facility seat, and getting into a small car. Most patients with a knee arthrodesis avoid these activities. If a patient *must* do any of them, an arthrodesis is not the best option.

Most patients are satisfied with their arthrodesis if it is solid. The un-united knee arthrodesis is not functional. Up to one third of patients who had severe pain before their arthrodesis continue to have pain, even with a solid arthrodesis.[26] On the other hand, between 80 and 95% of patients with a solid arthrodesis report that they are satisfied.[25,31] Many of these patients are satisfied because they had experienced the symptoms of an infected total knee replacement or another unsuccessful operation.

Gait analysis reveals a gait pattern that could have been predicted. The heel lifts off the floor early, weight is shifted to the forefoot, and the stance phase on the fused side is longer than on the unaffected limb.[23] In a comparison of patients with a normal knee, an above-knee amputation, or a rotationplasty, McClenaghan and associates showed that the patients with a knee arthrodesis consume more oxygen and have the slowest velocity.[38] Other authors report less of a difference in energy expenditure.[39]

A slight increase in the incidence of low back pain has been reported, but it is difficult to know what this means as there are no controlled studies. Certainly the lumbar spine must increase its motion to accommodate the loss of knee motion. The hip and ankle must do the same, but there is no mention in the literature of late ankle or hip difficulties.

There is at least one report of the conversion of a fused knee to a total knee arthroplasty, and the author has talked to a few surgeons who have tried this conversion.[40] A totally constrained endoprosthetic knee has been used and the patient usually does not have a functioning quadriceps muscle. This "take down" of knee arthrodesis has worked well early, but long-term function is doubtful. This conversion is not recommended except under experimental conditions.

Summary

There continue to be indications for arthrodesis of the knee although they are relatively few. The functional results are quite good, and in all likelihood, we should do more of these procedures than are currently being done. This is especially true for young, healthy, active patients.

References

1. Keith A, ed. *Menders of the Maimed.* Huntington, NY: Robert E. Kreiger; 1975;240.
2. Rand JA, Bryan RS, Chao EYS. Failed total knee arthroplasty treated by arthrodesis of the knee using the Ace Fischer apparatus. *J Bone Joint Surg Am.* 1987;69:39–45.
3. Hibbs RA. An operation for stiffening the knee joint with report of cases from the service of the New York Orthopaedic Hospital. *Ann Surg.* 1911;53:404–407.
4. Goddu LAO. Bone plates and clamps in excision of the knee joint. *Bost Med Surg J.* 1911;20:757–760.
5. Osgood RB. The end results of excision of the knee for tuberculosis with and without the use of bone plates. *Bost Med Surg J.* 1913;22:1–7.
6. Galloway HPH. The patellar bone-graft in excision of the knee. *Am J Orthop Surg.* 1917;15:704–710.
7. Key JA. Positive pressure in arthrodesis for tuberculosis of the knee joint. *South Med J.* 1932;25:909–915.
8. Charnley J. Positive pressure in arthrodesis of the knee joint. *J Bone Joint Surg Br.* 1948;30:478–486.
9. Charnley J, Baker SL. Compression arthrodesis of the knee. A clinical and histological study. *J Bone Joint Surg Br.* 1952;34:187–199.
10. Charnley J. Arthrodesis of the knee. *Clin Orthop.* 1960; 18:37–42.
11. Charnley J, Lowe HG. A study of the end results of compression arthrodesis of the knee. *J Bone Joint Surg Br.* 1958;40:633–635.
12. Rand JA, Bryan RS, Broderson MP. Arthodesis of the knee joint. In: Evarts CM, ed. *Surgery of the Musculoskeletal System.* 2nd ed. 1990;3692–3708.
13. Goldberg JA, Drummond RP, Bruce WJM, Viglione W, Lennon WP. Huckstep nail arthrodesis of the knee: A salvage for infected total knee replacement. *Aust NZ J Surg.* 1989;59:147–150.
14. Kaufer H, Matthews LS. Intramedullary knee arthrodesis using a curved nail. In: Evarts CM, ed. *Surgery of the Musculoskeletal System.* 2nd ed. 1990;3709–3723.
15. Lucas DB, Murray WR. Arthrodesis of the knee by double plating. *J Bone Joint Surg.* 1961;43:795–808.
16. Mazet R Jr, Urist MR. Arthrosdesis of the knee with intramedullary nail fixation. *Clin Orthop.* 1960;18:43–53.
17. Potter TA. Fusion of the destroyed arthritic knee. *Surg Clin North Am.* 1969;49:939–945.
18. Rand JA, Bryan RS. The outcome of failed knee arthrodesis following total knee arthroplasty. *Clin Orthop.* 1986;205:86–92.
19. Soudry M, Binazzi, Johanson NA, Bullough PG, Install JN. Total knee arthroplasty in Charcot and Charcot-like joints. *Clin Orthop.* 1986;208:199–204.
20. Drennen DB, Fahey JJ, Maylahn DJ. Important factors in achieving arthrodesis of the Charcot knee. *J Bone Joint Surg Am.* 1971;53:1180–1193.
21. Enneking WF, Shirley PD. Resection-arthrodesis for malignant and potentially malignant lesions about the knee using an intramedullary rod and local bone grafts. *J Bone Joint Surg Am.* 1977;59:223–236.
22. Sims FH, Beauchamp CP, Chao EYS. Reconstruction of the musculoskeletal defects about the knee for tumor. *Clin Orthop.* 1987;221:188–201.

23. Carugno C, Iacobellis C, Pedini G. Arthrodesis of the knee: A baropodometric evaluation of the long-term results. *Ital J Orthop Traumatol*. 1990;16:229–233.
24. Green DP, Parkes JC, Stinchfield FE. Arthrodesis of the knee. *J Bone Joint Surg Am*. 1967;49:1065–1078.
25. Rud B, Jense UH. Function after arthrosdesis of the knee. *Acta Orthop Scand*. 1976;19:217–219.
26. Siller TN, Hadjipavlou A. Knee arthrodesis: Long-term results. *Can J Surg*. 1976;19:217–219.
27. Campbell WC. *Operative Orthopaedics*. St. Louis: CV Mosby; 1939;278–284, 313.
28. Figgie HE III, Brody GA, Inglis AE, Sculco TP, Goldberg VM, Figgie MP. Knee arthrodesis following total knee arthroplasty in rheumatoid arthritis. *Clin Orthop*. 1987;224:237–243.
28. Knutson K, Hovelius L, Lindstrand A, Lidgren L. Arthrodesis after failed knee arthroplasty. *Clin Orthop*. 1984;191:202–211.
29. Vahvanen V. Arthrodesis in failed knee replacement in eight rheumatoid patients. *Ann Chir Gyn ecol*. 1979;68:57–62.
30. Rand JA. Knee arthrodesis. *Instruct Course Lect*. 1986;35:325–335.
31. Brattstrom H, Brattstrom M. Long-term results in knee arthrodesis in rheumatoid arthritis. *Acta Rheum Scand*. 1971;17:86–93.
32. Key JA. Arthrodesis of the knee with a large central autogenous bone peg. *South Med J*. 1937;30:574–579.
33. Bailey JD, Burkhalter WE. Knee fusion after severe injury to the knee joint. *J Trauma*. 1975;15:398–406.
34. Morris HD, Mosiman RS. Arthrodesis of the knee. A comparison of the compression method with the noncompression method. *J Bone Joint Surg Am*. 1951;33:982–987.
35. Cunningham JL, Richardson JB, Soriano PM, Kenwright J. A mechanical assessment of applied compression and healing in knee arthrodesis. *Clin Orthop*. 1989;242:256–264.
36. Brashear HR. The value of the intramedullary nail for knee fusion particularly for the Charcot joint. *Am J Surg*. 1954;87:63–65.
37. Chapchal G. Intramedullary pinning for arthrodesis of the knee joint. *J Bone Joint Surg*. 1946;30:728–734.
38. McClenaghan BA, Krajbick JJ, Pirone AM, Koheil R, Longmuir P. Comparative assessment of gait after limb-salvage procedure. *J Bone Joint Surg Am*. 1989;71:1178–1182.
39. Mazzetti RF. Effect of immobilization of the knee on energy expenditure during walking. Abstract. *J Bone Joint Surg Am*. 1960;42:533.
40. Holden DL, Jackson DW. Considerations in total knee arthroplasty following previous knee fusion. *Clin Orthop*. 1988;227:223–228.

23

Total Knee Replacement for Posttraumatic Arthritis

John M. Siliski and Frank X. Pedlow, Jr.

Primary total knee arthroplasty has become a commonly performed surgical procedure, with approximately 213,000 primary knee replacements done in the United States in 1992.[1] The results of primary knee arthroplasty have provided greater than 95% satisfactory initial results.[2-7] The long-term durability of primary knee arthroplasty has also been very gratifying, with a relatively low failure and revision rate. The success of primary knee arthroplasty is due to a number of factors, including improvements in implant design and materials, understanding of lower limb alignment, instruments and surgical techniques for bone preparation and ligament balancing, and postoperative management. Most primary total knee arthroplasties are done in patients with osteoarthritis or rheumatoid arthritis. Most commonly, these patients do not have surgical scars, malalignment, instability, and bone defects that can complicate and compromise knee arthroplasty. These types of problems are, however, encountered frequently in patients who have undergone previous major reconstructive surgery of the knee, such as osteotomy above or below the joint and previous knee arthroplasty that has failed for any of multiple reasons.[8-10] It is known that patients with previous osteotomy and arthroplasty require extra planning in preparation for surgery, and that the outcomes of these types of revision surgeries, especially major revision total knee arthroplasty, are not as good as for primary knee arthroplasty.[11-16]

Posttraumatic Arthritis

The term *posttraumatic arthritis* is often used to describe the development of arthritis in a joint with a specific history of prior trauma, minor or major, repetitive or single, causing damage to its ligamentous, cartilaginous, or osseous anatomy.[17] It is pathologically and radiographically similar to osteoarthritis.[17] Joint instability, osteoarticular damage, and skeletal malalignment may predispose the joint to the eventual and sometimes early development of arthritis. Although many injuries to the knee have been associated with a development of arthritic changes, the term *posttraumatic arthritis* here is reserved for those cases in which the development of arthritis follows direct joint damage or periarticular limb malalignment resulting from a major disruptive trauma to the knee. These injuries are usually intraarticular fractures or complete dislocations of the knee, which often have required operative treatment.[18] The knee is often left with permanent alterations in structure, stability, and alignment. The end result can be an arthritic knee with problems involving joint instability, stiffness, bony defects, malalignment secondary to intra- or extraarticular deformity, surgical scars, soft tissue abnormalities, and retained internal fixation devices. These patients may eventually require total knee arthroplasty to relieve pain and improve function. Although the first attempt at knee replacement in this group of patients may be considered a primary arthroplasty, the factors mentioned combine to make the use of total knee replacement in the treatment of posttraumatic knee arthritis a challenge often different from that of the osteoarthritic or rheumatoid knee. Consequently, primary knee arthroplasty for posttraumatic arthritis has similarities to revision total knee replacement.

There are limited reports in the orthopedic literature regarding the incidence of posttraumatic arthritis of the knee and the use of prosthetic arthroplasty for its treatment. The lack of knowledge pertaining to the incidence of posttraumatic arthritis is due partly to the limited availability of long-term follow-up studies. The lack of control groups, variations in fracture classification and treatment methods, and different diagnostic criteria for the development of significant arthritis also make comparison of reports difficult. Etiology and presentation of arthritic changes following fractures about the knee have received much attention. Gylling and Lindholm reported an incidence of degenerative changes in 55% of patients following fractures of the tibial condyles.[19] Apley believed the incidence of symptomatic arthritis was much less common and stressed the benefit of treatment by "traction and exercise" in the prevention of osteoarthritis.[20] Hohl and Luck reviewed 227 cases with a follow-up between 2 and 13 years. They concluded that early motion was most important in obtaining optimal results following tibial plateau fractures and stressed the reestablishment of articular surfaces perpendicular to the weight bearing axis.[21] Rombold,[22] as well as Shatzker and Lambert[23] and Shatzker et al,[24] have all advocated reestablishment of joint stability, joint surface congruity, and early motion.

Rasmussen reported a 21% incidence of arthritis in 192 patients with tibial condylar fractures examined an average of 7.3 years after injury.[25] He stated that biomechanical factors played a major role, the most important being an angular deformity of greater than 10°. Localized joint surface disruptions were given less importance in the development of osteoarthritis than angular deformity, joint instability, and condylar displacement. Lansinger et al presented a 20-year follow-up of 102 patients from the original series of Rasmussen, reporting 90% excellent or good results.[26] They supported the conclusions made by Rasmussen in 1973, promoting nonoperative treatment regardless of radiographic appearance of the fracture in patients without lateral or medial instability in extension.

Egund and Kolmert found that of 62 patients with distal femoral fractures followed for 5 years, only 3 patients developed tricompartmental arthritis, and 11 patients had patellofemoral arthritis.[27] Intercondylar and transcondylar joint surface displacement greater than 3 mm had a significant correlation with the development of arthritis. They concluded that arthritic changes developed earlier in patients in whom joint malalignment was caused by intraarticular deformity as opposed to extraarticular angular malalignment. In a series of 52 intraarticular fractures of the distal femur followed for 2 to 20 years, Siliski et al noted early arthritic changes in only 3 patients, and no patients underwent total knee arthroplasty during the follow-up.[28] There were no cases in this operatively treated series of joint stepoff greater than 2 mm or residual malalignment greater than 8°. Kettelkamp et al reviewed 15 limbs with degenerative arthritis of the knee and a history of tibial or femoral fractures.[29] They observed that degenerative arthritis could occur even after minimal malalignment and stressed the goal of anatomic alignment. They

noted a 31.7-year interval between fracture and degenerative changes as evidence of the tolerance of articular cartilage to prolonged excessive loading. In contrast, Merchant and Dietz, in a retrospective study of the 37 patients with tibial and fibular fracture evaluated an average of 29 years after injury, reported 92% clinical and radiographic results that were good or excellent regarding the knee.[30] Outcome was not affected by the degree of angular deformity or period of immobilization in this series.

Volpin et al studied 31 patients with osteoarticular fractures of the knee.[31] They found a 23% incidence of arthritis at an average follow-up of 14 years. Long-term results following conservative and surgical treatment were similar, and older patients had a higher incidence of arthritic changes.[31] Using total knee arthroplasty as an endpoint, Siliski et al noted that the development of posttraumatic arthritis following distal femoral or proximal tibial fractures is often a slow process.[32] The average interval between fracture and arthroplasty was noted to be 15 years (range 1–44 years). Chow and Hohl used survivorship analysis to study 693 proximal tibial fractures followed for 1 to 42 years.[33] Using radiographic criteria for the development of significant arthritis, they noted incidences of 16% at 5 years, 32% at 10 years, and 49% at 15 years after fracture. Their survivorship study using radiographic criteria is in agreement with a long delay between fracture and the need for total knee arthroplasty as noted by Siliski et al.[32]

Therefore, review of the literature reveals conflicting views regarding etiology and incidence of posttraumatic arthritis of the knee. There is not complete agreement on the contribution of intraarticular and extraarticular malalignment, joint instability, and joint surface displacement in the development of posttraumatic arthritis. The role of conservative and operative treatment in the prevention of subsequent degenerative changes has also been debated. In the management of intraarticular fractures, restoration and maintenance of joint surface congruity, normal anatomic alignment, joint stability, and early motion appear to offer the best chance for prevention of significant arthritic change. Even with these objectives, and regardless of the type of treatment, severe trauma to the knee will sometimes eventually result in an arthritic knee requiring prosthetic arthroplasty.

Total Knee Replacement

There are limited reports in the orthopedic literature of the use of total knee replacement in patients with posttraumatic arthritis. Most large series of primary total knee arthroplasty include a very small percentage with a preoperative diagnosis of posttraumatic arthritis. From these large series, it has not been possible to determine the outcome of this subgroup of patients with post-traumatic arthritis.[2,3,5-7]

Bomler and Arnoldi reported the use of polyethylene resurfacing of the tibia for posttraumatic arthritis in five patients with depressed lateral plateaus. Follow-up was short, averaging only 2 years, but initial results were reported as good.[34]

Marmor reported the use of his modular knee system for posttraumatic arthritis in a series of 18 cases.[35] In 15 of these cases, both the medial and the lateral compartments were resurfaced with the modular components. Nine of the eighteen patients had undergone previous open reduction and internal fixation. Osteotomy was not required to correct bony deformities in these patients selected for knee replacement. At 2-year follow-up, satisfactory results were noted in 78% of patients.

Siliski et al reported 21 cases of knee arthroplasty for posttraumatic arthritis, performed at the Massachusetts General Hospital and West Roxbury VA Hospital, during the period 1978–1988.[32] Seventeen of these injuries were tibial plateau fractures, and nine patients had undergone initial open reduction and internal fixation. An additional three were shrapnel injuries with open fractures treated by debridement and casting. An additional eight surgical procedures were subsequently performed in these patients for arthroscopy, ligament reconstruction, hardware removal, and high tibial osteotomy. The mean time from initial injury to total knee replacement (TKR) was 15 years (range 1–44 years). Early complications included one case of deep vein thrombosis, one case of wound dehiscence leading to arthrodesis, and three cases of patellar dislocation. Three patients required knee manipulation. Late complications included one case of loosening treated by arthrodesis, and one painful, although well-fixed, total knee replacement that also was ultimately treated by arthrodesis. Final knee score, using the Hospital for Special Surgery knee rating system, was only improved from 41 preoperatively to 66 postoperatively. Preoperative range of motion averaged 4° to 85°; postoperatively it was 10° to 95°. The conclusion in this study was that this group of patients did not do as well as those with rheumatoid and osteoarthritis. Soft tissue problems including previous incisions and scarring made wound healing more tenuous and recovery of knee motion more difficult. The patients had more problems with patellar maltracking than expected for primary TKR. The final motion was relatively poor, and these patients had more pain than expected for primary knee replacement.

Roffi and Merritt reported 17 cases of posttraumatic arthritis treated with total knee replacement.[36] One was treated with a distal femoral osteotomy before arthroplasty. Follow-up was short, averaging 27 months (range 1–4 years). Only five cases were considered to have successful clinical results. Five patients with unsuc-cessful results had a major intraoperative or postoperative complication. They emphasized the importance of assessing tibial tilt in both anteroposterior and lateral views. They recommended consideration of varus or valgus osteotomy for extraarticular fractures that had healed with a malunion. They also noted that incisions required careful planning, and that results may more resemble revision rather than primary knee arthroplasty.

Total knee arthroplasty for posttraumatic arthritis requires extra planning, longer and more complicated surgical procedures, and more concern about postoperative complications than primary knee arthroplasty. The major areas of planning and concern are those of exposure, correction of malalignment, filling of bony defects, provision of ligamentous stability, and postoperative management. Each of these areas is discussed in the remainder of this chapter. There is an interdependency requiring complete knowledge of all of these areas for the planning and surgical execution of arthroplasty in the patient with posttraumatic arthritis.

Surgical Exposure

The two main goals are to avoid wound healing problems and to achieve sufficient exposure to accomplish the knee arthroplasty.

Most knee arthroplasties are done with an anterior vertical skin incision, which leaves intact the medial and lateral subcutaneous vessels that supply the skin. As this skin incision is preferable for a knee arthroplasty, it can be argued that all significant incisions made for knee surgery be vertical anterior incisions, so that if subsequent total knee arthroplasty is required an appropriate incision already exists; however, many fractures of the distal femur and tibial plateau are approached through skin incisions placed elsewhere than the anterior surface. Many distal femoral fractures are approached laterally, with the skin incision curving down to the tibial tubercle. Many tibial plateau fractures are exposed through medial and/or lateral incisions. Consequently, the surgeon performing a knee arthroplasty may encounter preexisting skin incisions that are not ideally placed for knee arthroplasty.

In the setting of suboptimal preexisting skin incisions, three options exist. In some cases, the preexisting incision can be used, with or without extension proximally or distally and with or without alteration of the deep exposure. Examples of this approach include the following. A preexisting medial incision may be extended distally over the anteromedial surface of the tibia and proximally up to the midline over the quadriceps tendon; this may then be followed by a medial arthrotomy (Fig. 23–1). In such a case, the skin incision may actually be medial to the typical parapatellar arthrotomy; however, the skin flap required is usually minimal. If a flap is developed at the proximal portion of the incision, it is

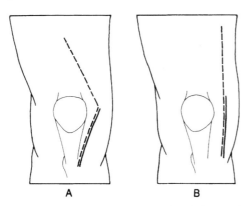

Figure 23-1. Preexisting medial incisions (—) extended proximally (---) and used for (**A**) medial subvastus or (**B**) parapatellar approach.

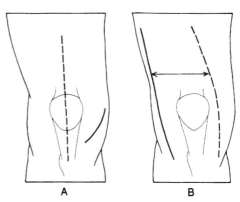

Figure 23-3. A. Preexisting medial incision (—) is avoided using an anterior vertical midline incision (---). **B.** Preexisting lateral incision (—) is far enough lateral to perform an anteromedial skin incision. The width of the flap between the old and new incisions is kept as wide as possible, preferably 10 cm or greater.

usually well tolerated as it is over the quadriceps muscle. A medial subvastus approach may also be used. With a preexisting lateral incision, this may in some circumstances be combined with a lateral parapatellar arthrotomy (Fig. 23-2). This may be an excellent solution particularly if the replacement to be done is a lateral unicompartmental replacement where limited exposure is required. Also, the lateral incision can be combined with osteotomy of the tibial tubercle (see Chapter 5) to provide extensile exposure of the knee.

Another option with preexisting incisions is to not use them for knee arthroplasty, but to make an entirely new skin incision (Fig. 23-3). The basic principle is to avoid creation of flaps or long pointed intersections where the new and old scars will meet. It is easiest to

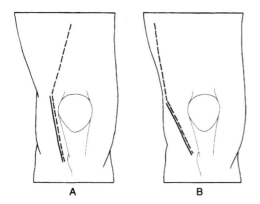

Figure 23-2. Preexisting lateral incisions (—) extended proximally (---) and used for (**A**) lateral subvastus or (**B**) parapatellar approach.

ignore preexisting incisions when they are short, placed far medially or laterally, and oriented horizontally as opposed to obliquely or vertically. If there is a long vertical incision, ideally the surgeon should try to leave a distance of 10 cm between the old and new incisions. Moving the new anterior vertical incision somewhat medially may help to create a wider space between an old lateral incision and the new incision.

Some of the most difficult incisions to deal with are those that are long and oblique and distally come into the region of the tibial tubercle (Fig. 23-4). The skin over the tibial tubercle is at most risk for wound healing problems. For such an old incision, one would prefer to use that portion over the tibial tubercle; however, the proximal extent of the old incision may not be ideally placed to reach the quadriceps tendon. If it is an oblique medial incision, there are two choices. The old incision can be used and a subvastus approach employed. The other option is to use the distal part of the old skin incision and extend at a 90° angle from the old incision a new skin incision that crosses back toward the quadriceps tendon. In general, the latter approach does not work with long oblique lateral incisions. When such incisions exist, it is usually better to use either the old lateral skin incision with some type of lateral approach or an anteromedial skin incision with a medial parapatellar arthrotomy.

Using these principles, the senior author has not encountered problems with wound healing.

The deep exposure may be limited by scarring of the extensor mechanism. An initial lateral release may be needed to evert the patella and gain adequate exposure. Patella baja may limit exposure and ultimately result in

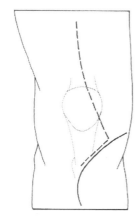

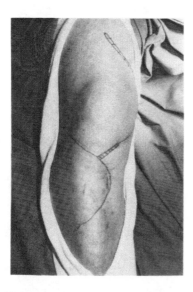

Figure 23–4. A. Preexisting curving anteromedial incision (—) is difficult to use in its entirety or to avoid. The portion over the proximal tibia can be used, with an extension (- - -) at right angles to the previous incision. **B.** Clinical example of previously operated knee about to undergo arthroplasty. The preexisting incisions over the proximal tibia and along the medial edge of the patella are marked with a solid line (—). These were connected and extended (ribbed lines). The final incision used was the shape of a "3".

improper relation of the patella to the femur (Fig. 23–5). Tibial tubercle osteotomy may improve exposure during total knee arthroplasty. As well, the tubercle can be shifted proximally by 1 to 2 cm to improve patellofemoral alignment.

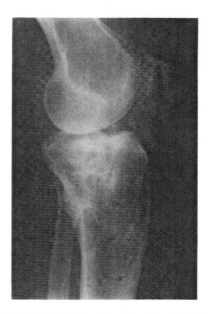

Figure 23–5. Patella baja after a bicondylar tibial plateau fracture treated by fixation and subsequent hardware removal. Lateral x-ray.

Malalignment

Malalignment after fracture may result either from bone loss and degenerative changes at the articular level or from altered anatomy from an extraarticular fracture line. Malalignment resulting from bone loss at the joint level is discussed in the next section.

Malalignment at the metaphyseal or diaphyseal level in the femur and tibia may cause deformities in multiple planes including shortening, malrotation, varus–valgus malalignment, flexion–extension malalignment, and translocation (Fig. 23–6). Careful clinical examination, combined with plain x-rays and a full-length extremity film, is essential in the workup and planning of the knee arthroplasty. The ultimate goal is to achieve a satisfactory knee replacement with normal alignment of the lower extremity. With minor degrees of malalignment, correction of leg alignment can be achieved by making somewhat eccentric cuts on the femur and tibia at the time of arthroplasty. The greater the degree of preoperative malalignment, the more eccentric bone cuts become. As bone cuts become more eccentric, ligaments become displaced from their normal relationship to the joint line. Consequently, the more eccentric the bone cuts, the greater the need to use increasing amounts of constraint in the knee prosthesis to provide stability. To use a less constrained prosthesis, it may be preferable

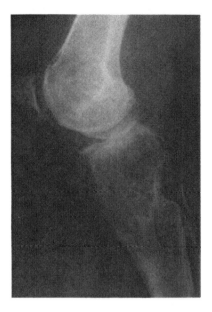

Figure 23–6. Tibial plateau malalignment on a lateral x-ray after a Shatzker type VI fracture.

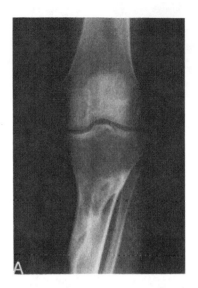

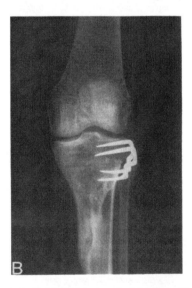

to correct the malalignment with an osteotomy before proceeding with a total knee arthroplasty. The reader is referred to Chapter 21 for more detail on preoperative planning and execution of corrective osteotomies of the lower extremity. If the arthritis is relatively mild and confined to a single compartment, the surgeon and the patient may choose to perform a corrective osteotomy as a separate procedure with the goal of improvement of symptoms from that operation alone (Fig. 23–7). If after osteotomy symptoms persist or recur, an arthroplasty may subsequently be performed (Fig. 23–8). If the arthritic changes in the knee are advanced, and it is very likely that an arthroplasty will be necessary, osteotomy and arthroplasty may be performed simultaneously (Fig. 23–9). If arthroplasty and osteotomy are performed simultaneously, fixation of the osteotomy should be secure enough that no restriction is required postoperatively during range of motion of the knee.

Figure 23–7. High tibial osteotomy for correction of malalignment in the frontal plane resulting from an old proximal tibial fracture with subsequent medial compartment pain and early arthritis. **A.** Preoperative x-ray. **B.** Postoperative x-ray.

Bone Defects

Loss of bone from the original trauma, subsequent debridements, or posttraumatic degenerative changes must be anticipated prior to arthroplasty; however, management of bone defects follows the same principles as used in revision total knee arthroplasty, where

defects are commonly encountered.[37,38] Tibial plateau fractures are the most common cause of posttraumatic arthritis of the knee, and consequently the most likely defect to be encountered is in the lateral tibial plateau. Wedges and other total knee systems for filling of cen-

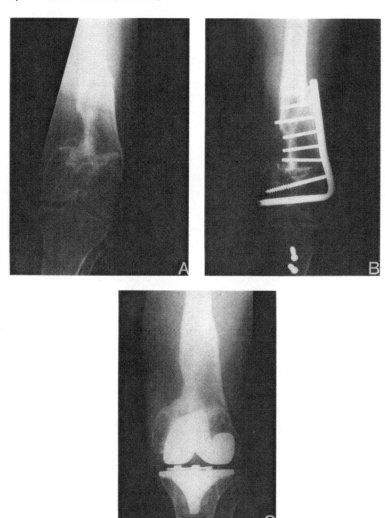

Figure 23–8. A. Posttraumatic arthritis of the knee after an open type C3 femoral fracture, with residual varus deformity of the femur. **B.** Alignment corrected with a distal femoral valgus osteotomy. **C.** Total knee replacement done several years later for progressive knee pain. (See Fig. 5–8 for surgical exposure.)

tral and rim defects of the plateau are available with many total knee systems (Fig. 23–10). Smaller defects, particularly in the lower-demand patients, can be adequately filled with polymethylmethacrylyte during cementing (Fig. 23–11). Defects may also be filled with bone graft, often taken from the resected portions of the femur or tibia (Fig. 23–12).

Implants

Most cases of posttraumatic arthritis of the knee can be treated with conventional primary knee replacement implants. The choice of posterior cruciate ligament sacrificing versus sparing designs will in most cases be determined by surgeon preference, as opposed to the rare

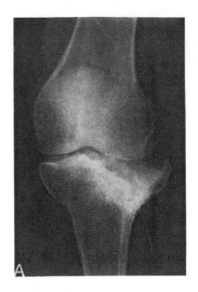

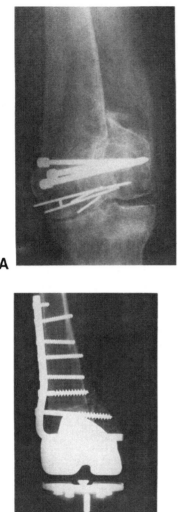

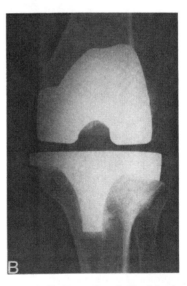

Figure 23–9. A. Posttraumatic arthritis of the knee after a closed type femoral fracture, with varus and flexion deformity of the femur. **B.** Supracondylar osteotomy and total knee replacement performed simultaneously. (See fig. 5–16 for surgical exposures.)

Figure 23–10. A. Posttraumatic arthritis of the knee after lateral tibial plateau fracture. **B.** Total knee replacement done with metallic wedge on tibial component to fill bone defect.

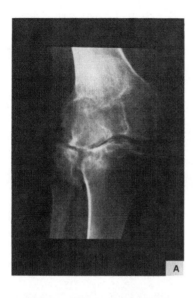

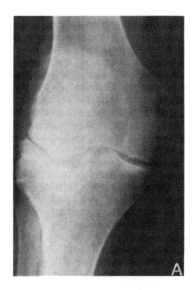

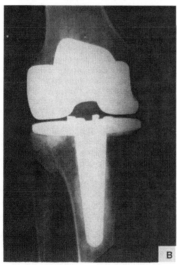

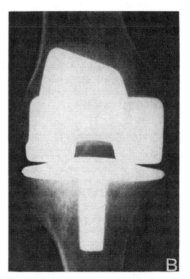

Figure 23–11. A. Posttraumatic arthritis of the knee after lateral tibial plateau fracture with nonunion of split fragment, in elderly woman. **B.** Total knee replacement performed with excision of prominent portion of ununited fragment and long-stem cemented tibial component.

Figure 23–12. A Posttraumatic arthritis of the knee after ateral tibia plateau fracture in a 50-year-old man. **B.** Total knee replacement performed with bone grafting of contained tibial defect and uncemented tibial component.

situation of preoperative absence of the posterior cruciate ligament. Use of wedges and other augmentation blocks has been described in the preceding section.

When bone quality is poor as a result of the previous fracture and disuse osteoporosis, stem extensions may be desirable on either the femoral or tibial components. Difficulty in using long stems may be encountered when bone deformity exists from the old fracture. Modular stems may not fit down the medullary canal and still maintain the component in proper position on the end of the bone. Several creative options are available to deal with this situation, including (1) use of bone graft to improve bone stock and eliminate the need for longer stems, (2) osteotomy to correct the malalignment, and (3) use of custom components with altered stem placement. Each of these options has its advantages and disadvantages and must be considered in light of the overall plan for arthroplasty.

Increasing constraint in the implant is required for two conditions. The first is loss of normal ligamentous structures as part of the original trauma. The surgeon should be able to plan for this option based on the nature of the original injury and the preoperative physical examination. The second need for increased constraint in the implant occurs where there is substantial malalignment of the joint line, and the surgeon chooses not to correct the malalignment with an initial osteotomy. The ends of the femur and tibia are simply used as bone stock for securing a prosthesis, and normal function of the ligaments is eliminated. If the surgeon chooses this approach, then an implant will need to restore both cruciate and collateral stability.

Postoperative Management

This group of patients requires intensive and carefully monitored therapy postoperatively. Because of potential problems with flap edema and wound healing problems, the soft tissues need to be inspected frequently. If any problems occur, the knee may need to be rested to allow soft tissue healing to proceed. If any significant problems develop with the wound sealing and healing, the patient may need to be returned to the operating room for appropriate wound management.

Even when no skin problems occur, this group of patients has been demonstrated to be at high risk for stiffness and a difficult postoperative therapy course. If a patient does not achieve satisfactory knee motion during the first 2 weeks, knee manipulation should be considered.

References

1. *Orthopaedic Network News*. 1993;4:1. (Mendall Associates, Ann Arbor, MI.)
2. Insall JN, Kelly M. The total condylar prosthesis. *Clin Orthop Relat Res*. 1986;205:43–48.
3. Knutson K, Lindstrand A, Lidgren L. Survival of knee arthroplasties: A nationwide multicenter investigation of 8,000 cases. *J Bone Joint Surg Am*. 1986;66:795–803.
4. Rorabeck CH, Bourne RB, Nott L. The cemented Kinematic-II and the non-cemented porous-coated anatomic prosthesis for total knee replacement: A prospective evaluation. *J Bone Joint Surg Am*. 1988;70:483–490.
5. Scott WN, Rubinstein M. Posterior stabilized knee arthroplasty. *Clin Orthop*. 1986;205:138–145.
6. Vince KG, et al. Long-term results of cemented total knee arthroplasty. *Orthop Clin North Am*. 1988;19:575–580.
7. Wright J, Ewald FC, Walker PS, Thomas WH, Poss R, Sledge CB. Total knee arthroplasty with the kinematic prosthesis. Results at five to nine years: A follow-up note. *J Bone Joint Surg Am*. 1990;72:1003–1009.
8. Staeheli JW, Cass JR, Morrey BF. Condylar total knee arthroplasty after failed proximal tibial osteotomy. *J Bone Joint Surg Am*. 1987;69:28–31.
9. Windsor RE, Insall JN, Vince KG. Technical consideration of total knee arthroplasty after proximal tibial osteotomy. *J Bone Joint Surg Am*. 1988;70:547–555.
10. Windsor RE, Insall JN, Sculco TR. Bone grafting of tibial defects in primary and revision total knee arthroplasty. *Clin Orthop Relat Res*. 1986;205:132–137.
11. Cameron HU, Welsh RP. Potential complications of total knee replacement following tibial osteotomy. *Orthop Rev*. 1988;18:39–47.
12. Friedman R, Hirst P, Poss R, Kelley K, Sledge C. Long-term results of revision total knee replacement. Presented at AAOS Annual Meeting; 1988: Paper 300.
13. Hanssen AD, Rand JA. A comparison of primary and revision total knee arthroplasty using the kinematic stabilizer prosthesis. *J Bone Joint Surg*. 1988;70:491–499.
14. Katz MM, Hungerford DS, Krackow KA, Lennox DW. Results of total knee arthroplasty after failed proximal tibial osteotomy for osteoarthritis. *J Bone Joint Surg Am*. 1987;69:225–233.
15. Rand JA, Bryan RS. Results of revision total knee arthroplasty using condylar prostheses. A review of fifty cases. *J Bone Joint Surg Am*. 1988;70:738–45.
16. Rand JA, Peterson LJA, Bryan RS, Ilstrup DM. Revision total knee arthroplasty. In: *AAOS Instructional Course Lectures*. St. Louis: CA Mosby; 1986;305–318.
17. Pinals RS. Traumatic arthritis and allied conditions. In: McCarty, ed. *Degenerative Arthritis and Allied Conditions. A Textbook of Rheumatology*. Philadelphia: Lea & Feibiger; 1989:1371.
18. Bowes DN, Hohl M. Tibial condylar fractures. Evaluation of treatment and outcome. *Clin Orthop Relat Res*. 1980;171:104–108.
19. Gylling U, Lindholm R. Fractures of the tibial condyle. *Ann Chir Gynaecol Fenn*. 1953;42:229.
20. Apley AG. Fractures of the lateral tibial condyle treated by skeletal traction and early mobilization: A review of sixty cases with special reference to long-term results. *J Bone Joint Surg Br*. 1956;38:699–708.
21. Hohl M, Luck J. Fractures of the tibial condyle: A clinical and experimental study. *J Bone Joint Surg Br*. 1956; 38:1001–1018.
22. Rombold C. Depressed fractures of the tibial plateau: Treatment with internal fixation and early mobilization: A preliminary report. *J Bone Joint Surg Am*. 1960;42:783–797.

23. Shatzker J, Lambert DC. Supracondylar fractures of the femur. *Clin Orthop Relat Res.* 1979;138:77–83.
24. Shatzker J, McBroom R, Bruce D. The tibial plateau fracture. The Toronto experience 1968–1975. *Clin Orthop Relat Res.* 1979;171:104–108.
25. Ramussen PS. Tibial condylar fractures as a cause of degenerative arthritis. *Acta Orthop Scand.* 1972;43:566–575.
26. Lansinger O, Bergman B, Korner L, Anderson GBJ. Tibial condylar fractures. A twenty-year follow-up. *J Bone Joint Surg Am.* 1986;68:13–19.
27. Egund N, Kolmert L. Deformities, gonarthrosis and function after distal femoral fractures. *Acta Orthop Scand.* 1982;52:963–974.
28. Siliski JM, Mahring M, Hofer HP. Supracondylar-intercondylar fractures of the femur. *J Bone Joint Surg Am.* 1989;71:95–104.
29. Kettelkamp DB, Hillbury BM, Murrish DE, Heck DA. Degenerative arthritis of the knee secondary to fracture malunion. *Clin Orthop Relat Res.* 1988;234:159–169.
30. Merchant TC, Dietz FR. Long-term follow-up after fractures of the tibial and fibular shafts. *J Bone Joint Surg Am.* 1989;71:599–606.
31. Volpin G, Dowd GSE, Stein H, Bentley G. Degenerative arthritis after intra-articular fractures of the knee. *J Bone Joint Surg Br.* 1990;72:634–638.
32. Siliski JM, Awbrey BJ, Tomford WW., Trippel SB, Bayley JC. Total knee replacement for post-traumatic arthritis. Presented at AAOS Annual Meeting; 1989: Paper 310.
33. Chow GH, Hohl M. Osteoarthritis of the knee following tibial plateau fracture: A survivorship analysis. Presented at AAOS Annual Meeting; 1992: Paper 52.
34. Bomler J, Arnoldi C. Resurfacing of depression fractures of the lateral tibial condyle. *Acta Orthop Scand.* 1981; 52:231–232.
35. Marmor L. The Marmor modular knee in traumatic arthritis. *Orthop Rev.* 1979;8:35–40.
36. Roffi RP, Merritt PO. Total knee replacement after fractures about the knee. *Orthop Rev.* 1990;19:614–620.
37. Brooks PJ, Walker PS, Scott RD. Tibial component fixation in deficient tibial bone stock. *Clin Orthop Relat Res.* 1984;184:302–308.
38. Dorr LD, Ranawat CS, Sculco TA, et al. Bone graft for tibial defects in total knee arthroplasty. *Clin Orthop Relat Res.* 1986;205:153–165.

24

Femoral Fractures Above Total Knee Arthroplasty

William L. Healy, Michael Schmitz, and John M. Siliski

Fractures of the distal femur above total knee arthroplasty are uncommon, with a reported incidence ranging from 0.3 to 2.5%[1-8]; however, the combination of an aging population, broadening indications for total knee arthroplasty, and increased levels of activity of patients after knee replacement suggests the incidence of these fractures may increase in the 1990s. Reported risk factors for ipsilateral fracture of the distal femur after total knee arthroplasty include osteopenia, rheumatoid arthritis, steroid therapy, and revision arthroplasty of the knee.[3,4,7,9] Neurologic disorders, most commonly seizure disorders and cerebral ataxia, are also risk factors.[10]

Notching of the anterior femoral cortex as a risk factor for fracture of the distal femur above a knee replacement is controversial. Some investigators suggested that notching is associated with an increased incidence of fracture, especially in the early postoperative period.[6,9-11] Culp et al offered a biomechanical model and suggested that a 3-mm defect yields a 29.2% decrease in torsional strength.[10] Aaron and Scott noted that the fracture lines of the distal femur appear to originate from the area of cortical notching[11]; however, while reviewing 670 total knee arthroplasties to determine the incidence and extent of anterior femoral cortical encroachment, Ritter et al noted no significant increase in the incidence of fracture in 180 patients with femoral notching.[12]

Although the design of the implant has not been shown conclusively to be a risk factor for these fractures, some authors have suggested that the design may predispose the distal femur to fracture.[10,13] Theoretically, a more constrained prosthesis is more likely to transfer torque to bone. Furthermore, the increase in stiffness associated with a stemmed femoral component may serve as a stress riser, predisposing the distal femur to fracture.[1]

A stiff knee with restricted range of motion may predispose the distal femur to fracture by transferring forces across the joint to periprosthetic bone. Bogoch et al found that range of motion in a series of fractures above a knee replacement was less than 85° flexion arc.[14]

Trauma is the primary cause of fractures of the distal femur above total knee arthroplasty. Minimal trauma can cause major fractures.[3,15,16] Most commonly, patients fall on the affected knee; however, these fractures have also been reported after a high-velocity motor vehicle accident,[3,7,14,17] after passive range-of-motion exercises to increase the postoperative range of motion,[7] and as an intraoperative complication.[1]

Evaluation and Classification

All patients with a fracture of the distal femur require evaluation to rule out other injuries to the head, spine, pelvis, and other long bones. In high-velocity injuries, cranial, spinal, thoracic, abdominal, and urologic problems must be evaluated and treated. Neurovascular injury is not common after fractures of the distal femur, but the neurovascular integrity of the limb must be evaluated thoroughly.

Fractures of the distal femur above total knee arthroplasty are usually extraarticular fractures in the A group of the comprehensive classification of fractures of long bones (types A1, A2, and A3).[18] Distal femur fractures without prostheses usually demonstrate a predictable pattern of displacement including shortening, posterior angulation, and external rotation. Displacement of fragments can be the reverse of what would be expected in a knee without total knee arthroplasty.[13,16] Wiedel attributed this finding to decreased muscular tone around the knee associated with disuse atrophy.[16]

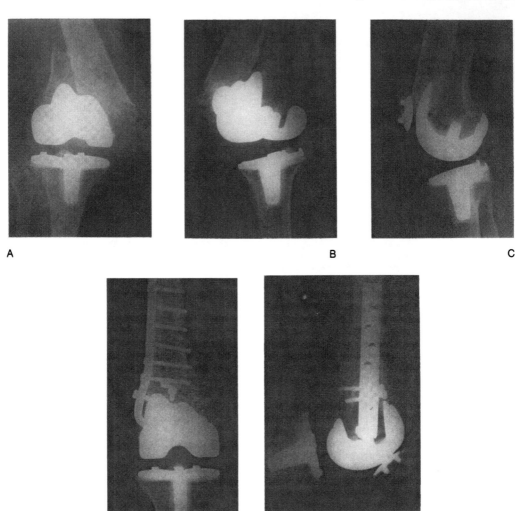

A   B   C

D   E

Figure 24–1. A 72-year-old woman with rheumatoid arthritis who had been receiving long-term steroid therapy fell and broke her femur just above a knee replacement. After unsuccessful treatment with traction followed by a cast brace for 4 months, the patient was referred for surgical repair. **A.** Antero-posterior view shows an oblique, displaced, malaligned, and malrotated fracture of the femur above the knee replacement. **B.** Although a routine lateral view shows the fracture well, it is not a true lateral view of the prosthetic components and, therefore, is not satisfactory for preoperative planning. **C.** An oblique view of the knee shows the joint in the lateral projection and is suitable for the evaluation of the bone–cement–prosthesis interfaces in the condylar fragment. This view also provides the information needed to plan reduction and insertion of fixation devices. **D.** Anteroposterior view of the healed fracture after open reduction and internal fixation using anterior-to-posterior interfragmentary screws and a lateral blade plate followed by allografts obtained from a femoral head. **E.** Lateral view of healed fracture. **F.** Tangential view of patellofemoral joint after fracture had healed. (Adapted with permission from Healy et al.[3])

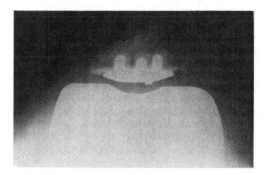

F   **Figure 24–18** (continued)

Appropriate roentgenographic studies must be obtained to evaluate the fracture in the presence of a knee replacement. Routine anteroposterior and lateral views of the fracture may not demonstrate the knee replacement satisfactorily. It is important to evaluate the bone–cement interface or the bone–prothesis interface for signs of loosening (Fig. 24–1). When the knee replacement is loose, it may not be appropriate to consider open reduction internal fixation.

Roentgenographic evaluation must be directed to the distal condylar fragment to determine how fixation of the fracture can be achieved. Tomography in the lateral projection may be helpful in evaluating the distal condyle. It should be determined whether stress shielding under the anterior flange of the femoral component has produced osteopenia. Furthermore, it should be determined whether fracture lines have extended into the condylar fragment and whether the design of the femoral component will interfere with or prevent placement of a specific fracture fixation device. The preoperative evaluation should include use of templates of implants for fixation of the fracture and the prosthetic components. The templates are used to plan fixation of the fracture so that anatomic alignment and rotation of the fragments of the fracture can be achieved and that fixation of the prosthesis to the bone is not disrupted.

History of Treatment

Recommendations for treatment of fractures of the distal femur above total knee arthroplasty vary. Both operative and nonoperative methods of treatment have been proposed. Studies of patients with these fractures have been retrospective for the most part.

Between 1981 and 1989, thirteen articles were published in the English literature that reviewed the results of treatment of fractures of the distal femur above total knee arthroplasty.[1,4–7,10,13,14,17,19–22] Of the 173 fractures reported, 78 fractures were treated operatively,

and 95 fractures were treated nonoperatively. In patients treated operatively, the results were excellent or good in 69%. In patients treated nonoperatively, the results were excellent or good in 68%. Nonoperative methods of treatment included immobilization in traction or a plaster cast in cast brace. Methods of operative fixation included blade plates, buttress plates, and intramedullary rod. In a few instances, patients were treated by external fixation or by revision of the knee replacement.

Early reports on these fractures recommended nonoperative treatment with skeletal traction or cast bracing as long as an accurate reduction of the fracture could be obtained or maintained.[1,14,13] Operative treatment was associated with a risk of disruption of the prosthetic component by the fracture implant and with the risk of infection.[13] Authors advocating nonoperative treatment suggested that surgical treatment was associated with the best results because anatomic reduction could be obtained[13,20]; however, operative treatment was also associated with the worst results, including above-knee amputation and arthrodesis. Authors supporting nonoperative treatment for these fractures conceded that operative treatment may be necessary when adequate alignment cannot be obtained with traction.[1,7,13,20]

Proponents of operative treatment of these fractures suggested that malalignment, loss of motion, nonunion, inability to hold fracture reduction, and problems with decreased patient mobility were indications for surgical treatment.[6,10] Operative treatment provides the best opportunity for anatomic fracture reduction. Furthermore, anatomic reduction and stable fixation maximize the potential of healing in an area of compromised blood supply, and early mobilization of the patient can limit the complications of prolonged bed rest.[5,10,14,21]

The results of the these reports published during the 1980s showed that neither operative treatment nor nonoperative treatment could produce a predictably successful outcome. Excellent to good results of 68 and 69% are not particularly encouraging for the patient who experiences this fracture.

Principles of Treatment

Fractures of the distal femur above total knee arthroplasty range from nondisplaced fissure lines to severely comminuted displaced fractures with angulation and malrotation. In our experience, patients with stable nondisplaced fractures can be treated successfully nonoperatively. In general, these fractures should be treated as if knee replacement components were not in place as long as no loosening of components is demonstrated. Nonoperative treatment using casts or cast braces can lead to restoration of prefracture range or motion levels, and functional activity can be restored when union and prefracture tibiofemoral alignment are obtained and maintained.

Operative treatment is recommended for patients with displaced, unstable, and poorly reduced fractures or for fractures for which functional treatment is not possible. Rapid mobilization of elderly patients after surgical procedures is beneficial. The keys to successful operative treatment are preoperative planning and appropriate surgical technique. As noted previously, preoperative evaluation with satisfactory roentgenographic views of the fracture and prosthetic components is essential.

A straight lateral approach is preferred when operative treatment is selected. We have not encountered problems with skin vascularity using this approach. An extended anterior approach through the previous incision for arthroplasty may also be used; however, the anterior approach may be difficult when the fracture or comminution extends more proximally. Intraoperative roentgenography or fluoroscopy is recommended to check the position of guidewires and fixation devices, fracture reduction, and limb alignment.

Fixation of the fracture can be achieved with several different implants, including blade plates, distal condylar screw plates, condylar buttress plates, and intramedullary devices. Intramedullary devices are best suited for more proximal fractures at or above the junction of the middle and distal thirds of the femur. Satisfactory locking of the intramedullary device in the distal condyle must be achieved for rotational stability. Furthermore, introduction of the intramedullary device must be well controlled so that the distal bone–prosthesis interface is not disrupted.

In our experience, extramedullary plate devices are the most predictable fracture implants for these fractures that are difficult to treat. We prefer the use of the 95° condylar blade plate. One advantage is that no bone is removed when the blade plate is implanted. Because it is relatively thin, the blade can be placed close to femoral component lugs; however, a blade plate can be unforgiving at the time of insertion and can be difficult to use. A distal condylar screw plate requires removal of bone, which is not desirable. A condylar screw has more volume than a blade, and thus, placement may be more difficult. Distal fixation depends on the purchase of the screw, and, therefore, flexion, extension, and rotation micromotion may not be controlled. When proximal screws placed through the plate capture the distal condylar fragment, this flexion–extension motion can be overcome. The condylar buttress plate has the least secure distal fixation, but it provides the greatest flexibility in placement for the comminuted fracture. All of these devices can provide stable fixation when applied correctly.

An anterior approach may be considered for very distal fractures or fractures associated with osteopenia, when the need for revision of the component is a possibility. Approaching the fracture through the original anteromedial arthrotomy, used for the knee replacement, allows several options for treatment. Revision of the femoral component (with allograft if indicated) may be performed, if the component is loosened from the distal femoral fragment. If the distal fragment and femoral component can be salvaged, this exposure permits sufficient exposure of the distal femur to double-plate the fracture. Plates applied to the anteromedial and anterolateral surfaces grasp the distal fragment like a vise, and do not rely solely on screw fixation (Fig. 24–2).

In some fractures, fixation of the fracture implant in the distal condylar fragment may be difficult because of osteopenia. One method for increasing stability of the fracture is to use anterior-to-posterior intrafragmentary lag screws. These screws are perpendicular to the plane of the lateral fracture implants, and these fractures frequently leave dense posterior cortical bone that is capable of holding lag screws in an anterior-to-posterior direction. In patients who have severe osteopenia of the distal condylar fragment, fixation may be augmented by using polymethylmethacrylate or corticocancellous strips of femoral head allografts (Fig. 24–3). Bone grafts or bone cement permits better purchase of a blade plate or a condylar screw in the distal condyle. In some patients, depending on the geometric design of the prosthesis, a blade plate may be wedged between the anterior flange of the femoral component and the distal lugs of the intramedullary stem to improve distal condylar fixation (Fig. 24–4).

Bone grafting of the fracture site is routinely recommended. The distal femur receives its blood supply from epiphyseal, metaphyseal, and nutrient artery sources. The initial knee replacement can injure the epiphyseal blood supply, and depending on how much methacrylate enters the medullary canal, the intramedullary blood supply can be injured. The fracture may disrupt both the intramedullary and extramedullary blood supply. The operative approach to the fracture may further disrupt the epiphyseal, metaphyseal, and intramedullary blood supply. Therefore, bone grafting is recommended to increase the chance for union.

We have used both autografts and allografts. Autogenous bone grafts are preferable because of their osteoinductive and osteoconductive properties. In elderly patients with osteopenia, however, it is not possible to harvest satisfactory amounts of autogenous cancellous bone for grafting. Bone chips from fresh-frozen allografts of the femoral head can be used to enhance osteogenesis of the site of the fracture.

After operation, patients with stable fixation can be treated with continuous passive motion, which permits early restoration of motion and quicker rehabilitation. In patients in whom fixation is not satisfactory for early

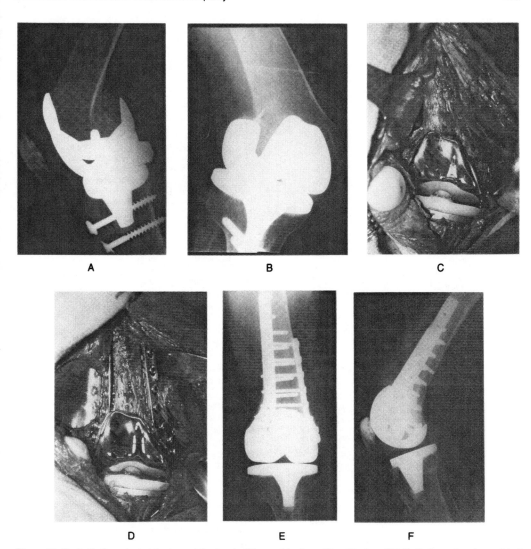

A   B   C

D   E   F

Figure 24–2. A, B. Comminuted fracture at the level of the trochlear flange in osteoporotic bone. **C.** Anteromedial exposure through original incision used for total knee replacement. **D.** Completed internal fixation with two AO/ASIF tibial plateau plates turned "upside down." **E, F.** Radiographs of completed internal fixation. She recovered prefracture motion and function.

motion, casting or bracing can be used. If immobilization is required, a position of 90° hip flexion and 90° knee flexion permits maintenance of quadriceps length and a maximal range of motion. This 90°–90° position is recommended only for 3 to 5 days.

Postoperative rehabilitation includes strengthening of the quadriceps muscles as soon as possible. Weight bearing should be spared until healing is evident.

Complications and Pitfalls

When displaced angulated fractures are treated nonoperatively, complications such as malreduction, malrotation, malalignment, and stiff knee are common. These complications become indications for operative treatment. Complications of operative treatment include those from anesthesia, infection, thromboembolic

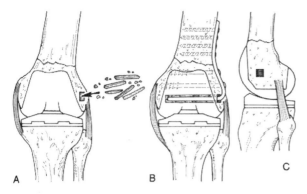

A   B

C

Figure 24–3. For patients with extreme osteopenia in the distal condylar fragment, polymethylmethacrylate or bone graft may be used to augment distal fixation of the fracture implant. **A.** A window is made in the lateral distal condyle, and bone graft is packed into the metaphysis. **B.** Fracture fixation with implant in place and augmentation of distal fixation with bone graft. **C.** Lateral view. (Reprinted by permission of the Lahey Clinic.)

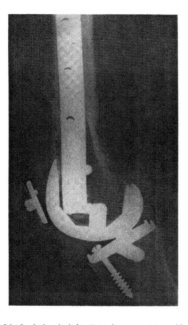

Figure 24–4. A healed fracture in a woman with severe osteopenia and ankylosing spondylitis 6 months after open reduction internal fixation and bone grafting. Fracture is healed. To achieve fixation of the blade plate in the distal condylar fragment, femoral head allograft was packed into the condyles and the blade plate was wedged between the anterior femoral flange and the lugs. The bone graft can be seen as sclerotic bone distal to the blade plate. (Reprinted with permission from Healy et al.[3])

disease, and delayed union. The potential for healing is clearly compromised because of insult to the blood supply at the time of arthroplasty, at the time of fracture, and at the time of operative treatment.

Results of Treatment

Published reports on the treatment of these fractures during the 1980s showed success rates of 69% after operative treatment and 68% after nonoperative treatment. These results are not spectacular. A recent series of operative treatment of fractures of the distal femur above a knee replacement has been presented by the New England Trauma Study Group.[3] A total of 20 patients with 20 fractures were treated operatively, and union was obtained in all patients.

In the New England Trauma Study Group series, 18 of 20 fractures healed after a mean of 12 weeks (range 6–40 weeks). The other two fractures had delayed union, but repeat open reduction internal fixation combined with autogenous bone grafting resulted in union. After operative treatment, these patients returned to their activities before fracture. Tibiofemoral alignment and range of motion of the knee were restored to their status before fracture. The average Knee Society knee and function scores[23,24] of the 20 knees were not decreased at follow-up examination.

Treatment of fractures of the distal femur above a knee replacement is controversial. The literature during the 1980s suggested that nonoperative treatment was acceptable for many patients and, although unacceptable for some patients, would lead to less severe complications. In the 1990s, this approach may not be justified. Operative treatment can provide union and restoration of prefracture activities when principles of anatomic reduction and stable fixation are applied. Patients with fractures of the distal femur above total knee arthroplasty should be treated functionally. When a functional result can be obtained without operation, that is the ideal treatment. When a functional result cannot be obtained without operation, surgical treatment should be offered.

References

1. Delport PH, Van Audekercke R, Martens M, Mulier JC. Conservative treatment of ipsilateral supracondylar femoral fracture after total knee arthroplasty. *J Trauma.* 1984;24:846–849.

2. Figgie MP; Goldberg VM, Figgie HE III, Sobel M: The results of treatment of supracondylar fracture above total knee arthroplasty. *J Arthroplasty.* 1990;5:267–276.

3. Healy WL, Siliski JM, and Incavo SJ. Operative treatment of distal femoral fractures proximal to total knee replacements. *J. Bone Joint Surg Am.* 1993;75:27–34.

4. Hirsh DM, Bhalla S, Roufman M. Supracondylar fracture of the femur following total knee replacement. Report of four cases. *J Bone Joint Surg Am.* 1981;63:162–163.

5. Nielsen BF, Petersen VS, Varmarken JE. Fracture of the femur after knee arthroplasty. *Acta Orthop Scand.* 1998; 59:155–157.

6. Short WH, Hootnick DR, Murray DG. Ipsilateral supracondylar femur fractures following total knee arthroplasty. *Clin Orthop.* 1981;158:111–116.

7. Sisto DJ, Lachiewicz PF, Insall JN. Treatment of supracondylar fractures following prosthetic arthroplasty of the knee. *Clin Orthop.* 1985;196:265–272.

8. Webster DA, Murray DG. Complications of variable axis total knee arthroplasty. *Clin Orthop.* 1985;193:160–167.

9. DiGioia AM III, Rubash HE. Periprosthetic fractures of the femur after total knee arthroplasty. A literature review and treatment algorithm. *Clin Orthop.* 1991;271: 135–142.

10. Culp RW, Schmidt RG, Hanks G, Mak A, Esterhai JL Jr, Heppenstal RB. Supracondylar fracture of the femur following prosthetic knee arthroplasty. *Clin Orthop.* 1987;222:212–222.

11. Aaron RK, Scott R. Supracondylar fracture of the femur after total knee arthroplasty. *Clin Orthop.* 1987;219:136–139.

12. Ritter MA, Faris PM, Keating EM. Anterior femoral notching and ipsilateral supracondylar femur fracture in total knee arthroplasty. *J Arthroplasty.* 1988;3:185–187.

13. Cain PR, Rubash HE, Wissinger HA, McClain EJ. Periprosthetic femoral fractures following total knee arthroplasty. *Clin Orthop.* 1986;208:205–214.

14. Bogoch E, Hastings Gross A, Gschwend N. Supracondylar fractures of the femur adjacent to resurfacing and MacIntosh arthroplasties of the knee in patients with rheumatoid arthritis. *Clin Orthop.* 1988;229:213–220.

15. Huo MH, Sculco TP. Complications in primary total knee arthroplasty. *Orthop Rev.* 1990;19:781–788.

16. Wiedel JD. Management of fractures around total knee replacement. In: Hungerford D, ed. *Total Knee Arthroplasty: A Comprehensive Approach.* Baltimore: Williams & Wilkins; 1984:258–267.

17. Hanks GA, Matthews HH, Rouston GW, Loughran TP. Supracondylar fracture of the femur following total knee arthroplasty. *J Arthroplasty.* 1989;4:289–292.

18. Müller ME, Allgöwer M, Schneider R, Willenegger H. *Manual of Internal Fixation: Techniques Recommended by the AO–ASIF Group.* 3rd ed. New York: Springer-Verlag, 1991;460–463.

19. Madsen F, Kjaersgaard-Andersen P, Juhl M, Sneppen O. A custom-made prosthesis for the treatment of supracondylar femoral fractures after total knee arthroplasty. Report of four cases. J Ortho Trauma 1989;3:332–337.

20. Merkel KD, Johnson EW Jr. Supracondylar fracture of the femur after total knee arthroplasty. *J Bone Joint Surg AM.* 1986;68:29–43.

21. Ritter MA, Stiver P. Supracondylar fracture in a patient with total knee arthroplasty. A case report. *Clin Orthop.* 1985;193:168–170.

22. Roscoe MW, Goodman SB, Schatzker J. Supracondylar fracture of the femur after Guepar total knee arthroplasty. A new treatment method. *Clin Orthop.* 1989;241:221–223.

23. Ewald FC. The Knee Society total knee arthroplasty roentgenographic evaluation and scoring system. *Clin Orthop.* 1989;248:9–12.

24. Insall JN, Dorr LD, Scott RD, Scott WN. Rationale of the Knee Society clinical rating system. *Clin Orthop.* 1989;248:13–14.

25

Patellar Fractures and Extensor Mechanism Disruptions in Total Knee Replacement

Roger H. Emerson, Jr.

Introduction

For total knee replacement, patellofemoral complications have been reported as the most common mode of failure leading tn revision, followed by aseptic loosening, infection, instability, and fracture.[1] The typical complications associated with patellar resurfacing include patellar fracture, component loosening, soft tissue catching or crepitation, and patellar instability.[2] In this chapter disruptions of the extensor mechanism after total knee replacement, including both fracture of the patella and patellar tendon failures, are presented.

Etiology

Although patellar fracture is relatively common, patellar tendon rupture is an uncommon mechanism of extensor mechanism failure, but is of clinical interest because the resulting disability for the patient is high and the outcome of routine repair unpredictable. Rand et al could find only 24 such ruptures reported in the orthopedic literature, mainly case reports and small series. They have reported a series of 18 ruptures in 17 patients treated with primary repair.[3] Emerson et al have reported a series of 10 patients with chronic patellar tendon rupture, treated with an extensor mechanism allograft.[4]

The reported incidence of patellar fractures after total knee replacement varies from 0 to 11%.[5–9] Although such fractures can be caused by obvious trauma, most are not associated with any specific traumatic event.[10,11] Similarly, most patellar tendon disruptions after total knee arthroplasty develop atraumatically, with a progressive extensor lag.[4]

Insall and co-workers noted more patellar fractures in knees that had undergone a lateral retinacular release,[8] and found avascular necrosis of the patella in a retrieval specimen. Scott and Goldstein have also speculated on an association between avascular necrosis of the patella and lateral retinacular release. They noted that five of six stress fractures of the patella were associated with a lateral release, and three of the five patellas had histologic evidence of avascular necrosis.[12] After a lateral release Scuderi et al have reported 9 of 16 knees (56%) demonstrating cold bone scans of the patella compared with 3 of 20 knees, 15%, with no lateral release. The abnormal scans had returned to normal by 3 months. There was one patellar fracture associated with a lateral release in this series, successfully treated nonoperatively.[13] Study of the blood supply of the patella as reported by Scapinelli reveals that incisions across the medial and lateral patellar retinaculum are likely to interrupt much of the blood flow to the patella[14] (Fig. 25–1).

The clinical significance of this avascularity is not clear. Leblanc recommended avoiding a lateral release if possible and staying 1 to 1.5 cm from the edge of the patella during surgical exposure and retinacular release, in an attempt to avoid disrupting the blood supply to the patella.[15] Brick and Scott urged preservation of the superior lateral geniculate vessels at the time of lateral release by dissecting the vessels free before releasing the retinaculum[6]; however, Ritter et al, looking at 48 patients undergoing bilateral simultaneous total knee arthroplasty, with only one knee having had a lateral release, found no difference in the rate of patella fractures between those with lateral releases and those without lateral releases.[16] In addition, Figgie et al studied a series of patellar fractures after total knee arthroplasty and found that out of 36 patellar fractures, only 6 had a lateral release. They concluded that lateral release played no causative role in most patellar frac-

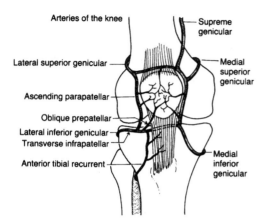

Arteries of the knee
Supreme genicular
Lateral superior genicular
Medial superior genicular
Ascending parapatellar
Oblique prepatellar
Lateral inferior genicular
Transverse infrapatellar
Anterior tibial recurrent
Medial inferior genicular

Figure 25-1. Blood supply to the patella. (Reprinted with permission from Scapinelli[14])

tures.[17] The literature suggests, therefore, that a vascular insult to the patella can occur after a lateral release, but is not the only cause of patellar avascularity at the time of total knee arthroplasty. By 3 months the patella has revascularized, and this transient avascularity infrequently results in any clinical problem for the knee.

Insall and co-workers noted that those knees with patellar fractures, using the posterior stabilized implant, had thicker patellar components, greater overall activity, and a greater range of motion (119°) compared with the series average (115°). With this design, they noted that patellar compressive forces are minimized below 95° of flexion, as a result of the cam effect of the tibial eminence.[10] Aglietti and Buzzi, in fact, have reported a patient series with this same implant, and found no fractures, although the average motion in this series was 98°, as the authors have pointed out.[5] Doolittle and Turner reported 3 patellar fractures out of a total of 350 arthroplasties with various designs, also in knees with a high range of motion (average 120°).[18] Knee motion is, therefore, one of the risk factors for patellar fractures.

Scott et al found a difference in the patellar fracture rate between rheumatoid arthritis and osteoarthritis. With the Duopatellar prosthesis the rates of fracture were 0.7% in 286 rheumatoid knees and 3.5% in 86 osteoarthritic knees.[11] The authors attributed this observation to the increased activity of the osteoarthritic patient. Grace and Sim have also noted an increase in patellar fractures in osteoarthritic patients, although not to the same magnitude as reported by Scott and co-workers.[19] These same authors also documented a statistically significant increase in patellar fractures in revision total knees, 0.61%, compared with primary knees, 0.12%, and in resurfaced patellae, 0.33%, compared with unresurfaced patellas, 0.05%, $P < 0.05$. They recommended preserving some of the patellar facet cortex

during preparation of the patella to maintain as much patellar strength as possible.

Certain implant design features predispose to patellofemoral problems. Hinged knee prostheses, which do not allow for rotation, have a higher incidence of patellar wear and dislocations, as reported by Mochizuki and Schurman. No patellar fractures or patellar tendon disruptions were reported in this series of 86 patients; however, Rand et al reported that 50% of the patellar tendon ruptures in their series were in fixed-hinge designs, although this series was from the era when hinged knee arthroplasties were more commonly used.[3]

MacCollum and Karpman have reported a series of knees with a 6% incidence of patellar fractures and an overall 16% patellofemoral complication rate, using a design with a constrained femoral trochlea and eccentrically shaped patella, the Porous Coated Anatomic knee.[21] They attributed this high rate of patellofemoral problems to the higher forces on the extensor mechanism in this design, if the patellar tracking was not perfect. Thirty-nine percent of the knees in this series required a lateral release to obtain patellar tracking. Two of the five patellar fractures in the report by MacCollum and Karpman had persisting lateral patellar subluxation. This compares, for example, with a patellar fracture incidence of 1.8% as reported by Thompson et al in a series of 1030 total condylar prostheses, with an unconstrained patellofemoral joint.[22]

Even in nonconstrained patellofemoral implant designs, patellar maltracking probably predisposes to patellar fracture, although patellar instability and patellar polyethylene dissociation are more common problems related to tracking.[9,18,21] Merkow et al reported one late patellar fracture out of 12 knees with patellar maltracking.[2]

Figgie and co-workers found that femoral and tibial component alignment correlated with patellar fractures.[17] They distinguished between major and minor component malalignments, described in an earlier study,[23] hypothesizing that the resulting component mismatch, or joint line shift, or "flexor/extensor imbalance" causes a fatigue fracture of the patella. The type and severity of the fractures correlated with the minor or major malalignment categories. They could find no vascular cause of patellar fractures.

Although the clinical evidence is convincing for a relationship between implant design and patellar fractures, the effect of design on patellar strain has been difficult to study. Andriacchi et al noted that a normal posterior cruciate ligament should diminish patellar strain by allowing rollback of the femur on the tibia, thereby maintaining a more favorable moment arm for the extensor mechanism.[24] McLain and Barger compared patellar strain in three different condylar designs: a posterior cruciate-retaining design, a posterior cruciate-substituting design, and a posterior cruciate-sacrificing design. Both the posterior cruciate-retaining and posterior cruciate-substituting implants were more protective of the extensor mechanism than the posterior cruciate-sacrificing implant; however, sectioning of the posterior cruciate ligament in the posterior cruciate-retaining design did not lead to as large an increase in patellar strain as expected. This was attributed to differences in the patellofemoral articulation between the two designs involved.[25]

Although it makes sense that design features that increase strain in the patella will also increase forces across the patellar tendon, the literature does not suggest a relationship between component design or alignment and patellar tendon rupture. The incidence of patellar tendon rupture is small, reported as a complication in 0.17% of total knee surgeries at the Mayo Clinic between 1973 and 1985.[3] Most patellar tendon ruptures occur late, prompting Gustillo and Thompson to speculate that impingement of part of the prosthesis on the patellar tendon, or removal of too much bone from the patella at the time of resurfacing, or a devascularization process from the surgical exposure is most likely the cause of most patellar tendon ruptures.[7] Laskin reported one patellar tendon rupture out of three instances in which he performed a complete excision of the fat pad and a simultaneous lateral release adjacent to the patellar tendon. He indicates, however, that in over 500 cases of fat pad excision alone, he saw no patellar tendon ruptures.[26] Acute patellar tendon avulsion at the time of surgery is very rare, but can certainly occur, prompting Rand et al to stress the importance of protecting the patellar tendon as much as possible during the actual surgery.[3]

Classification

There is no classification of patella fractures with total knee prostheses in common clinical use. Insall et al found that most patellar fractures were both comminuted and displaced.[10] MacCollum and Karpman described the five fractures in their series, two horizontally displaced and three vertically displaced.[21] Grace and Sim speculate that excessive resection of patellar bone predisposes the patella to transverse fracture (Fig. 25–2), and lateral subluxation predisposes to vertical fracture[19] (Fig. 25–3).

The exact location of most patellar tendon ruptures is difficult to determine. As most ruptures are chronic, even at surgery it is usually not clear where the actual disruption has occurred.

Principles of Treatment

There is no standard treatment regimen for patellar fractures after total knee replacement. With many of these fractures clinically asymptomatic,[10] conservative

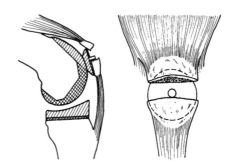

Figure 25–2. Transverse fracture pattern that may occur as a result of overresection of the patella.

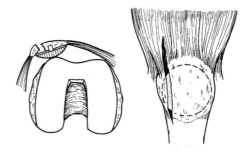

Figure 25–3. Vertical fracture pattern associated with lateral subluxation of the patella.

care seems appropriate for most. Grace and Sim recommend that treatment be based on the degree of displacement, the amount of comminution, the fracture location, and the fixation status of the patellar component.[19] Those fractures with greater than 5 mm of displacement (implying some disruption of the extensor mechanism), significant comminution, and a loose patellar component underwent operative treatment, usually a partial patellectomy or tension band or circumferential wiring. Aglietti et al reported 2 fractures of the patella in 87 knees, one posttraumatic and the other a stress fracture. Both fractures were treated nonoperatively with good results.[5] Doolittle and Turner reported three patellar fractures, all treated successfully in casts.[18] Scott et al advocated nonoperative management of patellar stress fractures, unless the patellar component is dislodged. Specifically they recommended splinting the knee in extension for 4 weeks, with daily gentle range-of-motion exercises to maintain motion. Their main indication for surgery was inadequate extension. Patellectomy, when necessary, gave good results in their experience.[11]

Figgie et al found in their study of condylar implants that the alignment of the components affects the type

A   B   C

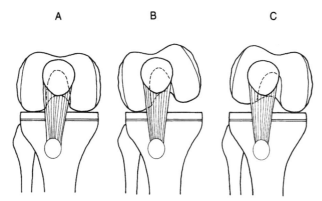

Figure 25-4. A. Normal patellar tracking with the femoral component in neutral rotation on the femur. **B.** Patellar tracking is still satisfactory with the femoral component in external rotation, as the patella can shift laterally without being displaced out of the groove in the femoral component. In addition, the resulting external rotation of the tibial component diminishes the Q-angle, which promotes better patellar tracking. **C.** Internal rotation of the femoral component rotates the trochlea out from under the patella and, by raising the lateral side of the femoral component, increases the patellofemoral compressive forces and increases the tension in the lateral retinaculum. Often a lateral retinacular release will compensate for this rotational mismatch, but malracking may persist. (Reprinted with permission from Figgie et al[17])

and prognosis of subsequent patellar fractures.[17] The role of rotational malalignment on patellar tracking is depicted in Figure 25-4. Most of the fractures in their series occurred less than 2 years from the date of surgery. No patients with patellar fractures were in the neutral range of alignment. The most severe fractures were seen in those knees with the most descrepancy in alignment. This neutral range was defined as (1) change of joint line by 8 mm or less, (2) lateral midline of the tibial component posterior to the midline of the tibial plateau, (3) patellar height between 10 and 30 mm from the tibial component, (4) tibial component centralized in the mediolateral direction, (5) femoral dimensions restored to within 5 mm, (6) femoral component restored to within $5 \pm 4°$ to the anatomic axis of the femur, (7) tibial component alignment at $90 \pm 2°$ in both the anteroposterior and lateral planes, (8) overall alignment of the leg passing from the femoral head through the center of the knee to the center of the ankle with no rotational mismatch between the femoral and tibial components, (9) patella coverage of 90 to 100%, and (10) 40% or less of patella height resected.

Patellar fractures associated with minor malalignments did well with nonsurgical treatment, if the components were well fixed and the extensor mechanism was intact. Minor malalignment was defined as meeting all of the criteria for neutral alignment with any of three deviations: (1) the tibial prosthesis not posterior to the lateral midline, (2) overresection of the posterior femoral condyles, or (3) joint line shift by 8 to 13 mm.

Patellar fractures associated with a major malalignment were more severe and required surgical management. A major malalignment was defined by the authors as failure to meet all of the neutral criteria, except for those making up a minor malalignment. Eighteen of twenty knees in this category underwent surgery, 15 of 18 with surgery to the extensor mechansim (including two patellectomies) and 3 with surgery to the knee components. No correlation in this series could be found between the degree of patellar coverage by the prosthe-

sis, amount of bone removed or final thickness of the patella after resurfacing, and subsequent patellar fractures.[17]

Treatment of patellar tendon rupture after total knee replacement has proved difficult, with no one technique universally successful. Permanent bracing can be the end result.[18] Of the 18 knees in the Mayo Clinic series, reported by Rand et al, 16 knees underwent repair, mostly by primary resuture, with only 4 of 16 (25%) achieving a healed repair. Staple fixation appeared to be the most successful technique.[3] Gustillo and Thompson have reported two patellar tendon repairs, both with primary suture and autograft augmentation and figure-eight wire support.[7] One of these two repairs ruptured (Fig. 25-5). Primary patellar tendon repair clearly has a continued role. The author has used the

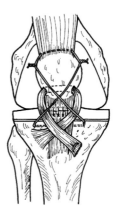

Figure 25-5. Example of primary patellar tendon repair with autogenous tissue augmentation (iliotibial band shown here) and additional figure-of-eight wire protection of the repair. If the patellar remnant is sufficient the tendon can be placed through a drill hole in the inferior pole. The wire should pass through the quadriceps tendon. (Adapted from *Total Arthroplasty of the Knee* by J.A. Rand and L.D. Dorr, eds., p. 43, with permission of Aspen Publishers, Inc., © 1987.)

technique of Gustillo and Thomspon when tendon rupture occurred at the time of total knee arthroplasty. There must be enough tendon substance to perform the repair, and simultaneous autogenous tissue augmentation seems sensible given the experience of Rand et al with primary repair alone. The literature supports a long period of bracing and protection from extremes of motion, for at least 6 months. Reruptures are likely to occur.

The treatment dilemma for patella tendon disruption comes about when there is not sufficient autogenous tissue remaining to carry out a tendon repair. Unfortunately, this is the most common clinical situation, typically encountered after a chronic tear or failed primary repair of an acute tear. In the setting of most chronic tears, at the time of surgery there is very little recognizable patellar tendon remaining, which explains the unreliable results of primary repair. In this setting the author has resorted to an allograft of the extensor mechanism, consisting of tibial tubercle, patellar tendon, patella, and quadriceps tendon, as decribed by Emerson et al[4] (Figs. 25–6 and 25–7). The underlying rationale is to return tissue to the patient, where there is a deficiency. No autogenous tissue should or need be removed with this tendon graft technique. As can be seen from the radiograph in Figure 25–8, the patient's patellar remnant is retained to maintain the integrity of the quadriceps and to provide coverage of the graft by as much host tissue as possible.

The author is following 15 patellar tendon allografts at this time, with 8 patients more than 3 years after reconstruction. Except for one young patient, age 36, the remainder have been elderly at the time of their surgery (average age 74 years). There have been no tibial tubercle nonunions. There was one quadriceps junction failure early in the series and one graft rupture at 6 months, attributed to surgical damage to the graft at the time of surgery. On the basis of this experience, no crushing or piercing instruments should be applied to the graft.

Using this technique, all patients were able to regain functional extensor function. The most difficult task with this technique is soft tissue tension and balance. Several early patients had persisting extensor lags, as a result of insufficient tensioning of the graft, and tilting patellar grafts. No dislocated grafts have occurred. With experience, the more recent extensor allograft patients have achieved full active extension, with better tracking of the grafts in the trochlea of the femur. With a chronic extensor rupture, the quadriceps muscle becomes shortened. At the time of surgery, therefore, the graft must be under tension, even at full knee extension. Sixty degrees of passive motion on the operating room table is all that is sought. With time, as the contracted quadriceps stretches to its more normal functional length, knee motion improves. All knees in the author's

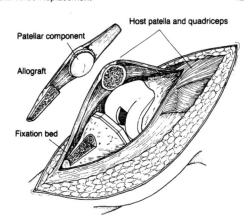

Figure 25–6. Extensor allograft overlying knee showing the fixation bed for the allograft tibial tubercle. The patellar component has been cemented to the allograft patellar.

series have gained at least 90° of motion. As a group, knees with a patellar tendon rupture have good motion before tendon reconstruction, flexing without the tethering effect of the quadriceps. No vigorous attempt was made to return motion to the patient, for fear of disrupting the graft–host junction.

Both freeze-dried and fresh-frozen grafts have been used with equal success in our experience to date. The sequence of surgical steps begins with preparation of the graft. The allograft patella is resurfaced on the back table, avoiding piercing or crushing clamps on the allograft. The facets are removed with a saw, and a polyethylene patellar prosthesis cemented in place. The bone resection should be conservative. The entire surface of the bony patellar remnant should be covered with the prosthesis. The patellar height should be around 25 mm after resurfacing (Fig. 25–6).

The allograft tibial tubercle is keyed into an appropriately sized slot cut from the proximal tibia, attempting to medialize the location slightly to enhance the tracking (minimizing the Q-angle) and to position the patella to articulate with the femoral flange in full extension. The allograft tubercle should be anatomically positioned in terms of tubercle elevation (see Fig. 25–6). Depressing the tubercle will increase patellar strain, which is undesirable. Elevating the tubercle would be theoretically advantageous, a "Maquet osteotomy" effect, but the skin in this area of the knee is invariably thin with little subcutaneous tissue with which to cover the graft. Wound closure with skin tension would predispose to a wound healing problem and likely failure of the surgery. The tubercle is rigidly fixed with bone screws and further supported with a tension band wire. (Figs. 25–7 and 25–8).

The quadriceps mechanism is sutured to the graft to

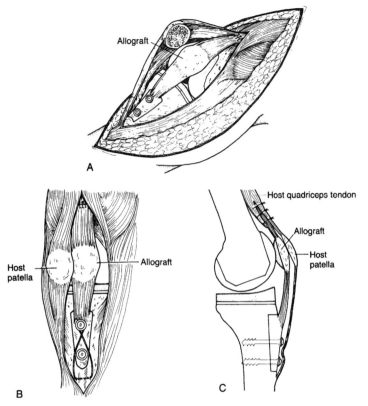

Figure 25-7. A. An extensor allograft in place with screw fixation to the distal graft to the host tibia. The quadriceps tendon has been sutured to the underside of the host quadriceps. The remnant of the host patella is still present with the patellar prosthesis removed. **B.** In this view, an additional figure-eight tension band wire has been added to the tibial fixation. Note how the scarred remnants of the patellar tendon has been lifted off of the host tibia to create better soft tissue coverage of the graft. **C.** A lateral view of the completed host–allograft composite showing the host soft tissue sleeve over the graft. This construct provides protection of the graft from a wound healing problem, probably provides some support of the graft, and may promote better healing of the graft which must come from the host tissues to the graft.

maintain a horizontal inclination of the graft with smooth tracking in the trochlea. The allograft should be placed under the host quadriceps muscle as much as possible, to provide a healthy vascularized bed for graft healing and to protect the graft from a superficial wound healing problem. In the few patients who had their own normal patella remaining, the prosthesis has been removed but the bony remnant has been left in situ, helping to anchor the quadriceps repair and serve as protection of the proximal allograft from the adjacent wound as discussed earlier (see Fig. 25–8). Ideally the entire graft should be covered by host muscle or joint capsule. However, this may be, anatomically impossible, and the allograft patellar tendon and tubercle may remain subcutaneous. Usually the autogenous patella has been re-

tracted proximally for a long time and cannot be brought down to the correct position on the femoral component.

Postoperatively the knee is placed in a hinged knee brace. The patient is allowed 60° of motion for the first 6 weeks. The brace is continued, with a 90° flexion stop for the next 6 weeks, allowing the patient to gradually increase range of motion as comfort allows. The patient is encouraged to stay on walking aids until the gait is smooth. The grafted leg should not be used to push up from a chair unless the patient cannot arise at all without use of the operated leg. Pushing up with the arms is an important long-term recommendation to protect the graft. Stair climbing should be one step at a time to protect the grafted knee.

References

1. Figgie HE, Goldberg VM. Some success rates of revision total knee arthroplasty. *Orthop Rev.* 1988;15:464–466.
2. Merkow RL, Soudry M. Insall JN. Patellar dislocation following total knee replacement. *J Bone Joint Surg Am.* 1985;67:1321–1327.
3. Rand JA, Morrey BF, Bryan RS. Patellar tendon ruptures after total knee arthroplasty. *Clin Orthop.* 1989; 224:233–238.
4. Emerson RH, Head WC, Malinin TI. Reconstruction of patellar tendon rupture after total knee arthroplasty with an extensor mechanism allograft. *Clin Orthop.* 1991;260: 154–161.
5. Aglietti P, Buzzi R. Posteriorly stabilized total condylar knee replacement. Three to eight years follow-up of 85 knees. *J Bone Joint Surg Br.* 1988;70:211–216.
6. Brick GW, Scott RD. Blood supply to the patella. Significance in total knee arthroplasty. *J Arthroplasty.* 1989; 4:575–79.
7. Gustillo RB, Thompson R. Quadriceps and patellar tendon ruptures following total knee arthroplasty. In: Rand JA, Dorr LD, eds. *Total Arthroplasty of the Knee.* Rockville, MD: Aspen; 1987:41.
8. Insall JN, Scott WN, Ranawat CS. The total condylar knee prosthesis. *J Bone Joint Surg.* 1979;61:173–180.
9. Lambardi AV, Engh GA, Volz RG, Albrigo JL, Brainard BJ. Fracture/dissociation of the polyethylene in metal-backed patellar components in total knee arthroplasty. *J Bone Joint Surg Am.* 1988;70:675–679.
10. Insall JN, Lachiewicz PF, Burstein AH. The posterior stabilized prosthesis: A modification of the total condylar design. A two- to four-year clinical experience. *J Bone Joint Surg Am.* 1982;64:1317–1323.
11. Scott RD, Turoff N, Ewald FC. Stress fracture of the patella following duopatellar total knee arthroplasty with patellar resurfacing. *Clin Orthop.* 1982;170:147–151.
12. Scott, RD, Goldstein W. Segmental osteonecrosis of the patella. *Am J Knee Surg.* 1988;1:67.
13. Scuderi G, Scharf SC, Meltzer LP, Scott WN. The relationship of lateral releases to patella viability in total knee arthroplasty. *J Arthroplasty.* 1987;2:209–214.
14. Scapinelli R. Blood supply of the human patella. Its relation to ischaemic necrosis after fracture. *J Bone Joint Surg Br.* 1967;49:563–570.
15. Leblanc J. Patella complications in total knee arthroplasty. A literature review. *Orthop Rev.* 1989;18:296–304.
16. Ritter MA, Keating EM, Faris PM. Clinical, roentgenographic, and scintigraphic results after interruption of the superior lateral genicular artery during total knee arthroplasty. *Clin Orthop.* 1989;248:145–151.
17. Figgie HE, Goldberg VM, Figgie MP, Inglis NE, Kelly M, Sobel M. The effect of alignment of the implant in fractures of the patella after condylar total knee arthroplasty. *J Bone Joint Surg Am.* 1989;71:1031–1039.
18. Doolittle KH, Turner RH. Patellofemoral problems following total knee arthroplasty. *Orthop Rev.* 1988;17:696–702.
19. Grace JN, Sim FH. Patellar fracture complicating total knee arthroplasty. *Complications Orthop.* 1988;3:149–155.
20. Mochizuki RM, Schurman DJ. Patellar complications following total knee arthroplasty. *J Bone Joint Surg Am.* 1979;61:879–886.
21. MacCollum MS, Karpman RR. Complications of the PCA anatomic patella. *Orthopedics.* 1989;12:1423–1428.

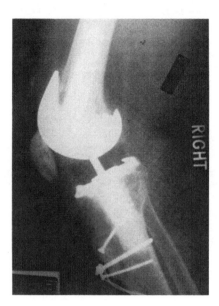

Figure 25–8. Lateral radiograph showing an allograft in position. Note the double patella, with the allograft patella deep to the remnant of the patient's original patella, as depicted in Figure 25–7C.

Results in the Literature

The results of patella fracture after total knee arthroplasty have not received the attention afforded to the study of the incidence. With greater than 2 years of follow-up, Grace and Sim noted an overall decrease in clinical knee scores, with some loss of motion, 96° to 87°, after patellar fracture treatment. Eight of twelve patients had no residual patellar pain after treatment.[19]

Figgie and co-workers have reported 22 of 36 knees achieving a good to excellent result, 4 a fair result, and 10 a poor or failed result.[17] Those with the good to excellent clinical rating had an arc of motion averaging 100° of motion, and those with a fair or poor result, an average arc of 80°. In addition, of 16 knees in their series that had been operated but did not have complete restoration of alignment, only 4 achieved a satisfactory outcome.

The short and intermediate follow-up results of the extensor allografts have been encouraging. There have been no late graft failures to date. It needs to be emphasized that the patient population with these grafts is very inactive, and the long-term durability has yet to be established.

22. Thompson RM, Hood RW, Insall J. Patellar fractures in total knee arthroplasty. Abstract. *Orthop Trans*. 1981; 5:516.

23. Figgie HE III, Goldberg VM, Heiple KG, Holler HS, Godgon NH. The influence of tibial-patellofemoral location on function of the knee in patients with the posterior stabilized condylar knee prosthesis. *J Bone Joint Surg Am*. 1986;68:1035–1040.

24. Andriacchi TP, Stanwyck S, Galante JO. Knee biomechanics and total knee replacement. *J Arthroplasty*. 1986; 1:211–219.

25. McLain RF, Barger WF. The effect of total knee design on patellar strain. *J Arthroplasty*. 1986;1:91–98.

26. Laskin RS. Total condylar total knee replacement in rheumatoid arthritis. *J Bone Joint Surg Am*. 1981;63:29–35.

Index

ISBN 0-387-94171-1

Lightning Source UK Ltd.
Milton Keynes UK

170934UK00007B/31/P